Conditions in Occupational Therapy

Effect on Occupational Performance

Conditions in Occupational Therapy

Fourth Edition

Effect on Occupational Performance

Ben J. Atchison, PhD, OTR/L, FAOTA
Professor
Department of Occupational Therapy
Western Michigan University
Kalamazoo, Michigan

Diane K. Dirette, PhD, OT
Professor
Department of Occupational Therapy
Western Michigan University
Kalamazoo, Michigan

 Wolters Kluwer | Lippincott Williams & Wilkins
Health
Philadelphia · Baltimore · New York · London
Buenos Aires · Hong Kong · Sydney · Tokyo

Acquisitions Editor: Kelley Squazzo
Product Manager: Kristin Royer
Marketing Manager: Allison Powell
Design Coordinator: Joan Wendt
Art Director: Jennifer Clements
Manufacturing Coordinator: Margie Orzech
Production Service: SPi Global

Library of Congress Cataloging-in-Publication Data
Conditions in occupational therapy: effect on occupational performance / [edited by] Ben Atchison, Diane Dirette. —
    p. ; cm.
Includes bibliographical references and index.
ISBN 978-1-60913-507-2
1. Occupational therapy. 2. Occupational therapy—Case studies. I. Atchison, Ben. II. Dirette, Diane K.
[DNLM: 1. Occupational Therapy. 2. Mental Disorders. 3. Nervous System Diseases. WB 555]
RM735.C66   2011
615.8'515—dc23

2011017373

10 9 8 7 6 5 4 3

CCS0413

To my wife, Marcia, my best friend.

— Ben Atchison

To Mom and Hervey, from whom I learned the meaning of hard work.

— Diane Dirette

Preface

The goals of this textbook were the same in previous editions: to provide a framework for students to learn about common conditions seen by occupational therapists and to facilitate the teaching and learning of conditions from an occupational therapy perspective. We thank Dr. Ruth Hansen for her significant contributions to the development of this framework and her significant contributions as first editor in the first and second editions of this textbook.

The original goals of this book have not changed in this fourth revised edition of *Conditions in Occupational Therapy: Effect on Occupational Performance*. Although not all conditions that an occupational therapist will encounter are included, we discuss those most common to our practice.

All chapters have the same basic structure, including sections on etiology, incidence and prevalence, signs and symptoms, course and prognosis, and medical/surgical management. The information is synthesized from an occupational performance perspective, using language included in the Occupational Therapy Practice Framework. It is important to begin the occupational therapy process with an understanding of client factors, including body structures and functions associated with a given condition, and to examine the potential effect on the occupational performance areas.

In this edition, the Occupational Therapy Practice Framework language, which is the most current "language of the profession," is inserted. We are pleased to announce the addition of several new chapters in this edition. These include Developmental Trauma Disorder, Infectious Diseases, Low Vision Disorders, and Muscular Dystrophy, as well as major revisions across all chapters to ensure current information on all aspects of these selected conditions. Case studies have been updated and are included for each chapter.

There is a continuing discussion in our profession about whether occupational therapists "treat diagnoses." We do not propose that there be an emphasis on the treatment of a diagnosis. We understand and support a patient-first philosophy. We do, however, argue that there are specific factors that impact on the ability to perform occupational roles and functions that are unique to a given condition. These factors must be understood and analyzed regarding their relative impact on the patient's ability to participate and engage in daily activity.

Each chapter in this fourth edition provides the authors' interpretations of the effects of the condition on occupational performance. This analysis is not absolute. Those who use this book may disagree about the importance of various disabilities and the secondary changes that might occur. That process, however, is the key to our goal for publishing this book. We expect it to be a starting point for discussion and analysis of the condition and its impact on occupational performance.

Ben Atchison
Diane Dirette

Contributors

Ben J. Atchison, PhD, OTR/L, FAOTA
Professor
Department of Occupational Therapy
Western Michigan University
Kalamazoo, Michigan

Ann Chapleau, DHS, OTR/L
Assistant Professor
Department of Occupational Therapy
Western Michigan University
Kalamazoo, Michigan

Carla Chase, EdD, OTR/L, CAPS
Associate Professor
Department of Occupational Therapy
Western Michigan University
Kalamazoo, Michigan

Gerry E. Conti, PhD, OTR/L
Assistant Professor
Department of Occupational Therapy
Wayne State University
Detroit, Michigan

Diane K. Dirette, PhD, OT
Professor
Department of Occupational Therapy
Western Michigan University
Kalamazoo, Michigan

Heather Javaherian-Dysinger, OTD, OTR/L
Assistant Professor
Department of Occupational Therapy
School of Allied Health Professions
Loma Linda University
Loma Linda, California

Joanne Estes, MS, OTR/L
Assistant Professor
Department of Occupational Therapy
Xavier University
Cincinnati, Ohio

Jennifer L. Forgach, MS, OTR/L
Children's Hospital of Michigan
Detroit, Michigan

Joyce Fraker, MS, OTR
Department of Psychiatry
Ann Arbor VA Medical Center
Ann Arbor, Michigan

Paula W. Jamison, PhD, OTR/L
Professor Emeritus
Department of Occupational Therapy
Western Michigan University
Kalamazoo, Michigan

Laura V. Miller, MS, OTR/L, CDI, CDRS
Private Practice
Livonia, Michigan

Brandon G. Morkut, MS, OTR/L
VanBuren Intermediate School District
Lawrence, Michigan
Clinical Faculty
Department of Occupational Therapy
Western Michigan University
Kalamazoo, Michigan

Karin J. Opacich, PhD, MHPE, OTR/L, FAOTA
School of Public Health
University of Illinois
Chicago, Illinois

David P. Orchanian, MPA, OTR
Master Clinical Faculty Specialist
Department of Occupational Therapy
Western Michigan University
Kalamazoo, Michigan

Sharon L. Pavlovich, M.A.M, COTA/L
Department of Occupational Therapy
Loma Linda University
Loma Linda, California

Elizabeth L. Phillips, PhD, RN
Bronson School of Nursing
Western Michigan University
Kalamazoo, Michigan

Kathryn M. Shangraw, MA, CCC-SLP
Grand Rapids Public Schools
Grand Rapids, Michigan

Michelle A. Suarez, PhD c, OTR/L
Assistant Professor
Department of Occupational Therapy
Western Michigan University
Kalamazoo, Michigan

Christine K. Urish, PhD, OTR/L, BCMH, FAOTA
Professor
Department of Occupational Therapy
St. Ambrose University
Davenport, Iowa

Andrea L. Washington, BS, OTR/L
Children's Hospital of Michigan
Detroit, Michigan

Mary Steichen Yamamoto, MS, OTR/L
Private Practice
Ann Arbor, Michigan
Davenport, Iowa

Contents

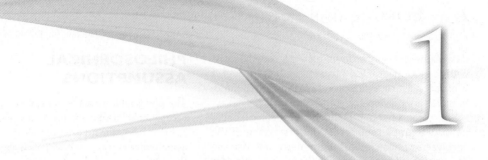

Thinking Like an OT

- *Diane Dirette*
- *Ben Atchison*

KEY TERMS

Altruism

Client factors

Context

Dignity

Equality

Freedom

Justice

Performance in areas of occupation

Performance patterns

Performance skills

Person-first language

Prudence

Truth

It is more important to know what kind of person has the disease than what kind of disease the person has.

—Sir William Osler (Address at Johns Hopkins University, February 1905)

Lindsey is finishing her course work in occupational therapy and is now beginning her first level II fieldwork experience. Throughout her education, she has learned the importance of evidence-based practice to guide her treatment decisions. Her challenge now is to develop her clinical reasoning skills to merge the science she has learned with the art of practice. To achieve this, she must understand the person's diagnosis, analyze the person's unique set of problems based on the person's individual characteristics and determine the impact on occupational performance. The first step of this process is the referrals she receives. Each referral gives her some basic information about the person including the person's diagnosis. Her job is to decide what to do next.

How does a student learn to correlate general information about a diagnosis with the needs of a particular person and to identify the problems that require occupational therapy intervention? How does a staff therapist set priorities for problems and decide which require immediate attention? How much problem identification can be done before the therapist actually sees the patient? How does a supervisor know when a student or therapist is doing a "good job" of screening referrals and anticipating the dysfunction that the patient might be experiencing? These are precursors to the actual intervention process and are essential to effective and efficient clinical reasoning (Benamy, 1996).

The clinical reasoning procedure used by each health care professional is somewhat different. The information that is the main focus of intervention for a speech therapist will differ from that of a psychologist or a nurse. What makes occupational therapy unique among health care professions is that practitioners gather and use information to help people become self-sufficient in their daily activities. Such data gathering and analysis provide the therapist with the foundation for a treatment plan through a prioritized list of anticipated problems or dysfunctions for an individual.

To comprehend the unique aspects of occupational therapy requires an understanding of the core values, philosophical assumptions, and domain of concern of the profession, as well as the language that is used to communicate information clearly and precisely.

CORE VALUES OF OCCUPATIONAL THERAPY

The core values of occupational therapy are set forth in the document "Core Values and Attitudes of Occupational Therapy Practice" (Kanny, 1993). Seven have been identified: **altruism, dignity, equality, freedom, justice, truth,** and **prudence**.

1. *Altruism* is the unselfish concern for the welfare of others. This concept is reflected in actions and attitudes of commitment, caring, dedication, responsiveness, and understanding.
2. *Dignity* emphasizes the importance of valuing the inherent worth and uniqueness of each person. This value is demonstrated by an attitude of empathy and respect for self and others.
3. *Equality* requires that all individuals be perceived as having the same fundamental human rights and opportunities. This value is demonstrated by an attitude of fairness and impartiality.
4. *Freedom* allows the individual to exercise choice and to demonstrate independence, initiative, and self-direction.
5. *Justice* places value on the upholding of such moral and legal principles as fairness, equity, truthfulness, and objectivity.
6. *Truth* requires that we be faithful to facts and reality. Truthfulness or veracity is demonstrated by being accountable, honest, forthright, accurate, and authentic in our attitudes and actions.
7. *Prudence* is the ability to govern and discipline oneself through the use of reason. To be prudent is to value judiciousness, discretion, vigilance, moderation, care, and circumspection in the management of one's affairs, to temper extremes, make judgments, and respond on the basis of intelligent reflection and rational thought (Kanny, 1993).

These values are the foundation of the belief system that occupational therapists use as a moral guide when making clinical decisions.

PHILOSOPHICAL ASSUMPTIONS

The philosophical assumptions of the profession guide occupational therapists in providing client-centered therapy that meets the needs of the client and society. These assumptions express our basic beliefs about the client and the context in which the client functions (Mosey, 1996). These assumptions are as follows:

- Each individual has a right to a meaningful existence: the right to live in surroundings that are safe, supportive, comfortable, and over which he or she has some control; to make decisions for himself or herself; to be productive; to experience pleasure and joy; to love and be loved.
- Each individual is influenced by the biologic and social nature of the species.
- Each individual can only be understood within the context of his or her family, friends, community, and membership in various cultural groups.
- Each individual has the need to participate in a variety of social roles and to have periodic relief from participation.
- Each individual has the right to seek his or her potential through personal choice, within the context of accepted social constraints.
- Each individual is able to reach his or her potential through purposeful interaction with the human and nonhuman environment.
- Occupational therapy is concerned with promoting functional interdependence through interactions directed toward facilitating participation in major social roles (areas of occupational performance); and development of biologic, cognitive, psychological, and social components (client factors) fundamental to such roles.
- The extent to which intervention is focused on the context, the areas of occupational performance, or on the client factors depends on the needs of the particular individual at any given time.

LANGUAGE

Although many language systems and mechanisms are available, we will discuss language from two perspectives. First is a philosophical discussion of using **person-first language.** Second is the use of the Occupational therapy practice framework: domain and process, 2nd edition (American Occupational Therapy Association [AOTA], 2008), which presents the professional language and the occupational therapy domain of concern.

Person-First Language

In many cases the literature and the media, both popular and professional, describe a person with a given condition as the condition—the arthritic, the C.P. kid, the schizophrenic, the alcoholic, the burn victim, the mentally retarded. All of these terms label people as members of a group rather than as a unique individual. The use of person-first language requires that the person be identified first and the disease used as a secondary descriptor. For example, a woman, who is a physicist, is active in her church and has arthritis; the fourth-grade boy, who is a good speller, loves baseball and has cerebral palsy. The condition does not and should not be the primary identity of any person.

Consider the following: a father is introducing his son to his coworkers. Which of the following is the best introduction:

"Hey, everyone, this is my retarded son, John."

"Hey, everyone, this is my son, John, who is retarded and loves soccer and video games."

"Hey, everyone, this is my son, John. He loves soccer and video games."

Of course, the third statement is the best choice. Yet it is common when describing a person who has a disability to emphasize the disability first. The consequence is a labeling process. "Although such shorthand language is commonplace in clinics and medical records, it negates the individuality of the person. Each of us is a person, with a variety of traits that can be used to describe aspects of our personality, behavior, and function. To use a disease or condition as the adjective preceding the identifying noun negates the multiple dimensions that make the person a unique individual" (Hansen, 1998).

THE OCCUPATIONAL THERAPY PRACTICE FRAMEWORK

The professional language for the profession of occupational therapy was revised in 2008 and presented in a document titled the "Occupational Therapy Practice Framework: Domain and Process," second edition (AOTA, 2008). The Practice Framework outlines the language and constructs that describe the occupational therapy profession's domain of concern. The domain defines the area of human activity to which the occupational therapy process is applied. The process facilitates engagement in occupation to support participation in life. The focus of the process is on the use of and the enhancement of engagement in occupation. The specific aspects of the domain are outlined in Table 1.1.

The Framework is organized into six aspects—performance in areas of occupation, performance skills, performance patterns, context, activity demands, and client factors. **Performance in areas of occupation** are broad categories of human activity that are typically part of daily life. The areas include activities of daily living, instrumental activities of daily living, education, work, and play, leisure, and social participation. **Performance skills** are features of what a person does during an activity. These skills are separated into the categories of motor skills, process skills, and communication/interaction skills. **Performance patterns** are the habits, routines, and roles that a person adopts. **Context** refers to the conditions that surround the person. Those conditions include cultural, physical, social, personal, spiritual, temporal and virtual contexts. **Activity demands** are the aspects of the task that influence the performance by the person. These demands include the objects used and their properties, space demands, social demands, sequencing and timing, required actions, required body functions and required body structures. **Client factors** are the body functions and the body structures that reside within the person (Fig. 1.1.) See Table 1.1 for an overview of the practice framework domains.

Each of these aspects has a relationship with and influence on the others. The outcome is, of course, the ability to function and engage in occupations. Although at a given time you may focus on areas of occupation or client factors, the ultimate concern is whether the individual is able to perform necessary and desired tasks in daily life. For example, a therapist may evaluate a person's attention span, but not in isolation. Attention span is evaluated within the realm of the performance patterns and context of the person—attention span required to work on an assembly line, to drive a car, to learn a card game, or to conduct a business meeting.

Once you know the diagnosis and age of the person, you can use this Practice Framework to examine systematically the deficits that occur in the client factors (described in Figure 1.1) as well as how these particular deficits can and do alter the person's ability to complete tasks in relevant areas of occupational performance. In other instances, you may focus primarily on the area of occupational performance or the contextual factors for the individual, without paying much attention to the underlying client factors that influence the performance areas.

EVIDENCE-BASED PRACTICE

There has been a call to action in the health professions to practice health care based on evidence of the effectiveness of each treatment approach (Gutman, 2010). High levels of evidence are based on studies that compare groups of

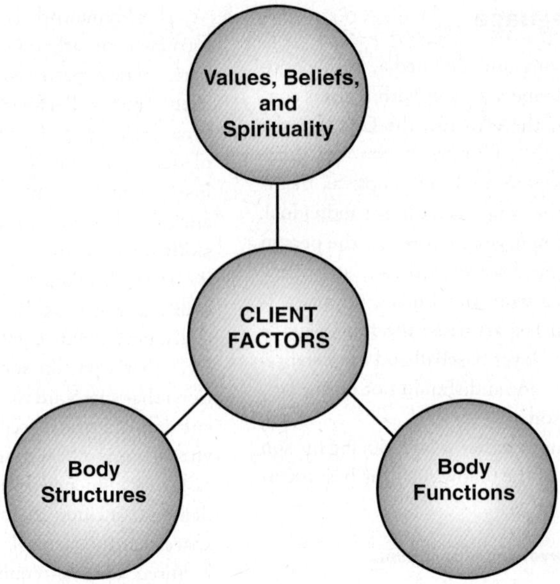

VALUES: *Principles, standards, or qualities by a person, organization, or population*	
BELIEFS: *Cognitive content held as true by a person, organization, or population*	
SPIRITUALITY: *"Personal quest for understanding answers to ultimate questions about life, about meaning, and the sacred" (Moyers and Dale, 2007, p 28)*	
BODY FUNCTIONS	*Includes mental, sensory, neuromusculoskeletal, cardiovascular, hematological, immunological, respiratory, voice and speech, digestive, metabolic, endocrine, genitourinary, reproductive, and skin and related functions.*
BODY STRUCTURES	*Structures of the nervous system, and those related to eyes, ear, voice and speech, cardiovascular, immunological, respiratory, digestive, metabolic, endocrine, genitourinary, reproductive, movement, and skin.*

Source: American Occupational Therapy Association (2008). Occupational therapy practice framework: domain and process, (2nd ed.). *American Journal of Occupational Therapy, 62,* 625–683.

Figure 1.1 Client factors.

people, usually with similar diagnoses. Evidence, especially high levels of evidence, on which to base one's practice, however, might be limited (Dirette, Rozich & Vau, 2009). First, it is limited by an insufficient number of resources to support specific treatment approaches with specific diagnoses. Second, it might be limited by the fact that groups of people with "average" results do not always represent the unique situation of the person with whom the therapist is working.

Therefore, while we support the idea of evidence-based practice in general, there is clearly a need for therapists to develop clinical reasoning skills that will not only help them decide which evidence to use with particular diagnoses but also help them decide what to do with the unique individual with whom they are working. Understanding the diagnosis with which the individual presents is often the first step in the clinical reasoning process. This textbook provides information about common diagnoses seen by occupational therapists and provides the first steps in the clinical reasoning process by providing ideas about the potential impact on occupational performance.

TABLE 1.1 Occupational Therapy Practice Domains

Areas of Occupation	Client Factors	Performance Skills	Performance Patterns	Context and Environment	Activity Demands
Activities of daily living (ADL)[a]	Values, beliefs, and spirituality	Sensory perceptual skills	Habits	Cultural	Objects used and their properties
Instrumental activities of daily living (IADL)	Body functions	Motor and praxis skills	Routines	Personal	Space demands
Rest and sleep	Body structure	Emotional regulation skills	Roles	Physical	Social demands
Education		Cognitive skills	Rituals	Social	Sequencing and timing
Work		Communication and social skills		Temporal	Required actions
Play				Virtual	Required body functions
Leisure					Required body structures
Social participation					

[a]Also referred to as basic activities of daily living (BADL) or personal activities of daily living (PADL).

Used with permission from American Occupational Therapy Association (2008). Occupational therapy practice framework: domain and process (2nd ed.). *American Journal of Occupational Therapy, 62,* 625–683.

ORGANIZATION AND FRAMEWORK OF THIS TEXTBOOK

Whereas the primary purpose of this book is to describe the potential impact of a condition on occupational performance, the descriptions should not be considered prescriptive or exhaustive. It is necessary to understand common facts of these conditions, including etiology, basic pathogenesis, commonly observed signs and symptoms, and precautions. However, it is equally important to recognize that the effects of a condition on occupational well-being will also be dependent on contextual factors such as age, developmental stage, health status, and the physical, social, and cultaural environment (Dunn, Brown, & McGuigan, 1994). Rather than viewing an individual as a diagnostic entity or as the sum of biologic cells, the condition must be personalized.

The general organization of each chapter is similar to previous additions. First, there are descriptions and definitions followed by information about the etiology, incidence and prevalence, signs and symptoms, course and prognosis, and medical/surgical management. This book is unique because the authors have used these details to generate a description of the various aspects of occupational performance that might be affected. At the end of each chapter is a discussion of at least one case study. Cases provide a beginning point to discuss specific details about how the condition might impact the daily functioning of a person.

Occupational therapists have a unique and valuable view of an individual as an occupational being. All

TABLE 1.2 Most Frequently Cited Conditions Treated by Occupational Therapists

Neurologic	Stroke 24%	Dementia 16%	Cerebral Palsy 12%	Traumatic Brain Injury 12%	Parkinson's 9%	Low Vision 5%
Development	Dev. delay 22.6%	Sensory integrative disorder 18.5%	Mental retardation 12.1%	Learning disorder 11%	Visual processing deficit 6.1%	
Cardiopul-monary	Congestive heart failure 26.1%	Chronic obstructive pulmonary disease 25.7%	Myocardial infarction 25.6%			
Orthopedic	Fractures 29%	Joint replacement 22%	Osteoarthritis 17%	Upper and lower ext. amputations 12%		
General Medical	Decond. debilit. 23%	Diabetes 20%	Cancer 16%	RA 15%		
Psychosocial	ASD 17%	Behavior disorders 17%	ADD HD 16%	Anxiety disorder 14%	Mood disorder 8.4%	Schizophrenia 7.1%

From National Board for Certification of Occupational Therapists (2008). *Executive summary: NBCOT 2008 practice analysis.* Retrieved January 3, 2011, from http://www.nbcot.org/pdf/Executive-Summary-for-the-Practice-Analysis-Study-OTR.pdf

of us attach meaning to our lives and the lives of others through the activities and occupations that are part of our daily existence. Occupation, then, means more than just work. It is a much broader concept that refers to human involvement in activities that will result in productive and purposeful outcomes. It also includes participation in leisure, rest, and self-care activities that some may not consider productive and purposeful. For example, the occupations of a 3-month-old infant include those that could be categorized under the general headings of play or activities of daily living. Activities such as play exploration, socialization, and functional communication are critical at this age.

The complexity of occupation changes dramatically as the infant progresses toward preschool and school age. It is interesting to observe the rapid addition of new occupational roles and expectations as the child enters school. Many aspects of occupational development are emerging. For example, a 7-year-old child participating in classroom activities is involved in a type of work. Being on time, turning in assignments that are completed properly, good grooming, and getting along with others are all behaviors that will be important as the child approaches adulthood.

Adults are expected to assume, independently pursue, and maintain relevant occupations. In general, adults spend the greater portion of their waking hours engaged in some type of work or instrumental activities of daily living. These occupations may be a job or vocation that is done for pay, organized volunteer activities, or home management. The percentage of time spent in each area is largely determined by the role the individual assumes. In addition, adults spend a portion of their time exploring and performing leisure and social activities. Activities of daily living, sexual expression, grooming, and eating are also important for adults.

The basic tenets regarding occupational performance are that these tasks are critical and must be performed by the person or by others to survive. By engaging in various occupations, the person develops, learns adaptive mechanisms, and meets individual needs. It is important to understand the influence of culture on adaptation. Cultural influences, such as institutions, rules, values, architectural design, art, history, and language, affect the ways and the extent to which a person uses adaptive mechanisms.

Conversely, illness, trauma, or injury can cause varying degrees of occupational dysfunction. The individual receiving occupational therapy is most often experiencing permanent, long-term changes in the ability to engage in everyday activities. The continuum between health and illness is dynamic. The individual's state of health or illness can be judged by the ability to engage in activities that meet both immediate and long-range needs, and to assume desired roles. Illness or disability is considered in relation to its effects on occupational performance and, therefore, the degree of occupational dysfunction that is experienced.

These precepts are the foundation for the reasoning process described in this book. The combination of these assumptions or beliefs and the occupational performance structure is the frame that provides a unique occupational therapy perspective.

This book of course cannot cover every condition that an occupational therapist will encounter in practice. In the three previous editions, conditions were selected conditions based on the AOTA Member Data Survey gathered in the late 1980s and on feedback we received from individuals who read and used the first three editions of this textbook. We selected conditions representing the broad range of occupational therapy practice—mental health, physical rehabilitation, geriatrics, and pediatrics. The most current published survey data regarding the highest frequency of conditions treated by occupational therapists were published in 2008 by the National Board for Certification in Occupational Therapy (NBCOT), which conducted a practice analysis survey. A total of 1,283 surveys were sent to practitioners across all practice settings jurisdictions, and 1,156 respondents completed the survey indicating a response rate of 90% with 96% of the respondents actively in practice.

Respondents were asked to indicate their top three diagnoses for six different client condition categories: neurologic, developmental, musculoskeletal/orthopedic, cardiopulmonary, and psychosocial conditions. The results of this survey were consistent with our selection of common conditions for this current edition. In addition, the results from a survey were similar between the data obtained by surveys of certified occupational therapy assistants, citing similar frequencies in diagnoses treated (NBCOT, 2008).

As an instructional tool, this book provides an opportunity to examine each condition closely. The reader is urged to use the information as a springboard for further study of the conditions included here and the many other conditions that occupational therapists encounter in practice. The analysis of the impact on occupational performance for a particular condition is dynamic, and the identification of the most important areas of dysfunction and, therefore, treatment will vary from practitioner to practitioner. In addition, factors such as secondary health problems, age, gender, family background, and culture contribute greatly to the development of a unique occupational performance profile for each individual served.

The occupational performance approach to the identification of dysfunction described in this book can be used to examine the effects of any condition on a person's daily life. This process will enable the therapist to identify and set a priority for problems in occupational performance, which, in turn, will serve as the foundation for creating an effective intervention plan.

REFERENCES

American Occupational Therapy Association (2008). Occupational therapy practice framework: domain and process (2nd ed.). *American Journal of Occupational Therapy, 62,* 625–683.

Benamy, B. C. (1996). *Developing clinical reasoning skills.* San Antonio, TX: Therapy Skill Builders.

Dirette, D., Rozich, A., & Viau, S. (2009). The Issue Is: Is there enough evidence for evidence-based practice in occupational therapy? *The American Journal of Occupational Therapy, 63,* 782–786.

Dunn, W., Brown, C., & McGuigan, A. (1994). Ecology of human performance: a framework for considering the effect of context. *American Journal of Occupational Therapy, 48*(7), 595–607.

Gutman, S.A. (2010). From the desk of the editor: AJOT publication priorities. *The American Journal of Occupational Therapy, 64*(5), 679–681.

Hansen, R. A. (1998). Ethical implications. In J. Hinojosa & P. Kramer (Eds.), *Evaluation: obtaining and interpreting data.* Bethesda, MD: American Occupational Therapy Association, p. 203.

Kanny, E. (1993). Core values and attitudes of occupational therapy practice. *American Journal of Occupational Therapy, 47,* 1085–1086.

Mosey, A. C. (1996). *Applied scientific inquiry in the health professions: an epistemological orientation* (2nd ed.). Bethesda, MD: American Occupational Therapy Association.

National Board for Certification in Occupational Therapy (2008). *Executive summary: NBCOT 2008 practice analysis.* Retrieved January 3, 2011, from http://www.nbcot.org/pdf/Executive-Summary-for-the-Practice-Analysis-Study-OTR.pdf

Cerebral Palsy

■ *Mary Steichen Yamamoto*

Jill's parents, who had been trying to conceive a child for several years, were thrilled when a family friend asked if they would be interested in adopting a baby girl that had just been born to a young unmarried woman in her church. The baby was born 6 weeks early and her weight was 4 pounds, but she appeared to be healthy. After initiating the paperwork for a private adoption, they brought the baby home and named her Jill. By the time of Jill's 6-month well-baby visit, her parents had become concerned. She appeared to be a bright baby who smiled and cooed and enjoyed reaching for and playing with toys, but her legs seemed stiff and she was not yet rolling over. They spoke with their family doctor about their concerns, but he assured them that Jill was developing normally and that they had nothing to be concerned about.

By the time of Jill's 9-month well-baby visit, her parent's concerns were only growing. Jill was still not sitting up and had not yet learned to roll over or crawl. Her doctor decided to refer Jill to the county early intervention program for a developmental assessment. Jill was assessed by the early intervention team that included an occupational therapist, physical therapist, and speech and language pathologist. The occupational therapist noted some mildly increased tone and incoordination in her upper extremities, which resulted in about a 2- to 3-month delay in fine motor and self-help skills. The physical therapist noted that Jill had **hypertonicity** and retained **primitive reflexes** in her lower extremities, which was causing significant delay in the acquisition of gross motor skills. The speech and language therapist found Jill's cognitive, language, and social skills to be at age level. The team suggested to the parents that they have a pediatric neurologist assess Jill, as she was demonstrating some of the signs and symptoms of cerebral palsy. Both the occupational and physical therapist recommended that therapy services begin as soon as possible. An IFSP (Individualized Family Service Plan) was developed at a subsequent meeting and Jill began weekly physical and occupational therapy sessions.

Jill's parents took her to a pediatric neurologist who diagnosed her with spastic **diplegia**, a type of cerebral palsy. Her parents were initially overwhelmed and devastated by the diagnosis. The next year was very difficult as they grieved the loss of so many dreams that they had for Jill and so much uncertainty about her future. They waded through an array of possible therapy approaches and medical and surgical interventions that were recommended trying to decide which would be right for Jill and their family. They struggled to find time to work on home exercises that had been prescribed for Jill. The strain became so great that they even separated for a while but eventually reconciled. By the time Jill turned 3 years old, she was walking with a walker and able to sit in a chair independently, although she needed assistance with changing positions. She was feeding herself but not yet dressing herself. They enrolled her in a preschool special education classroom where she received therapy services. By kindergarten, Jill was in a regular education classroom with a paraeducator for safety and support. Jill was a happy child, who had many friends and did well academically. Jill most likely will continue to need some type of additional support in order to be an independent adult, but all involved were optimistic about her future.

DESCRIPTION AND DEFINITION

Sigmund Freud, in his monograph entitled "Infantile Cerebral Paralysis," points out that a well-known painting by Spanish painter Jusepe Ribera (1588–1656), which depicts a child with infantile **hemiplegia**, proves that cerebral paralysis existed long before medical investigators began paying attention to it in the mid-1800s (Freud, 1968). Freud's work as a neurologist is not generally well known and at the time that his monograph was published in Vienna in 1897, he was already deep into his work in the area of psychotherapy. However, he was recognized at the time as the prominent authority on the paralyses of children. Today, cerebral paralysis is known as cerebral palsy.

Cerebral palsy is not one specific condition but rather a grouping of clinical syndromes that affect movement, muscle tone, and coordination as a result of an injury or lesion of the immature brain. It is not considered a disease. It is considered a developmental disability since it occurs early in life and interferes with the development of motor and sometimes cognitive skills. Historically, cerebral palsy has been classified as and is still sometimes diagnostically referred to as a static encephalopathy (Brooke, 2010). This is now considered inaccurate due to recognition of the fact that the neurological manifestations of cerebral palsy often change or progress over time. Static encephalopathy is permanent and unchanging damage to the brain and includes other developmental problems such as fetal alcohol syndrome, mental impairments, and learning disabilities. Many children and adults with cerebral palsy perform well academically and vocationally without any signs of cognitive dysfunction, which is associated with the term encephalopathy (Johnson, 2004).

A child is considered to have cerebral palsy if all of the following characteristics apply:

1. The injury or insult occurs when the brain is still developing. It can occur anytime during the prenatal, perinatal, or postnatal periods. There is some disagreement about the upper age limit for a diagnosis of cerebral palsy during the postnatal period, but it typically is up to 2 or 3 years of age (Thorogood & Alexander, 2009; United Cerebral Palsy Research and Educational Foundation, 1995).
2. It is nonprogressive. Once the initial insult to the brain has occurred, there is no further worsening of the child's condition or further damage to the central nervous system. However, the characteristics of the disabilities affecting an individual often change over time.
3. It always involves a disorder in sensorimotor development that is manifested by abnormal muscle tone and stereotypical patterns of movement. The severity of the impairment ranges from mild to severe.
4. The sensorimotor disorder originates specifically in the brain. The muscles themselves and the nerves connecting them with the spinal cord are normal. Although some cardiac or orthopaedic problems can result in similar postural and movement abnormalities, they are not classified as cerebral palsy.
5. It is a lifelong disability. Some premature babies demonstrate temporary posture and movement abnormalities that look similar to patterns seen in cerebral palsy but resolve typically by 1 year of age. For children with cerebral palsy, these difficulties persist (Little, 1862).

ETIOLOGY

Historically, birth asphyxia was considered the major cause of cerebral palsy. When British surgeon William Little first identified cerebral palsy in 1860, he suggested that a major cause was a lack of oxygen during the birth process. In 1897, Sigmund Freud disagreed, suggesting that the disorder might sometimes have roots earlier in life. Freud wrote, "Difficult birth, in certain cases, is merely a symptom of deeper effects that influence the development of the fetus" (1968). Although Freud made these observations in the late 1800s, it was not until the 1980s that research supported his views (Freeman & Nelson, 1988; Illingworth, 1985). Extensive research conducted in the United States has shown that only 5% to 10% of the cases of cerebral palsy were a result of birth complications (National Institute of Neurological Disorders and Stroke [NINDS], 2001). The birth complications resulting in cerebral palsy are related to **hypoxemia** because of a reduction of umbilical or uterine blood flow (Blickstein, 2003). Table 2-1 lists specific risk factors related to intrapartum hypoxemia.

TABLE 2.1 Cerebral Palsy: Contributing Risk Factors and Causes

Preconception (Parental Background)
Biological aging (parent or parents older than 35)
Biological immaturity (very young parent or parents)
Environmental toxins
Genetic background and genetic disorders
Malnutrition
Metabolic disorders
Radiation damage

First Trimester of Pregnancy
Endocrine: thyroid function, progesterone insufficiency
Nutrition: malnutrition, vitamin deficiencies, amino acid intolerance
Toxins: alcohol, drugs, poisons, smoking
Maternal disease: thyrotoxicosis, genetic disorders

Second Trimester of Pregnancy
Infection: cytomegalovirus, rubella, toxoplasma, HIV, syphilis, chicken pox, subclinical uterine infections
Placental pathology: vascular occlusion, fetal malnutrition, chronic hypoxia, growth factor deficiencies

Third Trimester of Pregnancy
Prematurity and low birth weight
Blood factors: Rh incompatibility, jaundice
Cytokines: neurological tissue destruction
Inflammation
Hypoxia: placental insufficiency, perinatal hypoxia
Infection: listeria, meningitis, streptococcus group B, septicemia, chorioamnionitis

Intrapartum Events
Premature placental separation
Uterine rupture
Acute maternal hypotension
Prolapsed umbilical cord
Ruptured vasa previa
Tightened true knot of the umbilical cord

Perinatal Period and Infancy
Endocrine: hypoglycemia, hypothyroidism
Hypoxia: perinatal hypoxia, respiratory distress syndrome
Infection: meningitis, encephalitis
Multiple births: death of a twin or triplet
Stroke: hemorrhagic or embolic stroke
Trauma: abuse, accidents

Adapted from United Cerebral Palsy Research and Educational Foundation. *Factsheet: Cerebral palsy: Contributing risk factors and causes.* Retrieved September 1995, from http://cpirf.org/stories/339

It is now known that in the majority of cases, the damage that results in cerebral palsy occurs prenatally. Congenital cerebral palsy that results from brain injury during intrauterine life has been reported to be responsible for approximately 70% to 80% of children who have cerebral palsy (Johnson, 2004; United Cerebral Palsy Research and Education Foundation Factsheet, 2001). In most cases, however, the specific cause is not known (United Cerebral Palsy Research and Education Foundation Factsheet, 2001). There are a large number of risk factors that can result in cerebral palsy, and the interplay between these factors is often complex, making it difficult to identify the specific cause. The presence of risk factors does not always result in a subsequent diagnosis of cerebral palsy. The presence of one risk factor may not result in cerebral palsy unless it is present to an overwhelming degree. Current thought is that often two or more risk factors may interact in such a way as to overwhelm natural defenses, resulting in damage to the developing brain. The strongest risk factors include prematurity and low birth weight (Lawson & Badawi, 2003). During the postpartum period, premature and low birth weight infants are at greater risk for developing complications, especially in the circulatory and pulmonary systems. These complications can lead to brain hypoxia and result in cerebral palsy. Intraventricular-periventricular bleeding and hypoxic infarcts that occur during this period also place the premature infant at increased risk (United Cerebral Palsy Research and Educational Foundation, 1995). The most common type of ischemic injury in the premature infant is periventricular leukomalacia, which occurs in the white matter adjacent to the ventricles. Sixty percent to 100% of premature infants with periventricular leukomalacia later show signs of cerebral palsy (Zach, 2010). Additional risk factors that have been more recently identified include intrauterine exposure to infection and disorders of coagulation (NINDS, 2001). Maternal infection is a critical risk factor for cerebral palsy, both during prenatal development and at the time of delivery. The infection does not necessarily produce signs of illness in the mother, which can make it difficult to detect. In a study conducted in the mid-1990s, it was determined that mothers with infections at the time of birth had a higher risk of having a child with cerebral palsy (Grether & Nelson, 1997). Table 2-1 shows a more thorough list of risk factors.

In approximately 10% of children with cerebral palsy in the United States, the condition was acquired after birth (United Cerebral Palsy Research and Educational Foundation, 2001). The most common causes in the perinatal and early childhood periods include cerebrovascular accidents (CVAs), infections such as meningitis or encephalitis, poisoning, trauma such as near-drowning and strangulation, child abuse, and illnesses such as endocrine disorders (Grether & Nelson, 1997; Marmer,

1997; United Cerebral Palsy Research and Educational Foundation, 2001). Closed-head injury that occurs during this period is now classified as traumatic brain injury, even though the resulting impairments are very similar to cerebral palsy (United Cerebral Palsy, 2009). The cause remains unknown in 20% to 30% of cases with an early onset of symptoms postnatally (Grether & Nelson, 1997; United Cerebral Palsy, 2009).

INCIDENCE AND PREVALENCE

Estimates of the incidence of cerebral palsy in the United States range from 1.5 to 4 per 1,000 live births (United Cerebral Palsy, 2006). The Centers for Disease Control and Prevention (CDC) has been monitoring the incidence of cerebral palsy in children in the Atlanta, Georgia area since the mid-1980s. In 2000, the prevalence was 3.1 per 1,000 children or 1 in 323 children (CDC, 2004). In the CDC study as well as in two other geographically diverse counties where data were collected, there was a 30% higher rate among African American children as compared to non-Hispanic white children. There was a 70% increase in prevalence in middle- and low-income areas as compared with upper-class areas (CDC; Cerebral Palsy International Research Foundation, 2009). The United Cerebral Palsy Association estimated in 2001 that 764,000 children and adults in the United States show one or more symptoms of cerebral palsy. They estimated that each year, 8,000 infants and 1,200 to 1,500 preschool-age children are diagnosed with cerebral palsy (United Cerebral Palsy Research and Educational Foundation, 2001).

There has been considerable advancement in obstetric and neonatal care during the past 2 to 3 decades. Many hoped these advancements would reduce the incidence of cerebral palsy. Unfortunately, the rate has remained relatively stable. This is probably a result of increased survival rates of very low birth weight and premature infants. Another factor may be the use of fertility treatments by older women that have resulted in an increase in the number of multiple births. Multiple births tend to result in infants who are smaller and premature and are at greater risk for health problems. On the average, they are half the weight of other babies at birth and arrive 7 weeks earlier (United Cerebral Palsy Research and Educational Foundation, 2001). There is a 400% increase in the probability of cerebral palsy in twin births than in a single birth (United Cerebral Palsy Research and Educational Foundation, 1997).

SIGNS AND SYMPTOMS

The early signs and symptoms common to all types of cerebral palsy are muscle tone, reflex and postural abnormalities, delayed motor development, and atypical motor performance (United Cerebral Palsy, 2006).

Tone Abnormalities

Tone abnormalities include hypertonicity, **hypotonicity**, and fluctuating tone. Fluctuating tone shifts in varying degrees from hypotonic to hypertonic. Muscle tone can be characterized as the degree of resistance when a muscle is stretched. For instance, when there is hypotonicity and the elbow is passively extended, there will be little to no resistance to the movement and hypermobility in the elbow joint. With hypertonicity, there will be increased resistance and it may be difficult to pull the elbow into full extension if the tone is strong. Most infants with cerebral palsy initially demonstrate hypotonia. Later, the infant may develop hypertonicity, fluctuating tone, or continue to demonstrate hypotonia, depending on the type of cerebral palsy.

Reflex Abnormalities

With hypertonicity, reflex abnormalities such as **hyperreflexia**, **clonus**, overflow, enhanced **stretch reflex**, and other signs of upper motor neuron lesions are present (United Cerebral Palsy, 2006). Retained primitive infantile reflexes and a delay in the acquisition of righting and equilibrium reactions occur in conjunction with all types of abnormal tone. When hypotonia is present, there may be areflexia, or an absence of primitive reflexes. These reflexes should be present during the first several months of life and it is of concern when they are not.

Atypical Posture

The presence of primitive reflexes and tone abnormalities causes the child to have atypical positions at rest and to demonstrate stereotypical and uncontrollable postural changes during movement. For instance, a child with hypertonicity in the lower extremities often lies supine with the hips internally rotated and adducted and the ankles plantar flexed. This posture is caused by a combination of hypertonicity in the affected muscles and the presence of the crossed extension reflex. A child with hypotonicity typically lies with the hips abducted, flexed, and externally rotated because of low muscle tone, weakness in the affected muscles, and the influence of gravity.

Delayed Motor Development

Cerebral palsy is always accompanied by a delay in the attainment of motor milestones. One of the signs that often alert the pediatrician to the problem is a delay in the child's ability to sit independently. While cerebral palsy is present at birth in all but the approximately 10% of cases, it is often not recognized until the child fails to achieve these early motor milestones.

Atypical Motor Performance

The way in which a child moves when performing skilled motor acts is also affected. Depending on the type of cerebral palsy, the child may demonstrate a variety of motor abnormalities such as asymmetrical hand use, unusual crawling method or gait, uncoordinated reach, or difficulty sucking, chewing, and swallowing.

TYPES OF CEREBRAL PALSY

Types of cerebral palsy are classified neurophysiologically into three major types: spastic, athetoid, and ataxia.

1. Spastic is characterized by hypertonicity. Deep tendon reflexes are present in affected limbs and motor control is affected by the hypertonicity. This type is the most common and accounts for approximately 70% to 80% of the cases of cerebral palsy (NINDS, 2001; Thorogood & Alexander, 2009). The **spasticity** is a result of upper motor neuron involvement (Porter & Kaplan, 2009). Within this category, types are further subdivided anatomically according to the parts of the body that are affected.
2. **Athetoid**, also known as **dyskinetic** type, is characterized by involuntary and uncontrolled movements. These movements are typically slow and writhing. This type accounts for approximately 10% to 20% of the cases of cerebral palsy (NINDS, 2001). This type results from basal ganglia involvement (Porter & Kaplan, 2009).
3. **Ataxia** is characterized by unsteadiness and difficulties with balance, particularly when ambulating. It results from involvement of the cerebellum or its pathways (Porter & Kaplan, 2009). It is much less common than the other two types, occurring in only about 5% to 10% of the cases of cerebral palsy (NINDS, 2001).

It is common for there to be mixed forms where two of the types occur together as a result of diffuse brain damage. The most common is combination is spastic with athetoid features. Persons with this type have signs of athetosis, and postural tone that fluctuates from hypertonicity to hypotonia. Athetoid combined with ataxia is less common (Porter & Kaplan, 2009).

Spastic

Spastic cerebral palsy is characterized by hypertonicity, retained primitive reflexes in affected areas of the body, and slow, restricted movement. The impact on motor function can range from a mild impairment that does not interfere with functional skills, such as not having isolated finger movement, to a severe impairment, where there is an inability to reach and grasp. **Contractures**, which are caused by permanent shortening of a muscle or joint leading to deformities, are common. It is categorized anatomically by the area of the body that is affected. Spastic hemiplegia, spastic diplegia, and spastic **quadriplegia** are the most common types. Spastic triplegia has similar features to spastic quadriplegia with three limbs involved. Typically, it is both lower extremities and one upper extremity. There are often mild coordination difficulties in the noninvolved upper extremity. Monoplegia, where one limb is affected, is rare and when it does occur is typically mild (Molnar & Alexander, 1998)

Spastic Hemiplegia

Spastic hemiplegia involves one entire side of the body, including the head, neck, and trunk. Usually, the upper extremity is most affected. Early signs include asymmetrical hand use during the first year or dragging one side of the body when crawling or walking. The initial hypotonic stage is short-lived, with spasticity developing gradually (United Cerebral Palsy, 2006). Most children begin walking after 18 months of age, with nearly all children walking by their third birthday (United Cerebral Palsy, 2006). When walking, the child typically hyperextends the knee and the ankle in **equinovarus** or **equinovalgus** position on the involved side. The child often lacks righting and equilibrium reactions on the involved side and will avoid bearing weight on this side. The shoulder is held in adduction, internal rotation; the elbow is flexed; the forearm is pronated; the wrist is flexed and ulnar deviated; and the fingers are flexed. Spasticity increases during physical activities and emotional excitement. Arm and hand use is limited on the involved side, depending on the severity. The child may use more primitive patterns of grasping and lacks precise and coordinated movement. In more severe cases, the child may totally neglect the involved side or use it only as an assist during bilateral activities. Parietal lobe damage occurs in about 50% of cases and results in impaired sensation, including **astereognosis**, loss or lack of kinesthesia, diminished two-point discrimination, decreased **graphesthesia**, and **topagnosia** (United Cerebral Palsy, 2006).

Spastic Diplegia

Spastic diplegia involves both lower extremities, with mild incoordination, tremors, or less severe spasticity in the upper extremities. It is most often attributed to premature birth and low birth weight and is, therefore, on the rise as more infants born prematurely survive as a result of medical advances. The ability to sit independently can be delayed up to 3 years of age or older because of inadequate hip flexion and extensor and adductor hypertonicity in the legs (Bobath, 1980). Frequently, the child will rely on the arms for support. The young child will move forward on the floor by pulling along with flexed arms while the legs are stiffly extended. Getting up to a creeping position is difficult because of spasticity in the lower extremities. Similarly, standing posture and gait are affected to varying degrees, depending on severity. Because of a lack of lower extremity equilibrium reactions, excessive trunk and upper extremity compensatory movements are used when walking. Lumbar lordosis, hip flexion and internal rotation (scissoring), plantar flexion of the ankles, and difficulty shifting weight when walking are common. Many of these problems result in contractures and deformities, including dorsal spine **kyphosis**, lumbar spine **lordosis**, hip subluxation or dislocation, flexor deformities of hips and knees, and equinovarus or equinovalgus deformity of the feet (Bobath). Approximately 80% to 90% of children with diplegia will walk independently, some requiring assistive devices such as crutches or a walker to do so (Sala & Grant, 1995). Walking will be slower and more labored with a crouched gait sometimes developing.

Spastic Quadriplegia

With spastic quadriplegia, the entire body is involved. The arms typically demonstrate spasticity in the flexor muscles, with spasticity in the extensor muscles in the lower extremities. Because of the influence of the tonic labyrinthine reflex (TLR), shoulder retraction and neck hyperextension are common, particularly in the supine position. This results in difficulty with transitional movements such as rolling or coming up to sitting. In the prone position, there is increased flexor tone, also a result of TLR influence, causing difficulty with head raising and bearing weight on the arms. Independent sitting and standing are difficult for the child because of hypertonicity, the presence of primitive reflex involvement, and a lack of righting and equilibrium reactions. Only a small percentage of children with quadriplegia are able to walk independently, and less than 10% ever walk in the community after adolescence (Bleck, 1975; Sala & Grant, 1995). Oral musculature is usually affected, with resulting dysarthria, eating difficulties, and drooling (Molnar & Alexander, 1998). Individuals are susceptible to contractures and deformities, particularly hip dislocation and **scoliosis**, and must be closely monitored.

Athetosis

Athetosis is the most common type of dyskinesia or dystonia, characterized by slow, writhing involuntary movements of the face and extremities or the proximal parts of the limbs and trunk. Abrupt, jerky distal movements (choreiform) may also appear. The movements increase with emotional tension and are not present during sleep. Head and trunk control is often affected as is the oral musculature, resulting in drooling, **dysarthria**, and eating difficulties. Whereas spasticity is characterized by hypertonicity in the affected muscle groups and restricted movement, athetosis is characterized by fluctuating tone and excessive movement. Contractures are rare, but hypermobility may be present because of fluctuating hypotonicity.

Ataxia

Ataxia is characterized by a wide-based, staggering, unsteady gait. Children with ataxia often walk quickly to compensate for their lack of stability and control. Controlled movements are clumsy. Intention tremors may be present. The ability to perform refined movements such as handwriting is affected. Hypotonicity is often present (Low, 2010).

ASSOCIATED DISORDERS

There are a number of disorders and difficulties associated with cerebral palsy, in addition to the motor impairment that can significantly affect functional abilities. In some cases, associated disorders can have a more significant impact on function than the motoric aspects of cerebral palsy.

Cognitive Impairment

Of all the associated disorders with cerebral palsy, cognitive impairment has the most significant impact upon functional outcomes. Estimates of the incidence of cognitive or intellectual impairment with cerebral palsy range from 30% to 50% (Molnar & Alexander, 1998). In about one-third of these instances, the cognitive impairment is mild. The most significant impairments most often occur with mixed types and severe spastic quadriplegia. Athetoid-type cerebral palsy has the least occurrence of cognitive impairment. Many children with spastic hemiplegia and diplegia have average intelligence (Molnar & Alexander; Porter & Kaplan, 2009).

Seizure Disorder

Reports of the incidence of seizures in people with cerebral palsy range from 25% to 60% (Porter & Kaplan, 2009). The incidence varies across the diagnostic categories. It is most common in spastic hemiplegia and quadriplegia, and rare with spastic diplegia and athetosis (CDC, 2004; Johnson, 2004; Molnar & Alexander, 1998; Porter & Kaplan). A population-based study published in 2003 found that the frequency of epilepsy in children with cerebral palsy was 38%. Partial seizures were the most common type and children with a cognitive impairment had a higher frequency of a seizure disorder (Carlsson, Hagberg, & Olsson, 2003).

Visual and Hearing Impairments

Visual and hearing impairments occur at a higher rate with cerebral palsy than in the general population. **Strabismus** is the most common visual defect, occurring in 20% to 60% of children with cerebral palsy, with the highest rates in spastic diplegia and quadriplegia (Hiles, Wallar, & McFarlane, 1975). Other visual and ocular abnormalities include **nystagmus**, **homonymous hemianopsia** associated with spastic hemiplegia, and difficulties with visual fixation and tracking (Molnar & Alexander, 1998). Some children with athetosis have paralysis of upward gaze, which is a clinical manifestation of **kernicterus** (Porter & Kaplan, 2009). Ataxia can be associated with nystagmus and problems with depth perception (Russman & Gage, 1989).

Hearing impairments most often include sensorineural hearing loss, due to congenital nervous system infections (Johnson, 2004). Conductive hearing losses, caused by persistent fluid in the ears and middle ear infections, occur when there is severe motor involvement in children who spend a lot of time lying down (Blackman, 1997).

Oral Motor

If the oral musculature is affected, the individual with cerebral palsy may have significant difficulty with speaking and eating. Dysarthria, if it is severe, may affect functional communication resulting in the need for alternative forms of communication. Eating difficulties can result in increased risk of aspiration, limited amount of foods consumed, and difficulty with chewing and swallowing. Drooling is a significant problem in about 10% of the cases of cerebral palsy (Stanley & Blair, 1994). It can be due to many factors including oral motor muscular control, impaired oral sensation, inefficient and infrequent swallowing, poor lip closure and jaw control, and poor head control.

Dental problems occur frequently in individuals with cerebral palsy. Motor problems and oral sensitivity can make tooth brushing more difficult. The combination of enamel dysplasia, mouth breathing, and poor hygiene leads to increased tooth decay and periodontal diseases (Molnar & Alexander, 1998).

Gastrointestinal

Gastrointestinal difficulties occur frequently in cerebral palsy. **Gastroesophageal reflux** can create much discomfort and can result in refusal to eat or difficulty transitioning to solid foods. It requires medical intervention such as medication or in more serious cases surgery. Constipation is common due to decreased mobility and exercise as well as inadequate intake of water or unusual diets due to difficulties with oral motor control (Molnar & Alexander, 1998).

Pulmonary

Individuals with more severe motor impairments such as spastic quadriplegia often develop scoliosis or other spinal deformities that can impact respiration. The respiratory muscles themselves may be affected, which results in poor respiration. These individuals are prone to frequent upper respiratory infections that can significantly impact their health. When difficulty chewing and swallowing is associated with poor breathing and inadequate or decreased ability to cough, this can result in increased aspiration pneumonia (Johnson, 1994). A barium swallow study can be conducted to rule out aspiration as a cause of frequent pneumonia. In cases where there is aspiration, a gastric feeding tube may need to be inserted. Premature infants who had **bronchopulmonary dysplasia** also have compromised pulmonary systems (Molnar & Alexander, 1998).

DIAGNOSIS

No definitive test will diagnose cerebral palsy. Several factors must be considered. Physical evidence includes a history of delayed achievement of motor milestones; however, delayed motor development can occur with a host of other developmental disabilities and genetic syndromes. The quality of movement is the factor that helps provide a differential diagnosis. The findings of atypical or stereotypical movement patterns and the presence of infantile reflexes and abnormal muscle tone point toward a diagnosis of cerebral palsy. However, other causes must be ruled out, such as progressive neurological disorders, mucopolysaccharidosis, muscular dystrophy, or a spinal cord tumor. Many of these disorders can be ruled out by laboratory tests, although some must be differentiated by clinical or pathological criteria. A magnetic resonance imaging (MRI) or computed tomography (CT) scan may provide evidence of hydrocephalus, help determine the location and extent of structural lesions, and help rule out other conditions. However, these scans are not definitive as far as making a diagnosis of cerebral palsy and are not predictive as far as the child's functioning (Miller & Bachrach, 2006). The yield of finding an abnormal CT scan in a child with cerebral palsy is 77% and for MRIs it is about 89% (Ashwal, Russman, Blasco, & Miller,

2004). An electroencephalogram (EEG) should not be used to determine the cause of cerebral palsy but should be obtained if there is an indication that the child may be having seizures. Because of the high occurrence of associated conditions, children with cerebral palsy should be screened for cognitive, visual, and hearing impairments, as well as speech and language disorders.

Cerebral palsy often is not evident during the first few months of life and is rarely diagnosed that early. Most cases, however, are detected by 12 months and nearly all can be diagnosed by 18 months (Miller & Bachrach, 2006). In some cases, early postural and tonal abnormalities in premature infants can resemble cerebral palsy, but the signs are transient with normal subsequent development.

COURSE AND PROGNOSIS

The course of cerebral palsy varies depending on type, severity, and the presence of associated problems. With mild motor involvement, the child will continue to make motor gains and compensate for motor difficulties. With more severe forms, little progress may be made in attaining developmental milestones and performing functional tasks. As the child grows older, secondary problems such as contractures and deformities will become more common, especially with spasticity. Adults with cerebral palsy experience musculoskeletal difficulties and loss of function at an earlier age than their nondisabled peers. One study found that 75% of individuals with cerebral palsy had stopped walking by age 25 due to fatigue and walking insufficiency (Murphy, Molnar, & Lankasky, 1995). Another study of young adults found clinical evidence of arthritis in 27% of the subjects with cerebral palsy as compared to 4% in the general population (Cathels & Reddihough, 1993).

The survival rate for adults with cerebral palsy is good but lower than the general population. A study in Great Britain found there was an 86% survival rate at age 50 for adults with cerebral palsy compared to 96% for the general population. After age 50, the relative risk of death was only slightly higher in women as compared to the general population. The risk for men with cerebral palsy was the same as the general population. Adults with cerebral palsy were more likely to die of respiratory disease than the general population but less likely to die from an accident or injury (Hemming, Hutton, & Pharoah, 2006).

MEDICAL/SURGICAL MANAGEMENT

Because of the complexity and diversity of difficulties affecting the individual with cerebral palsy, medical management requires a team approach using the skills of many professionals. Depending on the type of cerebral palsy and the presence of associated problems, team members typically include an occupational therapist, physical therapist, speech pathologist, educational psychologist, nurse, and social worker. The emphasis of intervention is usually on helping the child gain as much motor control as possible; positioning the child to minimize the effects of abnormal muscle tone; instructing the parents and caregivers on handling techniques and ways to accomplish various activities of daily living (ADLs); recommending adaptive equipment and assistive technology to increase the child's ability to perform desired activities; providing methods to improve feeding and speech if difficulties are present; and helping parents manage behavioral concerns and family stresses.

The primary physician treats the usual childhood disorders and helps with prevention of many health problems. Physicians with various medical specialties may also be involved. The usual specialists include a neurologist to assess neurological status and help control seizures, if present; an orthopaedist to prescribe orthotic devices and any necessary surgeries; and an ophthalmologist to assess and treat any visual difficulties.

Medical management includes both surgical and nonsurgical approaches, with much of the focus on techniques to decrease spasticity. Oral medications such as diazepam (Valium), dantrolene (Dantrium), and baclofen have been used to reduce spasticity in severe cases with mixed results (Albright, 1996; Johnson, 2004). Intrathecal caclofen infusion (ITB) administered through a pump implanted in the abdominal wall to the spinal cord fluid has shown to be more effective than oral medications in reducing severe spasticity and dystonia in cerebral palsy. There is, however, the potential for serious side effects and the long-term consequences are not yet known (Stempien & Tsai, 2000). Another treatment more widely used in recent years is the injection of botulinum toxin (Botox) into muscles. Spasticity is reduced for a period of 3 to 6 months after injection. Botox is injected into specific muscles, which, in addition to reducing tone, increases range of motion and reduces deformities as well as provides an opportunity to work on muscle strengthening. Minimal side effects have been reported; however, its long term effectiveness on function has not been demonstrated (Steinbok, 2006).

Orthotics and splinting are used to improve function and prevent contractures and deformities. Upper extremity resting or night splints are used to maintain range of motion. Soft splints, dynamic splints, and those allowing movement of the fingers and thumb are used during waking hours and functional activities to reduce tone and promote more typical patterns of movement. Ankle-foot orthosie (AFO) and variants are often prescribed to control spastic equinus, promote alignment of the hind foot,

and control mid foot and excessive knee extension when standing (Cusick, 1990; Molnar & Alexander, 1998). Inhibitory and progressive casting has gained acceptance as an alternative to bracing in recent years (Hanson & Jones, 1989; Lannin, Novak, & Cusick, 2007). A molded footplate is constructed that inhibits the primitive reflexes, thus reducing spasticity. The footplate is surrounded by a snug, bivalve below the knee cast. Inhibitory and progressive casting also is used with the upper extremities.

Surgical approaches are used to improve the function and appearance of affected areas of the body and to prevent or correct deformities. Tendon lengthening to increase range of motion and tendon transfers to decrease spastic muscle imbalances are done. These procedures, commonly used on the lower extremities, are performed more selectively in the upper extremities (Steinbok, 2006). Selective dorsal rhizotomy (SDR) is a neurosurgical technique that is used to reduce spasticity and improve function in carefully selected individuals (Berman, Vaughan, & Peacock, 1990; Cleveland Clinic Health Information Center, 2010; Kinghorn, 1992; Peackock & Staudt, 1992). The procedure involves dividing the lumbosacral posterior nerve root into four to seven rootlets. Each rootlet is stimulated electrically. The dorsal rootlets causing spasticity are cut, leaving the normal rootlets intact. This approach is highly successful for individuals who meet the selection criteria (Berman et al., 1990; Cleveland Clinic Health Information Center; Kinghorn, 1992). The most likely candidates are children with either diplegia or severe quadriplegia (Berman et al.; Cleveland Clinic Health Information Center; Kinghorn; Peacock & Staudt, 1991). For children with diplegia, the goal is to improve gait and leg function. For children with spastic quadriplegia who have very limited movement, the goal is to increase their independence by allowing them to sit for longer periods of time enabling them to use a wheelchair or potty chair as well as making daily care easier for their caregivers by reducing spasticity, which makes dressing and other daily living tasks more manageable (Cleveland Clinic Health Information Center, 2010). An essential part of this treatment approach includes intensive post-surgical physical and occupational therapy for a period of several weeks.

IMPACT ON OCCUPATIONAL PERFORMANCE

Virtually all of the body function categories can be affected in the individual who has cerebral palsy. Which of the categories are affected depends on the type of cerebral palsy, the severity of the condition, and the presence of associated disorders. Milder forms of cerebral palsy may have limited impact upon occupational performance.

Some individuals will require physical assistance, additional training, or assistive technology to participate fully in occupational performance areas, while individuals with severe forms of cerebral palsy will be limited in their performance of all areas of occupation.

The body function category that is always affected in individuals with cerebral palsy is neuromusculoskeletal and movement-related function. If spasticity is present, it affects joint mobility and results in limited active or passive range of motion or both. Joint stability is affected in all types of cerebral palsy. With spastic type, uneven muscle pull affects stability and joint cocontraction; fluctuating movement and tone affects stability in athetoid type; and ataxic type is characterized by a lack of joint stability. Underlying the tone abnormalities is decreased muscle power. Tone abnormalities affect muscle endurance. It requires much more effort to complete motor tasks with both hypotonia and hypertonia and endurance is often diminished. Endurance is also decreased if respiratory muscles are affected. In movement functions, primitive motor reflexes such as the stretch reflex, asymmetrical tonic neck reflex (ATNR), or grasp reflex are retained in the child with spasticity and continue to influence movement throughout life. Individuals with all types of cerebral palsy have impaired involuntary movement reactions such as decreased righting and equilibrium reactions. Involuntary movements impact individuals with athetoid cerebral palsy. Some individuals with ataxia have intention tremors. Gait patterns are affected in all types of cerebral palsy; however, in milder cases they may have little effect on occupational performance.

All sensory functions can be affected. All types of cerebral palsy have associated visual difficulties such as strabismus and visual tracking and fixation or hearing impairments. Some individuals with cerebral palsy demonstrate sensory processing difficulties with either hypersensitivity to sensory input or with their ability to discriminate sensory input.

Mental functions, both global and specific, can be affected, particularly if there is an associated learning disability, attention deficit hyperactive disorder, or cognitive impairment. Voice and speech functions can be affected if the oral motor and respiratory muscles have tonal abnormalities. Functions of the cardiovascular and respiratory system can be affected in a variety of ways, such as associated spinal deformities that can compromise respiration or decreased physical endurance or stamina as a result of the amount of effort that it takes to move. The digestive system can be affected by a number of different medical and physical factors such as reflux and feeding difficulties. Urinary functions are impacted by decreased control of muscles used in urination and in some cases cognitive factors.

It is important for the occupational therapist to be aware of all the client factors that can be affected in individuals with cerebral palsy but to not make any assumptions based upon the type of cerebral palsy and known associated disorders but to directly assess each factor and its impact on occupational performance. Each individual is unique and will have their own set of strengths and challenges.

Case Illustrations

Case 1

A.K. is a 2-year-old girl who lives with her parents and older brother. She was born at 37 weeks gestation at a birth weight of 5 pounds 10 ounces. Pregnancy and birth were unremarkable. She was healthy at birth but by her well-baby visit at 9 months of age she was not yet rolling, crawling, or sitting independently. Her pediatrician referred her to a pediatric neurologist who diagnosed her with spastic diplegia at 11 months of age. The neurologist referred her to a physiatrist (a physician and rehabilitation physician) at the local children's hospital as well as the local school district for early intervention services. The physiatrist signed a referral for her to the orthotics department to fit her with AFOs to help her with standing and walking. He has also recommended Botox injections and selective posterior rhizotomy for consideration as

future treatments. Through the early intervention program, she received a multidisciplinary team assessment that included physical, occupational, and speech and language assessments. Delays were noted in gross motor, fine motor, and self-help skills. Speech and language, social, and cognitive skills were all determined to be at age level. Weekly occupational and physical therapy home-based services were recommended.

Affected performance skills are in the motor area, which includes posture, mobility, coordination, and strength/effort. She demonstrates spasticity in all lower extremities and her trunk. Her movement patterns reflect significant spasticity in her legs. Her joint range of motion is significantly limited in her hamstrings and hip adductors with mild limitations in her heel cords bilaterally. A.K. can sit independently; however, it is difficult for her to sit on the floor with her legs extended in front of her as a result of hamstring and hip adductor tightness. She requires assistance moving in and out of sitting. In prone, she can push up to hands and knees and can crawl for short distances. She bears weight on her legs in supported standing with knees in a slightly flexed position, hips adducted, and feet plantar flexed and pronated. She has begun ambulating with a walker for short distances.

In her upper extremities, there is mildly increased muscle tone bilaterally as well as some incoordination. A.K. grasps pegs and small blocks and releases objects into a container. She can place a peg in a pegboard but is not yet able to stack objects or complete a shape sorter. Areas of occupation that are affected include ADLs and play. Because she is only 2 years old, instrumental ADLs, student, work, and leisure areas of occupational are not yet relevant areas for her. In ADL, because of her age she would not yet be expected to be independent. Given this, A.K.'s affected ADLs include bathing, dressing, feeding, and functional mobility. A.K. needs assistance with dressing skills such as undressing and removing shoes and socks. She is independent in feeding with some adaptations. She requires assistance with maintaining a stable sitting position in the bathtub and requires assistance getting in and out of the bath tub. She needs assistance with functional mobility, such as getting in and out of chairs and moving from one place to another.

Exploratory play skills are affected by A.K.'s difficulty with moving about her environment to obtain toys she wants to play with. Participation is affected by the need for a stable position in which to free up her upper extremities to manipulate toys. She uses a bench with a pelvis stabilizer and tray for refined fine motor tasks.

Case 2

L.N. is a 54-year-old woman with cerebral palsy, spastic quadriplegic type. She has lived alone in an apartment complex for the elderly and disabled for the past 15 years. She supports herself on supplemental security income (SSI) and disability payments from the state. A personal-care attendant provided by the Department of Social Services comes in each morning and evening to assist her with ADLs, such as meal preparation, bathing, and dressing. L.N. has never been employed but has done volunteer work. She writes articles for a newsletter on her computer and has worked in her church's Sunday school. She has no family support but has many friends. She enjoys learning and taking classes through continuing education.

Spasticity, fluctuating tone, and retained primitive reflexes severely restrict L.N.'s purposeful movement. She has limited range of motion in her left upper extremity and both lower extremities. When reaching with the left arm, she cannot bring it to shoulder height or behind her back. She has a gross grasp in her right upper extremity and can grasp a joystick to operate her electric wheelchair. She cannot write or perform other activities requiring fine motor dexterity. Her left upper extremity is used as an assist for bilateral activities, with no grasping ability present. She can maintain an upright position in sitting, but her weight is shifted to the left (with resulting scoliosis). She can bring her head to an upright position, but neck flexion increases with activities requiring effort. Oral motor muscles are affected, resulting in severe dysarthria, drooling, and difficulty eating. Endurance is a problem, and L.N. becomes easily fatigued.

Communication/interaction skills are also affected. Articulation and modulation when speaking is affected by L.N.'s oral motor control. Limited dexterity and restrictions in movement limit her ability to use gestures and to orient her body in relation to others when engaged in social interactions.

All areas of occupation are affected. In ADLs, L.N. needs assistance with bathing, personal hygiene and grooming, toilet hygiene, and dressing. She brushes her teeth and performs light hygiene, such as washing her face, independently. She can transfer herself between her wheelchair and her bed. She needs assistance transferring to the shower seat she uses for bathing. She can transfer on and off the toilet in her apartment with grab bars and the toilet seat at the proper height and position, although it takes her a while to do this. In eating, L.N. can feed herself with adaptations if the food is setup for her, but the process is slow and messy. She drinks from a straw. She takes her own medications if they are set out for her.

In instrumental ADLs, L.N. needs assistance in clothing care, cleaning her apartment, household maintenance, and meal preparation. She can use a handheld portable vacuum cleaner for small cleanups. She has a cat that she cares for. She shops independently but needs assistance in getting money out of her wallet at the cash register. All areas of ADLs are affected except socialization. L.N. uses a computer for written communication. She uses a speaker phone for telephone communication. If she falls or is in danger at home, she has an emergency alert system that she can activate. Because her speech is difficult to understand, she has an augmented output device for communication but uses it infrequently. She uses a motorized wheelchair for mobility. In the community, L.N. uses public transportation with no difficulty. She has some difficulty transferring herself to and from the toilet when using public restrooms, which sometimes results in incontinence.

In work activities, L.N. has never been employed but has worked as a volunteer for the past several years in the religious education program at her church. She enjoys the interaction with the children that are in the classes.

In leisure activities, L.N. has varied interests. She is an avid reader and enjoys computer games. Social activities include getting together with friends frequently and going out into the community, either alone or with friends. L.N. participates in church retreats as well as community-based trips through an independent living center.

RECOMMENDED LEARNING RESOURCES

Domans, J., & Pellegrano, L. (1998). *Caring for children with cerebral palsy: A team-based approach.* Baltimore, MD: Brooks Publishing. *An interdisciplinary reference for team-based, collaborative care of children with cerebral palsy.*

Geralis, E. (1997). *Children with cerebral palsy—A parent's guide* (2nd ed.). Bethesda, MD: Woodbine House. *Good reference for therapists and parents for young children with cerebral palsy. Contains comprehensive information on cerebral palsy including medical treatment information, and the effects of cerebral palsy on the child's development and education.*

Levitt, S. (2003). *Treatment of cerebral palsy and motor delay* (4th ed.). Oxford, England: Blackwell Science LTP. *Book was written for occupational and physical therapists working with children with cerebral palsy. Good discussion of treatment approaches, principles of treatment, and description of procedures.*

Morris, S., & Klein, M. (1987). *Pre-feeding skills.* Tucson, AZ: Therapy Skill Builders. *Excellent reference for oral-motor and feeding therapy for children. Very thorough and good overall approach to feeding issues.*

United Cerebral Palsy National Office
1660 L Street, NW Suite 700
Washington, DC 20036
Tel: (202) 776-0406; toll free: (800) 872-5827
www.ucp.org
Leading source of information on cerebral palsy and national advocacy group.

Children's Hemiplegia and Stroke Association (CHASA)
4101 West Green Oaks Blvd.
PMB #149
Arlington, TX 76016
Tel: (817) 492–4325
www.hemikids.org
A comprehensive, practical resource related to children with hemiplegia type cerebral palsy.

National Institute of Neurological Disorders and Stroke (NINDS). *Cerebral palsy information page.* Retrieved from www.ninds.nih.gov/disorders/cerebral_palsy. *Lists resources including organizations, publications, links, and general information about cerebral palsy.*

REFERENCES

Albright, A. (1996). Intrathecal baclofen in cerebral palsy movement disorders. *Journal of Child Neurology, 11,* S29.

Ashwal, S., Russman, B., Blasco, G., & Miller, A. (2004). Practice parameter: Diagnostic assessment of the child with cerebral palsy. *Neurology, 62,* 851–863.

Berman, B., Vaughan, C., & Peacock, W. J. (1990). The effect of rhizotomy on movement in patients with cerebral palsy. *American Journal of Occupational Therapy, 44,* 6.

Blackman, J. (1997). *Medical aspects of developmental disabilities in children birth to three* (3rd ed.). Iowa City, IA: The University of Iowa.

Bleck, E. (1975). Locomotor prognosis in cerebral palsy. *Developmental Medicine and Child Neurology, 17,* 18–25.

Blickstein, A. (2003). Cerebral palsy: A look at etiology and new task force conclusions. *OBG Management, 15,* 5.

Bobath, K. A. (1980). *Neurological basis for the treatment of cerebral palsy.* Philadelphia, PA: JB Lippincott.

Brooke, H. (2010). *Cerebral palsy as a cause of static encelopathy in infants.* Retrieved February 2010, from http://www.associatedcontent.com/article/2688287/cerebral_palsy_as_a_cause_of_static.html?cat = 5

Carlsson, M., Hagberg, G., & Olsson, I. (2003). Clinical and etiological aspects of epilepsy in children with cerebral palsy. *Developmental Medicine and Child Neurology, 45*, 371–376.

Cathels, B., & Reddihough, D. (1993). The health care of young adults with cerebral palsy. *The Medical Journal of Australia, 159*, 444–446.

Centers for Disease Control and Prevention. (2004). *Metropolitan Atlanta Developmental Disabilities Surveillance Program*. Retrieved August 4, 2004, from http://www.cdc.gov/ncbddd/dd/cp3.htm#common

Cerebral Palsy International Research Foundation. (2009). *Racial disparities in the prevalence of cerebral palsy*. Retrieved May 2009, from http://cpirf.org/stories/478

Cleveland Clinic Health Information Center. (2010). *Selective dorsal rhizotomy*. Retrieved June 17, 2010 from http://my.clevelandclinic.org/services/selective_dorsal_rhizotomy/ns_overview.aspx

Cusick, B. (1990). *Progressive casting and splinting for lower extremity deformities in children with neuromuscular dysfunction*. Tucson, AZ: Therapy Skill Builders.

Freeman, J., & Nelson, K. (1988). Intrapartum asphyxia and cerebral palsy. *Pediatrics, 82*, 240–249.

Freud, S. (1968). *Infantile cerebral paralysis*. Coral Gables, FL: University of Miami Press. (Original work published in 1897).

Grether, J., & Nelson, K. (1997). Maternal infection and cerebral palsy in infants of normal birth weight. *The Journal of the American Medical Association, 278*, 3.

Hanson, C., & Jones, L. (1989). Gait abnormalities and inhibitive casts in cerebral palsy: Literature review. *Journal of the American Podiatric Medical Association, 79*, 53–59.

Hemming, K., Hutton, J. L., & Pharoah, P. O. (2006). Long-term survival for a cohort of adults with cerebral palsy. *Developmental Medicine and Child Neurology, 48*, 90–95.

Hiles, D., Wallar, P., & McFarlane, F. (1975). Current concepts in the management of strabismus in children with cerebral palsy. *Annals of Ophthalmology, 7*, 789.

Illingworth, R. (1985). A pediatrician asks—why is it called birth injury? *British Journal of Obstetrics and Gnyaecology: An International Journal of Obstetrics & Gynaecology, 92*, 122–130.

Johnson, M. (2004). Encephalopathies. In R. Behrman, R. Kliegman, & H. Jenson (Eds.), *Nelson's textbook of pediatrics* (17th ed.). Philadelphia, PA: Saunders.

Kinghorn, J. (1992). Upper extremity functional changes following selective posterior rhizotomy in children with cerebral palsy. *American Journal of Occupational Therapy, 4*, 6.

Lannin, N., Novak, I., & Cusack, A. (2007). A systematic review of upper extremity casting for children and adults with central nervous system disorders. *Clinical Rehabilitation, 21*(11), 963-976.

Lawson, R. D., & Badawi, N. (2003). Etiology of cerebral palsy. *Hand Clinics, 19*(4), 547–556.

Little, W. (1862). On the influence of abnormal parturition, difficult labor, premature birth and physical condition of the child, especially in relation to deformities. *Transactions of the Obstetrical Society of London, 3*, 243–344. Retrieved August 15, 2010 from http://www.neonatology.org/classics/little.html

Low, J. (2010). *Ataxic cerebral palsy*. Retrieved September 26, 2010, from www.disabled-world.com/health/neurology/cerebral-palsy/ataxic.php

Marmer, L. (1997). ACDC tracks disability in kids ages 3 to 10. *Advance for occupational therapists*. King of Prussia, PA: Merion Publications, Inc.

Miller, F., & Bachrach, S. (2006). *Cerebral palsy: A complete guide for caregiving*. Baltimore, MD: John Hopkins Press.

Molnar, G., & Alexander, M. (Eds.). (1998). *Pediatric rehabilitation* (3rd ed.). University of California Davis, CA: Hanley & Belfus.

Murphy, K., Molnar, G., & Lankasky, K. (1995). Medical and functional status of adults with cerebral palsy. *Developmental Medicine and Child Neurology, 37*, 1075–1084.

National Institute of Neurological Disorders and Stroke. (2001). *Cerebral palsy: Hope through research*. Retrieved July 1, 2001, from http://www.ninds.nih.gov/health_and_medical/pubs/cerebral_palsyhtr.htm

Peacock, W., & Staudt, L. (1991). Functional outcomes following selective posterior rhizotomy in children with cerebral palsy. *Journal of Neurosurgery, 74*, 380–385.

Porter, R., & Kaplan, M. (Eds.). *The Merck Manual Online*. Rahway, NJ: Merck Sharp & Dohme Corp. Retrieved May 2009, from http://www.merck.com/mmpe/sec19/ch283/ch283b.html

Russman, B., & Gage, J. (1989). Cerebral palsy. *Current Problems in Pediatrics, 19*, 65–111.

Sala, D., & Grant, A. (1995). Prognosis for ambulation in cerebral palsy. *Developmental Medicine and Child Neurology, 37*, 1020–1026.

Stanley, F., & Blair, E. (1994). Cerebral palsy. In I. B. Press (Ed.), *The epidemiology of childhood disorders*, New York, NY: Oxford University Press.

Steinbok, B. (2006). Selection of treatment modalities in children with spastic cerebral palsy: Management options. *Neurosurgical Focus, 21*(2). Retrieved September 4, 2010 from http://www.medscape.com/viewarticle/550745_2.

Stempien, L., & Tsai, T. (2000). Intrathecal baclofen pump use for spasticity: A clinical survey. *American Journal of Physical Medicine & Rehabilitation, 6*, 536–541.

Thorogood, C., & Alexander, M. (2009). *Cerebral palsy*. Retrieved March 11, 2009, from http://emedicine.medscape.com/article/310740-overview

United Cerebral Palsy Research and Educational Foundation. (1995). *Factsheet: Cerebral palsy: Contributing risk factors and causes.* Retrieved September 1995, from http://cpirf.org/stories/339

United Cerebral Palsy Research and Educational Foundation. (1997). *Multiple births and developmental brain damage.* Retrieved May 1997, from http://cpirf.org/stories/364

United Cerebral Palsy Research and Education Foundation Factsheet. (2001). *Cerebral palsy facts and figures.* Retrieved October 2001, from http://www.ucp.org/ucp_channeldoc.cfm/ 1/11/10427/10427–10427/447

Zach, T. (2010) *Periventricular leukomalacia.* Retrieved March 18, 2010, from http://emedicine.medscape.com/article/975728-overview

Autism Spectrum Disorders

■ *Kathryn Shangraw*

Rachel was the beautiful first-born daughter to her parents, and during her first year of life, she appeared to be a typically developing child. She responded to people and objects in her environment with interest and enjoyment. Though slightly delayed in learning to walk, she mastered this skill between 14 and 16 months of age. In contrast, many of her language skills developed strongly during her first year. Rachel was exposed to three different languages in her home and learned several vocabulary words in each language by the time she was 14 months old.

When Rachel was approximately 14 months old, her parents noticed a startling change in her behavior. Eye contact became rare, and she no longer turned in response when her mother called her name. Because of this decreased responsiveness, her parents worried she was losing her hearing. However, an *audiologic* test indicated normal hearing abilities. Dressing this little girl also became a challenge. Suddenly, she did not easily tolerate the sensation of clothes against her skin. She became intensely distressed when her mother tried to brush her hair or clip her nails. The vocabulary of approximately 30 words that she had previously developed was replaced by silence or babbling. Upon reflection, her mother realized Rachel had never used specific communicative gestures such as waving to greet others or pointing. Engaging Rachel in daily activities became increasingly difficult for she appeared frustrated, unable to express her needs and wants, and unable to leave familiar, preferred activities without becoming highly agitated. During these episodes of tantrums, Rachel would hit herself or bang her head repeatedly against a wall while crying. Her mother described that overall, "she no longer seemed happy." When Rachel was 2 years and 6 months old, her parents brought their concerns to the attention of early intervention specialists. As a result, Rachel began receiving occupational therapy, speech-language therapy, and special education services. During her preschool class and therapy sessions, these specialists observed the same concerning characteristics her parents had described. Additionally, they noted she did not appear interested in the other children in her preschool class. Transitioning from room to room consistently distressed her, causing "meltdowns" during which she flung herself on the floor and cried inconsolably. She used only a few real words or echoed words of others but did not appear to understand what they meant. Many times, the classroom environment seemed to provide her with far too much sensory input. As a result, she would close her eyes or seek out places away from others. Yet Rachel still showed moments of attachment and joy, such as a strong, loving connection toward her parents and grandparents. Additionally, she smiled, laughed, and shared eye contact during specific activities, such as swinging, playing peek-a-boo, or singing. Despite these moments of engagement, the changes and gaps in her development caused her parents and therapists to seek further neurodevelopmental testing. Rachel was therefore assessed by a local neurologist, who confirmed the suspicions of her family and therapists: Rachel presented with **autistic disorder,** one of the disorders on the autism spectrum.

DESCRIPTION AND DEFINITION

Autism is a developmental disorder that impacts an individual's ability to socially interact, communicate, and relate with others. Though the precise cause of the disorder is unknown, autism is of **neurobiologic** origin (Lord & McGee, 2001). In other words, undetermined abnormalities in the structure and/or function of a child's brain cause the atypical behaviors seen in autism (Autism Society of America, 2004). Autism is not a single, homogeneous disorder; rather, it describes a spectrum of disorders that range in severity of symptoms, onset and course of development, and presence of features that differ from the typical course of child development (Lord & McGee). *The Diagnostic and Statistical Manual, Fourth Edition, Text Revision (DSM IV-TR)* lists five main disorders under the synonymous term pervasive developmental disorders (PDDs): autistic

disorder, **Asperger's disorder** (also known as **Asperger's syndrome**), **pervasive developmental disorder—not otherwise specified (PDD-NOS)**, **childhood disintegrative disorder (CDD)** and **Rett's disorder** (American Psychiatric Association, 2000).

The autism spectrum disorders (ASDs) (Fig. 3.1) share the following characteristics:

1. Impairment in social interaction
2. Impairment in communication
3. Unusual behaviors, including (a) restricted behavior—the child does not show new or creative ideas—(b) repetitive/stereotyped behavior—a child repeats a behavior to an extreme degree.

A child with ASD shows deviations from, and often delays in, typical patterns of development. Some children evidence problems from birth, such as making far less eye contact than other infants. However, in most cases the characteristics of autism noticeably emerge between 12 and 36 months of age because of the following reasons:

1. Because children with autism progress more slowly in several areas of development than typically developing children, a gap in skills becomes clear at this age when children normally expand their language and social skills rapidly.
2. Children may have appeared to meet developmental milestones before 12 to 36 months of age, with a sudden loss of previously acquired skills, presenting in some cases of children with ASD (Strock, 2004).

Autism cannot be "cured." For those with autism, intervention that targets behavioral, language, cognitive, social, adaptive, and sensory concerns is available. Though these individuals often improve their skills as a result of intervention, they usually struggle with the challenges of their disorder throughout their lives.

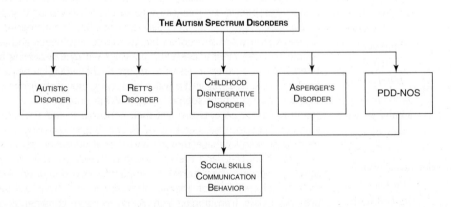

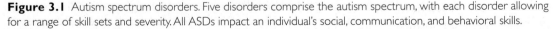

Figure 3.1 Autism spectrum disorders. Five disorders comprise the autism spectrum, with each disorder allowing for a range of skill sets and severity. All ASDs impact an individual's social, communication, and behavioral skills.

THE MANY NAMES OF AUTISM

The terms used in the autism field are confusing for many people, since some terms are used interchangeably or inconsistently in literature and by professionals. The most accurate and generally agreed-upon definitions are summarized as follows.

- The terms autism, ASDs, and PDDs are synonymous. Many professionals prefer using the term ASDs rather than PDDs, believing it more accurately reflects the variability that occurs both among the disorders and within an individual diagnostic category.
- This chapter will use autism and ASDs interchangeably, noting the term PDDs only when quoting another source that uses this phrase.
- Note that the similar term autistic disorder actually refers to one specific diagnostic category on the autism spectrum.

ETIOLOGY

Though researchers believe that certain factors (e.g., genetics) are more likely than others to cause autism, no one etiologic factor has clearly emerged. Therefore, autism is diagnosed based on observed behaviors, not by its cause. It was first described in literature in 1943 by Dr. Leo Kanner. Initial hypotheses that autism was caused by "cold" or unresponsive parents (Bettelheim, 1967) were dismissed as scientific evidence revealed that autism resulted from neurologic differences rather than the misguided assumption of aloof parenting (Lord & McGee, 2001).

Abnormalities in Brain Structure/ Function

Children with autism develop, process, and react differently to their world than children who are developing typically. This diversion from normal development means that children with autism begin life with brains that are physically different from nonautistic brains. Because the brain functions differently, the way in which life experiences are mapped onto the brain is altered as a result of the physical differences (Siegel, 2003). The precise distinctions are not yet entirely clear, since autism is not caused by a single obvious lesion in the brain. In fact, studies have indicated subtle differences in several areas of the brain, though researchers are not yet entirely certain which area, or combination of areas, results in the manifestation of autism (United Kingdom Medical Research Council, 2001).

Through the study of postmortem brain tissue and imaging studies such as positron emission tomography

scan and magnetic resonance imaging (MRI), consistencies have emerged in the research of brain abnormalities.

1. The brain is made up of about 100 billion **neurons,** or single cells, that interconnect and communicate information among the various brain regions and from other areas of the body. The behaviors of autism may result from abnormalities in the neural networking between the multiple areas of the brain, rather than in one area, as the brain processes complex information (Piven, Saliba, Bailey, & Arndt, 1997). With several areas of the brain affected, a constellation of deficits and neurologic differences occur, which would explain why many areas of a child's development are affected (Minshew, 2009). For instance, a recent study revealed lowered connectivity across networks relating to language, working memory, social cognition or perception, and problem solving (Fig. 3.2) (Levy, Mandell, & Schultz, 2009).

2. Though children with autism are born with normal head circumferences, acceleration in head growth often occurs between 9 and 12 months, with significant deceleration at 12 months. Interestingly, for children with autism, the gap in developmental skills often widens from 12 to 24 months and beyond, just following this period of noted head growth (Minshew, 2009). Meanwhile, individuals with Rett's disorder evidence smaller-than-usual brains (Bauman & Kemper, 1996).

3. There is a growing body of research that suggests that dysfunction of the **cerebellum** is a likely contributor to autism. This area of the brain has been traditionally known for its role in the coordination of movement. But the cerebellum, which sits over the brainstem, may also play a role in sensory discrimination, attention, emotions, mental imagery, problem solving, some aspects of language processing, visual-spatial orientation, spatial orientation, visuomotor function, and the speed, consistency, and appropriateness of mental and cognitive processes (Bauman, 2004; Kemper & Bauman, 1998). Neurons in the cerebellum known as **Purkinje cells** form a layer near the surface of the cerebellum and convey signals away from the cerebellum. In autistic individuals, an important deviation consistently noted is a decrease in the Purkinje cell number.

4. In the brainstem, the neurons in the **inferior olive** of individuals with autism also showed deviations depending on age. Cells were initially larger than normal but typical in appearance in young children; in adulthood, these cells were unusually small and pale (Kemper & Bauman, 1998; United Kingdom Medical Research Council, 2001).

5. Inferior olives are connected to Purkinje cells by climbing fibers, and this bond from the inferior olive

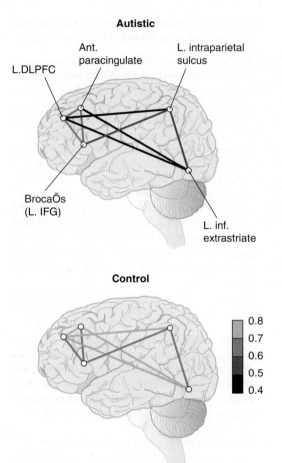

Figure 3.2 Autism: connectivity in the brain. The behaviors of autism may result from reduced connectivity among the different regions of the brain. This figure illustrates reliably lower functional connectivity for autism participants between pairs of key areas during sentence comprehension tasks. Darker end of scale denotes lower connectivity. (Slide courtesy of Marcel Just, Carnegie Mellon University.)

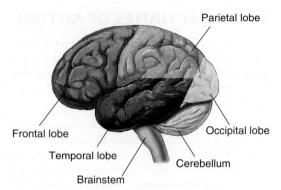

Figure 3.3 Cerebral cortex. Left lateral view of the brain, including the four lobes of the cerebrum and the cerebellum (From Bickley, L. S., & Szilagyi. [2003], P. *Bates' guide to physical examination and history taking* [8th ed.]. Philadelphia: Lippincott, Williams & Wilkins).

to the Purkinje cell is made at 28 to 30 weeks' gestation. Once this union occurs, if a Purkinje cell dies, the inferior olive will also deplete. As previously noted, Purkinje cells are reduced in number in children with autism, but the cells of the inferior olive are normal in quantity. The implication is that damage to the Purkinje cells in children with autism would have likely occurred in utero, prior to 30 weeks' gestation, before the bond was established (Bauman, 2004; Kemper & Bauman, 1998).

6. Imaging studies have indicated reduced activation of the **frontal lobe** in individuals diagnosed with autism (United Kingdom Medical Research Council, 2001).

Additionally, some areas of the frontal lobe appear markedly larger in children with autism compared with typically developing children (Carper & Courchesne, 2005). The frontal lobe's function is voluntary control of the body's movements. Specific regions of this lobe are also responsible for social behavior, spontaneous production of language, initiation of motor activity, processing sensory stimuli, and planning reactions as a result of the sensory input, abstract thinking, problem solving, and judgment (Kemper & Bauman, 1998). How the abnormalities affect the frontal lobe's ability to conduct these roles remains unclear, though many symptoms of autism appear related to problems in frontal lobe functioning (Fig. 3.3).

7. Within the **limbic system**, a network of structures that regulates emotion, structures known as the **amygdala** and **hippocampus** (Fig. 3.4), appear abnormal in the brains of individuals with autism. "Memories, the desire to produce language, feelings, and the emotional coloring of thought are all mediated by the limbic system. Anatomical systems necessary for cognitive functions, such as language, spatial concepts, understanding of meaning in life, and so forth are all intimately linked to the limbic system" (Helm-Estabrooks & Albert, 1991, p. 15). Since the functioning of these abilities is impacted in individuals with autism, it has been a logical step to focus research in this area. Thus far, anomalies include decreased size of the neurons that make up the structures of the limbic system, with a higher number of these neuronal cells packed into their respective spaces (Kemper & Bauman, 1998).

Scientists are persistently closing in on the differences in the brain structure and function of this population. In the meantime, the question arises: What has happened

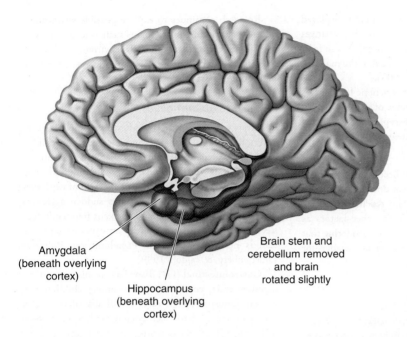

Figure 3.4 Amygdala and hippocampus. The limbic system is a group of subcortical structures in the brain that are responsible for learning, memory, and emotion. Deviations in the hippocampus and amygdala may contribute to autistic behaviors. (From Bear, M. F., Connors, B. W., & Parasido, M. A. [2001]. *Neuroscience: Exploring the brain* (2nd ed.). Philadelphia: Lippincott, Williams & Wilkins).

Amygdala
(beneath overlying
cortex)

Hippocampus
(beneath overlying
cortex)

Brain stem and
cerebellum removed
and brain
rotated slightly

in a child's system to cause these deviations in the brain to occur?

Hypothesized Causes of Autism

Parents of a child with autism, upon hearing the child's diagnosis, often exhaustively search for potential causes of this disability. The professionals who work with these parents must act as guides to discuss the most recent and accurate information in the autism field. Parents are likely to question professionals about many of the factors that will be discussed in the following sections. The scientific community has been delving into possible reasons for this disorder's occurrence, particularly as more and more children receive the diagnosis. It is important to share with parents those theories that are based on current scientific research and gently steer them away from invalid "trends."

Genetics

The differences in the neurobiology of children with autism are most likely accounted for by genetics. Genes are composed of DNA and, through heredity, determine each individual's unique characteristics. Genes are responsible for carrying the instructions for the brain. If these instructions are wrong, the brain deviates from a course of typical development (Siegel, 2003). No single gene has been found to cause these disorders; therefore, current research is focused on finding a combination of genes that may be responsible for an individual's susceptibility to autism (United Kingdom Medical Research

Council, 2001; Veenstra-VanDerWeele, Cook, & Lombroso, 2003). Rett's disorder is the only spectrum disorder that has a confirmed genetic mutation as its cause, occurring on the methyl-CpG-binding protein 2 gene (Webb & Latif, 2001).

Support for Genetic Etiology

- In sibling studies where one monozygotic twin was diagnosed with autism, the other was also diagnosed somewhere on the spectrum in up to 95% of cases. For dizygotic (fraternal) twins, both children received an ASD diagnosis in only 3% to 8% of cases studied (Centers for Disease Control and Prevention [CDC], 2010; Robledo & Ham-Kucharski, 2005). These statistics imply that shared genetic codes significantly increase the likelihood of autism (Rapin & Katzman, 1998; Veenstra-VanDerWeele et al., 2003).

- In the general population, an individual has an estimated 1% chance of having autism (CDC, 2010). Siblings of children with autism, however, are at a higher risk for presenting somewhere on the autism spectrum. For parents, the probability of having a second child with autism is 3% to 7% if the first child is male and autistic. If the first child is a female with autism, the likelihood of a second child with autism increases to approximately 7% to 14% (Rapin & Katzman, 1998). A higher rate of speech-language disorders has also been found among these families (Rutter, Silberg, O'Connor, & Simonoff, 1999), suggesting that these siblings received some, but not all, of the genes responsible for autism (Siegel, 2003).

- Relatives of these children more commonly displayed traits of autism (e.g., anxiety, aloofness) than relatives of other children. The presence of these traits in family members may be genetically linked to the manifestation of autism (Jick & Kaye, 2003).
- Additional weight is given to the genetic link since a disproportionately higher number of males are diagnosed with autism (with the exception of Rett's disorder), with four to five males diagnosed for every one female (CDC, 2010).

Because specific genes have not yet been identified as the cause of autism, and because autism does not appear to run in all families (Robledo & Ham-Kucharski, 2005), current research continues to explore other factors as possible etiologies. Researchers are also considering that autism may be caused by a different set of variables for each child on the spectrum.

Environmental Factors

Environmental factors may cause damage to a person's system if exposure to these external influences occurs during a period of critical development The United Kingdom Medical Research Council (2001) reviewed the following environmental risk factors as possible causes of autism: prenatal or postnatal exposure to viruses, infections, drugs/alcohol, endocrine factors, and carbon monoxide. Thus far, these factors are not significantly linked to ASDs. In terms of obstetric complications, most mothers reported entirely normal prenatal or perinatal experiences.

Researchers have paid particular attention to the measles-mumps-rubella (MMR) vaccination in recent years, with some researchers speculating that the mercury in this vaccination is responsible for causing changes in a person's system that lead to the symptoms of autism. When further investigated, a valid association between the MMR vaccine and autism was not found. For instance, many countries have discontinued the use of vaccines containing thimerosal, the preservative in vaccines containing mercury, yet autism in these countries has continued to rise at similar rates as countries whose vaccines continued to contain thimerosal (Madsen et al., 2003; Robledo & Ham-Kutcharski, 2005). In addition, the original study claiming to find a link between this vaccine and autism has been discredited. Though exposure to mercury may lead to impairments that look similar to those found in autism, children with autism have not consistently evidenced elevated levels of mercury in their systems. Therefore, while some parents feel they have seen a change in their child following administration of the vaccines, it appears no such link exists. Rather, the symptoms of autism tend to become more apparent around the same age that children receive vaccinations (Robledo & Ham-Kutcharski).

Research continues to explore possible environmental causes, including many toxins such as lead or plastics, though narrowing down potential environmental sources for this disorder is currently a daunting task with seemingly endless possibilities.

Physiologic Abnormalities

Children with autism need to be closely monitored for additional medical concerns, since many of these children are not able to clearly express a medical problem. For those children who are nonverbal, acting out with inappropriate behaviors may be their only form of expressing discomfort. If a child demonstrates sudden aggressive, severe, or unusual behaviors or awakens frequently from sleep, then medical attention by an experienced physician is necessary (Horvath, Papadimitriou, Rabsztyn, Drachenberg, & Tildon, 1999).

Gastrointestinal (GI) disorders, or disorders of the digestive tract, commonly occur among children with autism. Unusually high rates of GI disorders in children with autism have been documented in recent years, including GI reflux, gastritis, persistent gas, diarrhea, and constipation (Horvath et al., 1999; Levy, Mandell, Merhar, Ittenbach, & Pinto-Martin, 2003; McQueen & Heck, 2002). These problems should be treated by a gastroenterologist, a physician who specializes in GI disorders. A common, though unproven, theory hypothesizes that children with autism experience abnormal digestion of **gluten,** a mixture of proteins that may be found in wheat and other products (e.g., some snack foods or delicatessen meats), and **casein,** a protein found in cow's milk. This theory suggests that children with autism lack an enzyme that efficiently digests these substances. As a result, opioid or morphine-like substances accumulate and may be the reason these children socially withdraw or engage in repetitive behaviors (Levy & Hyman, 2003; McCandless, 2003). However, most medical professionals do not believe that food allergies cause autism; rather, these researchers believe that a child may experience both conditions, and experiencing discomfort from food allergies may exacerbate the symptoms of autism (Robledo & Ham-Kucharski, 2005).

The idea of a vulnerability to immune system disorders in children with autism has gathered interest and has been widely debated, but similar to theories of food allergies, there is currently a lack of research to prove or disprove this as a factor.

Combination of Factors

It is plausible that the interaction of gene susceptibility and environmental factors gives rise to autism. In other words, an individual may be genetically at risk for this disorder, but in order for characteristics to appear, an individual would also need to be exposed to a yet-to-be-identified environmental factor (United Kingdom Medical Research Council, 2001).

PREVALENCE AND INCIDENCE

The CDC (2010) estimates that 1 in 110 children in the United States has an ASD, diagnosed with autistic disorder, Asperger's syndrome, or PDD-NOS. CDD and Rett's disorder are less common, with CDD occurring in 0.1 to 0.6 children per 10,000 and Rett's disorder occurring in 1 in 10,000 to 1 in 15,000 children (United Kingdom Medical Research Council, 2001; Webb & Latif, 2001). Prevalence information for the adult population on the autism spectrum is not known.

Prevalence of autism has been on the rise since the early 1990s. Though this increase has raised speculation of a possible epidemic, the rise in prevalence results, at least in part, from better identification and availability of services. In addition, changes in diagnostic criteria now allow more children to fit the diagnosis of autism (Fombonne, 1999; Jick & Kaye, 2003; Rapin, 2002).

Incidence, or the measure of new cases per year, is best studied in disorders that have a clear onset. Because the age of onset in autism is usually unclear, accurate incident rates are difficult to measure. The incidence of ASDs is likely to be within the range of 30 to 60 cases per 10,000, which represents a huge increase over the original estimate 40 years ago of 4 cases for every 10,000 individuals (Rutter, 2005).

Autism affects children across all racial, ethnic, and socioeconomic groups. It is four times more likely to occur in boys than in girls, with the exception of Rett's disorder (CDC, 2010).

SIGNS AND SYMPTOMS

Each ASD is related to the other disorders in social, language, and behavioral deviations, and each differs in terms of age of onset, severity of symptoms, and presence of other features such as cognitive impairment (Lord & McGee, 2001). However, these core behaviors do not nearly encompass the entire picture of these complex human beings. Motor abnormalities, sensory processing disorders, and co-occurring medical disorders (e.g., seizures, sleep disturbances, GI problems) are only some of the additional concerns that arise in this population. Every child with autism displays a separate matrix of strengths and challenges; even two children who fall into the same diagnostic category on the spectrum (e.g., Asperger's syndrome) will exhibit individual differences resulting from personality and experiences (United Kingdom Medical Research Council, 2001).

The first of the core symptoms, difficulty in social interaction, includes limited use of eye contact, facial expressions, social gestures (e.g., pointing, waving, reaching arms up to be lifted by parent), and body postures. Additionally, children on the autism spectrum are usually challenged to accurately interpret the body language and facial expressions of other people. A child with ASD may not seek out others to share enjoyment, share interest in the same objects, or look for approval or reassurance from parents. Individuals may not frequently **gaze shift**; that is, sharing attention with another person by alternating gaze between an object and a person or following the gaze of another person. Maintaining continuous back-and-forth play or conversation with another person is often difficult for those with autism (Greenspan & Wieder, 2006). Moreover, individuals experience challenges in developing friendships with same-age peers. These obstacles range from showing a lack of interest in others to desiring friends but having difficulty understanding how to relate appropriately to peers. Problems with interaction may exist because children with autism are hypothesized to have limitations in **theory of mind,** which is the ability to understand another person's thoughts, feelings, or intentions. It is how an individual "reads" someone's thoughts, understands another person's perspective on an issue, and predicts another's feelings (Leslie & Frith, 1987). Without this ability, a person is not able to predict or understand the actions of others (Strock, 2004). Other social disturbances that manifest in children with autism include limited or repetitive play routines and limited or absent pretend play skills. A child may experience intense emotional outbursts if confused, frustrated, anxious, or overstimulated by the environment (Strock).

Language skills for those with autism are marked by abnormal characteristics and delays. Typically developing children progress through several communication milestones in their first few years. During a child's first year of life, a toddler gazes at others with interest, begins babbling, and reacts to sounds and voices. By 12 months, gestures and first words emerge, and a child shows recognition of his name and some familiar words and phrases. By 2 years of age, a child understands longer phrases and directions, has built a substantial vocabulary, and combines words into two- to three-word phrases (Strock, 2004). However, children with autism frequently show delays in learning to comprehend language and to speak.

Comprehension of a word must occur in order to produce that word in a meaningful way. In addition, as children develop, they begin to understand not just words but expressions, gestures, and social contexts. Many individuals with autism show challenges in comprehension, evidenced by

- Echoing back a speaker's words rather than showing understanding of the speaker
- Difficulty responding to questions or comments

■ Not responding to directions or requests to participate in an activity
■ Not attending to things that others are pointed out in
the environment
■ Not showing, looking at, or getting objects when
asked
■ Showing confusion, anxiety, and "falling apart" emotionally (dysregulation)
■ Not engaging, relating, or communicating as we might
expect (Gerber, 2009)
■ Struggling to understand social cues such as sarcasm,
humor, and facial expressions (Stark, 2004)

In the area of language production, many children
with autism are delayed in talking; some are unable to
use words until their school-age years. In severe cases
of autism, spoken language may not be acquired at all,
with recent studies estimating that about 20% to 25%
of those with autism remain nonverbal throughout
their lives (Tager-Flusberg, Paul, & Lord, 2005). Social
impairments further affect these children's communication because they may not be motivated to communicate
with others, are typically challenged to use or understand
social cues such as intonation and facial expressions to
interpret meaning, and have difficulty maintaining the
"give and take" of conversations (e.g., a child may discuss
only his topic of interest without allowing others to take
a turn).

For those children who develop spoken language,
conversation may appear peculiar because of the presence of **echolalia,** pronoun reversal, out of context
words, and odd vocal intonation patterns. Echolalia is
speech in which the child repeats what he has previously heard, including intonation similar to the speaker's (Luyster, Kadlec, Carter, & Tager-Flusberg, 2008;
Tager-Flusberg et al., 2005). Echolalia in not exclusive
to autism, as most young children use echolalia as they
are learning language. However, children with autism
retain this characteristic and often apply it in abnormal
ways. It likely results from poor **auditory processing**
(a child's ability to respond to sounds and comprehend
verbal language) while auditory memory remains intact
(Siegel, 1996). Echolalia may be immediate, meaning
that it occurs just after another speaker's utterance, or
delayed, occurring a significant period of time after hearing the spoken words (e.g., reciting an entire children's
book from memory an hour or day later) (Siegel, 1996).
Though echolalia may appear unusual in conversation,
children with autism frequently use this inappropriate
device in meaningful ways (e.g., a child may recite lines
from his favorite movie as a self-calming strategy when
he feels anxious or to help aid processing of what the
child just heard). Because children with autism often
fail to understand language, pronouns (e.g., "you" and

"me") are also often used incorrectly. Other times, these
individuals may use language that seems out of place for
the context. For instance, a child may say a pet's name
while pushing a toy train. Unusual intonation patterns
may include a monotone speech pattern, meaning that
the usual melody of speech sounds "flat" or unemotional.
Other children with autism may use a sing-song pattern
in their speech. Poor volume control and higher frequency of whispering for children who echo have also
been reported (Tager-Flusberg et al.).

In the area of repetitive behaviors, individuals with
ASD may exhibit an abnormal or intense preoccupation with routines or patterns. For instance, a child may
line up blocks or toy cars for hours without playing with
others or using these toys in pretend play. Rigidity in
this type of play may occur; for instance, the child may
scream or cry in reaction to someone joining his play
or moving the lined-up toys. Obsessions with specific
topics are common, such as showing an unusual interest in elevators or numbers and letters. Individuals with
autism are often successful with routines; however, disruption to that routine may be extremely disturbing
to that person (Strock, 2004). Many people diagnosed
with autism display abnormal, stereotyped behaviors
such as repetitive hand-flapping, body rocking, or looking at objects/people out of the corner of their eyes.
Another common feature of autism includes unusual,
nonfunctional preoccupation with parts of an object,
such as spinning the wheels of a toy car without showing
interest in any other type of play with this toy (American Psychiatric Association, 2000; Strock).

All children with autism demonstrate some combination of these social, language, and behavioral symptoms.
Additionally, specific characteristics are associated with
each disorder on the autism spectrum and are discussed
in the following sections.

Autistic Disorder

Autistic disorder is diagnosed when severe challenges
occur in each area of social, language, and behavioral characteristics. Marked delays and deviations are noted in language development, which are the most common initial
concerns of parents and pediatricians. Approximately half
of children with autistic disorder remain nonverbal or
struggle with severely impaired speech as adults (Rapin,
2002). Because both the comprehension and the use of
language are affected, these individuals are additionally
challenged to compensate for lack of verbal language
with another mode of communication, such as meaningful social gestures (pointing or acting out what they
want/need) or sign language (Lord & McGee, 2001).
Even those who develop verbal language may struggle in

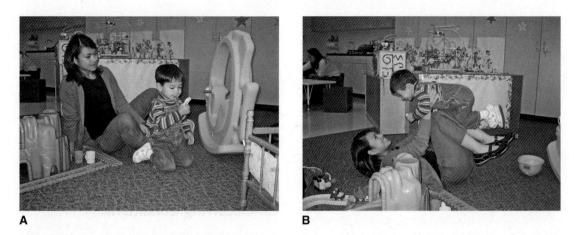

A   B

Figure 3.5 Young child with autistic disorder. **A,** Children with autism bear no obvious physical features that distinguish them from other children; rather, it is their behaviors that set them apart from their peers. Here, though a familiar adult approaches this little boy to play, he prefers gazing at an object for an unusual length of time. **B,** Initially, children with autism were thought to be incapable of any social interaction with others. This generalization no longer holds true. Though it requires more effort to engage this child in social interaction than it takes with typically developing children, he is clearly capable of sharing moments of joy with other people.

the initiation, maintenance, or relevance of conversation. Cognitive deficits are evident in the majority of children with autistic disorder, though these children often demonstrate a scattered pattern of skills (Rapin, 2002). For instance, a child may be exceptional at puzzles and matching colors but poorly comprehends time concepts. A child does not need to evidence cognitive challenges to receive a diagnosis of autistic disorder (Fig. 3.5).

Asperger's Syndrome

The hallmarks of this disorder include the social and behavioral challenges observed in other ASDs; however, children with Asperger's syndrome exhibit little or no delay in cognitive and language skills. Though early language milestones are met, children with Asperger's have difficulty using language appropriately in reciprocal interactions. Problems occur in the interpretation of others' gestures and nonverbal signals. Therefore, they may launch into a lengthy monologue on a topic, but not give their partner a conversational turn or observe their partner's signals of disinterest in a conversation (e.g., bored expression, fingers drumming on a table in exasperation). Unfortunately, because these children usually develop language at a typical age, their symptoms may not be immediately apparent, resulting in a diagnosis at a later age than children with autistic disorder (American Psychiatric Association, 2000). Though the term "high-functioning autism" is at times used synonymously with Asperger's syndrome, these two terms actually refer to two different diagnostic categories.

Pervasive Developmental Disorder— Not Otherwise Specified

This category is used when children demonstrate a significant impairment in social interaction, as well as impairment either in the use of language or with the presence of stereotypical behaviors (American Psychiatric Association, 2000). An individual does not need to demonstrate a language delay or deficiency to receive this diagnosis (DeBruin, Ferdinand, Meester, deNijs, & Verheig, 2007). Children given the diagnosis of PDD-NOS display less severe forms of ASD behaviors or show fewer of the symptoms of autism (Siegel, 1996). If symptoms first appear following the age of 36 months, a diagnosis of PDD-NOS is warranted (Matson, Wilkins, Smith, & Ancona, 2008).

Rett's Disorder

Rett's disorder primarily affects females who evidence a significantly deviant pattern of development. Individuals with Rett's disorder show an unusual progression of development. These children's prenatal and perinatal experiences are normal, and following birth, typical development progresses for several months. However, onset of unusual characteristics begins after this period of normal growth, as head growth decelerates between 5 and 30 months of age and hypotonia appears. Use of previously acquired functional hand skills diminishes between 5 and 48 months of age and is replaced by frequent, stereotyped hand movements, such as hand wringing (American Psychiatric Association, 2000). At the same time, dementia, autistic features, and possible onset of seizures appear (Dunn & McLeod, 2001). Poor coordination may be noted in gait or trunk movements. The pattern of social development is quite unusual. These children lose their previous ability to socially engage with others; however, social interaction is often later reacquired in a child's development. Expressive language, receptive language, and psychomotor skills are significantly impaired in this population (American Psychiatric Association, 2000; Dunn & McLeod). Rett's disorder stands alone as the only ASD with a known etiology caused by a single gene disorder (Webb & Latif, 2001).

Childhood Disintegrative Disorder

In this rare disorder, children with CDD develop normally for a minimum of 2 years following birth. Prior to 10 years of age, a loss of skills is noted in at least two of the following areas of development: receptive/expressive language, social/adaptive functioning, bowel/bladder control, play abilities, and motor skills (American Psychiatric Association, 2000). Skills disintegrate until the child exhibits features consistent with those in autism. However, before the loss of skills has occurred, children with CDD have usually acquired far more words, phrases, and even sentences than children with autistic disorder or PDD-NOS, meaning that the loss of language is more obvious in CDD than in autistic disorder (Siegel, 1996) (Table 3-1).

Co-Occurring Conditions

Autism has been associated with medical or genetic conditions in approximately 10% of its population. These conditions include, but are not limited to, Fragile X syndrome, tuberous sclerosis, metabolic disorders, rubella

TABLE 3.1 The Autism Spectrum Disorders

Disorder	Characteristics
Autistic disorder (classic autism)	Presence of ≥6 of 12 potential deficits involving all three behavioral domains that define the autistic spectrum ≥2 deficits in sociability, empathy, and insight into other person's feelings and agendas ≥1 deficit in communicative language and imagination ≥1 deficit in behavioral and cognitive flexibility Detectable before the age of 3 years Diagnosis not excluded by the level of cognitive competence or the existence of other handicaps
Asperger's disorder	Troublesome social ineptness Behavioral inflexibility with a narrow range of interests IQ ≥70 (affected children may be normally intelligent or gifted) No delay in the emergence of speech Often demonstrates clumsiness
Pervasive developmental disorder—not otherwise specified	Applies to less severely affected children who do not meet criteria for either autistic disorder or Asperger's disorder
Childhood disintegrative disorder	Early development entirely normal, including speech Severe regression between the ages of 2 and 10 years, affecting language, sociability, cognition, and competence in skills of daily life
Rett's disorder	Severe global regression in infant girls (rarely in boys), resulting in lifelong severe mental retardation, lack of language and purposeful hand use, and other neurologic deficits

syndrome, and *Haemophilus influenzae* meningitis (Fombonne, 1999).

Seizure disorders are not specific to autism but occur more frequently than in the general population. An estimated one-third of children are reported to have experienced at least two seizures before reaching adulthood. The probability of experiencing seizures is highest during adolescence and has been linked to causing or worsening cognitive and motor impairment (Rapin, 1997).

Diagnosis

Autism is now diagnosed at a younger age than ever before since characteristics of autism have become more defined and better recognized in recent years. Receiving a diagnosis at an early age is optimal because the sooner the disorder is recognized, the more likely the child can experience dramatic gains in learning and reduction in symptoms (Lord & McGee, 2001; Strock, 2004). In addition, parents are able to receive valuable support and education from professionals and other families.

Researchers have begun focusing on differences as early as the first year of life using families' home movies. One study that examined children diagnosed with autism reviewed home videotapes from their first birthdays and revealed interaction and behavioral differences clearly at 12 months of age. Consistent signs among these children included lack of the following skills: pointing, showing objects to others, looking to others, and responding to their names (Osterling & Dawson, 1994). In other studies that examined retrospective home videotapes, infants with autism also displayed hypotonia, poor visual attention, mouthing objects with extreme frequency, aversion to social touch, decreased or lacking babbling, and absence of shifting their attention from people to objects (Maestro et al., 2002). Researchers are now wondering if these initial characteristics may show that not as many children as originally thought have a "sudden onset" of autism but rather show these subtle signs early in life, with more significant signs appearing after 12 months (Osterling & Dawson, 1994).

A child is usually referred for an assessment because those who interact closely with him (e.g., family members, pediatrician, teachers) may observe warning signs either specific to autism or to a development delay in one or more areas. When these concerns become apparent, the child is initially screened, usually by primary care providers or early child care professionals, to look for the "red flags" that may indicate autistic behaviors. Published screening instruments for children with autism include

- The Checklist for Autism in Toddlers (Baron-Cohen, Allen, & Gillberg, 1992)

- The Autism Screening Questionnaire (Berumet, Rutter, Lord, Pickles, & Bailey, 1999)
- The Screening Tool for Autism in Two-Year-Olds (Stone, Coonrod, & Ousley, 2000)
- Australian Scale for Asperger's syndrome (Garnett & Attwood, 1998)
- Pervasive Developmental Disorders Screening Test—Stage 1 (Siegel, 1998a)
- The Modified Checklist for Autism in Toddlers (Robins, Fein, Barton, & Green, 2001)

If a child does not pass the screening, enough warning signs of autism are present to warrant a thorough assessment for autism. Since each child on the ASD displays a unique profile of strengths and weaknesses, no two children on the autism spectrum will look the same. Therefore, critical to an accurate diagnosis is an assessment with clinicians are experienced in identifying the characteristics of autism. Additionally, a thorough diagnosis with a team of professionals can gather insight into each child's skills across several areas of development, which, in turn, helps with intervention planning. The following elements should be included in every sensitive, comprehensive evaluation of a child with autism:

1. *History:* Though autism is not known to result from complications during pregnancy, it is important to discuss any unusual pre- or perinatal events to rule out other disorders. Because of autism's genetic implications, it is important to determine if other family members have been diagnosed with autism, psychiatric concerns, or developmental disorders. As noted previously, a child's history of development and behaviors is key in diagnosing this disorder. Therefore, questioning about autism-specific behaviors, including changes over time, in the areas of social, language, behavioral, play, cognitive, and sensory processing abilities is critical (Rapin, 1997).

2. *Medical history:* During this portion of the assessment, parents report when their child's developmental milestones were reached (e.g., what age their child said his first word, learned to walk), if regression of developmental skills occurred at any point, or if any other medical problems are occurring (e.g., psychiatric, sleeping, or eating problems) (Filipek et al., 1999).

3. *Physical/neurologic examination:* Other illnesses such as Fragile X syndrome, tuberous sclerosis, fetal alcohol syndrome, or congenital rubella need to be ruled out, since these disorders may look similar to autism (Rapin, 1997). The physician also checks for other medical illnesses (e.g., GI disorders, ear infections), measures head circumference, gives a general physical examination, examines mental status, verifies

that cranial nerves function normally, and performs a motor examination (Filipek et al., 1999).

4. *Parent interviewing:* Many diagnostic tools are available to gain parents' insight into their child's autism-specific behaviors. A clinician should also ask parents about their overall impression of their child, since more general questions may reveal further insight beyond the scope of these tools (Filipek et al., 1999; Lord & McGee, 2001). Parent interviewing tools include

   ■ The Autism Diagnostic Interview: Revised (Lord, Rutter, & LeCouteur, 1994)
   ■ Functional Emotional Assessment Scale (Greenspan, DeGangi, & Wieder, 1999)
   ■ The Gilliam Autism Rating Scale (Gilliam, 1995)
   ■ The Pervasive Developmental Disorders Screening Test—Stage 2 (Siegel, 1998b)

5. *Tests in developmental areas,* including language, social, motor, cognitive, and adaptive skills.

6. *Informal observation of the child* interacting with others. This is considered one of the most valuable pieces of the evaluation process, since it typically reveals the qualitative impairments of the child (such as lack of eye contact, limited initiation of interaction, or difficulty transitioning between tasks).

7. *Audiologic testing:* An audiologic evaluation is necessary to rule out hearing disorders. Children with autism are often unresponsive to verbal auditory stimuli, and it is important to determine that this behavior is not caused by a hearing impairment. If hearing loss co-occurs with autism, language comprehension may be further impacted than with a diagnosis of autism alone (Filipek et al., 1999).

8. *Other testing:* Certain tests may prove beneficial to specific circumstances. For instance, an electroencephalograph may be needed if the child is suspected of having seizures (Filipek et al.). Some children are assessed through university studies, and MRIs are typically included in these autism assessments (Bauman, 2004; Filipek et al.). Genetics testing may be appropriate for parents who are considering having another child. Some parents are also concerned about heavy metal contamination and wish to pursue a lead screening for their child.

During the comprehensive assessment, a diagnostic instrument should be used that examines autistic behaviors while the clinician observes the child's interests and interactions with others.

The instruments that are currently available include

■ The Autism Diagnostic Observation Schedule—Generic (Lord, Rutter, Goode, Heemsbergen, & Jordan, 1989)
■ The Childhood Autism Rating Scale (Schopler, Reichler, & Renner, 1998)

COURSE AND PROGNOSIS

Because each category in the autism spectrum presents with a range of abilities, the course of the disorder during one's lifetime depends on the child's diagnosis and individual differences. In addition, a diagnosis can change for an individual. For instance, a child with autistic disorder may show improvement in his symptoms, thereby displaying characteristics more similar to PDD-NOS (Siegel, 1996). Most individuals with autism tracked by longitudinal studies have retained ASD symptoms to some degree throughout their lives (Lord & McGee, 2001).

Autistic Disorder

A child displays traits of autism before the age of 3 years, and these symptoms are generally most apparent following the child's second birthday. In some cases, deviations in a child's developmental and interaction skills are noted shortly following birth (e.g., hypersensitivities, limited eye contact, difficulty imitating facial expressions), while other infants appear to develop normally and seem to lose skills between 12 and 36 months of age (Tager-Flusberg et al., 2005). Though gains may be made in developmental and social skills, these children are typically not able to catch up with their peers and remain autistic once the loss has occurred (Rapin, 1991). In some cases, behavioral challenges increase as a child reaches school age, while these challenges may decrease in other children. Longitudinal studies have found that few individuals with autistic disorder reach full independence as adults; many are not able to live on their own or find employment. Even those who evidence higher skills in this category (known as high-functioning autism) frequently struggle with social interactions throughout their lives. In fact, it is older children with higher-functioning autistic disorders who often make more attempts to socialize and may feel greater distress and loneliness than younger or lower-functioning children with ASD when they are unsuccessful in reciprocal interactions (Rapin, 1991). For the many individuals who do not reach independence in adulthood, families must continue to provide support or these adults may enter residential programs. These programs offer special education, developmental, and behavioral techniques to teach new skills and generalize those skills into functional community activities (Holmes, 1990).

Asperger's syndrome

A child with Asperger's syndrome typically exhibits strong verbal skills in the school-age years; however, professionals and peers should not let these skills be misleading in terms of the child's social impairments. These children may show a strong interest in having friends but lack the

understanding of the social rules that apply to these interactions. As a result, these individuals may appear more
comfortable with others either older or younger than
themselves. Longitudinal studies suggest that prognosis
is better for Asperger's syndrome than autistic disorder
because more individuals are able to function independently in employment and self-sufficient living (American
Psychiatric Association, 2000).

Pervasive Developmental Disorder— Not Otherwise Specified

Children with PDD-NOS are typically diagnosed
between the ages of 3 and 4 years old. Some individuals demonstrate an intellectual disability, and those with
lower IQ scores show more severely impaired social
development (Matson et al., 2008). However, those
children with higher developmental skills do not always
walk an easier path. Increased awareness of their own
differences from their peers can cause individuals with
PDD-NOS to feel isolated, anxious, and/or depressed.
During adolescence, children with PDD-NOS face
confusing hormonal changes while trying to understand
the intricate social subtleties their peers seem to have
mastered. Both friendships and dating may be difficult
for these individuals. A counselor with training in ASDs
may help these adolescents feel supported and understood and can navigate teenagers through some of their
social challenges. As an adult, if an individual with this
disorder experiences only mild symptoms, he will likely
be independent and able to live on his own. For some
with PDD-NOS, marriage, parenting, and friendship
may be too complex and overwhelming, but others have
found success in these relationships despite the additional challenges of the disorder (Autism Speaks, 2010).

Rett's Disorder

Rett's disorder is evident before a child reaches 4 years
of age and most frequently presents in the first or second
year of life following a period of typical development.
Challenges in communication and behaviors are typically continuous throughout the individual's life. Gains
in developmental skills are usually not significant in later
childhood or adolescence, though the child may show a
heightened desire to socially interact with others (American Psychiatric Association, 2000).

Childhood Disintegrative Disorder

Symptoms appear in this disorder following the age of 2
years but prior to the age of 10 years, and children progress through typical developmental milestones before
the onset of this disorder. Following the onset, a significant loss of skills is noted. If this disorder occurs in isolation, the loss of skills ceases and minimal improvement is
observed later in life. This disorder may co-occur with a
progressive neurologic condition, in which case, the child
will continue to lose skills (American Psychiatric Association, 2000).

General Prognostic Indicators

Overall, children's language levels and IQ scores are the
strongest indicators related to prognosis in independence
and appropriate functioning in adulthood, particularly in
the area of verbal IQ (Lord & McGee, 2001).

In terms of communication skills, a child's ability to
spontaneously, meaningfully, and consistently combine
words into phrases or sentences before 5 years of age
is a good prognostic indicator of cognitive, language,
adaptive, and academic achievement measures (Lord &
McGee, 2001). It is important to observe that the child
is able to spontaneously construct sentences rather than
echo others' utterances (echolalia) or use memorized
chunks of language to communicate. A child's use of **joint
attention** has been found to be a predictor of language
outcome. Joint attention is the ability to share experiences with others through social communication, including eye contact, gesture, and verbal language. Children
who fail to use early gestural joint attention (e.g., failing
to point at an object and to turn to his mother to determine if his mother shares his interest) seem to struggle
in the development of meaningful language. In Lord and
McGee's review of autism research (2001), one longitudinal research finding implied that early joint attention,
symbolic play, and receptive language were strong predictors of a child's future outcomes. Another study in this
review examined severity of repetitive, stereotyped behaviors and social symptoms and found that the severity later
predicted adaptive functioning.

Early success in hand-eye coordination may predict
vocational abilities later in life. Fine motor skills also predicted later leisure pursuits. Children with autism who displayed a definite hand preference performed significantly
better on motor, language, and cognitive tasks (Hauck &
Dewey, 2001). The ability to imitate body movements
has been linked to expressive language development, and
imitation of actions with objects predicted later levels of
play abilities. The more established behavioral challenges
become without intervention, the more these problems
persist and worsen (Lord & McGee, 2001).

Medical/Surgical Management

Overall, treatment for autism does not heavily rely on
medical intervention, and surgical interventions are not

practiced for this disorder. Intensive early intervention is most effective in reducing problem behaviors while increasing language, social, sensory, motor, and cognitive skills. A variety of approaches are available, ranging from highly structured to naturalistic. Because no two children with autism present with the same set of symptoms, no one treatment plan is successful for all children with autism. Effective intervention must account for the child's individual strengths and challenges and must consider functional skills to be generalized across a variety of settings in the child's life. Substantial literature supports early intervention for children younger than 3 years old as the most beneficial time to connect new pathways for more appropriate functioning and behavior, though an individual may continue to make substantial gains following this period of development (Lord & McGee, 2001; Rapin, 1997; Rogers, 1996). Because it is beyond the scope of this book to discuss these approaches, this chapter focuses on current knowledge of medical interventions meant to accompany intervention techniques.

Pharmacologic Therapies

Use of medication does not cure the core social, language, and repetitive behavioral deficits of autism because "in most cases, the brain has undergone atypical cellular development dating from the earliest embryonic stages" (Rapin, 2002, p. 303). Much of the research in this area is presently limited or inconclusive. In addition, many parents and clinicians are cautious because use of pharmacotherapy with children presents the risk of harmful side effects. Lindsay and Aman (2003) reviewed existing literature on pharmacologic intervention and found that when certain medications are used appropriately, behavioral dysregulations such as hyperactivity, irritability, anxiety, and perseveration may be reduced. For instance, risperidone, an atypical antipsychotic agent, shows promising results in emerging research for reducing tantrums, irritability, aggression, and self-injurious and repetitive behaviors (Gordon, 2002; Lindsay & Aman, 2003; Pediatric Psychopharmacology Autism Network, 2002). Because autism is likely a genetic disorder determined before the child is born, pharmacologic treatments could probably not "undo" this disorder. Therefore, these treatments are not intended to replace educational services but rather to supplement them. For those children who respond successfully to medication, behavioral and educational intervention may be even more beneficial since they do not struggle as greatly with challenging behaviors.

Medical Conditions

Medical intervention is necessary for any co-occurring medical conditions, such as seizures or GI disorders. Children with autism need to be monitored closely for behaviors that may reflect a medical condition and should receive a complete medical workup and treatment through a physician who specializes in the child's medical condition.

Complementary and Alternative Medicine

Complementary and alternative medicine has gained popularity in the past decade as a supplementary treatment to educational services. Complementary and alternative medicine is defined as "a broad domain of healing resources that encompasses all health systems modalities and practices and their accompanying theories and beliefs, other than those intrinsic to the politically dominant health system" (Panel of Definition and Description, 2002, as cited in Levy et al., 2003, p. 418). Those who support complementary and alternative medicine believe the methods target underlying medical difficulties, such as GI and sleep disorders, which are not addressed through educational intervention. The goal of many of the complementary and alternative medicine treatments is to aid in the associated problems of autism, rather than claim to cure the disorder. Statistics reveal that 30% to 50% of children with autism in the United States are using complementary and alternative medicine; however, approximately 9% are using potentially harmful treatments and 11% are using multiple complementary and alternative medicine treatments (Levy et al., 2003). Several studies are currently under way to examine the effectiveness and the risks of these treatments since many parents have reported a decrease in associated problems (e.g., GI problems) and an increase in developmental skills. Table 3-2 summarizes the potentially harmful side effects of these methods. The following sections describe commonly used complementary and alternative medicine treatments.

Supplements

The use of vitamins and minerals to address ASD concerns purports that because children with autism experience GI inflammation and intestinal disorders, their ability to absorb nutrients is thereby reduced. As a result, development that relies on nutrients such as vitamins A, B1, B3, B5; biotin; selenium; zinc; and magnesium is altered. Frequently used supplements include vitamin C, cod liver oil (for vitamins A and D), and the combination of vitamin B6 with magnesium (Autism Society of America, 2004).

Gluten-Free, Casein-Free Diet

Parents and professionals who support the theory that gluten and casein negatively impact a child's development recommend a diet that completely eliminates these products (McCandless, 2003). Parent reports of improvement

TABLE 3.2 Potential Side Effects of Complementary and Alternative Medicine

Proposed Mechanisms	Example	Potential Adverse Side Effects
Neurotransmitter production or release	DMG B6/magnesium Vitamin C Omega 3 Fatty acids Secretin	No reported side effects (excessive doses) B6: peripheral neuropathy; Mg: arrhythmia Renal stones No reports of side effects from excessive administration Unknown impact of long-term administration of secretin
Change in GI function	Gluten-free/casein-free diet Secretin Pepcid Antibiotics	If nutritional state not monitored by clinicians, at risk for inadequate calcium, vitamin D, protein intake Unknown impact of long-term administration Hepatotoxicity in high doses Superinfection or antibiotic resistance with long-term use, implications for population at large with resistance
Putative immune mechanism or modulators	Antifungal agents Intravenous Immunoglobulin Vitamin A/cod liver oil	Possible superinfections or resistance with long-term use Aseptic meningitis, renal failure, or infection Hypervitaminosis A or pseudotumor cerebri
Agents that might remove toxins	Chelation—DMSA, DMPA Other detox agents or protocols	Renal and hepatotoxicity of oral agents Possible magnesium intoxication from Epsom salts ingestion

Reprinted with permission from Levy, S. E., & Hyman, S. L. (2003). Use of complementary and alternative medicine for children with autistic spectrum disorders is increasing. *Pediatric Annals, 32*(10), 687.

have been inconsistent, as some parents claim to see significant improvements in their child's behavior and/or developmental skills (e.g., improved eye contact), while others report that no change occurs by implementing this diet. Data are currently limited and inconclusive. Anecdotal information comprises the majority of reports rather than controlled studies.

Other Common Complementary and Alternative Medicine Treatments for Autism

- *Secretin:* Secretin, a hormone naturally produced in the small intestine, stimulates secretions in the pancreas and liver. The use of extra secretin through injections became a popular complementary and alternative medicine treatment before it was scientifically analyzed, but studies now show few changes for children with ASDs

who have used the extra hormone injection (Levy & Hyman, 2003).
- *Chelation:* Because mercury poisoning produces symptoms similar to those seen in autism, mercury and other heavy metals have been suggested as causes of autism. Some parents who believe their children have experienced overexposure to metal have chosen chelation therapy, a process to remove toxins from a child's system (Levy & Hyman, 2003). However, this procedure is highly controversial since chelation can have long-lasting, damaging side effects such as kidney damage and congestive heart failure (Robledo & Ham-Kucharski, 2005).
- *Antibiotic treatment:* Immune system dysfunctions and antibiotic treatments have been targeted as possible causes of autism, and those who believe in these theories use further antibiotic treatment to alter the

course of the symptoms in autism (Levy & Hyman, 2003).

■ *Antifungal treatment:* Yeast overgrowth in the colon is hypothesized to cause many medical disorders, including autism, with a low-sugar diet and the use of probiotic agents (which encourage helpful intestinal bacteria) used as treatments (Levy & Hyman, 2003).

Conclusion of Complementary and Alternative Medicine Treatments

The effectiveness of complementary and alternative medicine stands largely unproven and highly controversial. Attempts are under way for further studies since many parents report positive results by using these methods. Complementary and alternative medicine treatments are intended to supplement educational services rather than to replace them. Clinicians are currently encouraged to use an empathetic stance, with families providing complementary and alternative medicine to their children, though no alternative method should be administered without the guidance of an experienced physician.

IMPACT OF CONDITIONS ON CLIENT FACTORS

Global Impairment

Autism is considered a global impairment, meaning that it does not reflect damage as a result of one specific lesion in the brain. Since autism likely affects several regions of the brain, this global impact means that autism impairs multiple areas of a child's development. As a result, even a child's ability to regulate basic functions is impaired, such as consistent sleep patterns or emotional stability.

Irregular sleeping patterns are common in children with autism, particularly in the quality rather than the quantity of their sleep. Disturbances include problems falling asleep, waking throughout the night, disoriented awakening, difficulty sleeping in an unfamiliar place, and nightmare-type disturbances such as screaming. Children may exhibit sleep disturbances as early as 2 years of age, and higher occurrence of sleep disorders seems to exist in children with more severe forms of autism (Hering, Epstein, Elroy, Iancu, & Zelnic, 1999; Hoshino, Watanabe, Yashima, Kaneko, & Kumashiro, 1984; Schreck & Mulick, 2000).

Children with autism often have difficulty regulating their own emotions and interpreting the emotions of others. These children often experience depression, a sense of loneliness, and a limited range of emotions that results in a flattened affect. For example, they may show they are happy or angry, but more subtle emotions such as worry, jealousy, or disappointment are less commonly seen in these children. Additionally, difficulty in reading facial expressions, body postures, and intonation of voices to infer another's feelings are common challenges. An unusual characteristic of autism is **emotional lability,** which is a child's use of laughing or crying for unclear reasons or during inappropriate situations. Some parents may describe their children as "laid back" or less reactive to emotional stimuli, while other parents note a tendency to frequently cry inconsolably. Heightened anxiety is evident in many children, as are temper tantrums that often result from disrupted routines (Rapin, 1991). Other children show a lack of fear during dangerous situations (Lord & McGee, 2001). Aggressive behaviors such as hitting, biting, self-injury (head banging, hitting self), or self-stimulatory behaviors (e.g., body rocking) may occur when the child does not get his way or his routine is disturbed.

Specific Mental Functions

Each child with autism manifests the symptoms in different ways; therefore, children with an ASD show various combinations of concerns in their mental skills. Attention deficits, however, are nearly universal in this population. Unique patterns of attention include distractibility, disorganization, intense preoccupation for preferred, self-initiated activities for unusual lengths of time, and lack of boredom for repeating same action or play schema (Rapin, 1991). The ability to focus jointly on an activity with another person is significantly impaired.

A child with autism often shows a scattered pattern of memory functions (Hill, Berthoz, & Frith, 2004). Overall, "memory performance of individuals with autism becomes increasingly impaired as the complexity of the material increases" (Minshew & Goldstein, 2001, p. 1099). Children with autism also use fewer organizational strategies, relying on stereotyped rules regardless of the task's complexity. Therefore, a child with autism performs more poorly on tasks with higher complexity. Word recall is more significantly impacted than digit recall, and these children often have difficulty recalling activities in which they have recently participated (Boucher, 1981). However, certain areas of memory remain intact, particularly in the areas of visual and **rote memory**. Rote memory describes the memorization and use of previously heard chunks of language rather than the spontaneous generation of language.

In the area of perceptual functioning, individuals with ASDs perceive sensory stimuli but often process and react abnormally to it. Integration of perceptual and sensorimotor information allows individuals to respond appropriately with physical and emotional responses. In autism, this integration does not occur in the same efficient way; therefore, this population of individuals has difficulty responding with typical emotional and physical responses to the sensory stimuli around them. Between 30% and 100% of individuals with autism demonstrate deviant sensory-perceptual abilities (Dawson & Watling, 2000).

Cognitive impairments are common in, though not universal to, the autism population. Approximately 75% of these individuals have IQ scores below 70 (American Psychiatric Association, 2000), indicating intellectual disability. Those with Asperger's syndrome, however, show IQ scores within the normal range. Individuals with cognitive deficits typically demonstrate scattered skills; in other words, they may present with strong skills in some areas with significant concerns in other areas. These children often have difficulty sequencing a series of items, imitating the actions and words of others meaningfully, generalizing concepts across a variety of situations, demonstrating theory of mind, and playing with toys appropriately and symbolically (Lord & McGee, 2001). In her 1991 literature review of autistic features, Rapin described that children with autism tend to have better visual-spatial skills than auditory verbal skills on IQ tests. Children in this population may show above-average skills in very specific areas, such as calculating numbers, completing puzzles, or demonstrating rote verbal memory, while demonstrating overall cognitive impairment. Some children with autism are able to read at a young age with minimal instruction, but they have little or no understanding of what they read. This unusual occurrence is known as **hyperlexia**.

Studies examining higher level cognitive functions have revealed that executive functioning skills such as forward planning, cognitive flexibility, and the use of assistive strategies (e.g., creating a mnemonic such as a rhyme to assist in remembering information) in learning are impacted for those who have autism (Gordon, 2002).

As previously described, children with autism typically show language delay, with the exception of those with Asperger's syndrome. Deviations from typical language are noted across all diagnostic categories. Children on the autism spectrum typically have limitations in using language in appropriate contexts and for social purposes.

Sensory Functions and Pain

"The experience of being human is imbedded in the sensory events of everyday life. When we observe how people live their lives, we discover they characterize their experiences from a sensory point of view" (Dunn, 2001, p. 608). If a child's sensory system does not interpret stimuli in a typical way, it is easy to understand why this individual may react to the world differently. These sensory disturbances appear to occur more commonly in children than adults, and since the severity of sensory impairment seems to be related to the severity of stereotypic and behavioral abnormalities, sensory processing problems should be addressed through

early intervention to reduce these abnormal behaviors (Dawson & Watling, 2000; Lord & McGee, 2001).

The prevalence of sensory impairments in children with autism is significantly higher than in the population of typically developing children, though each child with autism shows a different profile of hyper- and hyposensitivity to sensory stimulation. Despite the variability in sensory thresholds from child to child, some general patterns have emerged in research.

Visual perception is usually an area of relative strength and may be used to compensate for challenging areas. For instance, the integration of vestibular, visual, and somatosensory afferent systems is needed to maintain upright postural stability. Molloy, Dietrich, and Bhattacharya (2003) measured the postural stability in children with autism and found that these children relied on visual cues to help them maintain stability. When these visual cues were omitted, children had difficulty maintaining their upright balance and reducing their sway. In addition, children may use their visual processing strengths to help learn routines through the use of a picture schedule, or they may communicate using picture symbols if verbal language is challenging (Prizant, Wetherby, Rubin, Laurent, & Rydell, 2006). One area of visual processing that is consistently impaired is integrating details of a figure into a whole (Deruelle, Rondan, Gepner, & Tardif, 2004). For instance, if given a line drawing of a house made up of geometric shapes, these children focus on the shapes rather than seeing the image of a house. Children with autism often twirl themselves or spin objects obsessively while staring intently at the object; they may be fascinated with the visual effects these actions create (Hewetson, 2002). They may seek out areas of visual interest, such as lines on the floor of a gymnasium. Some show hypersensitivities to a busy environment or bright light.

Auditory processing is often a significantly challenging area for children with autism. Frequently, children with ASDs are unresponsive to some auditory stimuli while being oversensitive to others. For instance, a child may not respond when her name is called but screams in response to hearing a vacuum cleaner running. Furthermore, children with autism may be distracted or irritable or have difficulty functioning in activities in noisy environments (Kientz & Dunn, 1997).

These children also show mixed patterns of craving and/or avoiding vestibular sensations. Some children appear to seek out, others withdraw from, and some show mixed preferences for certain types of these sensations. Common vestibular movements include swinging, spinning on a sit-and-spin or merry-go-round, and playing with spinning toys (Kientz & Dunn, 1997).

Food tastes and textures are difficult for many children on the autism spectrum. Many parents note their child with autism has unusual taste preferences. Due to sensory issues, these individuals are frequently "picky eaters" and may have a limited repertoire of food preferences (Williams, Dalrymple, & Neal, 2000). They may be sensitive to certain textures, such as avoiding wet (e.g., oranges in fruit syrup), "goopy" (e.g., macaroni and cheese), and/or mixed textured foods (e.g., a casserole). Though nutritional intake generally appears adequate (United Kingdom Medical Research Council, 2001), it is often stressful for families to meet nutritional needs of these children who have very specific food preferences. Parents and clinicians typically observe these individuals to crave strong tastes, such as spicy or salty foods, and crunchy foods that give the child significant sensory input.

As with taste, many individuals with autism have abnormal smell interests. Unusual behaviors are observed in the person's inappropriate smelling of objects or unusual attachment to or aversion of certain smells (Rapin, 1991; Williams et al., 2000).

Reports of clumsiness are common for children who are higher functioning on the autism spectrum (e.g., children with milder cognitive impairment, such as those with Asperger's syndrome) (Ghaziuddin & Butler, 1998). Another study suggested that in children with Asperger's, this observed clumsiness may result from a deficit in proprioception, not from a motor disturbance (Weimer, Schatz, Lincoln, Ballantyne, & Trauner, 2001).

Tactile defensiveness is a hypersensitivity to certain touch situations that most people find nonthreatening. Children with this symptom frequently exhibit an avoidance-withdrawal response (e.g., rubbing/scratching, avoiding certain textures, or crying when exposed to a specific texture) (Baranek & Berkson, 1994). The presence of tactile defensiveness appears to co-occur with stereotyped behaviors such as rocking of the body, hand flapping, and unusual interest or focus on objects (Baranek, Foster, & Berkson, 1997). A significant relationship also appears between tactile defensiveness and rigid behaviors (e.g., child has difficulty breaking out of own agenda), repetitive verbalizations, visual stereotypes, and abnormally focused affections. Though these children experience significant tactile hypersensitivities, many also appear to have a reduced response to temperature or pain (Rapin, 1991).

Functions Related to the Digestive System

Children with autism may be at a higher risk for experiencing GI problems such as reflux or gastritis, with persistent gas, diarrhea, and constipation also frequently reported (Horvath et al., 1999; Levy et al., 2003; McQueen & Heck, 2002). Additionally, hypotheses exist regarding functioning of the digestive system, such as increased intestinal permeability that allows absorption of morphine-like compounds from gluten and casein.

The buildup of these substances theoretically results in the social withdrawal and stereotypical behaviors seen in autism, but as previously described, this theory is controversial and has not been proven (Levy & Hyman, 2003).

Urinary and Reproductive Functions

In children with autism, the urinary tract is usually typical in its structure and function. However, for those children with cognitive and sensory impairments, toilet training is often complicated. Children with autism often learn to toilet train at a later age than typically developing children; display problems such as fear, pain, confusion, frustration, and constipation when learning to train; urinate or defecate in inappropriate places; and experience difficulty when a change of routine occurs or when entering an unfamiliar bathroom (Dalrymple & Ruble, 1992).

Because individuals with autism have difficulty interacting, inappropriate sexual behavior is also a concern. Close relationships with others are often challenging for these individuals; therefore, fewer person-oriented behaviors may be noted. Additionally, discouraging inappropriate sexual behaviors may be difficult. The most frequently reported inappropriate sexual behaviors include public masturbation or public touching of one's own private parts (Ruble & Dalrymple, 1993; Van Bourgondien, Reichle, & Palmer, 1997).

Gross and Fine Motor Skills

Though individuals with ASDs often show relative strengths in movement functions, some abnormalities in motor skills have been observed, including overall motor joint laxity, hypotonia, clumsiness, apraxia, and chronic toe-walking (Rapin, 1997). Persistent toe-walking may be from hypersensitivity to certain walking surfaces (e.g., grass, sand) or to provide children with additional proprioceptive feedback as their muscles contract (Robledo & Ham-Kucharski, 2005). Females with Rett's disorder frequently demonstrate poor coordination in gait or trunk movements. In children with Asperger's syndrome, "clumsiness" has been more specifically defined as poor performance on tests of apraxia, tandem gait, one-leg balance with eyes closed, and repetitive finger-thumb apposition (Weimer et al., 2001).

Further fine and gross motor impairments include problems in skilled movement, hand-eye coordination, speed, praxis and imitation, posture, and balance (Dawson & Watling, 2000). A particularly debilitating abnormality in individuals with autism includes deficits in motor imitation skills despite intact perceptual and motor capacities, which is most apparent in younger groups of children (Williams, Whiten, & Singh, 2004).

Furthermore, these children perform poorly on tasks of executing a sequence of movements, such as a sequence of hand or facial actions in imitation (Hughes, 1996). Reduced stride lengths, increased stance times, increased hip flexion at toe-off, reduced knee extension at initial ground contact, abnormal heel strikes, and decreased knee extension and ankle dorsiflexion at ground contact were noted in an earlier study of children with autism (Vilensky, Damasio, & Maurer, 1981).

In addition, a disproportionate number of children with autism display **ambiguous hand preference** (~40%) long past the age that dominant hand preference typically develops. A person who is ambidextrous will usually choose one hand for a specific task (e.g., left hand for writing, right hand for throwing a football). An ambiguous hand preference, however, refers to switching hands within the same activity (Hauck & Dewey, 2001). When this behavior persists into the school-age years, it may indicate abnormal functioning of the brain.

Motor stereotypes are common in those on the autism spectrum and often manifest through hand flapping, pacing, spinning, running in circles, and flipping light switches. More severe, self-injurious forms include biting, hitting oneself, or head banging (Rapin, 1997).

Brain Structure

The most significant abnormalities in a child's body structure include the anomalies of the brain that are currently under investigation. Likely caused by genetic abnormalities, these deviations in the brains of individuals with autism are not yet clearly defined, nor is it clear precisely how the differences cause the characteristics of autism. Studies have found consistent abnormalities in head growth, the cerebellum, frontal lobes, and limbic system (Bauman, 2004; Bauman & Kemper, 1996; Carper & Courchesne, 2005; Helm-Estabrooks & Albert, 1991; Kemper & Bauman, 1998; Piven et al., 1997; United Kingdom Medical Research Council, 2001). Research is also examining potential deviations in the way different regions of the brain communicate (Piven et al.).

Case Illustration

Child with Autism

At 1 year of age, Jacob was brought to an early intervention clinic because of delays in motor and cognitive skills. An initial evaluation conducted by an occupational therapist, educator, and speech-language pathologist confirmed these concerns. In the area of gross motor skills, Jacob was delayed in learning to walk and demonstrated moderate hypotonia in his trunk. Fine motor concerns included tactile defensiveness of wet or sticky substances and delays in grasping and manipulating objects appropriately. Cognitively, Jacob showed little interest in playing with toys or imitating the words and actions of others. Language impairments were not yet observed since Jacob frequently vocalized, babbled, and expressed his feelings through behaviors such as smiling or crying. At this young age, ASD was not initially suspected. Jacob was clearly a delightful little boy who showed a strong attachment to his parents and was interested in watching children and other adults in his environment.

Jacob was placed in a playgroup at the clinic where his occupational therapist and educator worked directly with him, while a speech-language pathologist monitored his language. As time passed, further concerns became evident. His language skills failed to further develop; as a result, first words did not emerge. Nor was he using gestures to indicate what he wanted. At the age of 14 months, he evidenced limitations in language comprehension and speech production, and his use of eye contact decreased. As the months progressed, he showed frustration more frequently through crying, banging his head, throwing himself on the ground, and arching his back to pull away from a person trying to hold him. His feeding skills were limited since he was not able to bring his hand to his mouth, and he demonstrated extreme sensitivities to many tastes and textures. He did not show an interest in other self-help skills such as learning to bathe or dress himself. While other children his age learned to imitate motor movements in songs, Jacob seemed to content to only listen to the songs. He did not demonstrate typical play skills for his age such as exploring how toys worked, taking toys in or out of a container, or taking turns with others. However, musical or flashing toys captured his attention for long periods of time. While he was engrossed with these toys, he evidenced unusual, repetitive behaviors such as rocking his body back and forth.

Through early intervention by his therapists and parents, Jacob's gross motor skills improved during the following months, and he successfully learned to walk at 18 months. He delighted in walking through his home, through the early intervention center, and outside. His eye contact improved, becoming more spontaneous and consistent. His repertoire of sounds increased, and he vocalized to take a turn in songs or games; in addition, he began signing "more" to request something desirable to happen again. He learned to play with toys in a more functional manner, including stacking rings and blocks and taking toys in and out of containers. Yet other skills continued to be challenging. When he was left to play on his own, he repetitively turned the pages of books or walked aimlessly around a room. He showed hypersensitivities to touching or mouthing certain textures, limited motor or imitation skills, difficulty understanding others, a lack of verbal words, and repetitive behaviors during play.

Currently, at slightly older than 2 years of age, Jacob continues to struggle in several areas of development. However, he has made steady progress in these developmental skills, and his family and team are encouraged that he will continue to make significant gains. More importantly, despite being faced with more challenges than typically developing children, Jacob is a young boy who is often able to share and express joy with others.

Adult With Autism

Patrick is a 38-year-old man who was diagnosed with autistic disorder at 2½ years of age. His mother was first concerned he had a hearing impairment, as he did not seem to understand what people said to him, did not respond to a fire truck siren, placed his ear close to the refrigerator, and acted out with negative behaviors. Behavioral and developmental concerns persisted after testing ruled out a hearing impairment. A psychologist specializing in autism assessed Patrick's developmental skills and behaviors and diagnosed Patrick with autistic disorder.

Patrick communicated nonverbally for several years, usually by grabbing a person's hand and leading the person to an item he wanted. He had a very limited diet as a young child, eating only peanut butter, raisins, and yogurt. In time, he increased his repertoire of foods. When Patrick was 3, he began attending a local school for children with autism; at the age of 8, he attended a school for children with a variety of special needs. Patrick began using words at the age of 9. He transferred to a local public high school at the age of 18, participating in the school's autism program, and working in the school's kitchen to learn to work with others. He graduated high school when he was 26, receiving a diploma of completion for the school's autism program.

Following high school, Patrick moved into a condominium with two other men diagnosed with autism; he currently maintains this living situation. Patrick and his roommates receive 24-hour supervision. He also works 5 days per week at a therapy center that encourages functional skill-building. He works alongside eight or nine other adults with autism and receives supervision in his daily tasks, which include shredding legal documents and inserting newspapers into plastic sleeves. To prevent overwhelming stimuli, the room is kept dim and without extraneous sound.

As with all individuals diagnosed with autism, Patrick shows personal strengths and unique challenges, with his own personality shining through.

Patrick has achieved several goals in activities of daily living and continues to work toward independence. He dresses himself, with the occasional need for help with fasteners. He toilets independently, though requires assistance with wiping after a bowel movement. He washes himself with verbal prompting from a supervisor and climbs in and out of the tub independently. He applies deodorant and cologne and combs his hair when directed. Once a supervisor has prepared his toothbrush, Patrick brushes his teeth for 2 minutes, needing occasional reminders to not swallow the toothpaste. He carries groceries into the house, takes out the trash, and wipes the table after meals.

Patrick displays unusual and stereotypical behaviors, such as rapidly bouncing or tapping a small ball on a tabletop, spinning lids, and repeatedly blowing up balloons. He eats his food very quickly and needs verbal reminders to eat at a slower pace. In the car, he often bends down to play with the hardware beneath his seat. Recently, Patrick has shown negative behaviors, such as destruction of property or soiling himself. His family and staff believe these behaviors are likely Patrick's way of showing grief from his father's death last year.

Socially, Patrick gets along well with his family, supervisors, and roommates, though he has few verbal interactions with his roommates. His family frequently brings him to community outings such as sports events; Patrick shows interest and enjoyment during these outings. He reciprocates another person's smile easily. He occasionally initiates and maintains eye contact with another person, but not with typical duration or frequency. He often responds to a speaker, but does not engage in back-and-forth conversation.

Regarding other developmental skills, Patrick currently understands more language than he uses. He follows familiar one-step directions, though sometimes needs repetition from the speaker to complete the request. He comprehends simple questions that relate to his interests and daily routines. Patrick communicates through single words and phrases. He names familiar people and objects, answers simple questions, and requests desired items and actions. He greets when prompted by another person. In the area of fine motor skills, Patrick does not demonstrate a hand preference. He writes his first name, last name, and the word "love" to sign letters and cards. Patrick shows many strengths in his gross motor skills. He enjoys playing a variety of sports, including swimming and throwing a ball back and forth with a partner. He loves to shoot basketball hoops (dribbling is more difficult for him), which was a favorite activity he had shared with his father. He experiences some difficulty with coordination and motor planning. Cognitively, Patrick has recently learned the

days of the week and loves to look at calendars. He can recite the alphabet and recognizes a few familiar written words. He does not yet tell time.

Patrick lives a very active life, filled with family, supportive staff, and opportunities to contribute to his community. His mother and professional team continuously work together to create new goals for Patrick, and he meets these challenges. He is a delightful and admirable individual.

RECOMMENDED LEARNING RESOURCES

Organizations

Autism Society of America
7910 Woodmont Ave., Suite 300
Bethesda, MD 20814-3067
www.autism-society.org/site/PageServer
Autism Speaks
http://www.autismspeaks.org
Web site includes a "100 day kit" for families whose children have recently been diagnosed with autism.
Centers for Disease Control and Prevention
http://www.cdc.gov/ncbddd/autism/index.html
Web site includes fact sheets and other helpful information for families, individuals with autism, healthcare providers, etc.
First Signs
http://www.firstsigns.org/
Web site includes valuable information on autism and an ASD video glossary
National Alliance of Autism Research
99 Wall Street, Research Park
Princeton, NJ 08540
www.naar.org
National Institute of Mental Health Office of Communications
6001 Executive Blvd
Room 8184, MSC 9663
Bethesda, MD 20892-9663
www.nimh.nih.gov/publicat/autism.cfm

Books on Autism Spectrum Disorders

Attwood, T. (1998). Asperger's syndrome: A guide for parents and professionals. London, England: Jessica Kingsley.

Greenspan, S. I., & Wieder, S. (2006). Engaging autism: Using the Floortime approach to help children relate,

communicate, and think. Cambridge, MA: Da Capo Press.

Lord, C., & McGee, J. P. (Eds.). (2001). Educating children with autism. Washington, DC: National Academy Press.

Ozonoff, S., Dawson, G., & McPartland, J. (2002). A parent's guide to Asperger syndrome and high functioning autism. New York, NY: Guilford Press.

Quill, K. A. (2000). Do-Watch-Listen-Say: Social and communication intervention for children with autism. Baltimore, MD: Paul H. Brookes Publishing.

Robledo, S. J., & Ham-Kucharski, D. (2005). The autism book: Answers to your most pressing questions. New York, NY: Penguin Group.

Siegel, B. (2003). Helping children with autism learn: Treatment approaches for parents and professionals. New York, NY: Oxford University Press.

Volkmar, F. R. (Ed.). (2005). Handbook of autism and pervasive developmental disorders (pp. 335–364). Hoboken, NJ: John Wiley & Sons, Inc.

Wing, L. (1996). The autistic spectrum: A guide for parents and professionals. London, England: Constable & Company Limited.

Books on Sensory Integration Disorder

Ayres, A. J. (1998). Sensory integration and the child. Los Angeles, CA: Western Psychological Services.

Kranowitz, C. S. (1998). The out-of-sync child: Recognizing and coping with sensory integration dysfunction. New York, NY: Perigree.

Diagnostic Guidelines Online

Filipek, P. (2006). Autism diagnostic guidelines. Screening and Diagnosis of Autism. Retrieved from http://www.neurology.org/cgi/reprint/55/4/468.pdf

REFERENCES

American Psychiatric Association. (2000). *Diagnostic and statistic manual of mental disorders* (4th ed., text revision). Washington, DC: Author.

Autism Society of America. (2004). *Autism info* [Fact sheets]. Retrieved April 11, 2004, from http://www.autism-society.org

Autism Speaks. (2010). *PDD-NOS*. Retrieved from http://www.autismspeaks.org/navigating/pdd_nos.php

Baranek, G. T., & Berkson, G. (1994). Tactile defensiveness in children with developmental disabilities: Responsiveness and habituation. *Journal of Autism and Developmental Disorders, 24*(4), 457–471.

Baranek, G. T., Foster, L. G., & Berkson, G. (1997). Tactile defensiveness and stereotyped behaviors. *American Journal of Occupational Therapy, 51*(2), 91–95.

Baron-Cohen, S., Allen, J., & Gillberg, C. (1992). Can autism be detected at 18 months? The needle, the haystack, and the CHAT. *The British Journal of Psychiatry, 161,* 839–843.

Bauman, M., & Kemper, T. (1996). Neuroanotomic observations of the brain in autism: a review and future directions. *International Journal of Developmental Neuroscience, 23*(2–3), 183–187.

*Bauman, M. *Innovative interventions in autism/nonverbal learning disabilities.* Conference presentation, December 3–4, 2004, Seattle, WA.

Berument, S. K., Rutter, M., Lord, C., Pickles, A., & Bailey, A. (1999). Autism screening questionnaire: Diagnostic validity. *The British Journal of Psychiatry, 175,* 444–451.

Bettelheim, B. (1967). *The empty fortress: Infantile autism and the birth of the self.* New York, NY: Free Press.

Boucher, J. (1981). Memory for recent events in autistic children. *Journal of Autism and Developmental Disorders, 11,* 293–302.

Carper, R. A., & Courchesne, E. (2005). Localized enlargement of the frontal cortex in early autism. *Biological Psychiatry, 57*(2), 126–133.

Centers for Disease Control and Prevention. (2010). *Autism spectrum disorders (ASDs)*. Retrieved from http://www.cdc.gov/ncbddd/autism/index.html

Dalrymple, N. J., & Ruble, L. (1992). Toilet training and behaviors of people with autism: Parent views. *Journal of Autism and Developmental Disorders, 22*(2), 265–275.

Dawson, G., & Watling, R. (2000). Interventions to facilitate auditory, visual, and motor integration in autism: A review of the evidence. *Journal of Autism and Developmental Disorders, 30*(5), 415–421.

DeBruin, E. I., Ferdinand, R. F., Meester, S., deNijs, P. F. A., & Verheig, F. (2007). High rates of psychiatric co-morbidity in PDD-NOS. *Journal of Autism and Developmental Disorders, 37*(5), 877–886.

Deruelle, C., Rondan, C., Gepner, B., & Tardif, C. (2004). Spatial frequency and face processing in children with autism and Asperger syndrome. *Journal of Autism and Developmental Disorders, 34*(2), 199–210.

Dunn, H. G., & MacLeod, P. M. (2001). Rett syndrome: Review of biological abnormalities. *Canadian Journal of Neurological Sciences, 28*(1), 16–29.

Dunn, W. (2001). The sensations of everyday life: Empirical, theoretical, and pragmatic considerations. *American Journal of Occupational Therapy, 55*(6), 608–620.

Filipek, P. A., Accardo, P. J., Baranek, G. T., Cook, E. C., Jr., Dawson, G., Gordon, G., et al. (1999). The screening and diagnosis of autistic spectrum disorders. *Journal of Autism and Developmental Disorders, 29*(6), 439–484.

Fombonne, E. (1999). The epidemiology of autism: A review. *Psychological Medicine, 29:*769–786.

Garnett, M. S., & Attwood, A. J. (1998). Australian scale for Asperger's syndrome. In: T. Attwood (Ed.) *Asperger's syndrome: A guide for parents and professionals.* London, England: Jessica Kingsley.

Gerber, S. (2009). Understanding the development and derailment of comprehension: The impact on engaging, relating, and communicating. *Proceedings from Interdisciplinary Council on Developmental and Learning Disorders 2009. Autism spectrum disorders: What works and why?* Bethesda, MD.

Ghaziuddin, M., & Butler, E. (1998). Clumsiness in autism and Asperger syndrome: A further report. *Journal of Intellectual Disability Research, 42,* 43–48.

Gilliam, G. E. (1995). *Gilliam autism rating scale.* Austin, TX: Pro-Ed.

Gordon, B. (2002). Autism and autistic spectrum disorders. In A. K. Asbury, G. M. McKhann, W. I. McDonald, and P. Dyck. (Eds.). *Diseases of the nervous system* (3rd ed) (Vol. I, pp. 406–418). Cambridge, England: Cambridge University Press.

Greenspan, S. I., DeGangi, G, & Wieder, S. (1999). *The functional emotional assessment scale for infancy and early childhood: A manual.* Madison, WI: International Universities Press.

Greenspan, S. I., & Wieder, S. (2006). *Engaging autism: Using the Floortime approach to help children relate, communicate, and think.* Cambridge, MA: Da Capo Press.

Hauck, J. A., & Dewey, D. (2001). Hand preference and motor functioning in children with autism. *Journal of Autism and Developmental Disorders, 31*(3), 265–277.

Helm-Estabrooks, N., & Albert, M. L. (1991). *Manual of aphasia therapy.* Austin, TX: Pro-Ed.

Hering, E., Epstein, R., Elroy, S., Iancu, D. R., & Zelnic, N. (1999). Sleep patterns in autistic children. *Journal of Autism and Developmental Disorders, 29*(2), 143–147.

Hewetson, A. (2002). *The stolen child: Aspects of autism and Asperger's syndrome.* Westport, CT: Bergin & Garvey.

Hill, E., Berthoz, S., & Frith, U. (2004). Cognitive processing of own emotions in individuals with autistic spectrum disorder and in their relatives. *Journal of Autism and Developmental Disorders, 34*(2), 229–235.

Holmes, D. L. (1990). Community-based services for children and adults with autism: The Eden family programs. *Journal of Autism and Developmental Disorders, 20*, 339–351.

Horvath, K., Papadimitriou, J. C., Rabsztyn, A., Drachenberg, C., & Tildon, J. (1999). Gastrointestinal abnormalities in children with autistic disorder. *Journal of Pediatrics, 135*(5), 559–563.

Hoshino, Y., Watanabe, H., Yashima, Y., Kaneko, M., & Kumashiro, H. (1984). An investigation on sleep disturbance of autistic children. *Folia Psychiatrica et Neurologica Japonica, 38*(1), 45–51.

Hughes, C. (1996). Brief report: Planning problems in autism at the level of motor control. *Journal of Autism and Developmental Disorders, 26*(1), 99–107.

Jick, H., & Kaye, J. A. (2003). Epidemiology and possible causes of autism. *Pharmacotherapy, 23*(12), 1525–1530.

Kanner, L. (1943). Autistic disturbances of affective contact. *Nervous Child, 2*, 17–250.

Kemper, T. L., & Bauman, M. (1998). Neuropathology of infantile autism. *Journal of Neuropathology & Experimental Neurology, 57*(7), 645–652.

Kientz, M. A., & Dunn, W. (1997). A comparison of the performance of children with and without autism on the sensory profile. *American Journal of Occupational Therapy, 51*(7), 530–537.

Leslie, A. M., & Frith, U. (1987). Metarepresentation and autism: How not to lose one's marbles. *Cognition, 27*(3), 291–294.

Levy, S. E., & Hyman, S. L. (2003). Use of complementary and alternative medicine for children with autistic spectrum disorders is increasing. *Pediatric Annals, 32*(10), 685–691.

Levy, S. E., Mandell, D. S., Merhar, S., Ittenbach, R. F., & Pinto-Martin, J. A. (2003). Use of complementary and alternative medicine among children recently diagnosed autistic spectrum disorder. *Journal of Developmental & Behavioral Pediatrics, 24*(6), 418–423.

Levy, S. E., Mandell, D. S., & Schultz, R. T. (2009). Autism. *Lancet, 372*, 1627–1638.

Lindsay, R. L., & Aman, M. G. (2003). Pharmacologic therapies aid treatment for autism. *Pediatric Annals, 32*(10), 671–676.

Lord, C., & McGee, J. P. (Eds.). (2001). *Educating children with autism.* Washington, DC: National Academy Press.

Lord, C., Rutter, M., Goode, S., Heemsbergen, J., & Jordan, H. (1989). Autism diagnostic observation schedule: A standardized observation of communicative and social behavior. *Journal of Autism and Developmental Disorders, 19*, 185–212.

Lord, C., Rutter, M., & LeCouteur, A. (1994). Autism diagnostic interview-revised: A revised version of a diagnostic interview for caregivers of individuals with possible pervasive developmental disorders. *Journal of Autism and Developmental Disorders, 24*, 659–685.

Luyster, R. J., Kadlec, M. B., Carter, A., & Tager-Flusberg, H. (2008). Language assessment and development in toddlers with autism spectrum disorders. *Journal of Autism and Developmental Disorders, 38*, 1426–1438.

Madsen, K. M., Lauritsen, M. B., Pedersen, C. B., Thorsen, P., Plesner, A., Andersen, P. H., & Mortensen, P. B. (2003). Thimerosal and the occurrence of autism: Negative ecological evidence from Danish population-based data. *Pediatrics, 112*(3), 604–606.

Maestro, S., Muratori, F., Cavallaro, M. C., Pei, F., Stern, D., Golse, B., et al. (2002). Attentional skills during the first 6 months ofage in autism spectrum disorder. *Journal of the American Academy of Child and Adolescent Psychiatry, 41*, 1239–1245.

Marcel, J. Reliably lower functional connectivity for autism participants between pairs of key areas during sentence comprehension. Slide courtesy of Dr. Marcel Just, Carnegie Mellon University.

Matson, J. L., Wilkins, J., Smith, K., & Ancona, M. (2008). PDD-NOS symptoms in adults with intellectual disability: Toward an empirically oriented diagnostic model. *Journal of Autism and Developmental Disorders, 38*(3), 530–537.

McCandless, J. (2003). *Children with starving brains: A medical treatment guide for autism spectrum disorder* (2nd ed.). Paterson, NJ: Bramble Books.

McQueen, J. M., & Heck, A. M. (2002). Secretin for the treatment of autism. *The Annals of Pharmacotherapy, 36*, 305–311.

Minshew, N. (2009). The details are in the connections: Deciphering heterogeneity in ASD. Proceedings from Interdisciplinary Council on Developmental and Learning Disorders 2009: *Autism spectrum disorders: What works and why?* Bethesda, MD.

Minshew, N. J., & Goldstein, G. (2001). The pattern of intact and impaired memory functions in autism. *The Journal of Child Psychology and Psychiatry, 42*(8), 1095–1101.

Molloy, C. A., Dietrich, K., & Bhattacharya, A. (2003). Postural stability in children with autism spectrum disorder. *Journal of Autism and Developmental Disorders, 33*(6), 643–652.

Osterling, J., & Dawson, G. (1994). Early recognition of children with autism: A study of first birthday home videotapes. *Journal of Autism and Developmental Disorders, 24*(3), 247–257.

Panel of Definition and Description. Defining and describing complementary and alternative medicine. Paper presented at CAM Research Methodology conference, April 7–9, Washington, DC.

Pediatric Psychopharmacology Autism Network. (2002). Risperidone in children with autism and serious behavioral problems. *New England Journal of Medicine, 347*(5), 314–321.

Piven, J., Saliba, K., Bailey, J., & Arndt, S. (1997). An MRI study of autism: The cerebellum revisited. *Neurology, 49*(2), 546–551.

Prizant, B. M., Wetherby, A. M., Rubin, E., Laurent, A. C., & Rydell, P. J. (2006). *The SCERTS model: A comprehensive educational approach for children with autism spectrum disorders.* Baltimore, MD: Paul H. Brookes Publishing Co.

Rapin, I. (1991). Autistic children: Diagnosis and clinical features. *Pediatrics, 87*, 751–760.

Rapin, I. (1997). Autism. *New England Journal of Medicine, 337*, 97–104.

Rapin, I. (2002). The autistic spectrum disorders. *New England Journal of Medicine, 347*(5), 302–303.

Rapin, I., & Katzman, R. (1998). Neurobiology of autism. *Annals of Neurology, 43*, 7–14.

Robins, D. L., Fein, D., Barton M. L., & Green, J. A. (2001). The modified checklist for autism in toddlers: An initial study investigating the early detection of autism and pervasive developmental disorders. *Journal of Autism and Developmental Disorders, 21*, 131–144.

Robledo, S. J., & Ham-Kucharski, D. (2005). *The autism book: Answers to your most pressing questions.* New York, NY: Penguin Group.

Rogers, S. J. (1996). Brief report: Early intervention in autism. *Journal of Autism and Developmental Disorders, 26*(2), 243–246.

Ruble, L. A., & Dalrymple, N. J. (1993). Social/sexual awareness of persons with autism: A parental perspective. *The Archives of Sexual Behavior, 22*, 229–240.

Rutter, M. (2005). Incidence of autism spectrum disorders: Changes over time and their meaning. *Acta Paediatrica, 94*(1), 2–15.

Rutter, M., Silberg, J., O'Connor, T., & Simonoff, E. (1999). Genetics and child psychiatry: II Empirical research findings. *The Journal of Child Psychology and Psychiatry, 40*(1), 19–55.

Schopler, E., Reichler, R. J., & Renner, B. R. (1998). *The childhood autism rating scale.* Los Angeles: Western Psychological Services.

Schreck, K. A., & Mulick, J. (2000). Parental report of sleep problems in children with autism. *Journal of Autism and Developmental Disorders, 30*(2), 127–135.

Siegel, B. (1996). *The world of the autistic child.* Oxford, England: Oxford University Press.

Siegel, B. (1998a). *Early screening and diagnosis in autism spectrum disorders: The Pervasive Developmental Disorders Screening Test (PDDST).* Paper presented at the NIH State of the Science in Autism Screening and Diagnosis Working Conference.

Siegel, B. (1998b). *Pervasive developmental disorders screening test—Stage 2.* Bethesda, MD.

Siegel, B. (2003). *Helping children with autism to learn.* Oxford, England: Oxford University Press.

Stone, W. L., Coonrod, E. E., & Ousley, O. Y. (2000). Brief report: Screening tool for autism in two-year-olds (STAT): Development and preliminary data. *Journal of Autism and Developmental Disorders, 30*, 607–612.

Strock, M. (2004). *Autism spectrum disorders (pervasive developmental disorders).* Retrieved from http://eric.ed.gov/

Tager-Flusberg, H., Paul, R., & Lord, C. (2005). Language and communication in autism. In F. R. Volkmar (Ed.), *Handbook of autism and pervasive developmental disorders* (pp. 335–364). Hoboken, NJ: John Wiley & Sons, Inc.

United Kingdom Medical Research Council. (December, 2001). *MRC review of autism research: Epidemiology and causes.* Retrieved July 25, 2004, from http://www.mrc.ac.uk/pdf-autism-report.pdf

Van Bourgondien, M. E., Reichle, N. C., & Palmer, A. (1997). Sexual behavior in adults with autism. *Journal of Autism and Developmental Disorders, 27*(2), 113–125.

Veenstra-VanDerWeele, J., Cook, E., & Lombroso, P. J. (2003). Genetics of childhood disorders: XLVI. Autism, Part 5: Genetics of autism. *Journal of the American Academy of Child and Adolescent Psychiatry, 42*(2), 116–118.

Vilensky, J. A., Damasio, A. R., Maurer, R. G. (1981). Gait disturbances in patients with autistic behavior: A preliminary study. *Archives of Neurology, 38*(10), 646–649.

Webb, T., & Latif, F. (2001). Rett syndrome and the MECP2 gene. *Journal of Medical Genetics, 38*, 217–223.

Weimer, A. K., Schatz, A. M., Lincoln, A., Ballantyne, A. O., & Trauner, D. A. (2001). "Motor" impairment in Asperger syndrome: Evidence for a deficit in proprioception. *Journal of Developmental Behavioral Pediatrics, 22*(2), 92–101.

Williams, J. H. G., Whiten, A., & Singh, T. (2004). A systematic review of action imitation in autistic spectrum disorder. *Journal of Autism and Developmental Disorders, 34*(3), 285–299.

Williams, P. G., Dalrymple, N., & Neal, J. (2000). Eating habits of children with autism. *Pediatric Nursing, 26*(3), 259–264.

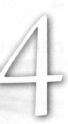

Intellectual Disability

■ *Michelle Suarez*
■ *Ben Atchison*

Jeffrey, aged 3 years, was brought to Early On at the local school district for a developmental evaluation. His parents report that his pediatrician is concerned about his language development. He smiled and interacted with examiners but was unable to express his wants and needs or follow single step directions. An interview with his parents revealed that Jeffrey was unable to dress or undress and was not self-feeding. He was diagnosed with an intellectual disability and enrolled in early childhood special education where he is working toward language and self-care goals. His family hopes he will eventually attend mainstream kindergarten with special education support.

Michael, now 2, was diagnosed by his pediatrician shortly after his birth as having **Down syndrome**. He exhibits the physical characteristics such as a round face, flattened nose bridge, abnormally small head, low-set ears, short limbs, and abnormally shaped fingers. His motor development is delayed, and his low muscle tone has made learning to walk difficult. Intellectual disability in children with Down syndrome is inevitable but varies in the degree of severity. Michael's early intervention program provides services for Michael as well as parent support and education.

Kelly, now in second grade, is pleasant and likable. Teachers have been concerned about her inability to write letters or sound out words since kindergarten, and as the curriculum becomes more challenging, she is falling further behind. She has trouble maintaining friendships and often struggles to join peers in play. School staff conducted multidisciplinary team evaluation and diagnosed Kelly with an intellectual disability. She was placed in a special education classroom where the material is appropriate for her cognitive ability and learning pace.

DEFINITION

The term intellectual disability (ID) has evolved from the previous diagnosis of mental retardation (MR). This terminology change reflects the shift from a view that classifies "MR" as a personal trait residing solely within the individual to a holistic perspective that includes the capabilities of the person within the context of the environment. The official definition of the disability is as follows and includes three specific criteria:

> *"Intellectual disability is characterized by significant limitations both in intellectual functioning and in adaptive behavior as expressed in conceptual, social, and practical adaptive skills. This disability originates before age 18."* (American Association on Intellectual and Developmental Disabilities [AAIDD], 2010)

Intellectual Functioning

The first component of this definition, intellectual functioning (or intelligence), is the general mental capability of an individual. This includes the ability to reason, plan, problem solve, think abstractly, comprehend complex ideas, and learn from experience. While it has its limitations, the accepted measure of intelligence is what is determined by an intelligence quotient (IQ) score, which involves administration of standardized tests given by a trained professional. In the 2010 publication of the AAIDD, a "significant limitation in intellectual functioning" was defined as two standard deviations below the mean, in the context of the standard error and strengths and limitations of the specific instrument (IQ test) used in assessment (AAIDD, 2010). The IQ score is not a complete representation of human functioning and must be considered in the context of adaptive behavior, health, participation and context. Therefore, clinical judgment must be used to

interpret scores when considering diagnosis or service provision (AAIDD).

Adaptive behavior

Adaptive behavior is the most related domain of concern among occupational therapists. Thus, it is our focus of assessment and intervention for persons with ID. As defined by the AAIDD, "adaptive behavior is the collection of conceptual, social, and practical skills that people have learned so they can function in their everyday lives" (American Association on Intellectual Disability, 2010). Significant limitations in adaptive behavior impact a person's daily life and affect the ability to respond to a particular situation or to the environment. Table 4-1 provides specific examples of these three areas, which are provided by the AAIDD.

Limitations in adaptive behavior can be determined by using standardized tests referenced to the general population, including people with disabilities and people without disabilities. On these standardized measures, significant limitations in adaptive behavior are operationally defined as performance that is at least two standard deviations below the mean. In contrast to IQ scores for determining intellectual abilities, adaptive behavior is measured with the focus on typical performance and not maximum performance. In other words, the criteria critical to measuring limitations in adaptive behavior is *how a person typically performs*, not performance potential.

Onset before the Age of 18

The final component of the definition of ID is that it begins early in life and therefore, a diagnosis of ID is usually made at or near birth. A diagnosis of ID is not considered in adult-onset degenerative diseases such

TABLE 4.1 Adaptive Skills

Conceptual Skills	Social Skills	Practical Skills
Receptive and expressive language	Interpersonal skills	Personal activities of daily living such as eating, dressing, mobility, and toileting
Reading and writing	Social responsibility	Instrumental activities of daily living such as preparing meals, taking medication, using telephone, managing money, using transportation, and doing housekeeping activities
Money concepts	Self-esteem	
Time concepts	Gullibility (likelihood of being tricked or manipulated)	
Number concepts	Naivete (wariness)	
	Following rules/obeying laws	Occupational skills
	Social problem solving	Maintaining a safe environment
	Avoiding victimization	

as dementia or those associated with traumatic brain injury.

In considering this definition, the AAIDD notes that there are five assumptions that need to be considered in the diagnostic process (American Association on Intellectual Disability, 2010):

1. Limitations in present functioning must be considered within the context of community environments typical of the individual's age peers and culture.
2. Valid assessment considers cultural and linguistic diversity as well as differences in communication, sensory, motor, and behavioral factors.
3. Within an individual, limitations often coexist with strengths.
4. An important purpose of describing limitations is to develop a profile of needed supports.
5. With appropriate personalized supports over a sustained period, the life functioning of the person with ID generally will improve.

ETIOLOGY

The causes of ID may be classified according to when they occurred in the developmental cycle (prenatally, perinatally, or postnatally) or by their origin (biomedical vs. environmental) (American Association on Mental Retardation, 1992; Yeargin-Allsopp, Murphy, Cordero, Decouflé, & Hollowell, 1997). There are hundreds of causes of ID (The Arc, 1993). Despite knowing the many factors that contribute to ID, in a large proportion of cases the cause remains unknown. The ability to determine the cause is highly correlated with the level of the retardation. The etiology of ID is much less likely to be known with individuals who are mildly intellectually disabled (IQs of 50–70) than with those who are severely affected (IQs of <50) (American Association on Mental Retardation, 2002; Matilainen, Airaksinen, & Monomen, 1995; Yeargin-Allsopp et al., 1997).

In a large U.S. population–based study describing probable causes of ID in school-aged children, the following results were obtained (Matilainen et al., 1995):

- No defined cause, 78.0%
- Prenatal conditions, 12.4%
- Genetic, 7.1%
- Perinatal conditions, 5.9%
- Intrauterine/intrapartum, 5.2%
- Postneonatal events, 3.6%
- **Teratogenic**, 2.9%
- Central nervous system (CNS) birth defects, 1.5%
- Other birth defects, 0.8%
- Neonatal, 0.7%

Prenatal factors that can cause ID include genetic aberrations, birth defects that are not genetic in origin, environmental influences, or a combination of factors (Matilainen et al., 1995). Up to 50% of the individuals diagnosed with ID may have more than one causal factor (American Association on Mental Retardation, 2002). With genetic aberrations, the problem is with either the genes, which are the basic unit of heredity, or the chromosomes, which carry the genes. Each nongerm cell (cells other than the ovum and spermatozoa) contains 23 pairs of chromosomes, including one pair of sex chromosomes that determine the sex of the person. Males have an X and a Y chromosome, and females have two X chromosomes.

In many cases of ID, the gene or chromosome that has caused the condition can be identified specifically. In fact, more than 350 inborn errors of metabolism that result from genetic changes have been identified. Many of these metabolic errors lead to ID (Scriver, 1995). The two most common genetic causes of ID are Down syndrome and **fragile X syndrome** (The Arc, 1996). Down syndrome is generally caused by an extra 21st chromosome, and fragile X syndrome is the result of a mutation at what is known as the fragile site on the X chromosome (Kaplan, Sadock, & Grebb, 1994). In other cases, the specific genetic aberration has not been identified. Factors such as higher incidences of a condition in specific families or increased recurrence rates among siblings suggest that the defect is genetic (Matilainen et al., 1995).

Birth defects that are not considered genetic in origin also can contribute to or cause ID. These could include such things as malformation of parts of the CNS (**cortical atrophy**, **hydrocephaly**, **spina bifida**, **craniostenosis**) (Yeargin-Allsopp et al., 1997), congenital cardiac anomalies (Rogers et al., 1995), or metabolic disorders not associated with a genetic defect (hypothyroidism) (Reuss, Paneth, Pinto-Martin, Lorenz, 1996).

Environmental factors may also be involved in prenatal development of ID. They may include exposure to chemical agents, such as alcohol or nonprescription drugs ingested by the mother during the pregnancy; maternal conditions such as **hyperphenylalaninemia** (Jardim, Palma-Dias, Silva, Ashston-Prolla, & Guigliani, 1996), **toxemia**, hypertension, and diabetes; or congenital infections such as **cytomegalovirus**, rubella, and syphilis (Yeargin-Allsopp et al., 1997).

Genetic Causes

Genetic causes can be divided into two types: single gene disorders and chromosomal abnormalities. In single gene disorders, there is a problem with the quality of the genetic material; a specific gene is defective. In chromosomal abnormalities, the problem is with the quantity of the material. There is either too much or too little genetic material in a specific chromosome (Gror & Shekleton, 1979).

TABLE 4.2 Single Gene Disorders

Type	Autosomal Dominant	Autosomal Recessive	Sex Linked
Transmission pattern	Either parent carries gene or spontaneous transmission	Both parents are carriers	Either parent can transmit gene: Mother is usually a carrier, father cannot be a carrier but can have the disorder
Risk factors	50% risk of child being affected with each pregnancy	25% risk of child being affected with each pregnancy	If mother has affected gene, 25% risk of having affected son or carrier daughter; if father has affected gene, all his daughters will be carriers and his sons will be normal
Sex distribution	Male and female children equally at risk	Male and female children equally at risk	Primarily male children at risk for having disorder, female children at risk for becoming carriers

SINGLE GENE DISORDERS

Single gene disorders follow specific patterns of transmission: autosomal dominant, autosomal recessive, or sex linked. Table 4-2 presents the transmission patterns and risk factors associated with each type.

The autosomal dominant type is caused by a single altered gene. Either parent may be a carrier, or there may have been a spontaneous mutation of the gene. Dominant inheritance occurs when one parent passes on the defective gene. This occurs even if the other parent passes a healthy gene. Because the defective gene can be passed by either parent, there is a 50% risk of the child being affected in each pregnancy (The Arc, 1996). An example of this type of inherited disorder is tuberous sclerosis.

In the autosomal recessive type, both parents are carriers but show no outward signs or symptoms of having the disorder. Inheritance occurs when both parents pass the defective gene to their offspring. Each pregnancy has a 25% risk of the child being affected (The Arc, 1996). Examples of this type of disorder are phenylketonuria and **Tay-Sachs disease**. With X-linked disorders, the affected gene is on the sex chromosomes, specifically the X chromosome, and can occur in either parent. Because males have only one X chromosome, if the father has an affected gene, he will always have the disorder and cannot be a carrier. Because the female has two X chromosomes, she can either be a carrier of the disorder (if only one X chromosome is affected) or have the disease herself (if both X chromosomes are affected). A carrier mother has a 25% risk of having an affected son. If the father has the affected gene, all his

daughters will be carriers, but his sons will not be affected (The Arc). Examples of X-linked disorders are Duchenne muscular dystrophy, fragile X syndrome, Lesch-Nyhan syndrome, and Hunter's syndrome.

Chromosomal Aberrations

Chromosomal aberrations include missing or extra chromosomes, either in part, such as a short arm, or the total chromosome, as is found in the trisomal types. Either the autosomes or sex chromosomes can be affected, with the autosomal type resulting in more serious neuromotor impairments (Harris & Tada, 1990). The most common are trisomy 21, 18, and 13. The patterns of transmission are not as readily identified as those of specific gene defects.

ENVIRONMENTAL INFLUENCES

Prenatal Factors

There are numerous environmental causes of ID in the prenatal period, including maternal infections such as rubella, cytomegalovirus, toxoplasmosis, and syphilis. Low birth weight that results from prematurity or intrauterine growth retardation can also be a contributing factor. Maternal factors associated with low birth weight include smoking, lack of prenatal care, infections, poor nutrition, toxemia, and placental insufficiency. Exposure to industrial chemicals or drugs, including certain over-the-counter prescriptions and illegal substances, also can affect birth weight, particularly during the first trimester of pregnancy.

Perinatal Factors

Two major causative factors of ID in the perinatal period are mechanical injuries at birth and perinatal **hypoxia**. Mechanical injuries are caused by difficulties of labor because of malposition, malpresentation, disproportion, or other labor complications that result in tears of the meninges, blood vessels, or other substances of the brain. Factors that cause perinatal hypoxia or anoxia include premature placental separation, massive hemorrhage from placenta previa, umbilical cord wrapped around the baby's neck, and meconium aspiration. Very premature infants also may have impaired respiration or an intracranial hemorrhage that can result in brain damage.

If a mother has an active case of herpes simplex II and is shedding the virus at the time of delivery, the baby can acquire the infection in the birth canal, which can cause severe developmental disability. This can be avoided by testing to determine whether the mother has an active case and, if so, delivering by cesarean section.

Postnatal Factors

Traumas or infections that result in injury or a lack of oxygen to the brain are a major cause of ID during the postnatal period. Traumas include near-drowning or strangulation, child abuse, and closed head injuries. Early severe psychosocial deprivation (i.e., attachment disorder, removal from the family home) can be part of the cause in the ID etiology (Shevell, 2008). Infections include encephalitis and meningitis. ID that results from meningitis caused by *Haemophilus influenzae* is now preventable, however, with the introduction of the *H. influenzae* type b (Hib) vaccine (Baraff, Lee, & Schriger, 1993).

Another major postnatal factor is sociodemographic characteristics or environmental influences. When an analysis of the relationship of sociodemographic characteristics and ID was completed for a large population of children with ID, it was found that boys, children with two or more older siblings, African American children, children whose mothers had not completed high school, and children of older mothers (with Down syndrome factored out) were more likely to experience ID (American Association on Mental Retardation, 1992).

INCIDENCE AND PREVALENCE

ID is the most frequently occurring developmental disability. Estimates of the prevalence of ID in the United States range from 1% to 3%. Most professionals associated with the AAIDD accept a prevalence of 2.5%, and they recognize that the prevalence varies with chronologic age (The Arc, 1996). A review of prevalence studies found that 2.5% to 3% is probably an accurate estimate of distribution in the general population (Frayers, 1993). Boys are 1.5 times more likely to experience MR than girls (Hauser & Ratey, 1994), which may be related to the sex-linked genetic disorders that result in MR (American Association on Mental Retardation, 2002).

SIGNS AND SYMPTOMS

ID often occurs in tandem with, or as a secondary manifestation of, another diagnosis. One study's results found that two-thirds of the children with severe ID (IQ < 50) had an additional neurologic diagnosis; <20% of children with mild ID were found to have an additional neurologic diagnosis. These diagnoses included conditions such as cerebral palsy, epilepsy, and hearing and visual impairments (The Arc, 2005). With certain genetic conditions, such as Down syndrome, MR is one of the clinical signs of the condition.

ID is defined by the AAIDD as a condition that is present from childhood (age 18 or younger), with (IQ) two standard deviations below the mean as measured on a standardized test and significant limitations in adaptive skills. Adaptive skills must be two standard deviations below the mean on a standardized test in conceptual, social, or practical skill areas (AAIDD, 2010). As previously stated, adaptive skill areas include communication, self-care, home living, social/interpersonal skills, leisure, health and safety, self-direction, functional academics, use of community resources, and work. Adaptive skills should be assessed in all of the individual's performance contexts. Someone with limited intellectual function who does not have adaptive skill deficits is not considered mentally retarded (AAIDD).

There are currently two major systems of classification for ID. The American Psychiatric Association uses the older, more traditional system of classifying ID based on performance on standardized intelligence tests using somewhat arbitrary cutoffs to assign levels of function. It is essentially used for diagnostic purposes (American Association on Mental Retardation, 1992). In 1992, the AAIDD (previously called the American Association on Mental Retardation) introduced a system of classification based on adaptive skills levels and supports needed to function (American Association on Mental Retardation, 2002). The AAIDD system, because it focuses on function and supports needed in adaptive skills across performance contexts, is more useful to the practice of occupational therapy.

In the traditional system, ID is classified according to the severity of the impairment in intellectual functioning. This is determined through standardized intelligence

TABLE 4.3   LEVELS OF INTELLECTUAL DISABILITY

Classification	IQ Range	When Identified	Adaptive Behavior as Adult
Profound	Less than 20/25	Infancy	Independent functioning • Requires total supervision • Dependent upon others for personal care Communication • Very minimal language • Occupation • Minimal participation
Severe	20/25–35/40	Early childhood	Independent functioning • Can contribute partially to self-care with total supervision • Communication • Care engage in simple conversation • Recognizes signs and selected words Occupation • May prepare simple foods, can help with simple household tasks, e.g., bed making, vacuuming, setting and clearing table • Requires much supervision
Moderate	35/40–50/55	Early childhood	Independent functioning • Feeds, bathes, and dresses self; prepares simple foods for self and others; able to care for own hair (wash and comb) • May function semi-independently in supervised living situation Communication • Carries on simple conversation, uses complex sentences; recognizes words, reads sentences, ads, and signs with comprehension Occupation • May do simple routine household chores (dusting, garbage, dishwashing); prepares food requiring mixing • May function in supported employment or sheltered workshop setting • Can learn some functional living skills: shopping, using post office, laundry
Mild	50/55–70/75	Elementary school	Independent functioning • Exercises care for personal grooming, feeding, bathing and toileting; may need health or personal care reminders; may need guidance and assistance when under unusual social or economic stress Occupation • Prepares meals, performs everyday household tasks • Can hold semi/skilled or simple skilled job

testing. To be considered intellectually disabled, the person's performance on these tests must be two standard deviation units or more below the mean. The levels of ID as identified by IQ tests are mild, moderate, severe, and profound. Approximately 85% of individuals with ID are in the mild range, 10% are in the moderate range, 3.5% are in the severe range, and 1.5% are in the profound range of function (Hauser & Ratey, 1994; Silka & Hauser, 1997). Table 4-3 presents the classifications, IQ levels, and general level of functioning as an adult. This information is adapted from *The Diagnostic and Statistical Manual of Mental Disorders, Fourth Edition (DSM-IV)*, which is the diagnostic standard for mental health care professionals in the United States. The *DSM-IV* classifies four different degrees of MR: *mild, moderate, severe,* and *profound*. These categories are based on the functioning level of the individual (American Association on Mental Retardation, 1992, 2002; Kaplan et al., 1994; Reiss, Goldberg, & Ryan, 2006). It is important to remember that not all individuals in a particular classification will function at exactly that level. The DSM 5, currently in development, is projected to use diagnostic criteria more in line with the American Association for Intellectual and Developmental Disabilities (American Psychological Association, 2011).

The classification system developed by the AAIDD involves a three-step process. The first step is to have a qualified person administer standardized intelligence and adaptive skills assessments that are appropriate for the individual's age, communication abilities, and cultural experience. The second step is to describe the individual's strengths and weaknesses across the dimensions of (1) intellectual and adaptive behavior skills, (2) psychological/emotional considerations, (3) physical/health/etiologic considerations, and (4) environmental considerations. The third step is to have the interdisciplinary team determine needed supports across these four dimensions. Supports are classified based on the level of intensity and include intermittent, limited, extensive, and pervasive. Intermittent support is provided on an "as-needed" basis. Limited support occurs over a limited time span. Extensive support is assistance provided on a daily basis in a life area. Pervasive support refers to the need for support in all life areas across all environments on a daily basis (American Association on Mental Retardation, 2002).

In addition to the performance deficits produced by ID and the associated conditions already mentioned, a high proportion of individuals with ID also have some form of mental illness. Estimates of prevalence of mental illness among people with ID range from 10% to 20% (Reiss et al., 2006) to 40% to 70% (Silka & Hauser, 1997). Some of the common types of mental illness seen in people with ID include personality disorders, affective disorders, psychotic disorders, avoidant disorders, paranoid personality disorders, severe behavior problems that may include self-injurious behavior (Zigman, Schupf, Zigman, & Silverman, 1993), and dementia associated with Down syndrome (Behrman, Kliegman, & Nelson, 1992). Several misconceptions about people with ID may complicate or prevent appropriate care for their mental illness, including the beliefs that people who are mentally retarded cannot also be mentally ill, do not experience normal feelings and emotions, and are not affected by changes in their environment. Substance abuse problems, especially with alcohol, may be overlooked, and there is controversy about the benefit of using antipsychotic drugs with individuals who are mentally retarded (Hauser & Ratey, 1994). Because of limited communication skills and limitations in abstract thinking caused by the ID, the diagnosis of mental illness and mental health problems can be a very difficult process and is frequently inexact. Good communication with caregivers and significant others in the life of the individual with ID is essential.

COURSE AND PROGNOSIS

ID is generally considered a lifelong condition, but the course and prognosis will vary depending upon the cause(s) of the retardation (Beers & Berkow, 1997; Behrman et al., 1992). In terms of life expectancy, people with mild ID live as long as the general population (Shevell, 2008). However, people with more profound ID are less likely to reach old age. This is likely due to more serious neurologic deficits and associated disorders.

Most cases of ID are nonprogressive; that is, once the initial insult to the brain occurs, there is no further damage (Beers & Berkow, 1997; Behrman et al., 1992). The emphasis is on managing the medical aspects of the condition and helping individuals to achieve their highest potential. However, certain genetic conditions (e.g., **muscular dystrophy** and Tay-Sachs disease) are progressive, with incremental loss of function and, in some cases, associated early death. The goal for these individuals is to help them achieve the highest level of independence and maintain it as long as possible. Those with Down syndrome experience degenerative changes in the brain, beginning at about age 40, that eventually result in progressive dementia similar to Alzheimer's disease (Zigman et al., 1993). On a positive note, it is possible for individuals with mild ID to gain adaptive behavior skills through remedial programs to the extent that they no longer meet the diagnostic criteria for being intellectually disabled, although their intellectual function has probably not changed significantly (American Association on Mental Retardation, 1992).

DIAGNOSIS

An evaluation must be performed to determine whether a person meets the criteria for being mentally retarded. Besides ascertaining that the onset of the condition occurred before age 18, there are two main aspects to this process. The first part involves administration of appropriate standardized intelligence tests by a qualified individual. The selection of the specific standardized instrument should be based on factors like the individual's social, linguistic, and cultural background (American Association on Mental Retardation, 1992). The individuals' IQ is interpreted in the context of their level of adaptive behavior (AAIDD, 2010).

The second aspect of the process is the evaluation of adaptive behavior as it related to the targeted adaptive life skill areas. Adaptive functioning is an individual's ability to cope with life demands and meet societal expectations for independence depending on age group (American Association on Mental Retardation, 1992). The skills needed for adaptive behavior become more complex and varied as the person ages. For instance, eating and dressing independently are major skills for the young child, but the child does not need to be able to use a telephone or manage money. Evidence for deficits and strengths in adaptive function should be gained from one or more independent, reliable sources who are familiar with the individual's abilities in different performance contexts. This information should be used to complete a standardized scale designed to provide a composite "picture" of the individual's adaptive function. As with the selection of an intelligence test, care should be taken that the adaptive behavior scale chosen is appropriate for the individual's sociocultural background, education, associated handicaps, motivation, and cooperation level (American Association on Mental Retardation, 2002). There are more than 200 adaptive behavior measures and scales. The most common scale is the Vineland Adaptive Behavior Scales—Second Edition (VAB-II) (Sparrow, Balla, & Cicchetti, 2005), which purports to assess the personal and social skills needed for everyday living. It is an indirect assessment in that the respondent is not the individual in question but someone familiar with the individual's behavior. The VAB-II measures four domains: communication, daily living skills, socialization, motor skills, and an optional maladaptive behavior index. An adaptive behavior composite is a combination of the scores from the four domains. A second scale frequently used to assess adaptive behavior is the Diagnostic Adaptive Behavior Scale (DABS) formerly titled the Adaptive Behavior Scale (AAIDD, 2010). This measure was developed by the AAIDD to assess conceptual, social, and practical skills and focuses on the critical "cutoff area" for the purpose of ruling in or ruling out a diagnosis of ID.

MEDICAL/SURGICAL MANAGEMENT

There is no drug treatment for the condition of ID; however, medications may be needed for some of the conditions that may occur in tandem. Concomitant mental health problems such as affective or psychotic disorders and severe behavior problems would all benefit from appropriate medical intervention; seizure disorders would require drug therapy. Neuromuscular aberrations (spasticity, rigidity, etc.) seen in cerebral palsy may also be helped by medication.

IMPACT OF CONDITIONS ON CLIENT FACTORS AND OCCUPATIONAL PERFORMANCE

Virtually all areas of occupational performance and many client factors can be affected by ID, depending on the cause and severity of the ID. As stated previously, the diagnostic criteria for individuals with ID included three categories of adaptive behavior (conceptual, social, and practical skills) (AAIDD, 2010). These areas (communication, language, interpersonal skills, social responsibility, recreation, friendships, daily living skills, work, and travel) impact all occupational performance areas including (basic) activities of daily living, instrumental activities of daily living, work, play, leisure, and social participation.

Although all of the occupational performance areas and client factors can be influenced by ID, those that are affected will depend on factors such as the presence of additional medical diagnoses and the severity of the diagnosis. It is imperative that the clinician be informed about the specific diagnosis that accompanies the identification of ID to determine the associated client factors that are involved. For example, occupational therapists often work with persons who have Down syndrome. Babies with Down syndrome often have hypotonia or poor muscle tone. Because they have a reduced muscle tone, which results in oral motor dysfunction such as protruding tongue, feeding babies with Down syndrome is often difficult. Hypotonia may also affect the muscles of the digestive system, in which case constipation may be a problem. Atlantoaxial instability, a malformation of the upper part of the spine located under the base of the skull, is present in some individuals with Down syndrome. This condition can cause spinal cord compression as well as craniovertebral instability (Brockmeyer, 1999). Additionally, half of children with Down syndrome are diagnosed with a congenital heart. In addition to hearing disorders, visual problems also may be present early in life. Cataracts occur in approximately 3% of children with Down syndrome but can be surgically removed.

Approximately half of the children with Down syndrome have congenital heart disease and associated early onset of pulmonary hypertension or high blood pressure in the lungs. Echocardiography may be indicated to identify any congenital heart disease. If the defects have been identified before the onset of pulmonary hypertension, surgery has provided favorable results. Seizure disorders, though less prevalent than some of the other associated medical conditions, still affect between 5% and 13% of individuals with Down syndrome, a 10-fold greater incidence than in the general population. Congenital hypothyroidism, characterized by a reduced basal metabolism, an enlargement of the thyroid gland, and

disturbances in the autonomic nervous system, occurs slightly more frequently in babies with Down syndrome. Recent studies indicate that 66% to 89% of children with Down syndrome have a hearing loss of >15 to 20 decibels in at least one ear, due to the fact that the external ear and the bones of the middle and inner ear may develop differently in children with Down syndrome (National Institutes of Health [NIH], 2006). Given that 85% of all ID cases fall in the mild range of cognitive impairment, global and specific mental functions will be most affected with this population. The following case studies illustrate how ID affects an individual's area of occupational performance in different stages of the life cycle.

Case Illustration

Case I

K.R. is a 21-year-old young woman with Down syndrome. Despite the fact that she has reached the legal age of adulthood, she is still in the process of transitioning from the developmental stage of adolescence to young adulthood. She still receives special education services but is also working on developing work and job skills through traditional vocational services. Her "disability" is expected to be lifelong.

K.R.'s condition was identified at birth. She has received continuous support and direct services to facilitate development of her abilities since then. She has always lived at home with her parents and still does so. She has her own room and bathroom at home and generally has exclusive use of the family room for her leisure pursuits. Her parents are professionals who are actively involved in their professions and the community. They are very realistic about her abilities and extremely supportive, allowing her to make most of her life choices. K.R. has a younger sister who is now away at college. K.R. has always been exposed to and involved in many social and cultural opportunities in the community, both with her family and on her own. Her social circle includes friends with and without disabilities, and she has several close friends as well as many social acquaintances.

K.R. has recently declared her life goals to be getting a job, getting an apartment of her own, and spending leisure time at the local community drop-in/recreational center for individuals with disabilities. Her mother feels that, with appropriate supports, all of these goals are attainable.

K.R. is independent in most areas of personal care. As a result of limited fine motor coordination that seems to be complicated by visual perceptual deficits, she needs assistance with regulating the water temperature for her bath, fastening zippers and buttons,

and tying her shoes. She also occasionally needs reminders to straighten her clothing and brush the back of her hair. She has a speech impediment that makes it difficult for individuals who are unfamiliar with her to initially understand her. K.R. has learned to adapt to this limitation and works very hard to make people understand what she is trying to communicate. When cued, she will slow down and work on enunciating her words. She is independent in functional mobility, but because of problems with depth perception, she is very cautious when climbing steps and negotiating between different surface levels. She is able to travel independently in community areas she is familiar with and can ride the community "Dial-a-Ride" bus if the ride is arranged for her. Her mother feels that K.R. would be aware of danger in her home, such as a fire, and would get out of the house. She does not consistently answer the phone when it rings, although she is capable of doing so. For this reason, she is generally not allowed to be at home alone because her parents have no way of checking in with her if she does not answer the phone.

K.R. is able to perform many home management tasks and has recently become motivated to attempt more activities given her desire to have an apartment of her own. She generally dislikes "housework" but knows it is necessary in order to be a good roommate. She folds laundry and puts it away and is learning to sort light and dark clothing and operate the washing machine. Her mother questions her ability to make judgments about what should or should not go into the dryer, however. She is able to sweep, vacuum, and dust but is not thorough, and this may be a result of her lack of interest and/or her visual-perceptual impairment. She keeps her bathroom clean and makes her bed. She is currently dependent in meal preparation, and this is the area that will probably require the most support for her to live in her own apartment. She cannot safely regulate stove and oven temperatures because of her fine motor problems. At the current time, K.R. attends school in a self-contained special education classroom in the local high school for half a day, focusing on vocational and prevocational skills, and spends the other half-day at Goodwill Industries in a work adjustment trial placement. K.R. has told her mother that she no longer enjoys going to school and would rather go to Goodwill. In addition to school and vocational activities, K.R. volunteers at the local community theater and at her church office doing clerical tasks. She is very interested in obtaining employment and would prefer to work at a video store, a music store, the mall, or Pizza Hut. She is very interested in clerical tasks and has been working at her father's medical practice putting monthly billings in envelopes to be mailed. K.R. has many leisure interests and activities. She enjoys music and videos, likes to eat out, participates in Special Olympics, goes to a community center for structured activities, and socializes with her friends. She prefers not to do strenuous physical activities, probably because of the difficulty she has as a result of generalized hypotonia. She has participated in team sports at the center but does so mostly for the social interaction. K.R. is very aware of her limitations and takes herself out of situations that she knows will be difficult or where she might not succeed.

Case 2

F.B. is a 60-year-old man who is intellectually disabled. He has a history of behavior problems, including **PICA** and obsessive-compulsive type behaviors of picking at his skin and clothing and stuffing toilets. He was retired from a sheltered workshop approximately 18 months ago when the emphasis of the program shifted to work readiness for community placement. It was determined that he would not be a good candidate for community work because of his age and lack of necessary supports (e.g., transportation). He currently attends a day program for social/leisure activities. F.B. has no known family and has spent most of his life in public residential institutions or in adult foster care (AFC) homes. He currently has a court-appointed guardian who makes most significant life decisions for him, including those regarding medical care and living arrangements. His guardian supports and encourages F.B. to make his wishes known about how he would like to spend his leisure time and allowed him input into his last housing change. In addition to his intellectual limitations, F.B. also experiences fairly frequent medical problems related to his obsessive-compulsive behaviors (e.g., skin infections). Medical problems, which may be age related, are emphysema and frequent fractures of bones in his lower extremities. F.B. currently lives in an AFC with 11 other adults who are developmentally disabled. His home is only required by law to provide basic care, and so it does not offer training in or support for participation in many home management tasks. His social groups generally consist of other adults with developmental disabilities or paid paraprofessional staff, either at home or the day program. His cultural experiences have been very limited because of his background.

F.B. is independent in most self-care tasks but needs supervision when using the bathroom because of his history of stuffing the toilet. He needs assistance and supports for taking medication owing to his cognitive limitations. He also needs very close monitoring of health status because he has a very high pain tolerance. He tends to prefer solitary activities but has become more verbal, social, and outgoing since going to the day program. He generally seeks out staff to interact with, and this usually takes the form of teasing. He will share activities with day program peers if prompted and has shown protective behaviors toward clients who are more limited and vulnerable than he is. Although he is verbal, he has a speech impediment that makes it difficult for people who are unfamiliar with him to understand what he is saying. He is independently ambulatory; however, he has reduced endurance as a result of an old hip fracture and neuropathy of the right lower extremity caused by a degenerative disease in the lumbar spine. He is dependent for all community mobility as a result of cognitive limitations and lack of experience and training. It is not clear whether he understands emergency situations, but he is cooperative with emergency drill procedures at the day program. It is likely that he would need ongoing supervision to maintain his personal safety.

Because of a lack of experience and opportunity, F.B. is dependent in all home management tasks. He has no responsibility for caring for others but seems to be very aware when one of his peers needs assistance or protection and alerts staff to these needs. He has been retired from the vocational arena for 18 months and now attends a day program that emphasizes social and leisure activities.

F.B. is generally not open to exploring new activities and has to be coaxed and teased by staff to try them. He generally prefers solitary activities and appears to enjoy assembly activities that result in a finished product like picture puzzles and building with Erector-Set components. He does not seem to be very interested in watching television or listening to music but does enjoy going on automobile rides with his guardian, especially when she drives her convertible with the top down.

RECOMMENDED LEARNING RESOURCES

American Association on Intellectual Disability. (2010). *Intellectual disability: Definition, classification, and systems of supports* (11th ed.). Washington, DC: Author.

Baker, B., Brightman, A., Blacher, J., & Heifetz, L. (2004). *Steps to independence: Teaching everyday skills to children with special needs* (4th ed.). Baltimore, MD: Paul H. Brookes.

Behrman, R., & Kliegman, R. (Eds.) (2002) *Nelson essentials of pediatrics* (4th ed.). Philadelphia, PA: WB Saunders.

Case-Smith, J. (2005). *Occupational therapy for children* (5th ed.). St. Louis, MO: Mosby.

American Journal on Intellectual and Developmental Disabilities
American Association on Intellectual and Developmental Disabilities
444 North Capitol St., NW, Suite 846
Washington, DC 20001

Education and Training in Mental Retardation and Developmental Disabilities
Division on Mental Retardation & Developmental Disabilities
The Council for Exceptional Children
1920 Association Drive
Reston, VA 22091–1589

Journal of the Association for Persons with Severe Handicaps ·
Division on Mental Retardation & Developmental Disabilities
The Council for Exceptional Children
1920 Association Drive
Reston, VA 22091

Advocacy Resources

American Association on Intellectual and Developmental Disabilities (AAIDD)
444 North Capitol St., NW, Suite 846
Washington, DC 20001

Tel: +1-202-387-1968; toll free: +1-800-424-3688;
Fax: +1-202-387-2193
The Arc
500 E. Border St., Suite 300
Arlington, TX 76010
Tel: +1-817-261-6003; TTY: +1-817-277-0553;
Fax: +1-817-277-3941
The Association for Persons with Severe Handicaps (TASH)
11201 Greenwood Ave.
North Seattle, WA 98133
Tel: +1-206-361-8870
Division on Mental Retardation & Developmental Disabilities
The Council for Exceptional Children
1920 Association Drive
Reston, VA 22091–1589
Tel: +1-703-620-3660
National Down Syndrome Congress
1605 Chantilly Dr., Suite 250
Atlanta, GA 30324
Tel: +1-800-232-NDSC
National Down Syndrome Society
666 Broadway
New York, NY 10012
Tel: +1-212-460-9330; toll free: +1-800-221-4602
People First International (self-advocacy group)
1340 Chemeketa St., NE Salem, OR 97301
Tel: +1-503-588-5288
President's Committee for People with Intellectual Disabilities
U.S. Department of Health & Human Services
330 Independence Ave., SW
Washington, DC 20201
Tel: +1-202-619-0634
Special Olympics International, Inc.
1350 New York Ave., NW, Suite 500
Washington, DC 20005
Tel: +1-202-628-3630

REFERENCES

American Association of Intellectual and Developmental Disabilities (AAIDD). (2010). *Diagnostic adaptive behavior scale*. Retrieved August 5, 2010, from http://www.aamr.org/content_106.cfm?navid=23

American Association on Intellectual Disability. (2010). *Intellectual disability: Definition, classification, and systems of supports* (11th ed.). Washington, DC: Author.

American Association on Mental Retardation. (1992). *Mental retardation: Definition, classification, and systems of supports* (9th ed.). Washington, DC: Author.

American Association on Mental Retardation. (2002). *Mental retardation: Definition, classification, and systems of supports* (10th ed.). Washington, DC: Author.

American Psychiatric Association (2011). *DSM-5 development: a intellectual developmental disorder.* Retrieved May 18, 2011 from http://www.dsm5.org/proposedrevision/pages/proposedrevision.aspx?rid=384

Baraff, L., Lee, S., & Schriger, D. (1993). Outcomes of bacterial meningitis in children: A meta-analysis. *Pediatric Infectious Disease Journal, 12,* 389–394.

Beers, M., & Berkow, R., (Eds.). (1997). *The Merck manual of diagnosis and therapy* (17th ed.). Rahway, NJ: Merck Sharp & Dohme Research Laboratories.

Behrman, R., Kliegman, R., & Nelson, W. (Eds.). (1992). *Nelson's textbook of pediatrics* (14th ed.). Philadelphia, PA: WB Saunders.

Brockmeyer, D. (1999). Down syndrome and craniovertebral instability: Topic review and treatment recommendations. *Pediatric Neurosurgery, 31*(2), 71–77.

Frayers, T. (1993). Epidemiological thinking in mental retardation: Issues in taxonomy and population frequency. *International Review of Research in Mental Retardation, 19,* 97–133.

Gror, M., & Shekleton, M. (1979). *Basic pathophysiology: A conceptual approach.* St. Louis, MO: CV Mosby.

Harris, S., & Tada, W. (1990). Genetic disorders. In D. Umphred (Ed.). *Neurological rehabilitation.* St. Louis: CV Mosby.

Hauser, M., & Ratey, J. (1994). The patient with mental retardation. In S. Hyman & G. Tesar (Eds.). *The manual of psychiatric emergencies* (pp. 104–109). Boston: Little Brown & Co. Retrieved December 27, 2005, from http://www.psychiatry.com

Jardim, L., Palma-Dias, R., Silva, L., Ashston-Prolla, P., & Guigliani, R. (1996). Maternal hyperphenylalaninemia as a cause of microcephaly and mental retardation. *Acta Paediatrica, 85,* 943–946.

Kaplan, H., Sadock, B., & Grebb, J. (1994). *Synopsis of psychiatry* (7th ed.). Baltimore, MA: Williams & Wilkins.

Matilainen, R., Airaksinen, E., & Monomen, T. (1995). A population-based study on the causes of mild and severe mental retardation. *Acta Paediatrica, 84,* 261–266.

National Institutes of Health. (2006). *Facts about Down syndrome.* Retrieved February 12, 2006, from http://www.nichd.nih.gov/publications/pubs/downsyndrome/down

Reiss, S., Goldberg, B., & Ryan, R. (1993). *Mental illness in persons with mental retardation.* Retrieved January 16, 2006, from http://www.psychiatry.com

Reuss, M., Paneth, M., Pinto-Martin, J., & Lorenz, J. (1996). The relation of transient hypothyroxinemia in preterm infants to neurologic development at two years of age. *New England Journal of Medicine, 334,* 821–827.

Rogers, B., Msall, M., Buck, G., Lyon, N., Norris, M., Roland et al. (1995). Neurodevelopmental outcome of infants with hypoplastic left heart syndrome. *Journal of Pediatrics, 126,* 496–498.

Scriver, C. (1995). *The metabolic and molecular bases of inherited disease* (7th ed.). New York, NY: McGraw-Hill.

Shevell, M. (2008). Global developmental delay and mental retardation or intellectual disability: Conceptualization, evaluation and etiology. *Pediatric Clinics of North America, 55,* 1071–1084.

Silka, V., & Hauser, M. (1997). Psychiatric assessment of the person with mental retardation. *Psychiatric Annals, 27,* 3.

Sparrow, S., Balla, D., & Cicchetti, D. (2005). *Vineland adaptive behavior scales.* San Antonio, TX: PsychCorp.

The Arc. (1993). *Introduction to mental retardation.* Retrieved January 10, 2006, from http://www.thearc.org

The Arc. (1996). *Genetic causes of mental retardation.* Retrieved December 19, 2005, from http://www.thearc.org

Yeargin-Allsopp, M., Murphy, C., Cordero, J., Decouflé, P., & Hollowell, J. (1997). Reported biomedical causes and associated medical conditions for mental retardation among 10-year-old children, metropolitan Atlanta, 1985 to 1987. *Developmental Medicine and Child Neurology, 39,* 142–147.

Zigman, W., Schupf, N., Zigman, A., & Silverman, W. (1993). Aging and Alzheimer disease in people with mental retardation. *International Review of Research in Mental Retardation, 19,* 41–70.

Mohod Disorders

■ *Ann Chapleau*

KEY TERMS

Affect
Anhedonia
Avolition
Cyclothymia
Dysphoria
Euphoria
Flight of ideas
Grandiosity
Hypomanic episode
Major depressive episode
Mania
Manic episode
Mixed episode
Prodromal
Psychomotor agitation
Psychomotor retardation
Psychosis
Unipolar depression

Helen sits in her rocking chair in her small living room, smoking a cigarette. The room is dimly lit by the television screen. Her silver hair is disheveled and her sweat suit is stained and dirty. She has several days' worth of Meals on Wheels containers on the coffee table, mostly uneaten. A picture of her deceased husband is on the end table, as are various photos of her grown daughter, who lives in another state. Helen has not left her home in over 6 months, except for doctor visits. She has early-stage emphysema, but has not been able to stop smoking. She no longer knits or bakes, two of her favorite hobbies. At her last doctor's visit, her physician asked her if she was feeling depressed, but Helen was too ashamed to tell him how sad and lonely she had been feeling for months. She wanted to tell him that there wasn't any point in living anymore, that her life doesn't have any meaning. But she remained silent. At home, she is overwhelmed by feelings of guilt. She had been raised to keep a tidy home and be active, and not to feel sorry for oneself, but she feels too tired to do anything except to watch television.

DESCRIPTION AND DEFINITION

Mood disorders are among the most disabling and prevalent illnesses worldwide. The World Health Organization (WHO) estimates that major depressive disorder (MDD) and bipolar disorder (BPD) are among the leading cause of disability, and that MDD is expected to become the second leading cause of disability by 2020, second only to cardiovascular disease (WHO, 2008). Despite the prevalence and impact on global health care costs, as well as quality of life for individuals and their families, mood disorders often go undetected and untreated.

Mood disorders represent a spectrum of mood disturbances, from the extremely low mood of depression to the extremely elevated mood of **mania** (Figure 5.1). The American Psychiatric Association (APA) provides a classification system (APA, 2000) to identify symptoms using universal terminology. Depressive disorders include MDD and dysthymic disorder, which are often referred to as **unipolar depression**, as they do not include mood variances

59

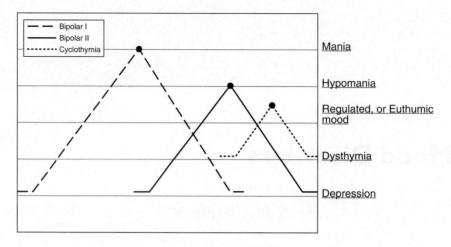

Figure 5.1 Mood spectrum.

on the other end of the mood spectrum. MDD, often referred to as major depression, is characterized by symptoms such as sadness, hopelessness, guilt, irritability, and cognitive impairments, like poor concentration and difficulty making decisions. A diagnosis of MDD requires the presence of a **major depressive episode,** which is a period of depressed or irritable mood, with additional symptoms lasting at least 2 weeks, resulting in severe impairments in functioning.

The BPD spectrum includes BPD I, BPD II, and **cyclothymia,** which all involve some degree of elevated mood and usually a history of at least one major depressive episode. BPD I is characterized by mood swings from extremely high (mania) to extremely low (depression). Manic behaviors include **euphoria,** irritability, **grandiosity,** decreased sleep, impulsivity, and distractibility, which significantly interfere with daily functioning. A diagnosis of BPD I is warranted when an individual presents with either a manic or **mixed episode.** A **manic episode** is a highly elevated or irritable mood lasting at least 1 week, with or without psychotic symptoms such as delusions and hallucinations. Severity of symptoms results in significant impairment in functioning which may require hospitalization. A mixed episode is characterized by the presence of both manic and major depressive symptoms almost daily for at least 1 week, resulting in rapid mood cycling with or without psychotic symptoms.

BPD II can be characterized by the presence or history of a major depressive disorder and at least one **hypomanic episode.** Hypomania involves similar but less intense mood and energy elevation than mania.

Cyclothymia represents a chronic (at least 2 years), but less severe mood disturbance involving both hypomanic behaviors and depressive symptoms that do not meet criteria for either a manic or major depressive episode (Fig. 5.1)

Terms to describe the clinical symptoms of mood disorders include

- **Affect:** the display of emotion, particularly facial expression
- **Anhedonia:** lack of interest in previously pleasurable activities
- **Avolition:** lack of drive or ambition to complete goal-directed tasks or activities
- **Dysphoria:** a depressed or negative mood state
- **Euphoria:** highly elevated, exaggerated mood
- **Flight of ideas:** rapidly changing, disconnected thoughts
- **Grandiosity:** inflated sense of self-esteem or importance
- **Hypomania:** elevated mood that is less intense than full mania
- **Psychomotor agitation:** increased physical movements that are purposeless and reflective of an agitated or anxious state, that is, wringing hands, fidgeting, pacing
- **Psychomotor retardation:** abnormally slowed or reduced movements or speech
- **Psychosis:** the presence of delusions or hallucinations without insight

ETIOLOGY

Despite ongoing research, there is still no one known cause of mood disorders.

Both MDD and BDP are widely believed to result from a complex combination of biologic, genetic, and psychosocial factors. Many factors can influence the development of mood disorders, including an individual's genetic makeup, biology, other co-occurring medical and psychiatric conditions, cognitive abilities, personality, support systems, personal history, particularly exposure to stress, and coping strategies. Additionally, mood disorders can be triggered by childbirth, seasonal changes, substance use, and other medical conditions.

Biologic Factors

Much of the research over the past 50 years has focused on biologic changes in brain function (U.S. Department of Health and Human Services, 1999). Current research using advanced technologies of brain imaging to examine structures and brain activity provides evidence that mood disorders are disorders of the brain. Magnetic resonance imaging (MRI) and positron emission tomography (PET) studies reveal abnormal functioning in regions of the brain that regulate mood, sleep, thinking, appetite, and behavior.

In studies of MDD, functional abnormalities have been found in the limbic system, including the amygdala, hippocampus, insula, regions of the anterior cingulate cortex, and the dorsolateral prefrontal cortex—brain regions that represent centers of emotion (Cole et al., 2010; Gos et al., 2010; McKinnon, Yucel, Nazarov, & MacQueen, 2009). Functional abnormalities of the limbic system have also been found in studies of BPD (Kruger, Seminowicz, Goldapple, Kennedy, & Mayberg, 2003). These abnormalities are consistent with studies in which both MDD and BPD subjects demonstrated blunted or decreased behavioral and physiologic reactivity to sad or negative stimuli, such as pictures and videos (Foti, Olvet, Klein, & Hajcak, 2010; Miklowski & Johnson, 2005; Rottenberg, 2005).

The role of neurotransmitters, such as serotonin, acetylcholine, and melatonin, in mood disorders has been studied for several decades. Neuroimaging and genetic studies have focused on the role of genes that may predispose an individual to dysregulated levels of neurotransmitters. Current research focuses on neurotransmitter systems, such as the effects of dysregulated dopamine and serotonin transporters and receptors in the brain (Miklowski & Johnson, 2005).

Biologic abnormalities of the brain, however, may not necessarily be the cause of a mood disorder, but can develop as a result of the disorder. For example, some researchers believe that chronic stress can trigger depression, as the body continually responds to stress through neurochemical changes (Hennessy, Schiml-Webb, & Deak, 2009; Miller & Blackwell, 2005). One such stress response is the excessive secretion of cortisol, which can interfere with the limbic-cortical systems. The challenge for researchers is to differentiate which abnormalities are causal factors and which develop in response to environmental factors that trigger neurochemical changes.

Both MDD and BPD are known to run in families as heritable traits, but researchers have had minimal success in isolating any specific, responsible genes. Genetic variations associated with both MDD and BPD support the growing belief among researchers that mood disorders involve a combination of altered genes that interact with environmental factors, such as stress, to explain why some family members with a known genetic risk develop either MDD or BPD while other family members do not (Caspi et al., 2003; McMahon et al., 2010).

Twin studies also support the genetic link in mood disorders. In studies of MDD, heritability was found to be 38%, with higher concordance rates among women than men (Kendler, Gatz, Gardner, & Pedersen, 2005). In studies of BPD, heritability is even higher; identical twins have a concordance rate of 57%, while the concordance rate for fraternal twins is 14% (Miklowitz & Johnson, 2005).

Psychosocial Risk Factors

In addition to the role of biologic and genetic factors in the development of mood disorders, the role of stressful life events has been widely studied. For example, traumatic events, such as childhood sexual, physical, or emotional abuse, increase the risk of both MDD and BPD (Hammen, 2005; Maniglio, 2010; Miklowitz & Johnson, 2005). Other risk factors include exposure to war, disaster, displacement, parental mental illness, domestic violence, physical or sexual assault, involvement in a serious accident, death of a loved one, chronic work stress, and caregiver stress (Maniglio, 2010; Wingo et al., 2010). However, it is important to remember that the majority of people who experience life stressors do not develop a mood disorder and that not all mood disorders are triggered by a traumatic event. For those who experience life events, it is estimated that 20% will develop MDD, perhaps higher for those who experience more profound trauma (Monroe & Reid, 2009).

INCIDENCE AND PREVALENCE

MDD is both common and widespread, with a lifetime prevalence of one in five, or 20%, and a relapse rate of more than 80% (Gotlib & Hamilton, 2008). The lifetime prevalence for BPD is much lower. Community samples can range from .4% to 1.5% (APA, 2000), or from 3.9% to 10%, based on inclusion criteria of the full bipolar spectrum (Miklowitz & Johnson, 2005).

In any given year, 20.9 million (9.5%) adults in the United States will experience a mood disorder, with 14.8 million suffering from MDD and 5.7 million suffering from BPD (Kessler et al., 2005). Women are more frequently diagnosed with MDD than men (Gavin et al.,

2010; Kessler et al., 2003). Additionally, lower socio-economic status is associated with both MDD and BPD (Everson, Maty, Lynch, & Kaplan, 2002; Schoeyen et al., 2010).

SIGNS AND SYMPTOMS

Both MDD and BPD are marked by a complex set of symptoms that interfere with daily functioning. Moreover, both disorders are associated with high rates of suicide (Moller & Henkel, 2005), making a proper diagnosis essential for treatment purposes.

Major Depressive Disorder

A diagnosis of MDD can be determined when an individual has experienced at least one major depressive episode, in the absence of any manic, mixed, or hypomanic episodes (APA, 2000). Symptoms must represent a significant change in typical functioning that interferes with daily living. According to the APA, a depressive episode must include at least five of the following symptoms during a 2-week period, and at least one of the symptoms observed must be either depressed mood or loss of interest or pleasure (APA, 2000).

- Depressed mood
- Anhedonia
- Weight loss
- Altered sleep
- Change in psychomotor behavior
- Fatigue/loss of energy
- Feelings of worthlessness or guilt
- Impaired cognition
- Thoughts of death or suicide

Children with depressive disorders may not exhibit the same set of symptoms as adults. Behaviors can include irritability, negativity, acting clingy or overly needy, behavioral problems in school, refusing to attend school, and fear of a parent's death (U.S. Department of Health and Human Services, 2008).

Bipolar Disorder

The bipolar disorders can be differentiated by the experience of either a depressive or manic episode. A diagnosis of BPD I is warranted when an individual has experienced at least one manic or mixed episode, with manic mood as the dominant presentation. The individual may have had at least one major depressive episode, as well. A classification of BPD II is determined when the individual has had at least one depressive episode and at least one hypomanic episode, but no manic or mixed episode. BPD II features a predominantly depressed mood. As in MDD, symptoms of BPD must represent a change from previous level of functioning. The disturbed mood must last a minimum of 1 week and include at least three of the following symptoms (APA, 2000):

- Grandiosity
- Minimal need for sleep
- Excessively talkative or having pressured speech
- Racing thoughts or flight of ideas
- Distractibility
- Excessive goal-directed activity or psychomotor agitation
- Impulsivity or participation in dangerous or risky activities

COURSE AND PROGNOSIS

The course of illness and prognosis of both MDD and BPD is varied and is complicated by co-occurring conditions such as anxiety, cardiovascular and pulmonary disease, diabetes, and obesity, which can be related to lifestyle, limited access to care, and the effects of long-term psychotropic medication use (Carnethon et al., 2007; Colton & Manderscheid, 2005; Egede & Zheng, 2003). In addition, individuals with mood disorders are more likely to abuse alcohol and/or drugs, which can negatively impact prognosis (Boschloo et al., 2010; Conway, Compton, Stinson, & Grant, 2005).

Major Depressive Disorder

Average age of onset for MDD is in the mid- to late-20s (Beesdo, et al., 2009). Approximately one-third of those diagnosed with MDD will develop a chronic course of the illness, often lasting throughout their lifetime (Arnow & Constantino, 2003). Although MDD is commonly regarded as an adult illness, there is growing evidence that depressive symptoms meeting diagnostic criteria can be present in adolescence, childhood, and even early childhood/preschool years (Hammen, 2009; Luby, 2010). Childhood depression carries a higher risk for recurrence (30% to 50%) during adolescent years and early adulthood (Costello et al., 2002) and can also be a risk factor for more severe depression in adulthood (Weissman et al., 1999).

During adolescence, rates for depression are equally common among boys and girls, but after age 13, the rate doubles or triples for girls. This higher rate continues into adulthood for women until after middle age (Costello et al., 2002). Adolescents who experience an initial depressive or manic episode are at a higher risk of conversion to BPD (Beesdo et al., 2009).

MDD among older adults is not uncommon. While the prevalence of diagnosed depression appears to decline with age, risk of depression and suicide increases when co-occurring physical illness or pain affects ability to function (National Institute of Mental Health, 2007). About one in three older adults with MDD develop a chronic course of the illness (Licht-Strunk et al., 2007).

Bipolar Disorder

Age of onset for BPD is earlier than in MDD, with an average age of 17.5 years (Beesdo, et al., 2009). BPD can occur in childhood and early adolescence, as well. A **prodromal** period, ranging from 1.8 to 7.3 years, before full onset of BPD, has been noted in a number of studies (Skjelstad et al., 2010). Symptoms of dysregulated mood and fluctuations in energy increase in intensity during this period.

Longitudinal studies of BPD indicate that a full, functional recovery from a first episode is uncommon. There is a high risk of relapse, recurring episodes, and mood cycling during the first 2 years of the illness. In addition, suicidal behavior is higher during this early phase (Salvatore et al., 2007). Sixty percent of people with BPD will experience a recurrence within the first 2 years, while as many as 75% will experience recurrences within the first 5 years. In addition, many will suffer residual symptoms, such as depression, between these episodes (Miklowitz, 2007).

Those who experience an initial depressive or mixed episode are at greater risk for more severe depression and morbidity later in the illness than those who initially experience a manic episode. In general, the course of the BPD is highly variable, but early treatment is associated with a better prognosis (Goldberg & Harrow, 2004).

Rates of suicide among people with BPD are higher than in any other psychiatric condition; four times higher than among those with MDD and 15 times higher than among the general population. As many as 50% of people with BPD attempt suicide at least once during the course of the illness and 11% die as a result of suicide (Angst, et al., 2005; Miklowitz & Johnson, 2006).

MEDICAL/SURGICAL MANAGEMENT

Pharmacology for Major Depressive Disorders

Antidepressant medications work to regulate neurotransmitters, particularly serotonin and norepinephrine. The newest and most widely prescribed category is the "second-generation" antidepressants called selective serotonin reuptake inhibitors (SSRIs) and serotonin and norepinephrine reuptake inhibitors (SNRIs). SSRIs and SNRIs are the current medications of choice due to lesser side effects than seen with "first-generation" tricyclics and monoamine oxidase inhibitors (MAOIs).

Unfortunately, side effects of all antidepressants can range from minor to life threatening depending on the individual, and can result in medication noncompliance. Side effects can include nausea, headache, agitation, sexual dysfunction or loss of drive, dry mouth, constipation, blurred vision, and sedation.

MAOIs require strict adherence to diet and medication restrictions, as certain foods and medicines can interact with the MAOIs, resulting in increased risk of stroke.

Pharmacology for Bipolar Disorder

Medications for mood stabilization can vary based on the need to treat acute symptoms versus maintenance treatment. Monitoring of medication use is important to ensure that the mood stabilizer does not cause an episode at the opposite end of the spectrum. Lithium was the first approved medication for BPD and has been the most commonly used medication for mood stabilization for decades. Extensive research has supported its efficacy (Miklowski & Johnson, 2005).

Other mood stabilizers found to be effective include Valproic acid or divalproex sodium (known as Depakote), and anticonvulsant medications, such as lamotrigine (Lamictal), gabapentin (Neurontin), topiramate (Topamax), and oxcarbazepine (Trileptal). Potential side effects include sedation, weight gain, tremors, dry mouth, excessive thirst, or polydipsia, restlessness, acne, gastric irritation, and kidney problems.

A treatment regime for acute mania may consist of a combination of either lithium, divalproex, or carbamazepine, and an atypical antipsychotic medication (McIntyre & Konarski, 2005). Atypical antipsychotic medication side effects can include sedation, dizziness, blurred vision, skin rash, and sun sensitivity (Table 5.1).

Electroconvulsive Therapy

Convulsive, or shock, therapy has been used in psychiatry for decades. Early use was often associated with tragic results, including permanent severe blunting of affect, permanent memory loss, and even death. Electroconvulsive therapy (ECT) has evolved over time, as medical advances have increased our knowledge of the intricacies of the brain. Currently, ECT is considered a safe, effective treatment for MDD and BPD, but is primarily used with those who are treatment resistant to pharmacology (Taylor, 2007). The mortality rate for ECT is about

TABLE 5.1 COMMON MEDICATIONS AND SIDE EFFECTS

Medications	Potential Side Effects
Mood Stabilizers	▪ Sedation
	▪ Weight gain
	▪ Tremors
	▪ Dry mouth
	▪ Excessive thirst (polydipsia)
	▪ Restlessness
	▪ Acne
	▪ Gastric irritation
	▪ Kidney malfunction
Atypical Antipsychotics	▪ Sedation
	▪ Dizziness
	▪ Blurred vision
	▪ Skin rash
	▪ Sun sensitivity
Antidepressants	▪ Sedation
–SSRIs	▪ Nausea
–SNRIs	▪ Headache
–"First-Generation" Trycyclics	▪ Agitation
–MAOIs	▪ Sexual dysfunction or loss of drive
	▪ Dry mouth
	▪ Constipation
	▪ Blurred vision
	▪ Increased risk of stroke (MAOI's)

2 deaths per 100,000 treatments and is associated with complications from anesthesia (Fink & Taylor, 2007).

The ECT procedure involves the use of anesthesia prior to induction of a controlled seizure. The seizure is evoked by administration of an electrical shock using electrodes attached to the scalp. ECT is usually administered in a series, over the course of several days or weeks, depending on the individual and severity of symptoms. Although effective, it is still not clear how ECT works. Researchers believe the antidepressive effects may result from an increase in monoamines and serotonin levels, increases in neurotrophic factors that can include cellular improvements and norepinephrine and serotonin receptor expression, and/or increases in anticonvulsant action which can increase opioids (Taylor, 2007).

Repetitive Transcranial Magnetic Stimulation

Repetitive transcranial magnetic stimulation (rTMS) is a newly emerging intervention for treatment-resistant depression. rTMS involves a noninvasive procedure of creating a magnetic field that passes through the skull inducing electrical currents in the brain that activate specific nerve cells. The procedure can be repeated daily over a period of days or weeks. It has proven successful in reducing depressive symptoms and improving remission rates (George et al., 2010; Gross, Nakamura, Pascual-Leone, & Fregni, 2007; Holtzheimer et al., 2010). Based on recent successful clinical trials, an rTMS device for the treatment of MDD has been recently approved by the U.S. Food and Drug Administration.

IMPACT ON OCCUPATIONAL PERFORMANCE

Mood disorders, particularly those at the extreme ends of the mood spectrum, can significantly interfere with daily functioning. Symptoms of both MDD and BPD interfere with one's ability to work, socialize, recreate, sleep, eat, and learn. The impact on occupational performance, however, can vary greatly based on factors such as severity of symptoms, responsiveness to treatment, number of episodes, co-occurring conditions and age of onset. For example, an adult with a high level of premorbid functioning, who experiences a single episode and responds well to intervention, may successfully return to work and family roles. For many individuals, however, there are numerous barriers to occupational performance once symptoms occur.

Basic Activities of Daily Living

The ability to care for personal health such as eating well, following a healthy diet, and sleeping and exercising regularly can be impaired. Previously maintained daily routines can be disrupted. Symptoms of avolition and anhedonia seen in depressive episodes can decrease motivation for exercise, proper nutrition, grooming, and hygiene. Symptoms of distractibility, impulsivity, and psychomotor disturbances that are characteristic of a manic or hypomanic episode can interfere with the quality of self-care. Additionally, sleep patterns are often disturbed, with individuals either not getting adequate sleep, sleeping excessively, or experiencing poor sleep quality. Weight gain or loss is common, and can be related to either changes in daily habits or long-term medication use.

Instrumental Activities of Daily Living

Early onset in childhood or adolescence, a time of developing skills and interests, coupled with high rates of recurrence throughout adulthood, can limit one's ability to develop educational, social, and work skills. For individuals who continue to experience residual symptoms between episodes, it can be even more difficult to reengage in meaningful life roles. The individual dealing with recurring depressed, manic, or cycling moods has great difficulty managing daily tasks that can include work, school, parenting/caregiving, home maintenance, and healthy leisure.

Many individuals with mood disorders lack the educational and training requirements needed for a successful career. Moreover, persons suffering from depressive episodes are likely to experience symptoms of anhedonia, avolition, and cognitive difficulties, which decrease motivation and ability to work. Studies reveal that those diagnosed with MDD or BPD are less likely to work outside the home, either full- or part-time (Substance Abuse and Mental Health Services Administration, 2009; Suppes et al., 2001), and those who do work, experience lowered productivity and increased absenteeism (Cook, 2005; Kessler et al., 2005).

Children and adolescents with early onset of a mood disorder may experience symptoms that can negatively impact school performance, such as lower scores on achievement tests and impaired peer interactions, including social withdrawal or fighting and disruptive behavior. Studies have shown that high school students with depression, particularly females, are more likely to drop out of high school and are less likely to enroll in college (Fletcher, 2007).

Involvement in healthy leisure activities is usually limited, as well. Those with MDD are likely to socially isolate and cease participation in activities due to symptoms of anhedonia and avolition. During a manic or hypomanic episode, an individual may experience an initial burst of creative, goal-directed energy, but is more likely to engage in risky or dangerous activities, and, over time, to become more unable to organize time and activities.

In general, those who experience recurring episodes, limited treatment success, co-occurring medical or psychiatric conditions, and lack of healthy support systems are more likely to demonstrate an overall decline in functioning. Early intervention and ongoing access to treatment and other support networks can improve one's ability to maintain meaningful and productive roles and to experience a greater quality of life through social participation.

Case Illustrations

Case 1

Phyllis spent excessive hours at her new human resources job, planning how to take over the company. She was visibly irritated with what she perceived as organizational inefficiencies and spoke about her concerns to her employers. Her grandiosity was evident by all her coworkers. She drafted numerous versions of detailed proposals to "take the company to the next level." Despite working long hours at her computer each day, she failed to complete the tasks she was hired to do. She was continually distracted by her big plans. In addition, she began shopping for new clothes that she felt would be in keeping with her elevated status. She ran up large credit card bills and was in financial trouble.

When she shared her business ideas with family members, they gave her feedback about how unrealistic she was being and urged her to focus on her job. She responded defensively, unable to recognize how her behavior was negatively affecting her work. Although she was highly talented in her field, she was fired after 3 months on the job.

Case 2

Justin is a 9-year-old boy who was admitted to the child and adolescent psychiatric inpatient unit at the local community mental health center. He had been living in a foster home since being removed from his biological parents' home at age 7, due to neglect.

His foster parents describe Justin as quiet and passive in his interactions with others. He avoids eye contact and wears his hair long, over his eyes. Justin spends most of his free time in his room, alone, watching television or playing video games. Schoolwork is a daily struggle for Justin's foster parents, as they indicate he is disinterested in school and avoids completing his assignments. They report he "throws temper tantrums" when they make him do homework. He frequently complains of having an upset stomach when it is time to get ready for school in the morning. During the initial interview with the occupational therapist, Justin shared that he felt he was "bad" and that was why he had been removed from his biological parents' custody.

RECOMMENDED LEARNING RESOURCES

National Alliance on Mental Illness (NAMI)
3803 N. Fairfax Dr., Ste. 100
Arlington, VA 22203
Phone: 703-524-7500
Fax: 703-524-9094
www.nami.org
National Institute of Mental Health (NIMH)
Science Writing, Press, and Dissemination Branch
5001 Executive Boulevard, Room 8184, MSC 9553
Bethesda, MD 20892-9553

Phone: 1-855-515-5454
Fax: 301-443-4279
www.nimh.nih.gov
NARSAD
50 Cutter Mill Road, Suite 404
Great Neck, NY 11021
Phone: 515-829-0091
Fax: 515-487-5930
www.narsad.org

REFERENCES

American Psychiatric Association. (2000). *Diagnostic and statistical manual of mental disorders* (4th ed., rev.). Washington, DC: Author.

Arnow, B. A., & Constantino, M. J. (2003). Effectiveness of psychotherapy and combination treatment for chronic depression. *Journal of Clinical Psychology, 59,* 893–905.

Beesdo, K., Hofler, M., Leibenluft, E., Lieb, R., Bauer, M., Pfenning, A. (2009). Mood episodes and mood disorders: Patterns of incidence and conversion in the first three decades of life. *Bipolar Disorders, 11,* 537–549.

Boschloo, L., Vogelzangs, N., Smit, J. H., van den Brink, W., Veltman, D. J., Beekman, A. T. F., et al. The performance of the Alcohol Use Disorder Identification Test (AUDIT) in detecting alcohol abuse and dependence in a population of depressed or anxious persons. *Journal of Affective Disorders, 125,* 441–445.

Carnethon, M. R., Biggs, M. L., Barzilay, J. I., Smith, N. L., Vaccarino, V., Bertoni, A. G., et al. (2007). Longitudinal association between depressive symptoms and incident type 2 diabetes mellitus in older adults: The cardiovascular health study. *Archives of Internal Medicine, 157,* 802–807.

Caspi, A., Sugden, K., Moffitt, T. E., Taylor, A., Craig, I. W., Harrington, H., et al. (2003). Influence of life stress on depression: Moderation by a polymorphism in the 5-HTT gene. *Science, 301,* 385–389.

Cole, J., Toga, A. W., Hojatkashani, C., Thompson, P., Costafreda, S. G., Cleare, A. J., et al. (2010). Subregional hippocampal deformations in major depressive disorder. *Journal of Affective Disorders, 125,* 272–277.

Colton, C. W., & Manderscheid, R. W. (2005). Congruencies in increased mortality rates, years of potential life lost, and causes of death among public mental health clients in eight states. *Preventing Chronic Disease, 3*(2), 1–14.

Conway, K. P., Compton, W., Stinson, F. S., & Grant, B. F. (2005). Lifetime comorbidity of DSM-IV mood and anxiety disorders and specific drug use disorders: Results from the National Epidemiologic Survey on Alcohol and Related Conditions. *Journal of Clinical Psychiatry, 57,* 247–257.

Cook, J. A. (2005). Employment barriers for persons with psychiatric disabilities: Update of a report for the President's Commission. *Psychiatric Services, 57,* 1391–1405.

Costello, E. J., Pine, D. S., Hammen, C., March, J. S., Plotsky, P. M., Weissman, M. M., et al. (2002). Development and natural history of mood disorders. *Society of Biological Psychiatry, 52,* 529–542.

Egede, L. E., & Zheng, D. (2003). Independent factors associated with major depressive disorder in a national sample of individuals with diabetes. *Diabetes Care, 25,* 104–111.

Everson, S. A., Maty, S. C., Lynch, J. W., & Kaplan, G. A. (2002). Epidemiologic evidence for the relation between socioeconomic status and depression, obesity, and diabetes. *Journal of Psychiatric Research, 53,* 891–895.

Fink, M., & Taylor, M. A. (2007). Electroconvulsive therapy: Evidence and challenges. *JAMA, 298,* 330–332.

Fletcher, J. M. (2007). Adolescent depression: Diagnosis, treatment, and educational attainment. *Journal of Health Economics, 17,* 1215–1235.

Foti, D., Olvet, D. M., Klein, D. N., & Hajcak, G. (2010). Reduced electrocortical response to threatening faces in major depressive disorder. *Depress Anxiety, 27,* 813–820. doi: 10.1002/da.20712

Gavin, A. R., Walton, E., Chae, D. H., Alegria, M., Jackson, J. S., & Takeuchi, D. (2010). The associations between socio-economic status and major depressive disorder among Blacks, Latinos, Asians and non-Hispanic Whites: Findings from the Collaborative Psychiatric Epidemiology Studies. *Psychological Medicine, 40,* 51–51.

George, M. S., Lisanby, S. H., Avery, D., McDonald, W. M., Durkalski, V., Pavlicova, M., et al. (2010). Daily left prefrontal transcranial magnetic stimulation therapy for major depressive disorder. *Archives of General Psychiatry, 57,* 507–515.

Goldberg, J., & Harrow, M. (2004). Consistency of remission and outcome in bipolar and unipolar mood disorders: A ten-year prospective follow-up. *Journal of Affective Disorders, 81,* 123–131.

Gos, T., Krell, D., Bielau, H., Steiner, J., Mawrin, C., Trubner, K., et al. (2010). Demonstration of disturbed activity of the lateral amygdaloid nucleus projection neurons in depressed patients by the AgNOR staining method. *Journal of Affective Disorders, 125,* 402–410.

Gotlib, I. H., & Hamilton, J. P. (2008). Neuroimaging and depression: Current status and unresolved issues. *Current Directions in Psychological Science, 17,* 159–153.

Gross, M., Nakamura, L., Pascual-Leone, A., & Fregni, F. (2007). Has repetitive transcranial magnetic stimulation (rTMS) treatment for depression improved? A systematic review and meta-analysis comparing the recent vs. the earlier rTMS studies. *Acta Psychiatrica Scandinavica, 115,* 155–173.

Hammen, C. (2005). Stress and depression. *Annual Review of Clinical Psychology, 1,* 293–319.

Hammen, C. (2009). Adolescent depression: Stressful interpersonal contexts and risk for recurrence. *Current Directions in Psychological Science, 18,* 200–204.

Hennessy, M. B., Schiml-Webb, P. A., & Deak, T. (2009). Separation, sickness, and depression: A new perspective on an old animal model. *Current Directions in Psychological Science, 18,* 227–231.

Holtzheimer, P. E., McDonald, W. M., Mufti, M., Kelley, M. E., Quinn, S., Corso, G., et al. (2010). Accelerated repetitive transcranial magnetic stimulation for treatment-resistant depression. *Depression and Anxiety, 27,* 950–953.

Kendler, K. S., Gatz, M., Gardner, C. O., & Pedersen, N. L. (2005). A Swedish national twin study of lifetime major depression. *American Journal of Psychiatry, 153,* 109–114.

Kessler, R. C., Akiskal, H. S., Ames, M., Birnbaum, H., Greenberg, P., Hirschfeld, R. M. A., et al. (2005). Prevalence and effects of mood disorders on work performance in a nationally representative sample of U.S. workers. *American Journal of Psychiatry, 153,* 1551–1558.

Kessler, R., Berglund, P., Demler, O., Jin, R., Koretz, D., Merikangas, K., Rush, A., Wang, P. S. (2003). The epidemiology of major depressive disorder: Results from the National Co-Morbidity Survey Replication. *JAMA, 289,* 3095–3105.

Kessler, R. C., Chiu, W. T., Demler, O., & Walters, E. E. (2005). Prevalence, severity, and comorbidity of twelve-month DSM-IV disorders in the National Comorbidity Survey Replication (NCS-R). *Archives of General Psychiatry, 52,* 517–527.

Kruger, S., Seminowicz, S., Goldapple, K., Kennedy, S. H., & Mayberg, H. S. (2003). State and trait influences on mood regulation in bipolar disorder: Blood flow differences with an acute mood challenge. *Biol Psychiatry, 54*, 1274–1283.

Licht-Strunk, E., van der Windt, D. A. W. M., van Marwijk, H. W. J., de Haan, M., & Beekman, A. T. F. (2007). The prognosis of depression in older patients in general practice and the community: A systematic review. *Family Practice, 24*, 158–180.

Luby, J. L. (2010). Preschool depression: The importance of identification of depression early in development. *Current Directions in Psychological Science, 19*, 91–95.

Maniglio, R. (2010). Child sexual abuse in the etiology of depression: a systematic review of reviews. *Depression and Anxiety, 27*, 531–542. doi: 10.1002/da.20587

McIntyre, R. S., & Konarski, J. (2005). Tolerability profiles of atypical antipsychotics in the treatment of bipolar disorder. *Journal of Clinical Psychiatry, 55*, 28–35.

McKinnon, M. C., Yucel, K., Nazarov, A., MacQueen, G.M. (2009). A meta-analysis examining clinical predictors of hippocampal volume in patients with major depressive disorder. *Journal of Psychiatry & Neuroscience, 34*, 41–54.

McMahon, F. J., Akula, N., Schulze, T. G., Muglia, P., Tozzi, F. Detera-Wadleigh, S.D., et al. (2010). Meta-analysis of genome-wide association data identifies a risk locus for major mood disorders on 3p21.1. *Nature Genetics, 42*, 128–131. doi: 10.1038/ng.523

Miklowitz, D. J. (2007). The role of the family in the course and treatment of bipolar disorder. *Current Directions in Psychological Science, 16*, 192–196.

Miklowitz, D. J. & Johnson, S. L. (2006). The psychopathology and treatment of bipolar disorder. *Annual Review of Clinical Psychology, 2*, 199–235.

Miller, G. E., & Blackwell, E. (2005). Turning up the heat: Inflammation as a mechanism linking chronic stress, depression, and heart disease. *Current Directions in Psychological Science, 15*, 259–272.

Moller, H. J., & Henkel, V. (2005). What are the most effective diagnostic and therapeutic strategies for the management of depression in specialist care? Copenhagen: WHO Regional Office for Europe. Retrieved November 5, 2010, from http://www.euro.who.int/en/home.

Monroe, S. M., & Reid, M. W. (2009). Life stress and major depression. *Current Directions in Psychological Science, 18*, 58–72.

National Institute of Mental Health. (2007). *Older adults: Depression and suicide facts* (NIH Publication No. 4593). Retrieved from http://www.nimh.nih.gov/health/publications/older-adults-listing.shtml

Rottenberg, J. (2005). Mood and emotion in major depression. *Current Directions in Psychological Science, 14*, 157–170.

Salvatore, P., Tohen, M., Khalsa, H. M., Baethge, C., Tondo, L., & Baldessarini, R. J. (2007). Longitudinal research on bipolar disorders. *Epidemiologia e Psichiatria Sociale, 15*, 109–117.

Schoeyen, H. K., Birkenaes, A. B., Vaaler, A., Auestad, B. H., Malt, U. F., Andreassen, O. A., et al. (2010). Bipolar disorder patients have similar levels of education but lower socio-economic status than the general population. *Journal of Affective Disorders*, doi: 10.1015/j. jad.2010.08.012

Schneck C. D., Miklowitz, D. J., Calabrese, J. R., Allen, M. H., Thomas, M. R., Wisniewski, S. R., et al. (2004). Phenomenology of rapid-cycling bipolar disorder: Data from the first 500 participants in the Systematic Treatment Enhanced Program. *American Journal of Psychiatry, 10*, 1902–1908.

Skjelstad, D. V., Malt, U. F., & Holte, A. (2010). Symptoms and signs of the initial prodrome of bipolar disorder: A systematic review. *Journal of Affective Disorders, 125*, 1–13.

Substance Abuse and Mental Health Services Administration. (2009). *The NSDUH Report: Employment and major depressive episode.* Retrieved from http://www.oas.samhsa.gov/2k9/152/Employment.htm

Suppes, T., Leverich, G. S., Keck, P. E. Nolen, W. A., Denicoff, K. D., Altshuler, L.L., et al. (2001). The Stanley Foundation Bipolar Treatment Outcome Network. II. Demographics and illness characteristics of the first 251 patients. *Journal of Affective Disorders, 57*, 45–59.

Taylor, S. (2007). Electroconvulsive therapy: A review of history, patient selection, technique, and medication management. *Southern Medical Journal, 100*, 494–498.

U.S. Department of Health and Human Services, National Institutes of Health, & National Institute of Mental Health. (2008). *Depression* (NIH Publication No. 08–3551). Retrieved from http://www.nimh.nih.gov/health/publications/depression/nimhdepression.pdf

U.S. Department of Health and Human Services, Substance Abuse and Mental Health Services Administration, Center for Mental Health Services, National Institutes of Health, & National Institute of Mental Health (1999). *Mental health: A report of the Surgeon General.* Retrieved from http://www.surgeongeneral.gov/library/mentalhealth/home.html

Weissman, M. M., Wolk, S., Goldstein, R. B., Moreau, D., Adams, P., Greenwald, S., et al. (1999). Depressed adolescents grown up. *JAMA, 281*, 1701–1713.

Wingo, A. P., Wrenn, G., Pelletier, T., Gutman, A. R., Bradley, B., & Ressler, K. J. (2010). Moderating effects of resilience on depression in individuals with a history of childhood abuse or trauma exposure. *Journal of Affective Disorders, 125*, 411–414.

Schizophrenia and Other Psychotic Disorders

■ *Ann Chapleau*

Joe, a thin, middle-aged man, can often be seen walking about downtown, wearing a cap fashioned out of aluminum foil, pulling a hand cart loaded with assorted household items and clothing. He is well-known to the mental health community and is a familiar sight to local residents. Joe grew up in a middle-class family, the only child of parents who were both accountants. His parents described him as a happy baby and a bright student, who had attended college to study engineering. But things began to change for Joe and his family when he moved one hour away to the state university when he was 19. Although his teen years were marked by a gradual withdrawal from friends and family, he began to demonstrate more socially bizarre behaviors while at college and when home on weekends, such as dressing in dark, heavy, hooded clothing even in warm weather, and an intense preoccupation with watching the CSPAN television channel. His parents were concerned about his behavior, but hoped it was a temporary phase of adapting to his changing life.

During winter break of his sophomore year in college, while his parents were vacationing in Mexico, Joe was seen by neighbors in the park near his family home, wearing camouflage and sleeping in a small pup tent. Police were called, and Joe hid in his tent, refusing to speak to them. He was forcibly removed and taken to the local psychiatric hospital for emergency admission. During his evaluation by the on-call psychiatrist, he revealed that he had moved out of his home because he had discovered "bugs" planted throughout the house. He believed that he was under surveillance by the Central Intelligence Agency (CIA) and was worried that his parents had been arrested. He reported that he had been suspicious of a plot against him for quite some time, but that this final "discovery" was the confirmation he was waiting for. When the staff arranged for him to speak to his parents, who reassured him they were only on vacation, Joe was convinced that CIA agents were impersonating their voices. A physical exam including blood testing was conducted to rule out any medical or drug-related cause of the psychosis. His parents were interviewed to obtain pertinent social and medical history. They shared that he had experienced some problems over the past 2 years in getting along with his roommates and was struggling with getting to all of his classes, resulting in low grades. Joe was diagnosed with paranoid-type schizophrenia and admitted to the inpatient program under court order. He was given antipsychotic medications and discharged to his parents upon their return home. He was not able to return to college as planned. He attempted to enroll at the local community colleges for various classes but was never able to complete the courses.

Joe has been in and out of the psychiatric hospital numerous times in the past 25 years. His admissions are typically preceded by his stopping his medications, which results in a return of delusions that he is under CIA surveillance. He has never been employed and has never had a significant-other relationship. He is suspicious of others, and so he will not consent to living in a room and board facility or group home. His attempts at independent living in community apartments are usually short-lived. He has been evicted for inability to pay rent as well as for unsafe conditions in the residence, such as hoarding and not cleaning. He resides for brief periods with his parents and has had numerous episodes of street homelessness.

DESCRIPTION AND DEFINITION

Schizophrenia is one of the most severe, complex, and debilitating of all mental health disorders. It is among the top 10 most disabling conditions worldwide (World Health Organization [WHO], 2008). Schizophrenia is a progressive disorder that can be treated, but not cured. This lifelong brain disorder is characterized by periods of **psychosis**, which is the presence of delusions or hallucinations without insight. It is also marked by a progressive decline in daily living skills, including work and education skills, social/relationship skills, and basic self-care abilities. To better understand the complex disorder of schizophrenia, one must understand the terms that describe the clinical symptoms.

■ **Delusions:** Fixed beliefs that, even in the face of contradictory evidence, are typically due to a misinterpretation of an event or experience. People with schizophrenia may experience more than one type of delusion at a time or at different points in time during the course of the illness. Delusions are categorized as bizarre or nonbizarre. Bizarre delusions

are characterized by beliefs of events that are clearly impossible and not related to everyday life experiences, such as a belief that aliens have impregnated the person while he or she was asleep. An example of a nonbizarre delusion is the belief that all coworkers are talking about the person. The individual may interpret that all private conversations observed at work to be about oneself. Delusional content can include any of the following types:

● *Persecutory:* The most common of all delusions; one believes himself or herself to be victimized, ridiculed, or placed under surveillance by known or unknown persons. Some people who suffer from persecutory delusions, such as **paranoia**, believe that someone is attempting to poison them, leading to a refusal to eat or drink. Another example is thought broadcasting, in which the individual is convinced that outside forces are able to transmit, or broadcast to others, their inner thoughts.

● *Referential:* These are also fairly common forms of delusions; one believes that common cues from the environment, such as facial expressions of celebrities on television, casual comments in daily conversations, or newspaper stories are specifically targeted to the individual, holding special meaning or a message for him or her.

● *Somatic:* This form of delusion is marked by beliefs that involve the person's body. For example, a person may believe they have received a secret operation while they were under anesthesia or that they are pregnant, despite evidence to the contrary.

● *Religious:* People who suffer from religious delusions may believe that they are Jesus Christ or are acting out direct orders from God.

● *Grandiose:* Examples include believing that one is all-powerful or important, that one is acting on secret orders from the president of the United States, or believing oneself to be a genius or multimillionaire.

■ **Hallucinations:** The experience of particular sensations that are not real to others and that are experienced while awake. The two most common forms include

● *Auditory hallucinations:* Hearing voices or sounds. The individual may perceive voices in the external environment, or inside his or her head, often more than one voice conversing or speaking directly to the person. Voices can be described as taunting and cruel, sometimes commanding the individual to perform certain acts, such as harming oneself or others, or can be familiar voices, which are perceived as friendly companions.

● *Visual hallucinations:* Seeing images of people or objects in the environment. Individuals may describe seeing shadowy figures or the image of a dead body.

- Other, less common forms of hallucinations include olfactory, tactile, and gustatory hallucinations.
- **Disorganized thinking:** Speech, which can provide clues about thought processes, may encompass any of the following:
  - *Loose associations:* Answers that begin to veer "off track" of the original questions.
  - *Tangential:* Unrelated comments or answers.
  - *Incoherent:* Often referred to as "word salad," seen in more severe cases.
- **Disorganized behavior:** Unpredictable, socially inappropriate behaviors that interfere with daily activities. Examples include agitated or angry outbursts with no known provocation; sexually acting out in public, that is, masturbation; and difficulties performing goal-directed tasks such as meal preparation or grooming.
- **Catatonic behavior:** Loss of responsiveness to environmental cues. The individual may assume rigid or bizarre postures and resist attempts made to move or reposition him or her. Excessive, nonpurposeful motor activity may also be observed. In extreme cases, the individual appears to be completely unresponsive, as in a catatonic stupor.

ETIOLOGY

There is no one single factor found to be the cause of schizophrenia. There are a number of models that attempt to explain the multiple factors that can contribute to the development of the disorder. Current research supports both a genetic vulnerability present at birth (Boos et al., 2007) and environmental triggers (Leask, 2004; McDonald & Murray, 2000). Findings from advanced neuropsychological and brain imaging suggest the presence of genetic markers, reduced brain activity in the frontal and temporal regions, and structural abnormalities in all regions of the brain, including enlarged ventricles, reduced volume of gray matter in the cerebral cortex, and decreased size of the hippocampus and thalamus (Lawrie & Abukmeil, 1998; Lieberman et al., 2008; Shenton, Dickey, Frumin, & McCarley, 2001; Velakoulis et al., 2006). The role of key neurotransmitters, including dopamine, glutamate, and serotonin, is being explored to determine their role in genetic alterations (Sawa & Snyder, 2002).

Complications in prenatal development or during delivery, affecting brain development, have also been associated with schizophrenia (Cannon, Jones, & Murray, 2002; Walker, Kestler, Bollini, & Hochman, 2004). Additionally, complications in later brain development, including chronic cannabis use, exposure to trauma, or other stress, have also been linked to schizophrenia (Veen et al., 2004).

Recent longitudinal studies have focused on the pattern of structural changes in the brain and have found progressive anatomical changes both prior to and following onset of the illness (Arango et al., 2008; Kempton, Stahl, Williams, & DeLisi, 2010; Sun et al., 2009; Velakoulis et al., 2006).

Despite major progress in research, the cause of schizophrenia and other psychotic disorders remains a mystery. With new technology including molecular genetics, in vivo brain imaging, and advancements in psychopharmacology, there is hope for discovering the cause or causes of schizophrenia that can ultimately lead to advancements in prevention and treatment.

INCIDENCE AND PREVALENCE

The incidence of schizophrenia is low, with a median value of 15.2 per 100,000 people. The lifetime prevalence is 4.0 per 1,000 (McGrath, Saha, Chant, & Welham, 2008). Schizophrenia crosses all racial, geographical, and socioeconomic boundaries. Some studies, however, indicate that migrant status, lower economic status, residing in a higher latitude, and male gender are factors associated with a higher incidence and prevalence (McGrath et al., 2008).

SIGNS AND SYMPTOMS

Despite scientific advancements that reveal neurobiological abnormalities of the brain, schizophrenia continues to be misunderstood by the general public. Negative stereotypes are reinforced by the unique nature of the signs and symptoms of this disorder. Schizophrenia affects the brain, which controls impulse, judgment, **affect**, and social skills. Perhaps most important, schizophrenia affects one's insight. As a result, people with schizophrenia are more likely to have difficulty recognizing and accepting that they have the disorder. This lack of insight can lead to resistance to treatment that can help reduce or eliminate symptoms.

Symptoms of schizophrenia vary greatly, but include the categories of positive, negative, cognitive, and affective symptoms, which are present to some degree in each person diagnosed with the disease (Jibson, Glick, & Tandon, 2004).

Positive Symptoms

Delusions, hallucinations, and disorganized thoughts are referred to as "positive" symptoms, as they involve an excess of behavior or experiences. Delusions are the most common type of **positive symptoms** observed, affecting 65% of people with schizophrenia, while hallucinations and disorganized thoughts each affect 50% of those with schizophrenia (Jibson et al., 2004). Positive symptoms may be continuously or intermittently present, but rarely abate completely.

Negative Symptoms

Flattened affect (facial and other nonverbal expression), **alogia** (impoverished speech), **avolition** (decreased motivation), **anhedonia** (loss of pleasure in previously enjoyed activities), and **associality** (decreased interest in socialization and maintenance of relationships) are referred to as "negative" symptoms, as they represent an absence of function or experience.

Cognitive Symptoms

Memory, attention, language, and executive function, such as abstract reasoning and planning skills, are affected by schizophrenia. In tests of sensory information processing, individuals with schizophrenia demonstrate reduced ability to process visual stimuli and to respond to environmental stimuli, due to motor skills deficits (Walker et al., 2004). Use of neuroimaging and cognitive tests have also revealed impaired neurocognitive functioning in completing tasks requiring use of frontal and temporal lobes (Lieberman et al., 2008).

Mean IQ scores range from 80 to 85, significantly lower than the norm of 100 for the general population (Jibson et al., 2004). People with schizophrenia also lack skills in identifying social cues and solving social problems. In general, research has not yielded any specific cognitive deficit present in all individuals with schizophrenia. Impairments appear generalized and vary greatly from person to person.

Affective Symptoms

Flattened or inappropriate affect is a common symptom of schizophrenia, and people with schizophrenia are more likely to demonstrate difficulties in identifying and expressing emotions. This, coupled with a limited ability to identify social cues, can lead to maladaptive social functioning.

Mood disturbances are also commonly seen. **Dysphoria** or depressed mood can be present during or following a psychotic episode and may require intervention. Individuals who develop insight into the severity of their illness are at greater risk of becoming depressed or experiencing demoralization.

The types and degree of symptoms present in an individual guide the diagnosis of one of five subtypes of schizophrenia: paranoid, disorganized, catatonic, undifferentiated, and residual types (American Psychiatric Association [APA], 2000). *Paranoid-type* schizophrenia is characterized by the presence of hallucinations or delusions, without disorganized thoughts or behavior or socially inappropriate affect. Persons with paranoid-type schizophrenia are believed to have a better prognosis. *Disorganized type* presents with disorganized behavior and speech and inappropriate affect. Those diagnosed with *catatonic type*, the rarest type, primarily experience abnormal posture and movement, with minimal speech or echolalia. A diagnosis of *undifferentiated type* is given when the individual does not meet criteria for any of the other types while still meeting the general diagnostic criteria for schizophrenia. *Residual type* reflects an absence of current psychosis, but continued **negative symptoms** or more mild impairments in social skills, affect, and thinking.

COURSE AND PROGNOSIS

Onset of symptoms can be gradual or acute, but there are usually earlier signs of dysfunction, in both **premorbid functioning**, the period from birth to the **prodromal phase**, and the prodromal phase, which can range from weeks or months to years before full onset of symptoms. Studies of premorbid functioning reveal subtle signs of problems in motor development, affect, and school performance. Impairments in cognitive functioning are often documented in school records and formal testing much earlier in life (Russell, Munro, Jones, Hemsley, & Murray, 1997). Some individuals do not present with significant premorbid "clues," but begin to show early signs of psychosis and unusual behavior in the prodromal phase. Nonspecific clinical symptoms seen in the prodromal phase can include affective changes such as depressed or anxious mood, irritability, insomnia, and cognitive changes such as impaired concentration and difficulty attending to tasks. Late-emerging symptoms in the prodromal phase can include suspiciousness, brief hallucinations, and perceptual difficulties (Kulhara, Banerjee, & Dutt, 2008).

Age of onset for schizophrenia is between 16 and 30 and is typically earlier for males than females. Diagnosis after age 45 is unusual (National Institute of Mental Health [NIMH], 2009). However, early-onset schizophrenia can be diagnosed in childhood or adolescence. Childhood onset refers to diagnosis of schizophrenia before the age of 13 and is characterized by an insidious onset, rather than a clear first episode, with multiple neurodevelopmental impairments present prior to the onset of psychotic or negative symptoms (Arango et al., 2008). Adolescent onset usually has a clear first episode, with a mean onset age of 15 (Arango et al.).

The criteria for a diagnosis of schizophrenia require the presence of symptoms for a period of at least 1 month, with some clinical signs present for at least 6 months (APA, 2000). The course of the illness varies greatly, with multiple episodes with changeable symptoms. The APA provides a classification of the longitudinal course that can be applied 1 year after initial onset (APA). The course can be classified as a single episode, episodic, continuous, or in partial or full remission.

Some individuals are able to maintain independent living and work competitively, whereas others experience a chronic decline in functioning, resulting in the need for 24-hour supervision and care. Approximately 10% to 20% of individuals are able to maintain remission for 5 years after the first psychotic episode, but the majority experience continued relapses (Jibson et al., 2004). Those who do not comply with an **antipsychotic medication** regime are five times more likely to relapse than those who are medication compliant. Relapses, which are associated with deterioration in daily functioning, can also be triggered by noncompliance with psychosocial treatment, environmental stressors, and substance abuse (Jibson et al.). Over time, with multiple psychotic episodes, negative and cognitive symptoms may become more prominent while positive symptoms are more likely to decrease in intensity in late middle age (Lieberman et al., 2008).

Other factors that can negatively impact prognosis include male gender, having a gradual and early onset of symptoms, a family history of schizophrenia, poor premorbid functioning, dysfunctional family relationships, and experience of abuse or neglect (Jibson et al., 2004; Walker et al., 2004).

Even when medication has been shown to reduce or even stop positive symptoms such as hallucinations and delusions, cognitive impairments, such as executive functions and abstract reasoning, are more likely to persist. Individuals with more severe cognitive loss are apt to experience decreased occupational performance and quality of life than those who demonstrate cognitive improvements (Jibson et al., 2004).

People with schizophrenia die, on average, 25 years earlier than those in the general population, related to pulmonary, cardiac, and infectious diseases (Colton & Manderscheid, 2006). Complications from antipsychotic medications, self-neglect, fear of health institutions, lack of access to health care, and increased suicide rate (Meltzer, 2002) are all contributing factors to this disparity in life expectancy.

Quality of life is also significantly lower for people with schizophrenia, as they represent lower socioeconomic status, are typically unemployed or underemployed, and are at higher risk of homelessness and incarceration (WHO, 2009). They are more likely to be victims of crime, especially violent crimes, and to abuse alcohol and/or drugs.

Approximately 50% of all people with schizophrenia have a co-occurring diagnosis of substance abuse or dependence (Volkow, 2009). Smoking rates are also high among those with schizophrenia, estimated as high as four times the general population (Kumari & Postma, 2005).

MEDICAL/SURGICAL MANAGEMENT

The focus of treatment is to reduce or eliminate symptoms and to provide environmental supports to enhance quality of life. The primary treatment for symptom reduction continues to be medication, although technological advances show promise for other medical or surgical approaches to treatment.

Pharmacologic Treatment

Prior to the 1950s, treatment consisted of institutionalization, including physical restraints and seclusion, even lobotomy. There was no medication for relief of clinical symptoms. Thorazine was the first antipsychotic medication introduced in the 1950s. Other similar medications, referred to as "first-generation" or "typical" antipsychotics, were also quickly developed. This first group of medications, which included Haldol, Prolixin, and Navane, proved effective in decreasing positive symptoms of schizophrenia by blocking dopamine receptors. Unfortunately, the side effects were often severe, including **extrapyramidal syndrome** (abnormal movements similar to Parkinson's disease), **tardive dyskinesia** (motor abnormalities such as writhing movements), cardiac problems, and heavy sedation.

The first atypical antipsychotics were introduced in the late 1980s. Atypical antipsychotics differ from the typical or first-generation antipsychotics in that they occupy different neurotransmitter receptors. Clozapine (Clozaril) was introduced in 1989, receiving FDA approval in 1990. It is considered to be highly effective in treating psychotic symptoms for individuals who were previously unresponsive to other first-generation medications. A major drawback, however, is the potential for serious side effects, including development of agranulocytosis, which requires regular blood work to monitor white blood cell count. Despite its effectiveness, it is not a favored medication among people with schizophrenia due to the medical risk, additional side effects, inconvenience, and excessive cost (Jibson et al., 2004).

Other atypical antipsychotics introduced since the 1990s include Risperdal (risperidone), Zyprexa (olanzapine), Seroquel (quetiapine), Geodon (ziprasidone), Aripiprazole (Abilify), and Paliperidone (Invego). They also are less likely to cause motor abnormalities such as extrapyramidal effects, but there can be other side effects including sedation, mild hypotension, weight gain, akathesia (restlessness), dry mouth, and constipation (Lieberman et al., 2005; NIMH, 2009).

Repetitive Transcranial Magnetic Stimulation

While medications have been successful in reducing positive symptoms of schizophrenia, there has been no proven treatment for negative symptoms. Transcranial magnetic stimulation (TMS) was developed in the 1980s to study brain function. It involves creating a magnetic field that passes through the skull, creating a current in the brain that activates nearby nerve cells. A coil of wire, wrapped in plastic, is held to the head while a capacitor is discharged to create the magnetic field. Researchers learned that repeated applications (repetitive transcranial magnetic stimulation [rTMS]) over the course of several days appear to affect brain activity. The magnetic field can be targeted to specific regions of the brain where nerve cells are associated with psychiatric symptoms. Recent studies of rTMS, while inconclusive, show promise in reducing negative symptoms of schizophrenia (Diabac-de Lange, Knegtering, & Aleman, 2010; Matheson, Green, Loo, & Carr, 2010). Other studies of rTMS have also shown effectiveness in reducing positive symptoms of auditory hallucinations, when used in conjunction with antipsychotic medication (Bagati, Haque Nizamie, & Prakash, 2009).

Electroconvulsive Therapy

Electroconvulsive therapy (ECT) is a medical procedure that consists of inducing a seizure by administration of electrical shock using electrodes attached to the scalp. Anesthesia is used for this brief procedure. It is generally administered in a series, over the course of days or weeks. The mortality rate for ECT is approximately 2 deaths per 100,000 treatments and is associated with anesthesia complications (Fink & Taylor, 2007). ECT is used for treating severe symptoms that do not respond to medication, particularly catatonia. Studies indicate some short-term benefits in global functioning when used in conjunction with antipsychotic medication (Tharyan & Adams, 2005). Side effects include confusion experienced immediately after the procedure as well as short-term memory loss for about 1 to 2 weeks.

IMPACT ON OCCUPATIONAL PERFORMANCE

Because schizophrenia typically presents in early adulthood, a period of developing new roles and responsibilities

such as career, life partnership, independent living, and parenthood, its lifelong effects are profound. Functional abilities vary greatly, but can be positively affected by environmental factors such as the presence of social support systems, financial assistance, and opportunities for housing or work.

Basic Activities of Daily Living

The ability to manage personal health is significantly compromised. Antipsychotic medications can cause weight gain, cardiac problems, and other health risks. Many individuals have impaired motor functioning and visual processing deficits, which, coupled with avolition and anhedonia symptoms, can limit interest or ability to participate in traditional exercise, nutrition, or smoking cessation programs.

Avolition, anhedonia, and disorganized behavior can also affect one's ability to initiate and complete self-care tasks such as grooming and hygiene. Impaired visual processing and difficulty interpreting visual stimuli can be associated with excessive application of makeup or ineffective attempts to bathe or shave thoroughly.

Instrumental Activities of Daily Living

The majority of people with schizophrenia do not live or work independently. The ability to work or succeed in school; manage a household including cooking, cleaning, laundry, and budgeting; or function as a caregiver requires multiple skills such as higher level cognitive processes, sensorimotor skills, and social nteraction skills, all of which can be affected by the positive, negative, affective, and cognitive symptoms of schizophrenia. Those who experience repeated relapses over time, which often involve hospitalization, demonstrate an overall decline in functioning, which limits opportunities for independent living.

Education

There is some evidence of impaired academic performance in premorbid functioning as well as during the prodromal phase, with standardized testing and general IQ scores in a significantly lower range than the general population (Fuller et al., 2002). Many individuals experience their first acute onset in young adulthood, which can derail plans for post–high school education or graduation. In fact, worldwide, about one-third of all people with schizophrenia do not graduate from high school (WHO, 2009). While antipsychotic medication can be effective in treating positive symptoms, there is no intervention that has been shown to create meaningful improvements in cognitive functioning. For the vast majority of those with schizophrenia, ongoing cognitive impairments persist and can have a major impact on academic success.

Work

Competitive work situations require multiple job-specific skills, the ability to learn new information quickly, and the ability to interact effectively with coworkers, customers, and superiors. Individuals with schizophrenia are more likely to lack college education or other technical or skilled trade certification. Even with supported employment assistance, they are more likely to be placed in minimum wage jobs such as fast food work, which requires the ability to process and respond very quickly while maintaining effective communication with coworkers. These work environments are often too demanding for the individual with active symptoms of schizophrenia. Successful work environments provide structured tasks, additional time allotted to complete work, the ability to work part-time hours, and opportunities for job coaching, particularly when new expectations are introduced.

Leisure and Social Participation

Symptoms of anhedonia and avolition can play a crucial role in limiting involvement in leisure activities. Psychosocial functioning may be impaired by both associality and affective symptoms, such as flattened affect and the ability to recognize and reciprocate appropriate social cues. People with schizophrenia typically have less financial and transportation resources for recreation, fewer social contacts, and less interest in leisure activities. As a result, they are more likely to be socially isolated.

OTHER PSYCHOTIC DISORDERS

In addition to schizophrenia, there are several other psychotic disorders as classified by the APA (2000). Schizophrenia and the following disorders all share the common feature of active psychosis.

Schizophreniform Disorder

Clinical features are nearly identical to schizophrenia with the exception of two differences: (1) Total duration of the illness is more than 1 month but <6 months, and (2) occupational performance deficits may not be present. About one-third of all people diagnosed with schizophreniform disorder will experience remission within a 6-month period, but the remaining two-thirds are likely to eventually be diagnosed with either schizophrenia or schizoaffective disorder.

Schizoaffective Disorder

Clinical symptoms of schizophrenia are present, including delusions or hallucinations, but at some point in the course of the illness, a major depressive, manic, or mixed episode occurs. There are two subtypes of schizoaffective disorder, depending on the mood presentation: bipolar type, which includes a manic or mixed episode, and depressive type. Age of onset is typically in early adulthood but can range from adolescence to late life.

Delusional Disorder

Symptoms include the presence of nonbizarre delusions lasting at least 1 month. Auditory or visual hallucinations may be present, but are not prominent. Olfactory or tactile hallucinations may be both present and prominent if they relate to the delusion. For example, if a person believes that he or she has an unknown infectious disease, he or she may experience related body sensations or odors. Activities of daily living skills are not significantly impaired, although work, social, and relationship problems can occur as a result of the delusional beliefs. For example, those who experience jealous or persecutory delusions may demonstrate angry or violent behavior. Age of onset for delusional disorders is highly variable, from adolescence to late life. The course of the illness can also be variable, from chronic to full remission within several months.

Brief Psychotic Disorder

Age of onset is typically in adolescence or early adulthood, with a sudden onset of positive psychotic symptoms or highly disorganized or catatonic behavior lasting between 1 day and 1 month. The brief episode is followed by a return to premorbid functioning. There may or may not be a precipitating stressor, such as death of a loved one or a traumatic experience in war combat. Individuals experience great confusion and dramatic mood shifts. Occupational performance can be significantly impaired, and there is an increased risk of suicide due to impulsivity.

Shared Psychotic Disorder

In this rarely seen disorder, the individual comes to believe in a nonbizarre or somewhat bizarre delusion held by a significant other, close friend, or family member. Although usually seen between two adults, it can occur among groups, particularly family members. For example, children may adopt a parent's delusional beliefs. The course of the illness can be varied but is usually chronic due to its occurrence in long-term relationships. When the individual is separated from the other person, the delusions abate.

Psychotic Disorder Due to a Medical Condition or Substance Use

Delusions or hallucinations are a direct result of a general medical condition, such as epilepsy, brain lesions, Huntington's disease, hepatic or renal disease, lupus, or auditory or visual nerve injuries. The course can be varied, from a single episode to recurrent. Even when the underlying medical condition is resolved, psychotic symptoms can continue, particularly in cases of brain injury.

Substance-Induced Psychotic Disorder

Clinical features include hallucinations or delusions directly due to effects of a drug or exposure to a toxin. In cases of intoxication or withdrawal from an abused drug, the hallucinations and delusions are more severe and present well beyond what would be expected during the intoxication/withdrawal/detoxification stages.

Psychotic Disorder NOS

Psychotic symptoms are present but do not meet the criteria for any specific psychotic disorder.

Case Illustration

Case 1

Megan is a 12-year-old girl, in the sixth grade at middle school. She was born in Texas, but moved with her mother and four siblings to Michigan when she was 5. Megan's father was jailed in Texas for running a methamphetamine laboratory in their family home. The family moved in with Megan's grandmother in the Detroit area, and her mother was able to find part-time employment in hotel housekeeping. Megan had difficulty adjusting to her new living situation and starting school for the first time. She had trouble following classroom rules such as sharing supplies and toys. In the second and third grades, she struggled with learning to read and write. Her IQ score was 85. She did not develop any close friendships. She struggled

academically with most subjects, but excelled in art, often drawing or painting very dark and strange images that she could not explain. She became increasingly withdrawn and disinterested in peer-related activities such as sports and going to the movies.

When Megan was 12, she was referred for psychological testing, which revealed that she had clinical symptoms of psychosis. Megan revealed to the psychologist that Satan had appeared to her on multiple occasions. She was tormented by voices telling her that she was evil and should commit suicide. She was seen by a psychiatrist who diagnosed her with early onset schizophrenia, admitting her to a local child and adolescent psychiatric hospital for medication and psychotherapy.

RECOMMENDED LEARNING RESOURCES

Torrey, E. F. (2001). *Surviving schizophrenia: A manual for families, consumers, and providers.* New York, NY: Harper Collins Publishing.

Organizations
National Alliance on Mental Illness (NAMI)
3803 N. Fairfax Dr., Ste. 100
Arlington, VA 22203
Tel: (703) 524-7600
Fax: (703) 524 9094
www.nami.org

National Institute of Mental Health (NIMH)
Science Writing, Press, and Dissemination Branch
6001 Executive Boulevard, Room 8184, MSC 9663
Bethesda, MD 20892-9663
Tel: (866) 615-6464
Fax: (301) 443-4279
www.nimh.nih.gov
NARSAD
60 Cutter Mill Road, Suite 404
Great Neck, NY 11021
Tel: (516) 829-0091
Fax: (516) 487-6930
www.narsad.org

REFERENCES

American Psychiatric Association. (2000). *Diagnostic and statistical manual of mental disorders* (Revised 4th ed.). Washington, DC: Author.

Arango, C., Moreno, C., Martinez, S., Parellada, M., Desco, M., Moreno, D., et al. (2008). Longitudinal brain changes in early-onset psychosis. *Schizophrenia Bulletin, 34*, 341–353.

Bagati, D., Haque Nizamie, S., & Prakash, R. (2009). Effect of augmentatory repetitive transcranial magnetic stimulation on auditory hallucinations in schizophrenia: Randomized controlled study. *Australian and New Zealand Journal of Psychiatry, 43*, 386–392.

Boose, E., Ellison, A. M., Osterweil, L. J., Podorozhny, R., Clarke, R., Wise, A., Hadley, J.L., & Foster, D. R. (2007). Ensuring reliable datasets for environmental models and forecasts. *Ecological Informatics, 2*, 237–247.

Cannon, M., Jones, P. B., & Murray, R. M. (2002). Obstetric complications and schizophrenia: Historical and met-analytic review. *The American Journal of Psychiatry, 159*, 1080–1092.

Colton, C. W., & Manderscheid, R. W. (2006). Congruencies in increased mortality rates, years of potential life lost, and causes of death among public mental health clients in eight states. *Preventing Chronic Disease, 3*. Retrieved from http://www.cdc.gov/pcd/issues/2006/apr/05_0180.htm

Diabac-de Lange, J. J., Knegtering, R., & Aleman, A. (2010). Repetitive transcranial magnetic stimulation for negative symptoms of schizophrenia: Review and metanalysis. *The Journal of Clinical Psychiatry, 71*, 411–418.

Fink, M., & Taylor, M. A. (2007). Electroconvulsive therapy: Evidence and challenges. *The Journal of the American Medical Association, 298*, 330–332.

Fuller, R., Nopoulos, P., Arndt, S., O'Leary, D., Ho, B. C., & Andreason, N. C. (2002). Longitudinal assessment of premorbid cognitive functioning in patients with schizophrenia through examination of standardized scholastic test performance. *The American Journal of Psychiatry, 159*, 1183–1189.

Jibson, M. D., Glick, I. D., & Tandon, R. (2004). Schizophrenia and other psychotic disorders. *Focus, 2*(1), 17–30.

Kempton, M. J., Stahl, D., Williams, S. C. R., & DeLisi, L. E. (2010). Progressive lateral ventricular enlargement in schizophrenia: A meta-analysis of longitudinal MRI studies. *Schizophrenia Research, 120*, 54–62.

Kulhara, P., Banerjee, A., & Dutt, A. (2008). Early intervention in schizophrenia. *The Indian Journal of Psychiatry, 50*, 128–134.

Kumari, V., & Postma, P. (2005). Nicotine use in schizophrenia: The self-medication hypotheses. *Neuroscience & Biobehavioral Reviews, 29*, 1021–1034.

Lawrie, S. M., & Abukmeil, S. S. (1998). Brain abnormality in schizophrenia: A systematic and quantitative review of volumetric magnetic resonance imaging studies. *The British Journal of Psychiatry, 172*, 110–120.

Leask, S. J. (2004). Environmental influences in schizophrenia: The known and the unknown. *Advances in Psychiatric Treatment, 10*, 323–330.

Lieberman, J. A., Drake, R. E., Sederer, L. I., Belger, A., Keefe, R., Perkins, D., et al. (2008). Science and recovery in schizophrenia. *Psychiatric Services, 59*, 487–496.

Lieberman, J. A., Stroup, S. T., McEvoy, J. P., Swartz, M. S., Rosenheck, R. A., Perkins, D. O., et al. (2005). Effectiveness of antipsychotic drugs in patient with chronic schizophrenia. *The New England Journal of Medicine, 353*, 1209–1223.

Matheson, S. L., Green, M. J., Loo, C., & Carr, V. J. (2010). A change in the conclusions of a recent systematic meta-review: Repetitive transcranial magnetic stimulation is effective for the negative symptoms of schizophrenia. *Schizophrenia Research*. Advance online publication. doi:10.1016/j.schres 2010.05 029

McDonald, C., & Murray, R. M. (2000). Early and late environmental risk factors for schizophrenia. *Brain Research Reviews, 31*, 130–137.

McGrath, J., Saha, S., Chant, D., & Welham, J. (2008). Schizophrenia: A concise overview of incidence, prevalence, and mortality. *Epidemiologic Reviews, 30*, 67–76.

Meltzer, H. Y. (2002). Suicidality in schizophrenia: A review of the evidence for risk factors and treatment options. *Current Psychiatry Reports, 4*, 279–283.

National Institute of Mental Health. (2009). *Schizophrenia* (NIH Publication No. 09-3517). Bethesda, MD: Author.

Pantelis, C., Velakoulis, D., Wood, S. J., Suckling, J., Phillips, L. J., Yung, A. R., et al. (2003). Neuroanatomical abnormalities before and after onset of psychosis: A cross-sectional and longitudinal MRI comparison. *Lancet, 25*, 281–288.

Russell, A. J., Munro, J. C., Jones, P. B., Hemsley, D. R., & Murray, R. M. (1997). Schizophrenia and the myth of intellectual decline. *The American Journal of Psychiatry, 154*, 635–639.

Sawa, A., & Snyder, S. H. (2002). Schizophrenia: Diverse approaches to a complex disease. *Science, 296*, 692–695.

Shenton, M. E., Dickey, C. C., Frumin, M., & McCarley, R. W. (2001). A review of MRI findings in schizophrenia. *Schizophrenia Research, 49*, 1–52.

Sun, D., Phillips, L., Velakoulis, D., Yung, A., McGorry, P. D., Wood, S. J., et al. (2009). Progressive brain structural changes mapped as psychosis develops in 'at risk' individuals. *Schizophrenia Research, 108*, 85–92.

Tharyan, P., & Adams, C. E. (2005). Electroconvulsive therapy for schizophrenia. *Cochrane Database of Systematic Reviews* (2), CD000076.

Veen, N. D., Selten, J. P., van der Tweel, I., Feller, W. G., Hoek, H. W., & Kahn, R. S. (2004). Cannabis use and age at onset of schizophrenia. *The American Journal of Psychiatry, 161*, 501–506.

Velakoulis, D., Wood, S. J., Wong, M. T., McGorry, P. D., Yung, A., Phillips, L., et al. (2006). Hippocampal and amygdala volumes according to psychosis stage and diagnosis: A magnetic resonance imaging study of chronic schizophrenia, first-episode psychosis, and ultra-high-risk individuals. *Archives of General Psychiatry, 63*, 139–149.

Volkow, N. D. (2009). Substance use disorders in schizophrenia—clinical implications of comorbidity. *Schizophrenia Bulletin, 35*, 469–472.

Walker, E., Kestler, L., Bollini, A., & Hochman, K. M. (2004). Schizophrenia: Etiology and course. *The Annual Review of Psychology, 55*, 401–430.

World Health Organization. (2008). *The global burden of disease: 2004 update.* Geneva: Author.

World Health Organization. (2009). *Discussion paper: Mental health, poverty and development.* Geneva: Author.

Anxiety Disorders

■ *Christine K. Urish*

As the occupational therapist arrives on the inpatient psychiatric unit, she finds April pacing up and down the hallway. April was admitted last evening as a result of her significant functional decline in all areas of occupational performance. She has been diagnosed with **generalized anxiety disorder** by her psychiatrist. "I know my psychiatrist has written a referral for me to attend occupational therapy, I know all about occupational therapy," she states. I have worked in this hospital on the pediatrics unit for quite some time." I know the occupational therapists come to the pediatrics unit and play with the children and try to get them to move and interact with their parents." I don't need to play." I am so anxious. I worry all the time and it seems as if I worry about everything. I don't really think occupational therapy and play will help me at all." I cannot sleep or rest and I am very worried that I will be fired because I'm not functioning as I should because I am anxious and tired."

The occupational therapist suggests April come with her to discuss occupational therapy services and to complete an initial interview. The occupational therapist wants to determine how April's anxiety is impacting her ability to do everyday things. As the occupational therapist walks down the hall, April responds by saying, "I'm not able to be a nurse anymore, then what will I do?" "This play therapy is not going to help my anxiety, I cannot do anything right and I am certain this is not going to help me." "What in the world was my psychiatrist thinking when he ordered me to attend occupational therapy groups?" "How in the world is this going to help me at all?"

April is obviously thinking that occupational therapy is one-dimensional. In her mind, occupational therapy is about play. The occupational therapist knows that she will have to explain to April how occupational therapy services on the pediatrics unit differ from an inpatient psychiatric setting. She also knows that she will have to do her best to try and convince April that occupational therapy can be beneficial to her. The occupational therapist feels that this information could assist April in improving her performance skills and decreasing her anxiety.

The occupational therapist looks forward to the challenge of working with April both individually and in a group of other patients diagnosed with mental illness. If April will learn relaxation techniques and develop her skill at using them, through participation in occupational therapy services, her level of anxiety may decrease. She may find that she is able to sleep at night, and thus her energy level and concentration may improve. The occupational therapist also has a feeling that April may be so focused on her success and performance at work that April's leisure lifestyle may be limited. As an occupational therapist she is concerned about April's ability to balance her work, activities of daily living, instrumental activities of daily living (IADLs), sleep and rest, leisure, and social participation. Although April thinks that all occupational therapy includes is play, this therapist will work with April to assist her in understanding that a balance of occupations and occupational performance is essential to being productive.

INTRODUCTION

This chapter discusses **anxiety disorders**: how they are classified, diagnosed, and differ from "normal" feelings. Evidence-based research on intervention will be presented throughout the chapter. The impact of anxiety disorders upon performance skills in occupation will be examined through the detailed case studies at the end of the chapter. Learning resources for development of additional knowledge are provided at the end of the chapter as well.

DEFINITION AND DESCRIPTION

Anxiety is defined as "apprehension of danger, and dread accompanied by restlessness, tension, tachycardia, and dyspnea unattached to a clearly identifiable stimulus" (Dirckx, 2001). It is important to distinguish fear from anxiety. Fear is similar in that it is an alerting response to a known, external, definite threat. Anxiety is a response to a threat that is unknown, vague, and internal and it can lead to conflicted feelings (Sadock & Sadock, 2007). It is normal to have some degree of anxiety in our lives: "Will I get a raise during my review with my boss?" "Will my dress be appropriate for the social occasion to which I am driving?" "Will I get a good grade on the test I recently completed?" Most often, even if we are nervous or anxious about a number of life events, we are able to perform daily activities and occupations without incident (Grey House Publishing, 2004). In our day-to-day existence we experience anxiety, whether or not we recognize it as anxiety. Anxiety can motivate us into action. For example, "I'm anxious about my performance review at work at the end of the month, so I will go in early or stay late this week to make sure I am caught up on things," or "I think my clothing is getting tighter, I seem to have put on a few pounds. I need to spend more time exercising to lose some weight and improve my physical appearance." Anxiety, however, can also be pathological, when we worry incessantly about things that we cannot control or change. When this incessant worry begins to negatively impact our ability to work, learn, or socialize, anxiety may be considered pathologic. Anxiety symptoms may vary from individual to individual (Sadock & Sadock, 2007).

Classification of Anxiety Disorders

The *Diagnostic and Statistical Manual of Mental Disorders IV-Text Revised (DSM IV-TR)* has established criteria to determine if anxiety or anxiety-related conditions are pathologic (American Psychiatric Association [APA], 2000). The criteria present both physical and psychological symptoms that must be met for a diagnosis to be made. Anxiety disorders are considered under Axis I in the *DSM IV-TR* multiaxial system. There are 11 anxiety disorders as classified by the *DSM IV-TR*. They include **panic disorder**, panic disorder with agoraphobia, agoraphobia without history of panic disorder, specific **phobia** (formerly known as simple phobia), **social phobia** (also known as social anxiety disorder), **obsessive-compulsive disorder** (OCD), **posttraumatic stress disorder** (PTSD), acute stress disorder, generalized anxiety disorder, anxiety disorder due to a general medical condition that is specified, and substance-induced anxiety disorder. In this chapter the anxiety disorders of panic disorder, phobia, social phobia, OCD, PTSD, and generalized anxiety disorder will be presented in a comprehensive fashion.

Occupational therapists treat clients diagnosed with these disorders in a variety of mental health settings including inpatient, partial hospitalization, and outpatient settings. Occupational therapists also treat clients in a variety of nonmental health settings in which they observe anxiety symptoms in the clients they treat across the lifespan. Although occupational therapists do not make psychiatric diagnoses, a thorough understanding of the criteria for making such a diagnosis is important for the clinician to facilitate clinical observations.

Panic Disorder

Panic disorder includes short, sudden attacks of fear; fear of losing control; or terror (John Hopkins, 2011).

The diagnosis of panic disorder without **agoraphobia** ("fear of the marketplace") includes having at least four **panic attacks** within the last month, an ongoing concern of having additional attacks or worry about the implications of having additional attacks (such as concern over health, having a "heart attack," or "going crazy"), and a change in behavior as a result of the panic attacks. The absence of agoraphobia and a panic attack cannot be a result of the physiologic effects of substance(s) and other general medical conditions or be attributed to another mental disorder such as social phobia or OCD, PTSD, or separation anxiety disorder (APA, 2000).

Phobia

Phobia refers to irrational fears that lead individuals to often avoid certain objects and specific situations all together (Substance Abuse and Mental Health Service Administration [SAMHSA], 2011). The diagnosis of phobia includes the individual presenting with marked and persistent fear, which is considered excessive or unreasonable in the face of, or when considering the anticipation of, a specific object (animals, seeing blood) or specific situation (preparing to fly on an airplane, having blood drawn, receiving an immunization or shot) (APA, 2000). Exposure to the feared stimulus produces an anxiety response that may present in the form of a situationally bound or situationally predisposed panic attack. According to one of the *DSM IV-TR* diagnostic criteria, individuals with phobia should be able to see the fear that they are experiencing is excessive or unreasonable. Individuals may often avoid environments or situations in which the feared stimulus will be present. If they feel compelled to put themselves in uncomfortable situations, they will endure the environment or situation with a great deal of anxiety and distress (APA, 2000). The avoidance of the feared stimulus, anticipation, or distress experienced as a result of the feared stimulus interferes with the individual's daily routine including occupational or academic functioning, social activities, or interpersonal relationships, and there is increased distress surrounding having the phobia.

In persons younger than 18 years of age, the duration of the phobia must be present for at least 6 months. Additionally, the anxiety present in phobias and the accompanying panic attacks (or phobic avoidance with a situation or object) cannot be better accounted for by another mental disorder such as OCD, PTSD, separation anxiety disorder, social phobia, or panic disorder with or without agoraphobia.

There are five different types of specific phobias found in adult clinical populations (Fadem, 2004). These phobias, in descending order of frequency seen in clinical settings, include situational, natural environment, blood-injection injury, animal, and other types. Situational phobias include fears of tunnels, bridges, using public transportation, flying in an airplane, and being in closed places. Situational phobias are usually more common in adults than children. Natural environment phobias include fear of natural occurrences such as lightening, thunder, heights, and deep water. These fears often present in childhood. Blood-injection injury phobias focus on the fear of receiving an injection or treatment, which requires some invasive bodily procedure. The specific phobia of animals is the fourth most frequently seen phobia in adult clinical populations. This phobia includes insects in addition to animals. The final type of specific phobia is categorized as other type that includes loud sounds, falling, contracting an illness, and choking. A fear of costume characters in children is also considered in this category (Fadem, 2004).

The diagnosis of social phobia, also known as social anxiety, is a marked, persistent fear in the presence of strangers. People fear being negatively judged by others. The individual experiences anxiety regarding his or her social interaction or performance and feels that his or her performance will be scrutinized by these people (Fadem, 2004). The person fears that he or she will act in a way that will embarrass or humiliate himself or herself. The person is concerned others will perceive him or her as weak, crazy, or stupid. If public speaking is an activity the individual must perform, he or she may fear others will see his or her hands and voice tremble and fear that he or she will appear inarticulate (APA, 1994). When an individual is exposed to the feared social or performance situation, he or she experiences anxiety that may appear as a situationally bound or situationally predisposed panic attack. The individual acknowledges and recognizes that his or her fear is excessive or unreasonable, yet feared performance or social situations are avoided. If the individual must attend a social event or perform, he or she endures this experience with a great deal of distress. Consequently, people with this disorder experience a marked impact on the quantity and quality of their daily activities. The individual expresses much distress about having the social phobia condition.

In persons younger than age 18, the duration of this condition must exist for at least 6 months for a diagnosis to be made. For the diagnosis of social phobia to be made, the fear or avoidance of the performance or social situations cannot be attributed to the effects of a substance (medication reaction or drug abuse), a general medical condition, or another mental disorder. In considering the diagnosis of social phobia, the consideration of avoidant personality disorder should be critically examined.

Obsessive-Compulsive Disorder

To be diagnosed with OCD, an individual must experience either **obsessions** or **compulsions** or both that he or she realizes are unreasonable, unnecessary, intrusive, and irresistible (APA, 2000; John Hopkins, 2011). Obsessions are recurrent persistent thoughts, impulses, or images that are experienced as intrusive and inappropriate and cause significantly increased anxiety and distress. The thoughts, images, or impulses are not excessive worries about day-to-day problems or events. The individual with OCD may attempt to suppress or ignore these thoughts, images, or impulses or try to counteract these thoughts with other thoughts or actions. The individual is aware that the obsessive thoughts, images, or impulses are created through his or her own mind, as opposed to thought insertion.

Compulsions are repetitive acts such as handwashing, straightening, or checking or mental activities such as prayer or silently repeating words (APA, 2000). The individual feels compelled to perform these acts in response to an obsession or according to specific rules that are typically rigidly applied. The behaviors or mental acts performed by the individual are targeted at preventing or decreasing distress or to prevent a negative (or dreaded) event or situation. Unfortunately, the thoughts and behaviors do not logically relate to the objects of distress the individual holds in his or her mind.

In addition to causing marked distress, the obsessions or compulsions must consume at least 1 hour or more of time daily and interfere in a significant manner with the individual's routine occupational functioning. The obsessive-compulsive behavior is not a result of a general medical condition or a result of the physiologic effects of a substance (APA, 2000).

Posttraumatic Stress Disorder

PTSD is a psychological stress disorder from exposure to traumatic events such as natural disasters, violent crime (e.g., rape, child abuse, and murder), torture, accidents, or war (John Hopkins, 2011). The diagnosis of PTSD is made when an individual has been exposed to a traumatic event in which he or she experienced, witnessed, or was confronted with situations that threatened or involved death or injury or a threat of death or serious injury to himself or herself or to others (APA, 2000). The individual's response to the event involved intense fear, helplessness, and horror. This traumatic event is reexperienced in a persistent fashion in one of five ways:

1. Intrusive, recurrent, and distressing recollections of the event that may include images, thoughts, or perceptions
2. Recurrent dreams that cause distress
3. Experiencing hallucinations, reliving the experience, illusions, or dissociative experiences

4. Psychological distress that is intense when experiencing internal or external cues that are symbolic of or are similar to a part of the traumatic event
5. Physiologic reactions upon exposure to internal or external cues that are symbolic of or are similar to a part of the traumatic event (APA, 2000)

Individuals with PTSD usually avoid stimuli associated with the traumatic event. They may appear numb, in an overall way, and demonstrate at least three of the following seven characteristics:

1. Attempts to avoid thinking about, feeling emotions related to, or discussing the trauma or anything associated to the trauma
2. Avoidance of activities, locations, or individuals who may facilitate recollection of the traumatic experience
3. Inability to recall events or aspects of the trauma
4. Significant decrease in interest or participation in activities that were once identified as meaningful
5. Feelings of estrangement or detachment from other people
6. Limitations in the individual's affective range
7. Limited ability to view future or viewing the future as shortened (APA, 2000)

Additionally, individuals may present with persistent symptoms of increased arousal as demonstrated by two or more of the following symptoms:

- Difficulty attaining or maintaining sleep
- Irritability or angry outbursts
- Concentration difficulties
- Hypervigilance
- Startle response, which is exaggerated

The duration of symptoms presented must be longer than 1 month, and the disturbance must cause significant functional impairment in all areas deemed important to the individual (APA, 2000).

Generalized Anxiety Disorder

This disorder is diagnosed when an individual has excessive worry and anxiety, which occurs more often than not for a period of at least 6 months. This excessive worry or anxiety can include a number of events or activities such as school or work performance or family concerns (APA, 2000). Individuals have difficulty controlling their worry, and they characteristically also have three or more of the following symptoms:

- Feelings of being on edge, restless, or keyed up
- Becoming easily fatigued
- Feeling as if his or her mind is going blank and difficulty with concentration

- Irritability
- Tension in muscles
- Difficulty with sleep, which can include falling asleep, staying asleep, or restless sleep

The concern of the individual with generalized anxiety disorder is not related to another *DSM IV-TR* Axis I disorder such as OCD (anxiety about contamination) or weight gain as in anorexia nervosa (APA, 2000). The anxiety, worry, and associated physical symptoms cause the individual difficulty in all areas of functioning important to the individual. The generalized anxiety disorder cannot be a result of the physiologic effects of substances or a general medical condition. This diagnosis cannot occur only during a mood disorder, pervasive developmental disorder, or a psychotic disorder. The *DSM IV-TR* does have a characterization for anxiety disorder due to a general medical condition as well as substance-induced anxiety disorder and anxiety disorder not otherwise specified (APA, 2000).

Anxiety disorders may coexist with other disorders such as depression, substance abuse, eating disorders, schizophrenia, personality disorders, or other anxiety disorders (National Institute of Mental Health [NIMH], 2011). Comorbidity of another mental illness was high when individuals were diagnosed with social phobia and generalized anxiety disorder (Brown, Campbell, Lehman, Grisham, & Mancil, 2001). Per the data from the Epidemiologic Catchment Area survey, there are high rates of comorbidity among Axis I disorders, including 46.5% phobic disorder, 31.7% major depression, and 24.1% substance abuse (most commonly alcohol abuse) (Karno, Golding, & Sorenson, 1998). Individuals diagnosed with social phobia also had high levels of comorbidity with avoidant personality disorder (Rettew, 2000). Data from the National Comorbidity Survey suggested close to 50% of persons diagnosed with PTSD also had three or more additional diagnoses, most commonly mood disorders, another anxiety disorder, and substance misuse (Kessler, Sonnega, Bromet, & Hughes, 1995). When considering anxiety disorders from a comprehensive perspective, it is important to note that anxiety disorders may coexist with cancer and heart disease as well (NIMH, 2011). It is important for clinicians to consider comorbidity to provide the best intervention for individuals with anxiety disorders and other coexisting conditions in everyday practice.

Etiology

The understanding of the causes of anxiety has increased in recent years as neurochemical and physical pathways of fear and anxiety have been critically examined (Brantley, 2007). Despite this, more research is needed as we are far from having a clear understanding of these complex conditions. In examining the causes of anxiety disorders, one must consider the powerful interaction between biology, cognitive/emotional influences, and stress. The likelihood of developing an anxiety disorder includes a combination of life experiences, psychological traits, and genetic factors. Anxiety disorders, such as panic disorder, have a stronger genetic basis than other disorders, although at this time specific genes have not been identified (United States Surgeon General [USSG], n.d.). Women are more at risk for being diagnosed with anxiety disorders than men, although it is not clear as to why. Some researchers suggest the role of gonadal steroid. Other researchers suggest women's response to stress and their exposure to a wider range of life events is different from those experienced by men (USSG, n.d.).

There are three major etiologic considerations in examining anxiety disorders. These include biological factors, genetic factors, and psychosocial factors. Three major schools of psychosocial theory have contributed to the understanding of the causes of anxiety: psychoanalytic, behavioral, and existential. Each of these frameworks presents conceptual and practice applications for the treatment of anxiety disorders.

According to the biological theories of anxiety, an excessive autonomic reaction is present with increased sympathetic tone. Increased catecholamines are released in addition to increased production of norepinephrine metabolites. **Aminobutyric acid (GABA)** levels are decreased, and this causes central nervous system hyperactivity. Additionally, a decrease in serotonin causes anxiety, and increased dopaminergic activity is related to anxiety. The temporal cortex activity in those with anxiety is decreased. The center of the brain, locus ceruleus, is hyperactive when anxiety is present, especially during a panic attack (Sadock & Sadock, 2001). Magnetic resonance imaging evidence indicates that individuals with panic disorder have pathology in the temporal lobes of the brain, in particular, in the hippocampus (Sadock & Sadock, 2007).

Research into the neurotransmitters of those diagnosed with OCD has indicated that dysregulation of serotonin is associated with formation of obsessions and compulsions. When critically examining data from brain imaging studies of individuals diagnosed with OCD, one can see altered neurocircuitry between the orbitofrontal cortex, caudate, and thalamus. Positron emission tomography scans have shown increased metabolism and blood flow in the basal ganglia and frontal lobe. Research indicates an altered noradrenergic system in individuals diagnosed with PTSD (Sadock & Sadock, 2001). Research has also suggested the possibility of opioid system hyperregulation in individuals with PTSD. Biological research into the etiology of generalized anxiety disorder has focused on GABA and serotonin receptors. There are also indications that genetics may play a role in the etiology of anxiety disorders.

Despite the fact that well-controlled research studies into panic disorder are limited, available genetic research has indicated nearly half the individuals with panic disorder have at least one relative affected with an anxiety disorder (Sadock & Sadock, 2007). Approximately 5% of individuals with high levels of anxiety have a variant of the gene associated with serotonin metabolism (Sadock & Sadock, 2001). Phobias also seem to be more common among family members. More specifically the blood-injection-type phobia has a significantly high familial tendency. Further, first-degree relatives with social phobia are three times more likely to be diagnosed with social phobia than those who have first-degree relatives without a mental disorder (Sadock & Sadock, 2007). When considering a genetic link in the diagnosis of OCD, available research supports the hypothesis that the disorder has a genetic component. However, the data at this time do not pinpoint the heritable factors from the influence of behavior and culture.

From a psychoanalytic perspective, anxiety is viewed as developmentally related to childhood fears of disintegration and is related to the fear of loss of a loved one or an object or the fear of castration. Clinicians critically examine possible triggers when working with individuals with anxiety disorders. In people diagnosed with phobias, from a psychoanalytic perspective, the individual attempts to repress. When this fails, other defense mechanisms such as avoidance are called upon (Sadock & Sadock, 2007).

Despite the significant biological underpinning of the diagnosis of OCD, one must consider the psychodynamic meaning associated with the obsessions and compulsions and the secondary gain that the individual may experience as a result of his or her behavior. Additionally, one must recognize the situations and experiences that precipitate or exacerbate the individual's obsessions and compulsions. In examining PTSD from a psychoanalytic perspective, the traumatic experience reactivates an unresolved psychological conflict (Sadock & Sadock, 2007). This results in the use of defenses including repression, regression, denial, splitting, dissociation, guilt, reaction formation, and undoing. Individuals diagnosed with generalized anxiety disorder, according to the psychoanalytic perspective, have unresolved unconscious conflicts.

Behavioral theories propose that anxiety is a response that is learned from exposure to parental behavior or through the process of classical conditioning. Anxiety disorders include faulty, distorted, or counterproductive thinking patterns (Sadock & Sadock, 2001). The success of treating individuals with anxiety disorders using a behavioral approach lends to the credence of this approach in intervention (Sadock & Sadock, 2007). Anxiety is acquired through classical conditioning and observational learning and maintained through operant conditioning. Learning theory is of significance in the treatment of phobias and provides clear explanation for many symptoms experienced by the phobic individual.

When examining OCD through the template of learning theory, obsessions are viewed as conditioned stimuli and are paired through fear and anxiety with an event that is noxious or anxiety producing. Compulsions are viewed as mechanisms that reduce anxiety attached to an obsessive thought. Over time, the compulsions become less effective in reducing the anxiety (Sadock & Sadock, 2007).

From a cognitive behavioral perspective an individual with PTSD cannot process or rationalize the traumatic experience that caused the diagnosis. The individual continues to experience and reexperience the extreme stress and ineffectively use avoidance as a mechanism for dealing with the stressful experience. Some individuals with PTSD may obtain secondary gain related to their diagnosis such as monetary compensation, increased attention, and others fulfilling their dependency needs. These gains need to be critically examined by the health care practitioner.

According to the cognitive behavioral school of thought, an individual with generalized anxiety disorder has an incorrect and inaccurate perception of danger. This inaccuracy is facilitated by selective attention to negative information within the environment, distortion in information processing, and an inability to cope.

From an existential perspective, there is no one specifically identifiable stimulus that facilitates the feeling of chronic anxiety in an individual. Anxiety, according to an existential approach, occurs when the individual becomes aware of profound feelings of a lack of meaning in his or her life. This lack of meaning for some individuals is more fear provoking than thoughts of death. With increased concerns of bioterrorism and nuclear attacks, existential concerns in society have been noted to be increasing (Sadock & Sadock, 2007). Occupational therapy professionals are well suited to address anxiety from an existential perspective as we critically examine meaning and occupation in an individual's day-to-day existence.

Stress is the prime cause of PTSD. However, not every individual will experience PTSD after exposure to a traumatic event. The stress experience in and of itself is not sufficient to cause the disorder. Preexisting biological and psychological factors before, during, and after the trauma must be taken into consideration (Sadock & Sadock, 2007). The cumulative and long-term effects of stress contribute to the development of anxiety and anxiety disorders. Chronic stress places an individual at serious risk for physical illness, emotional, social, and spiritual dysfunction. Clearly, unmanaged chronic stress needs to be identified and addressed (Brantley, 2007).

INCIDENCE AND PREVALENCE

In the United States more than 18.1% of adults are diagnosed with an anxiety disorder in 1 year. Another 48.4% of adults experience mood (9.5%), substance abuse (3.8%), impulse control (8.9%), or other mental disorder (26.2%). When considering comorbid disorders, 55% of individuals experienced one disorder whereas 22% experienced two diagnoses and 23% experienced three or more diagnoses (Kessler, Chiu, Demler, & Walters, 2005). Less than 30% of individuals who suffer from anxiety disorders, however, seek treatment (Lepine, 2002). When considering gender, women are 60% more likely to experience the diagnosis of an anxiety disorder than are men (Kessler et al., 2005). The annual cost of anxiety disorders is estimated to be $42 to $47 billion dollars per year (DuPont et al., 1996). Of the total cost, $23 billion (54% of cost) is spent in nonpsychiatric medical costs (physician office visits, emergency room costs). Approximately $4.1 billion (10%) is spent in indirect workplace costs, $1.2 billion (3%) in mortality costs, and $0.8 billion (2%) in pharmaceutical (prescription) costs. Costs to the workplace are attributed more to lost productivity rather than absenteeism. Other than phobia, all anxiety disorders were found to be associated with impairment in work performance.

Panic Disorder

This diagnosis affects 5 million American adults (NIMH, 2011). Women are twice as likely to be diagnosed with panic disorder as men. An underdiagnosis of panic disorder in men however may skew this distribution (Sadock & Sadock, 2007). The male-to-female ratio for panic disorder without agoraphobia is 1:1 and agoraphobia is 1:2 (Sadock & Sadock, 2001). The ethnic differences present in panic disorder are small. One social factor contributing to the development of a panic disorder is relational, for example, experiencing separation or divorce. The mean age for diagnosis of a panic disorder is 25 years of age (Sadock & Sadock, 2007). This disorder often begins in late adolescence or early adulthood (NIMH, 2011).

Phobia

Overall, phobias are the most common mental disorder in the United States with 19.2 million American adults being diagnosed with a specific phobia (NIMH, 2011). Specific phobia is considered to be more common than social phobia. In women, specific phobia is the most common mental disorder. In men the most common mental disorder is substance-related disorders with specific phobia being the second most common mental disorder (Sadock & Sadock, 2007). Despite the fact that phobias are the most common mental disorder, a significant number of persons do not seek help for their phobia(s) or are misdiagnosed upon seeking medical attention (Sadock & Sadock, 2007). In considering social phobia, 15 million American adults are diagnosed with this disorder. Men and women are equally likely to experience social phobia that usually begins in childhood or early adolescence (NIMH, 2011).

Obsessive-Compulsive Disorder

This diagnosis can occur in children, adolescents, or early adulthood. The National Institute of Mental Health (2011) estimates that more than 2% of the U.S. population or 1 in 40 individuals will experience OCD at some point during their lives. In adulthood both men and women are likely to be diagnosed with OCD. In adolescence, however, boys appear to be more frequently affected than girls. OCD has a male-to-female ratio of 1:1. The mean age of diagnosis for OCD is 20 years of age. However, this diagnosis can occur as young as 2 years of age. Individuals who are single are more frequently affected with OCD than individuals who are married. Limitations in the access to health care may be a factor as to why OCD occurs less often in blacks than whites (Sadock & Sadock, 2007).

Generalized Anxiety Disorder

Studies indicate 6.8 million American adults experience this disorder (NIMH, 2011), with twice as many men as women impacted (Sadock & Sadock, 2007). The lifetime prevalence for this diagnosis is 5%. In anxiety disorder clinics approximately 25% of the clients treated are diagnosed with generalized anxiety disorder (Sadock & Sadock, 2007).

Posttraumatic Stress Disorder

The diagnosis of posttraumatic stress disorder is estimated to occur between 2 and 9% of the population (NIMH, 2011). Approximately 30% of individuals who served in the Vietnam War experienced PTSD (Sadock & Sadock, 2007). This is of significant concern given recent events, such as the Gulf War and the extended United States conflicts in Afghanistan and Iraq. Men's and women's experiences differ in relation to the trauma to which they are exposed. The lifetime prevalence of PTSD is higher for women than men. Individuals who are diagnosed with PTSD are more likely to be single, divorced or widowed, withdrawn socially, and have low socioeconomic status. The most significant risk factor for this disorder is the duration, severity, and proximity of the trauma to the individual (Sadock & Sadock, 2007). Lifetime prevalence rate for anxiety disorder is 28.8% (Kessler et al., 2005).When considering individuals older than age 55, the best estimate prevalence rate based on ECA data for anxiety disorders was 11.4% (USSG, 2005). Prevalence of simple phobia in those older than 55 years of age was 7.3%, OCD was 1.5%, and panic disorder was 0.5% (USSG, 2005). The prevalence rates reported indicate that anxiety disorders are common in the general population, with anxiety disorders having the earliest age of onset of mental disorders (Kessler et al., 2005). Prevalence rates for anxiety disorders according to gender are between one third to two thirds higher in women. Rates of anxiety disorders in women could be due to the perception women hold regarding stressful life events (USSG, 2005). Further, the World Health Organization (WHO) identified gender-specific risk factors, which include gender-based violence (including sexual violence), subordinate social status, socioeconomic disadvantages specific to women, and responsibilities to care for others (WHO, n.d.)

SIGNS AND SYMPTOMS

It is important to consider the messages presented by society as we examine the signs and symptoms of anxiety disorders. Messages such as "Don't Worry, Be Happy" abound. It is something that individuals may subscribe to in trying to keep their symptoms "under control," so no one will recognize they are experiencing a great deal of internal turmoil and distress (Roth & Fonagy, 2004). In making a diagnosis of an anxiety disorder, presenting symptoms are the primary consideration. Many anxiety disorders may present with similar physical symptoms. In some disorders, however, the symptoms are more severe, whereas in others the symptoms are not as severe. Although all individuals may experience some degree of fear, worry, and anxiety, health care providers need to critically examine the diagnostic criteria relative to the degree of symptoms present and the duration of symptoms.

Panic Disorder

The diagnosis of panic disorder includes experiencing a panic attack. Symptoms of a panic attack include heart pounding, increased sweating, feelings of trembling or shakiness, feeling short of breath, feeling as if choking will occur, chest tightness, pain, discomfort, abdominal discomfort, distress or nausea, feeling faint, lightheaded or dizzy, feelings of unreality or depersonalization, fear of going crazy or losing control, fear of death, sensation of tingling or numbness, hot flashes, or chills. Individuals who experience at least four of these symptoms, which appear quickly and peak within 10 minutes, are said to

have experienced a panic attack. To obtain the diagnosis of panic disorder, an individual must have experienced four attacks within 4 weeks or one attack within the last month with ongoing worry or concern of when another attack will strike (SAMHSA, 2011). Panic attacks typically are short lived but can last up to 10 minutes in duration. Rarely, attacks will last up to 1 hour and can occur while sleeping.

Panic attacks are considered according to three categories: unexpected, situationally bound, and situationally predisposed Copeland, 2003). Unexpected panic attacks typically come "out of the blue" without warning and for no specific reason. Situationally bound panic attacks are just that—situational. Individuals may experience a panic attack each time they are exposed to a particular situation such as driving over a bridge, seeing a snake, or visiting the dentist's office (APA, 1994; Copeland). Predisposed panic attacks are situations in which an individual may have a panic attack, but the attacks are not consistent. An example of this would be when an individual experiences panic attacks when driving (Copeland). Individuals with panic disorder who reported childhood physical abuse were more likely to have additional comorbid Axis I diagnoses including depression and had a higher likelihood of attempting suicide (Friedman et al., 2002).

Phobia

Symptoms of a phobia include many of the physical symptoms previously presented when discussing panic disorder, including sweating, increased heart rate, and trembling (SAMHSA, 2010). Phobias are traditionally classified by the specific fear through the use of Greek or Latin prefixes. For example, acrophobia is the fear of heights, ailurophobia is the fear of cats, pyrophobia is the fear of fire, and xenophobia is the fear of strangers (Sadock & Sadock, 2007). Diagnosis of a phobia should indicate which type of phobia (animal, natural environment, blood injection, situational, other) (APA, 2000). If the person experiences extreme anxiety when faced with the feared situation or object, the individual's daily routine, social activities, and interpersonal relationships are impacted, and, because of these fears, a diagnosis may be made by a qualified and trained professional. Phobias may impact many different areas of occupation depending on the specific feared stimulus of the individual.

In social phobia, the symptoms present are similar to those for specific phobia. In addition the extreme anticipatory anxiety regarding performance or social situations negatively impacts cognition and leads to actual or perceived poor performance in the situations evoking fear, which only further perpetuates the cycle of anxiety (APA, 1994).

Obsessive-Compulsive Disorder

OCD is characterized by an individual's repetitive thoughts (obsessions) or behaviors (compulsions), or both (SAMHSA, 2010). Individuals may verbalize obsessions as recurrent thoughts, ideas, or images (which can be aggressive or violent in nature) that occupy the individual's consciousness (e.g., arm being attacked by flesh-eating bacteria, obsessing about germs). As much as the individual may try to counteract these thoughts, ideas, or images, they remain ever present. Compulsions are repetitive behaviors that are ritualistic and performed according to rules or stereotypical patterns. Excessive behavior (e.g., hand washing to counteract previously presented obsession) may temporarily relieve the tension brought about by the obsessions (John Hopkins, 2011). Common obsessions include fears of germs and contamination; fear of harm to self or others; excessive concern for orderliness; fear of making a mistake or losing a valuable item; constant thoughts of a number, sound, word, or image; or fears of social embarrassment (John Hopkins, 2011).

Symptoms presented by an individual with OCD can range from mild to severe. Some individuals may only experience obsessions and may be able to control their obsessions and associated compulsions for a short period of time, thus hiding the condition from friends, family, and coworkers. This diagnosis is characterized by symptoms that the client perceives as excessive or unreasonable. However, there is a wide range of insight that individuals have in relation to their obsessive-compulsive symptoms. Therefore, a subtype of OCD, "poor insight," has been introduced to the *DSM IV-TR* criteria for the diagnosis (Friedman et al., 2002). Clients who demonstrate poor insight tend to overestimate the likelihood of harm and are less likely to benefit from behavioral interventions but can benefit from pharmacologic interventions (Matsunaga et al., 2002).

Although a common societal misperception exists that OCD focuses exclusively on hand washing, this is only one of many potential compulsive behaviors. Common compulsive behaviors include hand washing and excessive cleanliness of the skin, checking and rechecking of appliances to assure they are turned off and of doors to assure they are locked, counting to a specified number repeatedly, repeating words or specific actions several times in a row throughout the day, arranging of items in a rigid and specific order, and hoarding and collecting items that are no longer needed such as mail or newspapers (John Hopkins, 2011).

Posttraumatic Stress Disorder

People with PTSD may relive the traumatic event over and over to the point of becoming emotionally numb. They can experience chronic anxiety, exaggerated startle response, trouble with concentration on tasks, nightmares, and insomnia. Individuals with this diagnosis may vehemently avoid situations that would remind them of the traumatic event as this will cause increased distress and could cause a panic attack (SAMHSA, 2010). Symptoms that last

<3 months are considered acute PTSD. Symptoms that last longer than 3 months are considered chronic in nature (APA, 2000). Individuals with PTSD may use alcohol or drugs to self-medicate and try to "forget" about the traumatic experience. This compounds the problems experienced in the areas of occupation for the person as not only are they dealing with the symptoms of PTSD, but they are also dealing with the negative effects of drug and alcohol use. Depression is comorbid with PTSD, and suicide risk associated with this diagnosis is one to which practitioners need to be attentive (Sadock & Sadock, 2000).

Generalized Anxiety Disorder

Symptoms of generalized anxiety disorder include chronic tension, exaggerated worry, and irritability. These symptoms that do not appear to have a cause present as more intense than a situation would warrant. Physical symptoms can include restlessness, difficulty with sleep (both falling asleep and staying asleep), increased headaches, trembling, muscle twitches, tension, and sweating. A diagnosis can be made when an individual has been worried excessively about everyday problems for >6 months (SAMHSA, 2010).

The *DSM IV-TR* diagnostic criteria are most commonly used in examining the signs and symptoms of anxiety disorders to make a diagnosis. Other psychological tests that may be used include Rorschach test, thematic apperception test, Bender-Gestalt, draw a person, the Minnesota multiphasic personality inventory II, state-trait anxiety inventory, Hamilton anxiety rating scale, and the Zung self-rated anxiety scale (Sadock & Sadock, 2001). At present there are no specific laboratory tests that can be used to diagnose anxiety.

COURSE AND PROGNOSIS

Panic Disorder

The age of onset for panic disorder is typically early to middle adulthood (Stekette & Pigott, 2003). However, onset can occur at childhood, early adolescence, or midlife (Sadock & Sadock, 2007). Panic disorder is associated with increased risk of agoraphobia and depression. One relationship factor identified as contributing to panic disorder is the history of a recent divorce or separation (Sadock & Sadock, 2007). Comorbidity of depression, substance abuse, and other anxiety disorders are associated with poor prognosis.

Considered a chronic condition, the course of panic disorder is variable across clients as well as within a single individual. Studies that have examined intervention for panic disorder are not easily interpreted because of the inability of researchers to control for the effects of treatment (Sadock & Sadock, 2007). However, 30% to 40% of individuals have presented as symptom free after long-term follow-up. One half of individuals with this diagnosis continue to have symptoms, but these symptoms are mild enough to not significantly impact their lives. Approximately 10% to 20% of individuals continue to have symptoms despite treatment (Sadock & Sadock, 2007).

It is important that clinicians use a psychometrically sound instrument such as the Panic Disorder Severity Scale to monitor clients and determine if symptoms are reoccurring to facilitate treatment modification. By responding to recurrence of symptoms, a complete relapse may be avoided (Rouillon, 1996). Full remission of all symptoms is the goal for individuals diagnosed with panic disorder, and individuals are considered to have met this standard when they no longer meet the diagnostic criteria in the *DSM IV-TR* for 6 months or longer (Rouillon).

Phobia

The most common phobia among women is a fear of animals and among men is a fear of heights (Shear & Clark, 1998). Phobias are the most common anxiety disorder. Individuals may commonly avoid the feared stimulus and may go to extreme lengths to avoid the feared stimulus (Sadock & Sadock, 2007). Depression is a comorbid condition in approximately one third of people with phobia. Animal phobia, natural environment phobia, and blood-injection phobia appear to peak at childhood. Other phobias have a peak onset at early adulthood. Phobias have been found to run in families, especially blood-injection phobia (Sadock & Sadock, 2001).

Limited data exist regarding the course of specific phobia despite being the most common anxiety disorder. Individuals frequently do not seek treatment for this condition and may live with anxiety for many years. The condition appears to remain constant and does not appear to have the waxing and waning progression that is seen in other anxiety disorders. For individuals who do seek treatment, a positive response to intervention was associated with better long-term outcomes (Curtis, Magee, Eaton, Wittchen, & Kessler, 1998). One study that examined outcomes of individuals diagnosed with phobia 10 to 16 years after treatment challenged the notion that recovery from this diagnosis is characterized by complete and lasting remission from symptoms (Curtis et al., 1998).

Social Phobia

The most misunderstood and least studied of the anxiety disorders is social phobia (Lipsitz, Mannuzza, Klein, Ross, & Fyer, 1999). The age of onset for individuals with social phobia is childhood or adolescence, and the individual may experience symptoms of the disorder for many years. Parental psychopathology, including social phobia, depression, and parenting style (overprotection or rejection), have been associated with development of social phobia in youth (Judd, 1994). This disorder is commonly associated with substance dependence, depression, avoidant personality disorder, panic disorder, and generalized anxiety disorder (Lieb et al., 2000).

Social phobia is more common in women than in men. Social phobia has onset before other psychiatric conditions (Long, 2011). Additionally, psychiatric conditions complicate approximately one third of those diagnosed with social phobia. Early intervention of social phobia may prevent the onset of other psychiatric conditions (Long). Without intervention the course of social phobia is chronic and unremitting. A significant concern relative to this disorder is the strong tendency of society, including mental health professionals, to trivialize this disorder (Lipsitz et al., 1999).

Obsessive-Compulsive Disorder

OCD is typically diagnosed in adolescence or early adulthood. Over half of the individuals with OCD experience sudden onset of symptoms. Between 50% and 70% of the symptoms occur after a stressful event such as death of a loved one, pregnancy, or sexual problems (Sadock & Sadock, 2007). If untreated, however, as the condition progresses individuals may become so consumed by obsessions and compulsions that they are unable to function in work or complete daily living activities because so much time is spent engaged in rituals (Weissman et al., 1994). Because of the desire of the individual to "hide" their condition, diagnosis and treatment are challenging. Individuals with OCD often do not receive intervention until as many as 5 to 10 years after the initial onset of symptoms (Sadock & Sadock, 2007). Between 20% and 30% of individuals can experience significant improvement in their symptoms, 40% to 50% may experience moderate improvement, and the remaining 20% to 40% may have continuation or worsening of symptoms (Sadock & Sadock, 2007). One third of individuals diagnosed with OCD also are diagnosed with depression. Suicide is a significant risk for this comorbidity (Sadock & Sadock, 2007).

OCD can be accompanied by depression, eating disorders, substance abuse, attention deficit hyperactivity disorder, and other anxiety disorders. Effective intervention for these conditions is essential for the successful treatment of OCD (NIMH, 2011). Poor prognosis is associated with the following characteristics: yielding to compulsions, childhood onset, bizarre compulsions, delusional beliefs, and comorbid personality disorder. The content of an individual's obsessions does not appear to be related to prognosis (Sadock & Sadock, 2007).

Posttraumatic Stress Disorder

The course of PTSD can be from as short as 1 week after exposure to a trauma to as much as 30 years after exposure.

Therefore, PTSD can be diagnosed at any age at which an individual experiences an extreme trauma. The male-to-female ratio for this diagnosis is 1:2 (Sadock & Sadock, 2007). Symptoms may vary with time and may be most extreme in cases of increased stress. Without treatment, 30% of individuals who would have been diagnosed with PTSD will recover, whereas 40% will continue to experience mild symptoms, 20% moderate symptoms, and 10% will remain the same or experience a worsening of symptoms (Sadock & Sadock, 2001). Of individuals diagnosed with PTSD, 50% will recover within 1 year.

Individuals who are very young and individuals who are very old have more difficulty with traumatic events than do those at midlife (Sadock & Sadock, 2007). This is associated with the fact that the young person may not have yet developed effective coping strategies to deal with the trauma and the older individual may have more rigid coping strategies that may be ineffective when presented with a traumatic experience. Individuals who experience rapid onset of symptoms of short duration, who had good premorbid functioning, and who experience positive social supports are more apt to experience a good prognosis. Furthermore, individuals who do not have a coexisting physical disability, substance-related disorder, or other medical condition are also more likely to have a good prognosis (Sadock & Sadock, 2007).

Generalized Anxiety Disorder

The age of onset for generalized anxiety disorder is variable and difficult to pinpoint. It can occur as early as childhood (Sadock & Sadock, 2007). Individuals, when questioned about their symptoms, often recall feeling anxious as long as they can remember. This condition tends to worsen without treatment and especially during times of increased stress (Fadem, 2004). One third of individuals with generalized anxiety disorder symptoms seek psychiatric intervention. More often these individuals present to family practitioners, cardiologists, internists, or gastroenterologists from whom they are seeking relief for the somatic concerns that they are experiencing as a result of this condition (Sadock & Sadock, 2007). Because of a high incidence of comorbidity of generalized anxiety disorder with other psychiatric conditions, a specific course and prognosis are difficult to identify. Generalized anxiety disorder can be viewed as a chronic condition in which the individual may experience symptoms that can be lifelong (Sadock & Sadock, 2007).

MEDICAL/SURGICAL MANAGEMENT

Society has become more aware and accepting of identification and treatment of mental illness over the last several years. This is apparent through public health initiatives targeted at addressing mental health concerns such as national mental illness awareness week, anxiety screening day, and depression screening day as well as through the increasing amount of information regarding mental illness, diagnosis, and treatment available via the Internet (Hwang, 1998; Wang, Berglund, & Kessler, 2000).

Current guidelines for treatment of severe mental illness can be found in four different categories (Richards, Klein, & Carlbring, 2003). These categories vary depending on the score and stringency for which the guidelines rely on research evidence. The categories include

- Recommendations
- Comprehensive treatment options
- Algorithms
- Expert consensus guidelines

In 1998, comprehensive treatment options were developed for panic disorder by the APA (Mellman et al., 2001). However, the strength of evidence presented in support of these treatment options is less stringent than Patient Outcomes Research Team (PORT) recommendations. PORT treatment recommendations for schizophrenia were developed by the U.S. Agency for Health Care Policy and Research. The PORT project critically examined literature, which was then followed by expert review. The PORT recommendations contain very specific evidence of efficacy of treatment interventions that supported the utilization of these interventions. The APA guidelines developed for panic disorder were by a professional organization and did not require the evidence considered for inclusion to be as stringent as the guidelines used for the development of PORT. As a result, the APA treatment guidelines are less prescriptive than the PORT treatment recommendations. Treatment guidelines have also been developed for PTSD by the International Society for Traumatic Stress Studies. These guidelines strongly endorse the use of specific serotonin reuptake inhibitors (SRIs) as a first-line medication for the treatment of PTSD (Mellman et al., 2001).

Algorithms, a single rule or set of rules, are used when solving a problem. Medication algorithms are considered within practice guidelines. Algorithms provide practitioners with a step-by-step approach to clinical decisions considering medications. At present the Texas Medication Algorithm Project has the most extensive collection of medication algorithms for persons with mental illness. Unfortunately, there are no algorithms for anxiety disorder treatment. Algorithms do exist, however, for schizophrenia, bipolar disorder, and major depressive disorder (Mellman et al., 2001).

The last category includes expert consensus guidelines. These are recommendations based upon surveys completed by a comprehensive array of experts in the treatment of identified conditions. These guidelines do not rely on critical analysis of research literature. The rationale provided for the development of these expert guidelines is related to the fact that research literature at times does not address specific points in treatment decision making. At present, expert treatment guidelines exist for panic disorder (APA, 2009), OCD, and PTSD (Foa, Davidson, & Frances, 1999; March, Frances, Kahn, & Carpenter, 1998). In addition to expert treatment guidelines for practitioners, guidelines have been developed for patients and families regarding these diagnoses (March et al., 1998).

People with anxiety disorders are three to five times more likely to seek the care of a physician and six times more likely to be hospitalized for a psychiatric disorder (Copeland, 2003). From an occupational therapy perspective their functional abilities would be assessed, and it would be determined how their anxiety was impacting activities of daily living, IADLs, sleep/rest, education, work, play, leisure, and social participation (American Occupational Therapy Association [AOTA], 2008). The occupational therapist may consider administering an activity configuration, role checklist, interest checklist, or self-assessment of occupational functioning to determine functional deficits (Reed, 2001).

The most common treatments for anxiety disorders include a combination of pharmacologic and psychological interventions with the exception of specific phobia for which there is no good pharmacologic treatment (Fadem, 2004). Remission is the ultimate goal for the treatment of anxiety disorders (Kjernistad & Bleau, 2004). Occupational therapy intervention is targeted at changing performance deficits in areas of occupation as a result of the symptoms experienced by the person (Reed, 2001). Occupational therapy intervention may also examine activity demands and modifications that could be made to the activity or environment to assist the individual in independence in areas of occupation (AOTA, 2008). Individuals with anxiety disorders may experience dysfunction in performance skills: emotional regulation, cognitive skills, and communication and social skills (AOTA, 2008). Although some individuals may continue to experience symptoms of anxiety throughout their lives, occupational therapy intervention can be focused toward the development or reestablishment of meaningful daily routines. Engagement in meaningful occupation can serve to facilitate adaptation, which can lead to improved health and wellness, quality of life, and positive life satisfaction. It is important to remain client centered as interventions that may reduce anxiety in one individual may prove ineffective for another.

Medications utilized to treat anxiety disorders include anxiolytics and antidepressants, specifically SRIs (Sadock & Sadock, 2007). One should be cautious when working with clients who are on benzodiazepines who have addiction concerns as these medications are highly addictive. Further, older adults are at risk of falls when on benzodiazepines because of side effects impacting balance as a result of the half-life of the medication. Side effects of benzodiazepines include sedation and fatigue, cognitive and memory impairments, delayed reaction time, impaired balance and coordination, hangover effects, withdrawal, and abuse potential.

For individuals diagnosed with panic disorder, antidepressant medications such as paroxetine hydrochloride (Paxil), which is a selective SRI, or benzodiazepines such as alprazolam (Xanax) are approved by the Food and Drug Administration and are often prescribed (Fadem, 2004; Sadock & Sadock, 2007). Paxil has been shown to be effective with individuals diagnosed with social phobia. Benzodiazepines may be used for social phobia on a very short-term basis. For the pharmacologic treatment of OCD, antidepressant medications such as fluvoxamine maleate (Luvox) and clomipramine hydrochloride (Anafranil) have been shown to be effective interventions (Fadem, 2004). Caution should be exercised when pharmacologic interventions are considered with individuals diagnosed with PTSD as substance abuse disorder can complicate the pharmacologic choices (Read, Brown, & Kahler, 2004). Antidepressants such as sertraline hydrochloride (Zoloft), anticonvulsants such as carbamazepine (Tegretol), and antipsychotic medications such as olanzapine (Zyprexa) are considered for individuals with PTSD (Fadem, 2004). With the use of consistent and ongoing antidepressant therapy, the remission rate of anxiety disorders is improved. However, response to medications is very individualized, and many clients may need extended time in treatment before a benefit is obtained (Kjernisted & Bleau, 2004).

Some research has indicated cognitive behavioral interventions are superior to pharmacologic approaches whereas other research indicates the contrary (Sadock & Sadock, 2007). In considering cognitive behavioral interventions for anxiety disorders, a variety of interventions exist. Findings from one study indicated when treating individuals with panic disorder, progress can be obtained through the use of a self-help workbook and brief therapist contact (Hecker, Losee, Robertson-Nay, & Maki, 2004). An emphasis on family and client psychoeducation, focusing on symptomatology, nature and course of panic disorder, and lifestyle modifications have been suggested as evidence-based interventions that cost less (in Australia) than the cost of drug therapy over a 1-year period of time (Andrews, Oakley-Browne, & Castle, 2003). The efficacy of cognitive behavioral therapy (CBT) has been examined through evidence-based research. It is important to note that CBT interventions are often coupled with pharmacotherapy; however, within individuals diagnosed with panic disorder, use of medications may interfere with CBT intervention approach (Shearer, 2007).

The APA's comprehensive treatment guidelines for panic disorder indicate most individuals can be treated on an outpatient basis and may rarely require hospitalization (APA, 2009). Cognitive behavioral interventions suggested by the APA include the use of psychoeducation, panic monitoring, breathing monitoring, anxiety management skill development, cognitive restructuring, and in vivo exposure. Establishing and maintaining a therapeutic alliance with the individual diagnosed with panic disorder is viewed as a key element in successful intervention as well as educating the individual on the early signs of relapse.

Panic Disorder

From an occupational therapy perspective, individuals with panic disorder may need assistance in the area of IADLs. People may be fearful of leaving the house and therefore community mobility may be impaired. Systematic desensitization can be useful, but very stressful for individuals in addressing this fear (Andrews et al., 2003). Relaxation training including deep breathing, progressive muscle relaxation, visualization, and autogenic training are effective interventions utilized by occupational therapy practitioners for individuals with panic disorder and phobias (Bonder, 2010). Although relaxation therapies such as visualization, deep breathing, meditation, and progressive muscle relaxation have been shown to decrease anxiety, there is limited research (Conrad & Roth, 2007).

Phobia

When considering other available interventions for phobia, 70% to 85% of individuals responded with clinically significant improvement when exposure was used as a behavioral intervention. The addition of cognitive components appeared to add little efficacy (Roth & Fonagy, 2004). Therapist-directed exposure was suggested rather than self-directed exposure to the feared stimulus. Although some studies have used virtual reality techniques as intervention for the treatment of phobias, this may be cost prohibitive and technically challenging but could provide a clinic with the ability to expose the client to a wide range of feared stimuli (North, North, & Coble, 1998).

Social Phobia

When considering evidence-based intervention for social phobia, five cognitive behavioral treatments including exposure therapy, cognitive restructuring, exposure coupled with cognitive restructuring, social skills training, and relaxation were compared and found to be moderately effective with no differences obtained at the end of the study or at the follow-up (Federoff & Taylor, 2001). Further, both individual and group interventions were found to be equally beneficial to individuals with this diagnosis. Some obstacles to effective treatment for social phobias are as follows:

- The individual's avoidance of treatment because of fear, shame, or stigma.

- Limited screening to assess social phobia is available at present.
- Assessment and intervention may be directed toward somatic complaints expressed by the individual rather than the social phobia syndrome.
- Physicians lack knowledge of effective treatment options or they trivialize the client's concerns or view them as unchangeable (Bruce & Saeed, 1999).

Despite these facts, cognitive behavior therapy is useful when treating social phobia (NIMH, 2011). Both cognitive therapy and exposure therapy present good efficacy, and the combination presents the largest effect sizes in meta-analytic reviews (Taylor, 1996). There is limited research on the efficacy of social skills training with social phobia.

Obsessive-Compulsive Disorder

Expert treatment guidelines exist for the treatment of OCD (March et al., 1998). These guidelines address specific cognitive behavioral strategies, medications, maintenance of treatment, treatment of comorbidities, and minimizing medication side effects. Guidelines for families and patients have also been developed. Treatment for OCD commonly combines medication and behavioral intervention to achieve effectiveness.

Exposure and response prevention has been identified as the most useful intervention in treating this condition. In this approach the individual is deliberately and voluntarily exposed to what triggers his or her obsessive thoughts. The individual is then taught techniques to avoid performing the compulsive behaviors and how to cope with the associated anxiety (NIMH, 2011). Although exposure and response prevention has been shown to be effective, it is important to note it may facilitate a reduction in symptoms, rather than a removal of symptoms. Some individuals continue to display ongoing distress even after intervention (Roth & Fonagy, 2004).

Posttraumatic Stress Disorder

Medications are used with caution in individuals with PTSD because of the concern of self-medication and the potential for substance abuse. Specific SRIs are suggested for individuals with this diagnosis (Fadem, 2004; Mellman et al., 2001). Expert consensus guidelines exist for the treatment of PTSD. These guidelines provide insight into recommended treatment interventions based on the most prominent symptoms present. For example, if an individual experiences intrusive thoughts, exposure therapy is suggested. If irritability and/or angry outbursts are present, cognitive therapy and anxiety management are suggested. Anxiety management training as specified in the guidelines includes relaxation training, breathing retraining, positive thinking and self-talk, assertiveness training, and thought stopping (Foa et al., 1999).

Cognitive therapy focusing on assisting people in modifying their unrealistic assumptions, beliefs, and automatic thoughts can be implemented by trained professionals. Exposure therapy, play therapy, and psychoeducation are examples of effective intervention for individuals with PTSD. Group therapy in which the individual can talk with others who have had similar experiences has been found to be effective intervention. Opportunities to express emotion are valuable. Activities including drawing emotions and experiences can be viewed by the individual as both relaxing and cathartic (Bonder, 2010). Journaling has been found to assist the individual in gaining insight, understanding, and acceptance of the occurrence (Pennebaker & Chung, 2007; Ullrich & Lutgendorf, 2002). Individuals may need assistance in reestablishing social relationships, work, and leisure participation.

Limited research has been completed examining the link between sensory defensiveness in adults and increased anxiety (Kinnealey & Fuiek, 1999). It is hypothesized that many symptoms of sensory defensiveness may be interchangeable with psychiatric disorders including generalized anxiety disorder. Research has explored the use of sensory integration interventions for decreasing anxiety levels by using deep pressure, tactile, and proprioceptive activities (Kinnealey, Oliver, & Wilbarger, 1995).

Generalized Anxiety Disorder

Generalized anxiety disorder can be addressed using cognitive therapy focusing on education and lifestyle alterations focusing on how the external environmental influences internal feelings. Addressing diet (caffeine intake), medication use (over-the-counter medications may increase anxiety), and the need for regular exercise can also be helpful in addressing generalized anxiety disorder (Kjernisted & Bleau, 2004). Rational/cognitive approaches that focus on assisting the person in replacing negative self-statements with more positive ones can be effective with individuals diagnosed with generalized anxiety disorder. Time management activities that assist the individual in prioritizing activities may assist in decreasing anxiety as well. Expressive activities such as journal writing, drawing, or other craft activities can provide a mechanism for the individual to communicate his or her feelings and may assist in the development of coping skills (Reed, 2001).

Clinicians should be mindful regarding the length of intervention provided to individuals with anxiety disorders. Outpatient sessions between 6 and 7 weeks were deemed too short by clients in two different studies (Prior, 1998; Rosier, Williams, & Ryrie, 1998). Structured course content should include opportunities for skill development, communication, and practice with ongoing monitoring by the clinician. Cognitive aspects of intervention such as relaxation training and assertiveness were found to be most beneficial per client report. An 8-week course was felt to allow more time for learning and practice of the cognitive aspects of the course deemed most important by those diagnosed with anxiety disorders (Rosier, Williams, Ryrie, 1998).

IMPACT OF CONDITIONS ON OCCUPATIONAL PERFORMANCE

The impact of anxiety disorders on client factors is dependent on the specific disorder with which the client is diagnosed. In the area of mental functions, specifically global mental functions, sleep, temperament, and energy can be impacted by the diagnosis of an anxiety disorder. In the area of specific mental functions, the following areas are impacted:

- Attention
- Reduced recall (memory)
- Impaired ability to make associations
- Time management
- Problem solving
- Decision making
- Emotional functions in the area of self-control (Sadock & Sadock, 2007)

From a sensory perspective, individuals with an anxiety disorder may demonstrate increased startle response. Physical signs present in anxiety disorder from a neuromuscular and movement-related perspective include feeling shaky, muscle tension, backache, headache, and fatigue. From a cardiovascular and respiratory perspective, symptoms include tachycardia and hyperventilation, which can lead to syncope (passing out). From a gastrointestinal perspective, clients may experience signs of diarrhea and have the feeling of an upset stomach or "butterflies" in the stomach. When considering the genitourinary system and reproductive functions, clients may experience urinary frequency and decreased libido, which could relate to reproduction or lack of desire for sexual relationships (APA, 2000; Fadem, 2004; Sadock & Sadock, 2007).

Panic Disorder

The symptoms an individual may experience during a panic attack can have a negative impact upon the many different areas of occupation, including care of others, care of pets, child rearing, community mobility, safety and emergency maintenance, shopping, sleep/rest, formal educational participation, job performance, and leisure and social participation (AOTA, 2008). A common concern of individuals who experience panic disorder is anticipation of *when* the next attack will occur. This fear can significantly alter daily roles, habits, routines, and rituals. This can have a negative impact upon their ability to initiate performance in daily activities. The individual who experiences a panic disorder and has children may worry about the well-being of his or her children. He or she may feel as if he or she is dying while having an attack. Those experiencing symptoms of panic disorder may begin restricting themselves to their residence for fear of having a panic attack while in public, and this behavior can facilitate agoraphobia.

Phobia

Social phobia impacts the areas of educational participation, such as having to get up in front of class and give a presentation. Job performance, as well as other social roles and responsibilities, may be impaired (Fischler & Booth, 1999). Communication skills may be negatively affected because of the individual's significant level of anxiety. Individuals with social phobia may experience low self esteem due to their inability to perform up to self-imposed standards, yet they frequently do not seek assistance for their concerns. Individuals with this disorder may be characterized by others as "nervous" or "ineffective" in social situations.

To increase the potential for individuals with social phobia to experience success, the occupational therapist should work toward establishing environmental control to reduce anxiety regarding the unknown. Individuals may benefit from working alone initially to reduce self-consciousness and at their own pace. Positive feedback for effective performance is essential. Working with individuals diagnosed with social phobia to self-disclose diagnosis to supportive individuals may assist in reducing self-consciousness and embarrassment when symptoms arise (Fischer & Booth, 1999).

Obsessive-Compulsive Disorder

Areas of occupation impacted by OCD can include activities of daily living, IADLs, sleep/rest, education, work, play, leisure, and social participation. OCD has a negative impact upon the individual's cognitive skills and emotional regulation skills. Motor and praxis skills are not typically affected (Thomsen, 2000). The obsessive and compulsive rituals engaged in by the individual can occur indirectly in any of these areas or can indirectly negatively affect another area. For example, a client who obsesses about turning off all the lights in the house prior to leaving for work may be frequently late to work, which

will most likely have a negative impact on his or her work performance. The obsession and compulsion are related to home management but may negatively impact job performance because of the poor work habit of arriving late. Strategies for occupational success include predictable and consistent expectations, setting a work pace, the option of working alone if working with others is distracting, and ongoing positive feedback for performance that is well done (Fischler & Booth, 1999). Occupational therapy interventions can assist the individual with OCD to develop improved coping skills and to explore issues related to the obsessive thoughts and compulsive actions. Performance patterns are seriously impacted in individuals diagnosed with OCD. Occupational therapy interventions can work to facilitate change in this area (Thomsen, 2000). Client motivation is a significant factor in the success of behavioral interventions for OCD (Prior, 1998).

Posttraumatic Stress Disorder

PTSD can impact activities of daily living to the point where the person does not care about his or her personal hygiene and grooming. Sleep/rest is of significant concern as the person may experience nightmares and flashbacks. IADLs can be negatively impacted in the areas of care of others, care of pets, child rearing, financial management (especially if alcohol and drug use/abuse are present), health management/maintenance, home establishment and management, meal preparation and cleanup, religious observance, safety and emergency maintenance, and shopping (AOTA, 2008). Further, formal educational participation, job performance, leisure performance, and all aspects of social participation are impacted by this diagnosis. Roles, routines, rituals, and habits can be negatively impacted through flashbacks and reexperiencing the trauma. Cognitive skills and emotional regulation skills are negatively impacted because of intrusive thoughts experienced by the individual (Levitt, 2005). Family and friends may notice these problems and try to provide assistance. Denial, however, is common and the person may refuse assistance or treatment.

Generalized Anxiety Disorder

Any area of occupation can be impacted by generalized anxiety disorder. The individual may express excessive worry about himself or herself and his or her own health and well-being (IADLs) or his or her educational participation, job performance, as well as social participation. This anxiety disorder is one that many people express as similar to the gray cloud of worry that follows them everywhere and as such impacts every area of occupation.

Case Illustrations

Generalized Anxiety Disorder

April is a 44-year-old registered nurse. She has worked in nursing for 20 years on a hospital pediatrics unit. For the last 7 months, for more days than not, April finds it difficult to control her level of anxiety and worry. She is worried about getting along with coworkers, pleasing the physicians with whom she works, and interacting appropriately with the parents of the children for whom she is providing care. Additionally, April has been worrying about her children's school performance and the fact that many companies in her community are downsizing. Although her husband has frequently reassured her that his position is stable, she cannot help but worry that he will lose his job or be demoted. With the economy being on a downhill slide, this serves to increase April's fears regarding employment and finances.

April also worries about her difficulty attending to her tasks as a nurse. She finds her mind going blank, and she has difficulty concentrating on what a physician is saying to her while she is doing rounds. Three times during the last month she has recorded physician's orders incorrectly. The unit secretary has caught these errors and brought them to April's attention. April is demonstrating difficulty responding in an appropriate fashion to safety concerns, which are typically presented in her workplace such as "Code Blue." She feels others know of her problems. She is concerned about her relationships with her coworkers since she is so preoccupied by her anxiety and she finds herself irritable at work and has "snapped" at a several coworkers over the last few months.

April has been having extreme difficulty falling and staying asleep. She has been awakening 2 to 3 hours early and is not able to fall back to sleep. As a result she feels fatigued and has been experiencing increased muscle tension, backaches, and frequent headaches. April describes her ongoing *keyed-up* feelings of restlessness like "walking on eggshells." April expresses frustration in her lack of ability to relax and inability to decrease her anxiety. April expresses little appetite and has experienced noticeable weight loss over the last 7 months.

At home, April has not been preparing meals for her family as she had in the past, rather has been relying solely on frozen dinners and takeout food for family dining. April *picks up* the house but does not clean per se. She used to keep her house immaculate, but for the past several months she has verbalized feelings of fatigue and lack of desire to keep things clean in her home. Although she expresses numerous interests including scrapbooking, cooking, reading, and walking, she has not been able to participate in these leisure activities because of her anxiety level and accompanying fatigue. April had previously been active as a volunteer at her church and involved in activities of her son's football league, but at this time she feels so overwhelmed that she is unable to complete these tasks. She has been caring for her children marginally. She has experienced difficulty helping them with their school work and has been distant or short with them in her communication.

April's husband and friends too have noticed a change in April's behavior. Although they have been supportive of and encouraging April, they do not know what to do or how to assist her in diminishing her level of worry. April agrees to go on family outings in the community with her husband and children, but at the last minute, she backs out. When asked why, she provides little to no explanation for the last minute change of plans. Infrequently she will speak to friends on the phone but has not gone to social activities with her friends in months.

Financially, April and her family have money in their savings, live comfortably, and have been saving for their children's college education and their retirement. Despite these facts, April spends between 4 and 6 hours each weekend reviewing the financial status of the family and constantly worrying about expenses that are considered by many others to be routine expenditures.

April has seen a psychiatrist who has prescribed medication and supportive psychotherapy 1 week ago. Despite April's complaints of fatigue, the psychiatrist encouraged her to try to walk one to two times per week as physical exercise is beneficial to those with generalized anxiety disorder. Additionally, deep breathing exercises were reviewed in attempts to decrease her level of anxiety. April plans to continue to pursue therapy on an outpatient basis with a psychologist and occupational therapist for relaxation training and to critically examine life stressors and develop effective coping mechanisms to deal with her current level of anxiety.

Obsessive-Compulsive Disorder

Lisa is a 28-year-old female who ruminates about the potential for her car and other valuable items in her possession to catch fire. In preparing to leave to go anywhere she repeatedly walks around the car and opens and closes the hood several times before getting in the car. Once she starts the car, she allows the car to idle for a few minutes but then turns off the car, walks around the car, and then again opens the hood. She repeats this routine at least three times before she is able to drive anywhere. It is not uncommon for Lisa to pull off the road and repeatedly turn her car off and on and open the hood to make sure the car is not on fire. Lisa is constantly late to work and social engagements because of her obsessive and compulsive routine regarding transportation. Lisa vehemently refuses to ride with others because they will not stop when she wants to stop to allow her to get out and check their car for signs of fire. Recently the police followed Lisa and pulled her over for her erratic behavior in driving and her frequent stops on the side of the road to check her car for signs of fire.

In her home, Lisa is constantly plugging and unplugging electrical appliances because she is fearful that if she leaves them plugged in, her home will catch fire. Lisa lives alone in a single-family home. Her family is unaware of her behavior as she is estranged from her parents and is an only child. Lisa frequently stares at light bulbs to make sure that the light is off despite the fact that she had turned off the light switch. This delays Lisa's ability to leave her home in a timely fashion.

As a result of being home a great deal of time, Lisa has become a compulsive shopper using television shopping channels for leisure and entertainment. She has numerous items that she has ordered and not taken out of the boxes that are piled in the corner of her living room. Lisa is also experiencing difficulties in the area of financial management because of her compulsive shopping behaviors and her inconsistent employment status. She has recently begun a new job as a customer service representative for a telemarketing company. She has been recently reprimanded several times for spending excessive time speaking with older adult customers who call in to the center.

Lisa does not eat healthy meals and does not like to leave her house to purchase food. As a result she is gaining weight, and her blood pressure is elevated. In the area of self-care, Lisa is meticulous about her personal appearance spending great lengths of time to make sure her hair, makeup, nails, and clothing are coordinated and appropriate for the event.

After 7 years of college, Lisa graduated with a bachelor of arts degree in English from a private college. She has never been able to secure the type of employment she desires, which would be creative writing. It took Lisa longer to graduate as she would frequently drop classes midsemester if she did not attain the grade that she felt she should have been receiving from the course instructor. Lisa has held seven jobs since she graduated from college 2 years ago. She is often fired for absenteeism, tardiness, or decreased productivity on the job because of her obsessive-compulsive behavior at work.

Socially, Lisa does not participate in community activities, is estranged from her family, and relies on her coworkers as friends. As a result of her frequent job changes she has a limited number of friends. Lisa has alienated herself from college friends and roommates who have tried to provide caring feedback about her behavior.

Post-traumatic stress disorder

Richard is a 35-year-old male who served in the war in Iraq. He is a member of the U.S. Marine Corps Reserve and was responsible for delivering equipment and supplies along various routes in Iraq. During his 18 months in Iraq, he was in several convoys that were shot at by insurgents. On one occasion, despite orders to not leave his vehicle, Richard ran to a vehicle in need of emergency assistance. Upon arrival at the vehicle that was engulfed in flames, Richard removed two of the four passengers who were already deceased as a result of an insurgent attack. After this event, Richard began having flashbacks, seeing the faces of his dead comrades in his dreams. Each time Richard would leave his base for a delivery of supplies after the event, he would be hypervigilant because of his fears of his convoy being attacked. While in Iraq, he reported auditory flashbacks of the attack on his convoy in which he tried to rescue his fellow soldiers. As a result of this experience, Richard reported decreased ability to sleep while in Iraq, and now that he is home he continues to demonstrate an inability to obtain a restful night's sleep. This is an ongoing complaint as he is extremely tired, and this makes him feel irritable and overwhelmed when faced with daily tasks. After this incident, Richard was noticed to be isolated from the other members of his unit. His superior noticed this behavior and attempted to get assistance for Richard, but he vehemently refused. Upon arrival in the United States, Richard's family and friends hosted numerous celebrations for him. Prior to his tour of duty in Iraq, Richard was a social, friendly, and outgoing individual. Since his return, he does not like to have attention drawn to himself, and his family is concerned about his "loner" behavior as he has been isolative since his return from Iraq. Richard has not been participating in community activities at this time. Prior to going to Iraq, Richard was active in his church and was a member of the Lion's club. However, at present, he rarely goes out with "the gang from work," an activity in which he participated regularly prior to going to Iraq. When friends call and ask him to participate in social activities, he states he will but then fails to follow though and attend these events.

In the area of work, upon his return to civilian life, Richard has returned to his position as an electrician. Richard has been home nearly 2 months. The attack he continues to reexperience occurred 4 months ago. He has experienced difficulty on the job in the areas of concentration, exaggerated startle response, and irritability with his coworkers. Richard has been calling in sick as a result of his excessive drinking behavior, has been showing up for work late, and has gotten into arguments with supervisors and coworkers who have expressed concerns about his behavior. Richard has not been completing tasks as assigned, rather he is verbalizing "he knows a better way" to do things. Richard has experienced difficulties in the area of safety and emergency maintenance response during the fulfillment of his duties as an electrician.

Richard is single and lives on his own. Prior to leaving for Iraq, he was in a relationship with Amber; however, he ended the relationship prior to his departure to Iraq. Amber maintained contact with Richard via email, Facebook, and Skype while he was in Iraq and came to his welcome-home event. She has made attempts to reach out to him, to engage him socially with their group of friends, but he does not return her phone calls and at times will agree to participate in social activities only to show up late and leave early. He refuses to accompany Amber, to attend a social gathering; rather he will drive himself. His parents and siblings reside in the same community. Richard has expressed his difficulty with sleep to his mother who is a nurse. He states he has difficulty falling asleep and often wakes up with vivid dreams of the attack on his convoy in which his comrades were killed. Richard has been lifting weights by himself at home. If he does participate in leisure activities, he often does so alone and has a couple of beers while playing darts at a local tavern. After the attack, Richard was noted to be using alcohol on an increased basis to cope with the stressful event he experienced.

RECOMMENDED LEARNING RESOURCES

Bourne, E. J. (2011). *The Anxiety and phobia workbook* (5th ed.). Oakland, CA: New Harbinger Publications.

Hyman, B. M., & Pedrick, C. (2010). *The OCD workbook: Your guide to breaking free from obsessive-compulsive disorder* (3rd ed.). Oakland, CA: New Harbinger Publications.

Kase, L., Antony, M. M., & Vitale, J. (2006). *Anxious 9 to 5: How to beat worry, stop second guessing yourself and work with confidence.* Oakland, CA: New Harbinger Publications.

Neziroglu, F., Bubrick, J., Yaryura-Tobias, J. A., & Perkins, P. B. (2004). *Overcoming compulsive hoarding: Why you can save and how you can stop.* Oakland, CA: New Harbinger Publications.

Reinecke, M. A. (2010). *Little ways to keep calm and carry on: Twenty lessons for managing worry, anxiety and fear.* Oakland, CA: New Harbinger Publications.

Anxiety Disorders Association of America. http://www.adaa.org/

Expert Consensus Guidelines Treatment of Obsessive-Compulsive Disorder. http://www.psychguides.com/ocd

Expert Consensus Guidelines Treatment of Obsessive-Compulsive Disorder for Patients and Families. http://www.psychguides.com/content/obsessive-compulsive-disorder-guide-patients-and-families

Expert Consensus Guidelines Treatment of Post-traumatic Stress Disorder. www.psychguides.com/ptsd

Expert Consensus Guidelines Treatment of Posttraumatic Stress Disorder for Patients and Families. http://www.psychguides.com/sites/psychguides.com/files/docs/ptsdhe.pdf

International OCD Foundation. http://www.ocfoundation.org/

International Society for Traumatic Stress Studies. http://www.istss.org/Home.htm

National Center for PTSD. http://www.ptsd.va.gov/public/pages/PTSDcoach.asp

T2 Virtual PTSD Experience. http://www.t2health.org/vwproj/

REFERENCES

American Occupational Therapy Association (AOTA). (2008). *Occupational therapy practice framework: Domain & process* (2nd ed.). Bethesda, MD: Author.

American Psychiatric Association. (1994). *Diagnostic and statistical manual of mental disorders* (4th ed.). Washington, DC: Author.

American Psychiatric Association. (2000). *Diagnostic and statistical manual of mental disorders IV* (4th ed., text revision). Washington, DC: Author.

American Psychiatric Association. (2009). *Practice guideline for treatment of patients with panic disorder* (2nd ed.). Washington, DC: Author.

Andrews, G., Oakley-Browne, M., & Castle, D. (2003). Summary of guidelines for the treatment of panic disorder and agoraphobia. *Australasia Psychiatry, 11*, 29–33.

Bonder, B. (2010). *Psychopathology and function* (4th ed.). Thorofare, NJ: Slack Inc.

Brantley, J. (2007). *Calming your anxious mind* (2nd ed.). Oakland, CA: New Harbinger Publications.

Brown, T. A., Campbell, L. A., Lehman, C. L., Grisham, J. R., & Mancil, R. B. (2001). Current and lifetime comorbidity of the *DSM-IV* anxiety and mood disorders in large clinical sample. *Journal of Abnormal Psychology, 110*, 585–599.

Bruce, T., & Saeed, A. (1999). Social anxiety disorder: A common underrecognized mental disorder. *American Family Physician, 60*, 2311–2320.

Conrad, A., & Roth, W. T. (2007). Muscle relaxation therapy for anxiety disorders: It works but how? *Journal of Anxiety Disorders, 21*(3), 243–264.

Copeland, M. E. (2003). *The worry control workbook.* Dummerston, VT: Peach Press.

Curtis, G. C., Magee, W. J., Eaton, W. W., Wittchen, H. U., & Kessler, R. C. (1998). Specific fears and phobias. Epidemiology and classification. *British Journal of Psychiatry, 173*, 212–217.

Dirckx, J. H. (2001). *Stedman's Concise Medical Dictionary for the Health Professional.* Philadelphia, PA: Lippincott Williams & Wilkins.

DuPont, R. L., Rice, D. P., Miller, L. S., Shiraki, S. S., Rowland, C. R., & Harwood, H. J. (1996). Economic costs of anxiety. *Anxiety, 2*, 167–172.

Fadem, B. (2004). *Behavioral science in medicine.* Philadelphia, PA: Lippincott Williams & Wilkins.

Federoff, I. C., & Taylor, S. (2001). Psychological and pharmacological treatments of social phobia: A meta-analysis. *Journal of Clinical Psychopharmacology, 21*, 311–324.

Fischler, G. L., & Booth, N. (1999). *Vocational impact of psychiatric disorders: A guide for rehabilitation professionals.* Gaithersburg, MD: Aspen Publication.

Friedman, S., Smith, L., Fogel, D., Paradis, C., Viswanathan, R., Ackerman, R., & Trappler, B. (2002). The incidence and influence of early traumatic life events in patients with panic disorder: A comparison with other psychiatric outpatients. *Journal of Anxiety Disorders, 16*(3), 259–272.

Foa, E. B., Davidson, J. R., & Frances, A. (1999). The expert consensus guideline series: Treatment of post-traumatic stress disorder. *Journal of Clinical Psychiatry, 60*(16 Suppl), 1–69.

Hecker, J. E., Losee, M. C., Roberson-Nay, R., & Maki, K. (2004). Mastery of your anxiety and panic and brief therapist contact in the treatment of panic disorder. *Journal of Anxiety Disorders, 18*, 111–126.

Grey House Publishing. (2004). *The Complete Mental Health Directory.* New York: Sedgwick Press.

Hwang, M. Y. (1998). I can't stop myself: The devastation of obsessive-compulsive disorder. *Journal of the American Medical Association, 280*, 1806.

John Hopkins. (2011). *Conditions we treat: Anxiety disorders.* Retrieved from: http://www.hopkinsmedicine.org/psychiatry/specialty_areas/anxiety/conditions.html

Judd, L. L. (1994). Social phobia: A clinical overview. *Journal of Clinical Psychiatry, 55*(Suppl), 5–9.

Karno, M., Golding J. M., & Sorenson, S. B. (1998). The epidemiology of obsessive-compulsive disorder in five US communities. *Archives of General Psychiatry, 45*, 1094–1099.

Kessler, R. C., Berglund, P., Demler, O., Jin, R., Merikangas, K. R., & Walters, E. E. (2005). Lifetime prevalence and age-of-onset distributions of *DSM-IV* disorders in the National Comorbidity Survey Replication. *Archives of General Psychiatry, 62*(6), 593–602.

Kessler, R. C., Chiu, W. T., Demler, O., & Walters, E. E. (2005). Prevalence, severity, and comorbidity of twelve-month *DSM-IV* disorders in the National Comorbidity Survey Replication (NCS-R). *Archives of General Psychiatry, 62*(6), 617–627.

Kessler, R. C., Sonnega, A., Bromet, E., & Hughes, M. (1995). Posttraumatic stress disorder in the national comorbidity survey. *Archives of General Psychiatry, 52*, 1048–1060.

Kinnealey, M., & Fuiek, M. (1999). The relationship between sensory defensiveness, anxiety, depression and pain in adults. *Occupational Therapy International, 6*, 195–206.

Kinnealey, M., Oliver, B., & Wilbarger, P. (1995). A phenomenological study of sensory defensiveness in adults. *American Journal of Occupational Therapy, 49*, 444–451.

Kjernisted, K. D., & Bleau, P. (2004). Long term goals in the management of acute and chronic anxiety disorders. *Canadian Journal of Psychiatry, 49*(Suppl 1), 51S–63S.

Lepine, J. P. (2002). The epidemiology of anxiety disorders: Prevalence and societal costs. *Journal of Clinical Psychiatry, 63*(Suppl 14), 4–8.

Levitt, V. B. (2005). Anxiety disorders. In E. Cara & A. MacRae (Eds.). *Psychosocial occupational therapy: A clinical practice* (2nd ed). New York: Delmar Learning.

Lieb, R., Wittchen, H. U., Höfler, M., Fuetsch, M., Stein, M. B., & Merikangas, K. R. (2000). Parental psychopathology, parenting styles, and the risk of social phobia in offspring: A prospective-longitudinal community study. *Archives of General Psychiatry, 57,* 859–866.

Lipsitz, J. D., Mannuzza, S., Klein, D. F., Ross, D. C., & Fyer, A. J. (1999). Specific phobia 10–16 years after treatment. *Depression & Anxiety, 10,* 105–111.

Long, P. W. (2011). *Anxiety disorders.* Retrieved from: http://www.mentalhealth.com/

March, J. S., Frances, A., Kahn, D. A., & Carpenter, D. (1998). *Expert consensus guidelines: Treatment of OCD.* Retrieved from: http://www.psychguides.com/content/treatment-obsessive-compulsive-disorder

Matsunaga, H., Kiriike, N., Matsui, T., Oya, K., Iwasaki, Y., Koshimune, K., et al. (2002). Obsessive-compulsive disorder with poor insight. *Comprehensive Psychiatry, 43,* 150–157.

Mellman, T. A., Miller, A. L., Weissman, E. M., Crismon, M. L., Essock, S. M., & Marder, S. R. (2001). Evidence-based pharmacologic treatment for people with severe mental illness: A focus on guidelines and algorithms. *Psychiatric Services, 52,* 619–625.

National Institute of Mental Health (NIMH). (2011). *Anxiety disorders.* Retrieved from: http://www.nimh.nih.gov/health/topics/anxiety-disorders/index.shtml

North, M. M., North, S. M., & Coble, J. R. (1998). Virtual reality therapy: An effective treatment for psychological disorders. *Virtual reality in neuro-psycho-physiology.* Amsterdam, the Netherlands: IOS Press.

Pennebaker, J. W., & Chung, C. K. (2007). Expressive writing, emotional upheavals and health. In H. S. Friedman & R. C. Silver (Eds.). *Foundations of health psychology* (pp. 263–284). New York: Oxford University Press.

Prior, S. (1998). Determining the effectiveness of short term anxiety management course. *British Journal of Occupational Therapy, 61,* 207–212.

Read, J., Brown, P., & Kahler, C. (2004). Substance use and posttraumatic stress disorders: Symptom interplay and effects on outcome. *Addictive Behaviors.* 29:1665–1672.

Reed, K. L. (2001). *Quick reference to occupational therapy* (2nd ed.). Frederick, MD: Aspen Publishers.

Rettew, D. C. (2000). Avoidant personality disorder, generalized social phobia, and shyness: Putting the personality back into personality disorders. *Harvard Review of Psychiatry, 8,* 283–297.

Richards, J., Klein, B., & Carlbring, P. (2003). Internet based treatment for panic disorder. *Cognitive Behavioral Therapy, 32,* 125–135.

Rosier, C., Williams, H., & Ryrie, I. (1998). Anxiety management groups in a community mental health team. *British Journal of Occupational Therapy, 61,* 203–206.

Roth, A., & Fonagy, P. (2004). *What works for whom: A critical review of psychotherapy research* (2nd ed.). New York: Guilford Press.

Rouillon, F. (1996). Epidemiology of panic disorder. *Encephale, 5,* 25–34.

Sadock, B. J., & Sadock, V. (2007). *Kaplan & Sadock's synopsis of psychiatry: Behavioral science & clinical psychiatry* (10th ed.). Philadelphia, PA: Lippincott Williams & Wilkins.

Sadock, B. J., & Sadock, V. A. (2001). *Kaplan & Sadock's pocket handbook of clinical psychiatry* (3rd ed.). Philadelphia, PA: Lippincott Williams & Wilkins.

Shear, M. K., & Clark, D. (1998). The road to recovery in panic disorder: Response, remission and relapse. *Journal of Clinical Psychiatry, 59*(Suppl 8), 4–8.

Shearer, S. L. (2007). Recent advances in the understanding and treatment of anxiety disorders. *Primary Care Clinics in Office Practice, 34,* 475–504.

Stekette, G., & Pigott, T. (2003). *Obsessive-compulsive disorder: The latest assessment and treatment strategies.* Kansas City, MO: Compact Clinicals.

Substance Abuse and Mental Health Services Administration (SAMHSA). (2010). *Handout: Anxiety disorders,* Retrieved from: http://www.ncsacw.samhsa.gov/files/TrainingPackage/MOD3/AnxietyDisorders.pdf

Taylor, S. (1996). Meta-analysis of cognitive-behavioral treatments for social phobia. *Journal of Behavior Therapy and Experimental Psychiatry, 27*(1), 1–9.

Thomsen, P. H. (2000). Obsessive-compulsive disorder: Pharmacological treatment. *European Child and Adolescent Psychiatry, 9,* 76–84.

Ullrich, P. M., & Lutgendorf, S. K. (2002). Journaling about stressful events: Effects on cognitive processing and emotional expression. *Annuals of Behavioral Medicine, 24*(3), 244–250.

United States Surgeon General (USSG) (n.d.). *Mental health: A report of the surgeon general.* Retrieved: http://www.surgeongeneral.gov/library/mental-health/home.html#topper

Wang, P. S., Berglund, P., & Kessler, R. C. (2000). Recent care of common mental disorders in the United States prevalence and conformance with evidence based recommendations. *Journal of General Internal Medicine, 15,* 284–292.

Weissman, M. M., Bland, R. C., Canino, G. J., Greenwald, S., Hwu, H. G., et al. (1994). The cross national epidemiology of obsessive compulsive disorder: The cross national collaborative group. *Journal of Clinical Psychiatry, 55*(3, Suppl), 5–10.

World Health Organization. (n.d.). *Gender and women's mental health.* Retrieved: http://www.who.int/mental_health/prevention/genderwomen/en/

Dementia

■ *Joyce Fraker*

Corrine slowly entered Roland's room and gently awakened him for his morning activities of daily living (ADLs). Roland opened his eyes and looked at her with an expression of disorientation and fear. Corrine had known him for almost a year, and though he could never remember her name, he usually greeted her with a smile of recognition. Today was different. Roland appeared tense, with agitated movements of his arms and legs. Corrine sat next to him, stroked his arms rhythmically, and told him her name. "It is such a beautiful day, let's open the curtain and look at the view," she told him. She opened the curtains and handed him his glasses. Roland put them on without difficulty and turned his vacant gaze toward the window. Within moments, Roland relaxed, and his limbs calmed.

Corrine said, "Let's get dressed. I will help you put on your clean pants." She lightly touched a leg to cue him to lift it so she could place his foot in the pant leg. Roland looked at her, anxious and bewildered. "What do you want me to do?" he cried. Corrine lightly touched his foot, directing him to lift it. Roland tightly gripped his upper thighs and began to shake. He pleaded, louder this time, "I can't move them, what do you want me to do?" Corrine gently took his hand and began stroking his arm. "Let's just rest for a moment," she said. After he had visibly calmed, Corrine gently lifted each foot and placed them into the pant legs. She positioned his walker and said, "You can help us stand." She lightly guided him by the elbow, and he came to a stand. "Thank you for doing such a good job," Corrine told him and helped him pull on the pants. "Now all we need are shoes, and then we can get some breakfast." Roland looked at her, again without recognition, the fear now replaced with calm.

spectroscopy

Magnetic resonance volumetry

Neurofibrillary tangles

Neuroleptic

Paraphasia

Paratonia

Personal episodic memory

Positron emission tomography

Procedural memory

Prodromal

Recent memory

Remote memory

Semantic memory

Short-term memory

Sundowning

Tau

Topographical orientation

COGNITIVE DISORDERS

Dementia, as defined by the *Diagnostic and Statistical Manual of Mental Disorders (DSM-IV-TR)* in 2000, is a condition characterized by multiple cognitive deficits, with the main deficit being impairment of memory. Alzheimer's disease (AD) is the most prevalent form of dementia. Dementia, an often misunderstood disorder, has been variously identified in the past as organic brain syndrome, organic mental disorder, or senile dementia. The American Psychiatric Association no longer classifies dementia as an organic disorder, because "organic" implies that only dementia, and not other mental disorders, has a biological basis (American Psychiatric Association, 2000). Senile dementia is a term that was used when the medical community believed that memory loss was a normal part of the aging process. "Senile" literally means age 65 or older, but the term conjures up negative images of one who is weak and incompetent. Some memory loss may occur as a normal part of aging; this varies from person to person and should not interfere with occupational performance. In fact, well into late old age, individuals can learn new things (Van Wynen, 2001). Memory loss that impairs function is a serious concern that calls for medical investigation.

Serious and persistent memory loss is the hallmark, or most significant symptom, of dementia. However, because memory loss is a symptom seen in other disorders as well, it is useful to review cognitive disorders in general. The *DSM-IV-TR* (American Psychiatric Association, 2000) includes dementia in the chapter "Delirium, Dementia, and Amnestic and Other Cognitive Disorders." These disorders are grouped together because they share the symptom of a significant deficit in cognition or memory that represents a decline from a previous level of occupational function.

Delirium and dementia are the cognitive disorders most commonly seen by occupational therapists. Although they differ greatly in their course and prognosis, they can easily be mistaken for each other. Therefore, the occupational therapist must be able to differentiate between them.

Delirium

The diagnostic criteria for delirium are as follows: (a) disturbed consciousness (reduced level of arousal) with decreased ability to focus, sustain, or shift attention; (b) change in cognition (such as memory loss, disorientation, language disturbance) or the development of perceptual disturbance (hallucinations, paranoid thoughts) that cannot be explained by a preexisting, established, or evolving dementia; (c) the disturbance quickly develops, usually within hours or days, and symptoms fluctuate throughout the course of a day; and (d) there is medical evidence that the disturbance is either caused by a medical condition or developed during intoxication or withdrawal from a substance, including alcohol, illegal substances such as cocaine or hallucinogens, or prescription medications (American Psychiatric Association, 2000).

It is not unusual for delirium to occur when a person is being treated, or is in need of treatment, for an acute physical condition. A high fever can bring on delirium, causing the person to be confused, to misinterpret shadows, to be disoriented (especially in a hospital environment, which is unfamiliar and possibly frightening), and to be unable to express thoughts and needs clearly. These symptoms might fluctuate, just as the degree of a fever might fluctuate during the course of a day. An asymptomatic urinary tract infection is often suspected when a delirium occurs without clear signs of a medical problem. The delirium ends as the acute medical condition clears.

Etiology of Delirium

Delirium is caused by one or more underlying medical conditions. Although a fever can bring on a delirium, the rise in body temperature is merely a symptom of an underlying medical condition. Medical conditions associated with delirium are many and varied. They include infection, burns, and metabolic disturbances. Delirium can also be the result of an adverse reaction to medication or the use of a toxic substance, including alcohol or illegal substances. Risk factors for delirium include increased severity and complexity of physical illness, use of many prescription medications, extremes of age (older or younger), and the presence of a baseline cognitive impairment, such as dementia (Hales & Yudofsky, 2003). Delirium can manifest in confusion and disorientation following surgery. In fact, delirium is a frequent finding during recovery from hip fractures, stem cell transplant, (AIDS), and terminal cancer (Hales & Yudofsky).

Incidence and Prevalence of Delirium

Estimating the incidence and prevalence of delirium is difficult because it is often overlooked or left untreated. Neugroschl and Samuels state that delirium is commonly underrecognized by health care workers and may be present in as many as 1% of community-dwelling adults, 10% of emergency department patients, 40% of terminally ill patients, and 50% of hospital patients (Samuals & Neugroschel, 2008). According to a more conservative estimate, 10% to 15% of inpatients are delirious at some point during hospitalization. For acutely ill geriatric patients, that number increases, to 30% to 50% (American Psychiatric Association, 2000; Samuals & Neugroschel).

Signs and Symptoms of Delirium

The **prodromal** symptoms of delirium can include restlessness, anxiety, sleep disturbance, and irritability. Clinical features of delirium include altered arousal and disturbance of the sleep-wake cycle. The person may be easily awakened, quickly fall asleep, or sleep restlessly. Perception may be altered, with misperceptions, illusions, delusions, or hallucinations. The wrinkled pattern of a blanket may appear to be an object; a shadow in the corner seems to move and is perceived as threatening. The person will likely have decreased attention, impaired memory, disorientation to time or place, and disorganized thinking and speech (Hales & Yudofsky, 2003). Neurologic abnormalities can include dysgraphia (inability to write a sentence); constructional apraxia (evidenced by inability to draw a clock face); **dysnomic aphasia** (difficulty naming objects); motor abnormalities (tremor, **asterixis**, or hand-flapping tremor); myoclonus or muscle spasms; and reflex and tone changes (Hales & Yudofsky). Additionally, there can be psychomotor agitation, psychomotor retardation, sadness, irritability, anxiety, anger, or euphoria.

Course and Prognosis of Delirium

Delirium has a rapid onset. For persons who have delirium, many meet diagnostic criteria within the same day that they developed their first symptoms, and most meet criteria within 48 hours of emergence of symptoms. The course usually fluctuates. There can be lucid intervals as well as periods of confusion and anxiety within the course of a day or even hours. It is not unusual for symptoms to worsen in the evening or at night, and this phenomenon is known as **sundowning** (Samuals & Neugroschel, 2008).

Delirium usually has a brief duration of days to weeks. It is a transient condition that ameliorates as the underlying medical condition resolves, although it is possible for posttraumatic stress symptoms or persistent cognitive dysfunction to emerge in its wake (Schneider & Levenson, 2008). The possible outcomes for delirium range from full recovery to death (Hales & Yudofsky, 2003).

It should be noted that a person does not die from delirium. For a person who is declining with a terminal illness, it is not uncommon for delirium to develop as the body's life-sustaining systems begin to fail. It is also important to note that there is a risk for falls that accompanies delirium. The person hospitalized postoperatively or for a serious illness may attempt to get out of bed even though he or she may not have the needed strength, balance, or coordination. Disturbed thought processes including impulsivity, emotionality, confusion, and fear may also lead a person with delirium to remove lines and tubes necessary for his or her medical treatment or engage in other, potentially dangerous, behaviors (Schneider & Levenson).

Medical Management of Delirium

Treatment for delirium involves treating any underlying cause or medical condition. It is important to withdraw any sedatives or most medications that act on the central nervous system (CNS). One exception to this rule is when the delirium is related to withdrawal from alcohol or sedatives, in which case the use of anxiolytics is indicated. In other patients with delirium, treatment may include the **neuroleptic** haloperidol (Schneider & Levenson, 2008). The person with delirium requires extra supportive physical care, including attention to nutrition and hydration, and maintenance of a safe and quiet environment. If hospitalized, it is also helpful for the person to have positive, orienting cues, such as familiar pictures or things nearby, and frequent contact with family or loved ones (Samuals & Neugroschel, 2008).

For a person who is normally alert with intact memory, the symptoms of delirium are significant cause for concern. If the person is recovering from a medical condition that resulted in delirium, care should be taken that long-term decisions, such as guardianship and nursing home placement, be avoided until the delirium has cleared. Consider the possibility of an individual who has a delirium caused by a prescribed medication, such as a sedative. If the delirium is not accurately diagnosed and the medication routine changed, the person could be assessed as being unable to live independently. Delirium is a temporary condition whose course usually ends as the person becomes medically stable.

Dementia

Memory impairment is the first and most prominent symptom to emerge in most cases of dementia. **Recent memory** is affected first, often manifested as the person uncharacteristically misplaces things. In addition to memory impairment, other cognitive deficits may emerge. These include **aphasia**, **apraxia**, **agnosia**, or a disturbance in executive functioning. For an individual to be diagnosed as having dementia, these deficits must be severe enough to impair occupational performance and represent a decline from a previous functional level (American Psychiatric Association, 2000).

A person who has dementia may experience other cognitive and personality disturbances as well. **Topographic orientation** may be affected, which, compounded by memory loss, can result in the person easily becoming lost. A disturbance in spatial relations creates difficulty with spatial tasks. The person with little or no awareness of memory loss, and who has other impairments, often displays poor judgment or poor insight. One who has awareness of cognitive deficits may become anxious or defensive. Dementia may be associated with gait disturbances that lead to falls, disinhibited behavior such as making inappropriate jokes, and psychotic symptoms such as delusional thinking or hallucinations (American Psychiatric Association, 2000).

The *DSM-IV-TR* (American Psychiatric Association, 2000) differentiates between the types of dementia based on their etiologies. Table 8-1 lists numerous potential causes of dementia. Dementia of the Alzheimer's type is more commonly known as Alzheimer's disease (AD). The cause of AD is the subject of much debate, and the diagnosis is made after ruling out other types of dementia. Vascular dementia was formerly referred to as multi-infarct dementia. Dementias that result from other general medical conditions may be diagnosed when one of the following medical conditions is present: HIV, head trauma, Parkinson's disease, Huntington's disease, Pick's disease, Creutzfeldt-Jakob disease, normal pressure hydrocephalus, hyperthyroidism, brain tumor, vitamin B12 deficiency, and intracranial radiation. Substance-induced dementia may be diagnosed when there is evidence that cognitive deficits are related to the effects of substance use, such as a drug abuse or a medication. The *DSM-IV-TR* (American Psychiatric Association) lists alcohol, inhalants, sedatives, hypnotics, and anxiolytics as substances that may induce dementia.

This chapter will focus on the most commonly seen dementias. According to the Alzheimer's Association, AD is the most common form of dementia and accounts for about 70% of all cases of dementia in people over the age of 70. Vascular dementia is the second most common form of dementia and comprises about 17% of dementia cases (Alzheimer's Association, 2009). However, these figures are likely an oversimplification that fail to account for cases of "mixed" AD and vascular dementia, which some researchers believe are very common (Szoeke, Campbell, Chiu, & Ames, 2009). This chapter

also briefly discusses frontotemporal dementia (FTD), otherwise known as Pick's disease, and dementia with Lewy bodies (DLB). Recent research has focused attention on these forms of dementia and the possibility that they may be more commonly occurring than was previously understood (Frank, 2003; Mosimann & McKeith, 2003).

Alzheimer's Disease

Etiology of Alzheimer's Disease

The cause of AD is poorly understood, and, at present, there is no perfect biological marker that is diagnostic of AD in a living person (Minati, Edinton, Bruzzone, & Giaccone, 2009). The clinical diagnosis is made after ruling out alternate etiologies, such as cardiovascular disease or Parkinson's disease. The best diagnostic tools for confirming a diagnosis of AD, such as **magnetic resonance volumetry** and **magnetic resonance spectroscopy**, **diffusion-tensor imaging**, **cerebrospinal fluid assays**, **positron emission tomography**, and **electroencephalography**, can be difficult and expensive. But even these advanced tests yield specificity and sensitivity of between 60% and 90% (Minati et al.). Development and utilization of superior diagnostic tools has not been a priority to researchers due to the lack of highly effective treatment options following a positive diagnosis (Minati et al.). However, much research has focused on associated features and laboratory findings relevant to AD in an attempt to discover its origin(s). This chapter will review some of the major findings now being studied.

Neuropathology of Alzheimer's Disease

Neuroimaging tools, such as **magnetic resonance imaging (MRI)**, are being used to detect the earliest changes of AD or to differentiate AD from other forms of dementia (DeCarli, 2001). Some of these physical findings are cortical atrophy, widened sulci, and ventricular enlargement (Hales & Yudofsky, 2003). This shrinking of brain structure is a result of neuronal loss, which seems to be caused by **neurofibrillary tangles** and **beta-amyloid plaques.**

Beta-amyloid plaques are caused by a chemical accident or the defective breakdown of a benign substance known as **amyloid precursor protein (APP)**. APP lives in various parts of the body, including the brain, and its role in cellular function is unknown. As part of its mysterious function, APP regularly gets broken down into much smaller soluble components and is washed away with other decomposed tissues and chemicals (Revesz, et al, 2006). Under some conditions that are not understood, the breaking apart does not proceed correctly. The outcome produces sticky, insoluble shards of beta-amyloid. These shards stick to each other, attracting

TABLE 8.1 Potential Causes of Dementia

Disorder	Pathology	Clinical Features
Alzheimer's disease (AD)	Cortical atrophy of the frontal, parietal, and temporal lobes as well as the hippocampal region; amyloid-beta senile plaques and tau protein neurofibrillary tangles	Progressive impairment of memory, executive function, attention, language, visual processing, and praxis; behavioral disturbances are common
Argyrophilic grain disease (AGD)	Cortical and subcortical granular changes in the neuropil related to tau protein	Memory disturbance and personality change similar to AD
Corticobasal degeneration (CBD)	Asymmetric parietofrontal or frontotemporal cortical atrophy, lightening of substantia nigra, astrocytic plaques, thread-like lesions, oligodendroglial bodies, and ballooned neurons; similar to FTD-17	Progressive asymmetrical rigidity and apraxia, sensory loss, alien limb phenomenon, dystonia, myoclonus, and tremor; often with progressive aphasia, FTD, or Alzheimer-type dementia
Creutzfeldt-Jakob disease (CJD) (familial, sporadic, or iatrogenic)	Diffuse spongy degeneration of brain tissue and presence of prion protein	Rapidly progressive dementia and myoclonus; motoric dysfunction, visual disturbance, and akinetic mutism also possible; often fatal within 1 year
Dementia lacking distinctive histopathology(DLDH)	Neuron loss, gliosis and spongiosis not caused by beta-amyloid, tau, ubiquitin, alpha-synuclein, or prion abnormalities	FTD or progressive aphasia; corticobasal syndrome and co-occurring motor neuron disease have also been observed
Dementia pugilistica	Associated with TBI in boxers; beta-amyloid deposition and widespread neurofibrillary tangles involving tau protein, similar to AD	Amnestic, cortical dementia with parkinsonism
Down's syndrome (DS)	Extra copy of chromosome 21 leads to overexpression of APP, accumulation of amyloid-beta plaques beginning around age 40	Cognitive decline consistent with AD detected in about one-third of people with DS who reach the age of 55; signs of dementia often confounded by preexisting cognitive disability

(Continued)

TABLE 8.1 Potential Causes of Dementia *(Continued)*

Disorder	Pathology	Clinical Features
Familial British dementia (FBD)	Widespread cerebral amyloid angiopathy, amyloid deposition in the parenchyma, and neurofibrillary tangles; caused by autosomal dominant mutation on chromosome 13	Progressive dementia, spastic tetraplegia, and ataxia
Familial Danish dementia (FDD)	Similar to FBD with neocortex and parenchyma more severely affected	Begins with cataract and ocular hemorrhages in the third decade of life followed by severe perceptive hearing loss 10–20 years later; after age 40, ataxia, psychiatric disturbance, and progressive dementia begin
Familial encephalopathy with neuroserpin inclusion bodies (FENIB)	Four different genetic mutations lead to neuroserpin inclusion bodies (Collins bodies) within the neurons of the deep cortex and substantia nigra (Miranda & Lomas, 2006)	Dementia, tremor, seizures, progressive myoclonus, epilepsy, dysarthria; age of onset varies from teens to age 50 depending on mutation type
Familial or sporadic fatal insomnia	Thalamic disturbance and possible cerebellar or cerebral atrophy caused by prion protein	Insomnia and autonomic dysfunction; dementia late in course; typically fatal within 13–15 months
HIV-associated dementia	Viral infection of microglia and astrocytes leads to neuroinflammation, myelin pallor, microglial nodules, synaptic pruning, and neuron loss primarily in the frontal and parietal lobes	Cognitive, motor, and behavioral dysfunction seen in approximately 10% of people with HIV, usually in the late stages
Inclusion body myopathy, Paget's disease of the bone, and frontotemporal dementia (IBMPFD)	Autosomal dominant mutation on chromosome 9 leads to degeneration of muscle, brain, and bone tissue	Proximal and distal muscle weakness and atrophy; FTD in about 30% of affected individuals

Frontotemporal dementia and parkinsonism linked to chromosome 17 (FTD-17) with progranulin mutation	Neuronal, intranuclear inclusions	FTD, progressive aphasia, corticobasal syndrome, or symptoms similar to AD or Parkinson's disease
Frontotemporal dementia and parkinsonism linked to chromosome 17 (FTD-17) with tau mutation	Neuronal or glial inclusions involving tau protein; specific features vary	FTD, progressive aphasia, or both, beginning around middle age or sooner (30–50)
Frontotemporal lobar degeneration with ubiquitin-positive inclusions (FTLD-U)	Abnormal neurites and/or cytoplasmic inclusions in the frontal or temporal cortex or dentate granule cell layer; frontotemporal gliosis and neuronal loss	FTD, progressive aphasia, or both; motor neuron disease co-occurs in about half of cases
Gerstmann-Strausser-Schenker syndrome (GSS)	Spongiform changes, neuronal loss, astrogliosis, deposition of prion protein plaques mainly in the cerebellum	Cerebellar dysfunction including ataxia, nystagmus, and dysarthria; course may progress over several years; dementia occurs late in course
Hippocampal sclerosis (HpScl)	Neuronal loss and astrocyte gliosis of the hippocampus, specifically the cornu ammonis and subiculum; lesions may extend to other nearby structures	Often accompanies another form of dementia, complicating clinical picture; deficits in episodic memory and language similar to AD; less executive and visuospatial impairment than AD
Huntington's disease	Striatal degeneration and variable neocortical atrophy	Parkinsonism, abulia, akinesia, eventual chorea, possible dysfunction in psychomotor speed, attention/concentration, learning, and memory; possible depression, hallucinations, delusions, disinhibition, and behavioral dyscontrol; typically 10–20 year course

(Continued)

TABLE 8.1 Potential Causes of Dementia *(Continued)*

Disorder	Pathology	Clinical Features
Kuru	Dense prion protein plaques (kuru plaques) transmitted via contact with infected human brain	Ataxia followed by dementia
Lewy body disease (dementia with Lewy bodies [DBL] or Parkinson's disease with dementia)	Lewy body proteins present in brain, usually predominant in limbic or neocortical areas; decrease in acetylcholine and dopamine levels	Progressive deficits in attention and executive function, memory impairment, fluctuating cognition, visual hallucinations, parkinsonism, autonomic dysfunction, and falls; REM sleep behavior disorder may be prodromal symptom
Multiple sclerosis	Autoimmune reaction causes inflammatory destruction of myelin, oligodendrocytes, and axons of the CNS	Variable neurologic disability consistent with the location of lesions; lengthy course may initially wax and wane but usually becomes progressive
Multiple system atrophy (rarely associated with dementia)	Neuron loss, gliosis, and intracellular cytoplasmic inclusions involving alpha-synuclein protein found throughout the basal ganglia, brain stem, cerebellum, and spinal cord	Sporadic parkinsonism and other movement-related dysfunction, autonomic insufficiency, and deficits in learning, recognition memory, and verbal fluency; REM sleep behavior disorder may be a prodromal symptom
Multisystem tauopathy with corticospinal tract degeneration	Tau protein inclusions in the oligodendrocytes of the motor cortex and corticospinal tract	Parkinsonism and features similar to PSP and CBD
Neuronal intermediate filament inclusion disease	Frontotemporal and caudate atrophy; extensive changes seen in many cortical areas, deep gray matter, cerebellum, and spinal cord	Behavior and personality change followed by executive dysfunction, language impairment, perseveration, hyperreflexia, and primitive reflexes
Neurosyphilis	Sexually transmitted bacterial infection spreads to the cerebrospinal fluid, leading to generalized cerebral atrophy and enlarged ventricles; meningeal, vascular, and parenchymal pathology may be present (Timmermans & Carr, 2004).	Variable; possibilities include psychosis, delirium, dementia, CVA, vision loss, spinal cord dysfunction, seizures, and brain stem or cranial nerve signs

Name	Pathology	Symptoms
Normal pressure hydrocephalus	Buildup of excess fluid in the brain; may be reversed with shunt placement	Difficulty walking, memory loss, and urinary incontinence
Pick's disease	Accumulation of hyperphosphorylated tau protein; thinning of affected gyri; lightening of substantia nigra	FTD, progressive aphasia, semantic dementia, or corticobasal syndrome (rarely)
Progressive supranuclear palsy (PSP)	Neurofibrillary tangles and neuropil threads in the basal ganglia, diencephalon, and brainstem	Supranuclear gaze palsy, postural instability and falls, parkinsonism; dementia in middle-late stages
Spinocerebellar degeneration (Machado-Joseph disease, other spinocerebellar ataxia types, dentatorubral-pallidoluysian atrophy, and Friedreich's ataxia)	Degeneration of the cerebellum, brainstem, spinal cord, and basal ganglia; different pathologies result from various heritable genetic mutations; other structures including the thalamus and cerebral cortex may be affected	Ataxia, dysarthria, dysphagia, and autonomic dysfunction; variable cognitive symptoms including impaired executive functioning, difficulty with spatial reasoning, personality changes, and language deficits
Systemic lupus erythmatosus (SLE)	Small focal lesions often accompanied by cortical atrophy, ventricular enlargement, and cerebral edema among other findings; highly variable; related to microvascular autoimmune disease (Kozoro, E., Hanley, J., Laptiva, L., & Filley, C. M., 2008).	Variable cognitive and neuropsychiatric syndromes observed in about 25%–75% of individuals with SLE; deficits in processing speed, attention, and executive function; fluctuating, chronic course
Vascular dementia	Cerebrovascular disease (often a series of small strokes) leads to focal lesions on the brain and neurotransmitter disruption	Cognitive decline similar to AD but often with less severe memory involvement; Gait disturbance is common; abrupt or stepwise (rather than continuous) decline

fragments of dead and dying neurons, and slowly decline into dense, misshapen plaques (Shenk, 2003). Beta-amyloid plaques collect outside and around the neurons. It is believed that this accumulation causes physical damage to axons and that prolonged neuronal response to this injury ultimately leads to the development of neurofibrillary tangles and neuronal death (Vickers, Dickson, & Adlard, 2000).

Neurofibrillary tangles are made up of another contaminated protein called **tau**. Tau normally serves as connectors or "railroad ties" for a track-like structure that transports nutrients and other important molecules throughout the cell body of every neuron (Josephs, et al., 2005). The contaminated or tangled tau somehow becomes hyperphosphorylated, a corruption resulting in several extra molecules of phosphorous. Without the stabilizing railroad ties of normal tau, the tracks bend into a twisted mess. Under the weight of the nutrients being transported, the tracks buckle, and the damage increases. Inside the neuron, this twisted debris gets worse as the filaments of track keep twisting around each other. As cell communication and nourishment is lost, the neuron begins to wither. The cell body, axons, and dendrites disintegrate, and as a result, thousands of synapses vanish (Bear, Connors, & Paradiso, 2001; Shenk, 2003). It is well documented that the brains of persons with AD have an abundance of the abnormal structures of beta-amyloid plaques and neurofibrillary tangles (Shenk). Filamentous structures known as "Hirano bodies" found primarily in the hippocampus are also associated with the disease (Neugroschl, Kolevzon, Samuels, & Marin, 2004).

The structural changes just described do not cause AD, but are the end product of a pathological process. The challenge for researchers is to discover what causes this degeneration. The loss of neurons occurs throughout the brain but is significant in the cerebral cortex. The cerebral cortex is responsible for higher brain functions, including thinking, judgment, reasoning, speech, and language. Plaques and tangles are also dense in the hippocampus, which plays a role in attention and memory (Cohen & Eisdorfer, 2001).

It is possible that amyloid has a function as a repair protein. Amyloid levels have been noted to increase when there is some injury to the brain. Some researchers contend that beta-amyloid plaques do not lead to AD, but in fact might be a by-product of the AD process (Shenk, 2003).

Genetic Predisposition of Alzheimer's Disease

Unlike some diseases, AD is not caused by a single gene. More than one gene mutation is seen in AD, and genes on multiple chromosomes are involved. In most cases, genes alone are not sufficient to cause AD. The two types of AD are early onset and late onset. Early onset refers to AD that manifests before the age of 65, and late onset

refers to AD seen at or after age 65. Less than 5% of AD is early onset, and this form of the disease is often inherited (Alzheimer's Disease Education & Referral Center, 2003a; Rocchi, Pellegrini, Siciliano, & Murri, 2003).

Three genes have been identified as responsible for the rare, early-onset, familial form of AD. Mutated chromosome 21 causes an abnormal APP to be produced. Mutated chromosome 14 causes an abnormal protein called presenilin 1 to be produced. Mutated chromosome 1 causes yet another abnormal protein, presenilin 2, to be produced (National Institute on Aging, 2003). It appears that these mutations increase the likelihood that beta-amyloid will be snipped from the APP, forming more of the sticky beta-amyloid (Cohen & Eisdorfer, 2001). Even if only one of these genes inherited from a parent is mutated, the person will almost certainly develop early-onset AD. This means that in these families, children have a 50% chance of developing early-onset AD if one parent has this disease.

In the more common, late-onset AD, a polymorphism in the apolipoprotein E gene is associated with increased susceptibility (Tanzi & Bertram, 2001). The apolipoprotein E gene is found on chromosome 19. This gene codes for a protein that helps carry cholesterol in the bloodstream. The apolipoprotein E gene comes in several forms, called alleles. The three most common alleles are apolipoprotein E 2, apolipoprotein E 3, and apolipoprotein E 4. A person inherits one apolipoprotein E allele from each parent. One or two copies of the 4 allele increases the risk of getting AD. However, having the 4 allele does not mean that AD is certain, as some persons with even two of the 4 allele do not develop the disease. The rarer 2 allele may be associated with having a lower risk for AD (Alzheimer's Disease Education & Referral Center, 2003a; Blazer, Steffens, & Busse 2004). AD may also be linked to mutations in the gene that encodes for insulin-degrading enzyme, which helps to break down beta-amyloid. Other genes related to AD include those involved in intracellular APP trafficking and the creation of apolipoprotein neural receptors and transmembrane proteins that influence calcium levels and beta-amyloid production (Minati et al., 2009).

Down syndrome (DS) is a risk factor for AD. Individuals with DS carry an extra copy of chromosome 21, which contains the APP gene. As a result, researchers believe that APP processing in neuronal membranes is abnormal, leading to the formation of beta-amyloid plaques and eventual AD neuropathology. In fact, the brains of almost all individuals with DS over the age of 40 show anatomical changes associated with AD, and as many as 66% will develop clinically detectable dementia in their 50s (Beacher et al., 2009). In another study, it was reported that 32.1% of a sample of individuals with DS between the ages of 55 and 59 had dementia, 17.7% between the ages of 50 and 54, and 8.9% between the ages of 45 and 49 (Coppus et al., 2006). Due to preexisting learning disabilities, AD is more difficult to detect and treat in this population (Beacher et al., 2009).

More recently, a possible link between environmental conditions in early brain development and future manifestation of AD has been proposed. The "latent early-life associated regulation (LEARn)" model posits that factors such as diet, toxin exposure, and hormones early in one's development may disrupt DNA structure in a manner that influences the way certain genes are regulated. In support of this model, animal studies have shown that exposure to lead early in life may upregulate the expression of APP in old age (Lahiri, Zawia, Sambamurti, & Maloney, 2008; Wu et al., 2008).

Neurotransmitter Abnormalities in Alzheimer's Disease

There is some evidence that the neurotransmitter acetylcholine is implicated in the progression of AD. Neurons that contain acetylcholine are known as cholinergic neurons, and many of these are bunched together to form tracts. Cholinergic tracts radiate throughout the entire brain. Autopsy shows that for a person with AD, many cholinergic tracts throughout the entire brain have been destroyed. The enzyme choline acetyltransferase (CAT), which is needed to form acetylcholine, is seriously reduced in the brains of persons with AD. This reduction of CAT is greatest in areas of the brain where there is a dense amount of plaques and tangles (Alzheimer's Disease Education & Referral Center, 2003a). Other neurotransmitter systems found to be altered in people with AD include norepinephrine, GABA, and glutamate (Neugroschl et al., 2004).

Cardiovascular Risk Factors in Alzheimer's Disease

Although vascular dementia accounts for 15% to 25% of all dementia cases, there is now a concern that cardiovascular disease is also linked to AD. As people are living longer with AD, and living long enough to be diagnosed with AD at ages 80 and 90, these groups are also at risk for developing cardiovascular disease. Some see this group as having a "mixed dementia" or a combination of AD and vascular disease (Cohen & Eisdorfer, 2001). Epidemiologic studies suggest that risk factors for cardiovascular disease and stroke are associated with cognitive impairment and AD and that the presence of these factors intensifies the severity of symptoms in AD (Alzheimer's Disease Education & Referral Center, 2003a). In autopsy studies, 60% to 90% of AD cases exhibit variable cerebrovascular pathology (Kawas & Brookmeyer, 2001). Researchers have also found that the use of statins, the most common type of cholesterol-lowering drug, is associated with a lower risk of developing AD (Rocchi et al., 2003).

Other Potential Causes of Alzheimer's Disease

One of the theories of aging suggests that over time, damage from a kind of molecule called a free radical can build up in neurons and cause a loss of function. Free radicals can be helpful in fighting infection, but too many can injure cells by changing other nearby molecules, such as those in the neuron's cell membrane or in DNA. This process can lead to a chain reaction, releasing more free radicals, and causing more damage. This is called oxidative damage and may contribute to AD by upsetting the proper flow of substances in and out of cells; by disrupting cell metabolism; and/or by interfering with other cell processes such as protein synthesis, stress response, and enzyme-catalyzed reactions (National Institute on Aging, 2003; Reed, Sultana, & Butterfield, 2010). Some researchers are focusing on a possible connection between oxidative stress and beta-amyloid, the principle component of plaques found in the brain of the person with AD (Varadarajan, Yatin, & Aksenova, 2000). To support the role of oxidative stress in contributing to AD, researchers have found that antioxidant defense is altered in the brains of persons with mild cognitive impairment (MCI), a condition that is often a precursor to AD (Reed et al., 2010).

Researchers are also studying the possible role of inflammation, because cells and compounds that are known to be involved in inflammation are found in AD plaques. Some scientists think that inflammation is harmful and sets off a cycle of events that lead to the death of neurons. Others believe that some aspects of the inflammatory process may be a helpful part of the brain's natural healing efforts (National Institute on Aging, 2003).

Research is focused on even more factors that may be related to AD, including trace elements, the role of the immune system, and the possibility of a viral connection. The role of numerous misfolded proteins in the neuropathology of AD along with other neurodegenerative diseases such as Parkinson's disease, Huntington's disease, and amyotrophic lateral sclerosis (ALS/Lou Gherig's disease) is also a topic of scientific inquiry (Kanehisa, Limviphuvadh, & Tanabe, 2010).

Incidence and Prevalence

In the next 50 years, the prevalence of AD in the United States is expected to nearly quadruple. This means that 1 in every 45 Americans would meet the diagnostic criteria (Kawas & Brookmeyer, 2001). This phenomenon is largely a result of the fact that the baby-boom generation will be elderly and that life expectancies are increasing with medical advances. The *DSM-IV-TR* (American Psychiatric Association, 2000) states that, while the prevalence increases with age, women tend to have a higher incidence of AD. Based on the large-scale, longitudinal "Framingham study," the estimated lifetime risk for developing AD is about 1 in 5 for women and 1 in 10 for men. This study also indicates that while the risk of developing dementia between the ages of 65 and 75 is about 1%, it rises sevenfold in the following 10 years and 20-fold by the age of 85. By 2050, it is estimated that between 11 million and 16 million older Americans will have AD unless preventative treatment becomes available (Alzheimer's Association, 2009).

In addition to age, there are numerous factors that appear to create a higher risk for AD (Hales & Yudofsky, 2003; Neugroschl et al. 2004; Reitz et al., 2010; Shah et al., 2009). These factors include the following:

1. Low educational level
2. History of head trauma with loss of consciousness
3. History of depression
4. Late maternal age
5. Environmental and occupational exposure (e.g., to aluminum)
6. History of electroconvulsive therapy (ECT)
7. Alcohol abuse
8. **Analgesic** abuse
9. Long-standing physical inactivity
10. Vascular risk factors (e.g., hypertension, high cholesterol)
11. Type II diabetes
12. Black or Hispanic ethnicity
13. High waist to hip ratio

Minati et al. (2009) state that traumatic brain injury (TBI) is increasingly believed to be a risk factor for the development of AD due to the accumulation of beta-amyloid and tau pathology that follows neural degeneration. They also indicate that cerebrovascular abnormalities may increase the chances of being diagnosed with AD. However, they assert that the most important risk factors are advanced age and genetic predisposition.

Related to these risk factors, there also appear to be several variables that may reduce the risk of developing AD (Breitner & Albert, 2009; Neugroschl et al., 2004; Shah et al., 2009). These include

1. Exposure to antioxidants (such as vitamin E)
2. Regular consumption of fish
3. Estrogen replacement therapy in postmenopausal women
4. Use of nonsteroidal antiinflammatory drugs
5. Use of specific antihypertensive drugs
6. Use of statins
7. Use of specific histamine blockers
8. Physical activity
9. Exposure to education, cognitive training, and mental stimulation

However, the effectiveness of some of these agents is still a matter of scientific debate.

Signs and Symptoms of Alzheimer's Disease

Although the hallmark symptom of dementia is memory impairment, the signs and symptoms of AD impact virtually all performance skills. Because AD is a progressive disease, the first signs can be mistaken for normal aging. Even though there are small changes in process skills with normal aging, a healthy older adult can continue to learn and problem solve at any age. Researchers are generating new information on normal aging versus MCI. A person with MCI will have more impairment of process skills than is expected with normal aging, but will not yet meet the diagnostic criteria for dementia.

Defining the progressive stages of AD is an arbitrary process, and various researchers use different ideologies. Reisberg, a prominent researcher in the study of AD, has proposed seven stages (Reisberg & Sclan, 1992). These stages range from stage 1, in which there is no impairment, to stage 7, which is very severe decline. Most researchers use a three-stage approach (Goldman, Wise, & Brody, 2004; Samuels & Neugroschl, 2004; Shenk, 2003). The Clinical Dementia Rating (CDR) is used to measure dementia (Hughes, Berg, & Danziger, 1993). This scale defines three levels of dementia as mild, moderate, and severe.

This chapter will use the three-stage approach, with the stages being defined as early, middle, and late. We will also briefly review MCI, as it is possibly a precursor to dementia. It is important to remember that each person with AD is a unique individual, with unique concerns, needs, and strengths. Although such individuals do not always fit into a rigid classification system, using the three stages will give the reader general guidelines for better understanding the problems facing the person with AD and his or her caregivers.

Mild Cognitive Impairment

MCI is defined as the clinical state of individuals who are memory impaired but are functioning well and do not meet the criteria for dementia (Peterson, Stevens, & Ganguli, 2001). MCI appears to be a prodromal stage of AD. It is a stage of mild but persistent memory loss and is often seen with word naming difficulties. According to Cohen, the diagnosis of MCI includes five criteria:

1. The individual complains of memory problems.
2. Memory loss is abnormal for the person's age.
3. ADLs are not affected.
4. Other cognitive abilities are intact.
5. There is no dementia.

For individuals given a diagnosis of MCI, approximately 15% will progress to AD each year compared with 1% of age-matched controls (Neugroschl et al., 2004).

Early Stage

The early and mild stage usually lasts 2 to 3 years (Gauthier, 2002). The cognitive changes in the early stage can be divided into three groups: memory, language, and visuospatial.

Memory **Short-term memory** is significantly impaired, which makes new learning very difficult. The person forgets tasks, loses the thread of a conversation, and misplaces things. **Long-term memory** begins to be impaired (Hales & Yudofsky, 2003). The person might be able to remember a phone number long enough to repeat it, but will forget it if there is any delay in using it. **Procedural memory**, such as knowing how to write, will remain intact. However, other types of memory begin to show deficits, including **personal episodic memory**, which is time-related information about one's self, such as where and if one ate breakfast; **semantic memory**, such as remembering the name of a common object; and general knowledge, such as remembering the name of the highest mountain in the world (Alzheimer's Disease Education & Referral Center, 2003a).

Language Aphasia, an abnormal neurologic condition in which language is impaired, appears in the early stage. The person can usually maintain sentence structure, though it becomes less complex. Poor semantic memory leads to difficulty with word retrieval (the ability to name an object when shown a picture of it) and word list generation (e.g., being able to quickly name words in a common category or beginning with the same letter). When forgetting a word, the person may substitute inappropriate words, making sentences incomprehensible (Alzheimer's Disease Education & Referral Center, 2003a). This would be an example of **paraphasia**, which means saying the wrong word, substituting a word that sounds alike, or using a word in the same category as the intended word. **Anomia** is the phenomenon in which a person searches in vain for a word and says "thing-a-ma-jig" or just gives up. **Circumlocution** may occur, in which the person tries to express an idea by talking around the intended word with extensive description and elaboration (Liu, McDowd, & Lin, 2004).

Visuospatial Skills Visuospatial abilities decline in early AD. The person starts to get lost in a familiar neighborhood or does not recognize a familiar intersection. There may be some disorientation within the home, such as putting the frying pan in the freezer or the wallet in the dishwasher (Bear et al., 2001).

Executive Functions In addition to these classic symptoms, the person in the early stage of AD begins to have difficulty with instrumental activities of daily living (IADLs). Balancing the checkbook is impossible, and bills may be forgotten. The family notices that the person is more rigid and irritable and less spontaneous or adventurous. Problems with planning, organizing, sequencing, and abstracting become apparent as the person begins to have difficulty in the workplace or following a recipe. The person may begin to prepare a meal, become distracted, and forget to complete it (Hales & Yudofsky, 2003).

The person may recognize that memory has become impaired or may not have the judgment necessary for such insight. It is not unusual to see personality changes. Some persons with AD become suspicious, thinking that one's things are being stolen or that his or her spouse is being unfaithful. Depression is seen in up to 25% of people in the early stage of AD. Confusion or anxiety may lead to withdrawal from routine social activity. In some cases, delusional thinking may emerge (Kovach, 1997).

Middle Stage

In the middle stage of AD, which can last from 2 to 10 years, there is continued decline in memory, visuospatial skills, and language. All areas of performance skills begin to show deficits, psychiatric symptoms increase, and behavior disturbances arise.

Memory Recent and **remote memory** worsens. The person may think he or she is back at an earlier stage of life and become focused on a past worry, such as getting the children to school on time. The person is no longer bothered by the memory loss. There is disorientation to place and time, and at times the person may not recognize his or her own face in the mirror, much less friends or family members. New information is not retained for more than a few moments. There is difficulty organizing thoughts and thinking logically and inability to cope with new or unexpected situations. Thinking is concrete, with no ability to take into account ideas or objects that are not present (National Institute on Aging, 2003; Shenk, 2003; Zgola, 1999).

Language Aphasia worsens, and the person loses fluent language. Language is limited to the concerns of the moment or reminiscing about the past. There may be diminished verbal responsiveness, or verbalizations may be impulsive and inappropriate. There is difficulty understanding simple questions or instructions. The person has trouble following a conversation and may be unable to keep track of his or her own thoughts or words (Frank, 2003).

Internal speech is part of the complex process used when an individual makes plans or mentally solves problems. A person who can no longer use words effectively loses this ability of rational planning and problem solving. His or her actions will become impulsive and disorganized, requiring step-by-step direction and supervision for any occupation (Zgola, 1999).

Visuospatial Skills Visuospatial abilities continue to decline. Visual inattention, which is seen in the early stage, begins to seriously limit function in the middle stage (Liu et al., 2004). The person gets lost in familiar environments and is unable to become oriented if he or she moves to a new environment. Constructional skills are compromised, and the person is unable to sort out the arms and legs of garments while trying to get dressed. There is a loss of ability to judge depth and distance. The person may step highly over a mark on the ground or choose to walk around it. He or she may not be able to distinguish furniture from designs on the carpet or interpret changes in flooring. These visuospatial impairments can lead to falls. Judging direction and distance is problematic, resulting in knocking things over when trying to grasp them or grasping at thin air (Zgola, 1999).

Psychiatric Symptoms Psychiatric symptoms that emerged in the early stage worsen. Depression and anxiety are frequently seen, and the presence of depression is associated with increased mortality. The person may lose control over his or her emotions, having outbursts of fear or anger. Visual hallucinations are not uncommon, and auditory hallucinations can also occur. Sleep is disturbed, with increased daytime napping and frequent nighttime wakefulness (Kovach, 1997).

Behavior Disturbances Behavior disturbances increase the likelihood that the individual will need nursing home placement. It is in the middle stage of AD that wandering and agitation become a problem (National Institute on Aging, 2003). The person paces, seemingly without a goal or destination. Pacing could be a sign of stress or anxiety, or perhaps it is the person's need for activity and exercise. Agitation could be the person's only way to respond to fear or frustration (Kovach, 1997). Loss of impulse control manifests in sloppy table manners, undressing at inappropriate times or places, and vulgar or rude language (Vickers et al., 2000). There is a loss of social propriety and inhibition, a failure of the filtering system that determines which thoughts to keep to one's self and which thoughts to act upon. This inability to inhibit impulses can cause offense to others or become dangerous if the person with AD acts upon aggressive impulses (Zgola, 1999).

Late Stage

The late stage of AD can last from 8 to 12 years. At this stage, the person with AD is fully dependent on others for basic ADLs, such as bathing, dressing, and eating. Motor skills are affected, and the person becomes immobile and incontinent.

Memory There is no ability to create new memories and little or no recognition of close family members. All process skills are seriously impaired, and purposeful, goal-directed occupation is lost.

Language Speech is limited to one or two words, or speech and vocabulary may be totally unintelligible. Over time, speech will decline to the point where there is none. The person no longer smiles or communicates with facial expression (Shenk, 2003). There can be instances of moaning or crying, and since these are universal sounds of distress, it is important for caregivers to explore the possible causes of discomfort. Receptive language is also seriously impaired. The person cannot process the meaning of words but may respond to a calm and soothing tone of voice.

Motor Skills The person becomes bed-bound with eventual loss of postural control. Neurologic symptoms develop, including **hyperflexia**, apraxic gait, and frontal release signs (grasp and snout reflexes). **Paratonia** is a primitive reflex in which there is involuntary resistance in an extremity in response to a sudden passive movement. Thus, if a caregiver quickly moves the person's arm, he or she automatically resists the movement (Goldman et al., 2004).

Seizures may occur, and contractures, pressure ulcers, urinary tract infections, and pneumonia may develop from immobility. There is incontinence of bladder and bowel. Appetite decreases, and eventually the person develops **dysphagia** or the loss of ability to chew and swallow (Kovach, 1997).

Psychiatric Symptoms The sleep cycle is very disturbed as the person spends 60% of time sleeping, including much of the daytime. Hallucinations persist for some (Kovach, 1997).

Course and Prognosis

The course of AD tends to be slowly progressive, with the loss of about 3 points per year on the Mini Mental State Examination, a standard cognitive assessment instrument (Neugroschl et al., 2004). The stages outlined in the previous section of this chapter illustrate the progression of the signs and symptoms of AD. A 2004 study reported the average survival time following diagnosis of AD to be 4 to 6 years. On average, those who are newly diagnosed live approximately half as long as people of the same age without AD. However, some people can survive as long as 20 years after the first appearance of symptoms (Alzheimer's Association, 2009; Varadarajan et al., 2000).

This disease progresses until death. Death is usually a result of complications, such as infection, or the eventual inability of the individual to maintain nutrition and hydration. Despite suspected underreporting, AD was the sixth leading cause of death in the United States in 2006 (Alzheimer's Association, 2009).

Medical Management

Diagnosis

There are three primary criteria in the diagnosis of AD. First, there is the development of multiple cognitive deficits manifested by both memory impairment and at least one other cognitive disturbance. These cognitive disturbances include aphasia, which is language disturbance; apraxia, which is impaired ability to plan motor activities despite intact motor function; agnosia, which is failure to recognize or identify objects despite intact sensory function; and disturbance in **executive function**, such as problems with planning, organizing, sequencing, and abstracting.

The second criterion for AD is the finding that the multiple cognitive deficits cause significant impairment in social or occupational functioning and represent a significant decline from a previous level of functioning. The third criterion is having a course characterized by gradual onset and continuing cognitive decline (American Psychiatric Association, 2000).

The *DSM-IV-TR* (American Psychiatric Association, 2000) uses the first two criteria in diagnosing all other dementias. In addition to the aforementioned criteria, the clinician must eliminate other possible causes of dementia for the diagnosis of AD to be made. A definitive diagnosis of AD is possible only after death, when an autopsy can reveal the physical findings of plaques and tangles in the brain.

The diagnosis is a time-consuming process, but an important one, as the thorough medical investigation may reveal a condition that can be treated. The possibility of reversible dementia will be discussed later.

The National Institutes of Health (NIH) (National Institute on Aging, 2003) has outlined the following steps in diagnosing AD:

1. A detailed patient history should include a description of how and when the symptoms developed, the patient's and family's medical condition and medical history, and an assessment of the patient's emotional state and living environment.
2. Interviewing family members or close friends, which can provide information on how behavior and personality have changed.
3. Physical and neurologic examinations and laboratory tests, which help determine neurologic functioning and identify possible non-AD causes of dementia.
4. A computerized tomography (CT) scan or an MRI test, which can reveal changes in the brain's structure and function that indicate early AD.
5. Neuropsychologic tests that measure memory, language skills, and other cognitive functions, which help indicate what kind of cognitive changes are occurring.

General Treatment Approach

Goldman et al. (2004) describe the following four pillars of complete dementia care:

1. Supportive care for the patient
2. Supportive care for the family and/or caregiver
3. Disease treatment
4. Symptom treatment, including cognitive, mental, and behavioral symptoms

Supportive care includes assessing the environment for aspects of safety as well as looking at how the environment can improve function and well-being. Very early in the disease process, the person with AD needs to discuss financial and medical concerns such as wills and advance directives. It is important to determine the level of care that is needed, who will provide the care, and additional supports such as day programs. The family may need to help make decisions regarding ability to drive and work. Maintaining the person's dignity and privacy is always important. The person with AD will also need ongoing medical care and evaluation of vision and hearing.

Minati et al. (2009) summarizes a number of evidence-based interventions that may be helpful in the treatment of persons with AD. These include individual and group-based structured activities, psychological therapy, and cognitive rehabilitation. Cognitive strategies based on implicit learning include spaced retrieval, vanishing cues, and errorless learning. However, it is important to note that this type of "learning" depends on implicit aspects of cognition not as rapidly affected by the disease; such treatments should be used only to the extent that they are therapeutic for the individual. Other cognitive interventions include cognitive stimulation, reminiscence therapies, and external memory aids. These authors assert that "person-centered therapeutic interventions" are helpful in addressing emotional issues that underlie much of the problem behavior and distress associated with AD for both the patient and the caregiver (Minati et al., 2009).

Support for the caregiver is critical. Approximately 80% of people with dementia are cared for by their families in the community (Neugroschl et al., 2004). Caring for someone who is progressively losing memories and skills can be stressful, sad, and frightening. Care giving can become a 24-hour-a-day job. Complicating the stress of caring for a person with AD is the tendency of caregivers to withhold the diagnosis from friends and family and the social isolation that may result from embarrassing behavior or functional decline (Neugroschl et al.). The stress of caregiving leads to increased risk of depression, sleep disturbance, and substance abuse in caregivers and may result in patient neglect (Neugroschl et al.). The Alzheimer's Association can refer caregivers for support, resources, and advocacy.

Disease treatment is meant to target the etiology or cause of the progressive decline in AD. The etiology of AD is still unknown. Former President Ronald Reagan brought national attention to the disorder when, in 1994, he announced that he had been diagnosed with AD. Since his death, his widow, Nancy Reagan, has publicly campaigned for increasing dementia research funds and for limiting obstacles to stem cell research. Until the causes of AD are better understood, medical management of the vascular process continues to be important not just for persons with vascular dementia but also for AD.

Symptom treatment targets cognitive decline, psychiatric symptoms (including psychosis or depression), and behavior disturbances. Pharmacotherapy is useful for these symptoms. The use of medications will not stop the disease process, but relieving the associated symptoms can comfort the person with AD and improve the quality of life for both patient and caregivers. In addition to pharmacotherapy, behavioral and environmental strategies can provide support for more positive experiences as the disease progresses.

Pharmacotherapy

Prescription drugs are frequently used in managing symptoms such as impaired cognition, depression, delusions and hallucinations, and agitation or aggression. Some of the newest medications are those used in treating cognitive symptoms and work as cholinesterase inhibitors. These include donepezil (Aricept), rivastigmine (Exelon), and galantamine (Reminyl). Inhibiting acetylcholinesterase leaves more acetylcholine in the synapse, which facilitates the activity of remaining neurons. The various cholinesterase inhibitors tend to perform equally in comparison group studies, but it is possible for individuals to respond more favorably to one drug than another (Farlow & Boustani, 2009). These medications do not inhibit cell loss, but research does show that there is modest cognitive improvement in about a third of the persons who take them. This improvement is seen in increased function in ADLs and in delayed placement in nursing homes (Peterson et al., 2001). Some studies show that treatment with cholinesterase inhibitors can restore cognition to the level seen about 6 months prior to the start of treatment (Liu et al., 2004). This means that the person may be able to again do the things he or she could do half a year ago, such as dressing with verbal prompts only. However, these treatments cannot halt the progression of AD, and cognitive decline will continue. Common side effects of cholinesterase inhibitors include nausea, vomiting, diarrhea, and loss of appetite (Farlow & Boustani, 2009).

Memantine (Namenda) is another medication used in an attempt to slow the progression of AD. It works by blocking excess glutamate, a chemical involved in memory function (National Institute on Aging, 2003). Memantine has few long-term side effects but may cause temporary confusion or sedation while the dosing is being adjusted. A combination of Memantine and a cholinesterase inhibitor is the preferred treatment for moderate to severe AD. However, as AD progresses and the person is no longer able to share meaningful interactions, medication may be discontinued (Farlow & Boustani, 2009).

At the present, pharmacologic advances in the treatment of AD include large-scale clinical trials of an antihistamine drug called Dimebon (Latrepirdine). This agent appears to have mitochondrial stabilization properties that promote neuronal function and inhibit cell death, leading to improved cognition in people with AD. Investigators are also exploring drug treatments that target amyloid-beta production and aggregation, but so far success has been minimal (Massoud & Gauthier, 2010).

Depression is seen in as many as 25% to 30% of persons with dementia. Depression can occur in the early stage of AD and, if untreated, can lead to earlier institutionalization and death, aside from the emotional suffering. Select serotonin re-uptake inhibitors (SSRIs) are the first line of treatment for depression, followed by the use of agents with dual effects on the serotonin and norepinephrine systems (Peterson et al., 2001). Many SSRI's have anticholinergic side effects, so fluoxetine (Prozac) and sertraline (Zoloft) are usually most appropriate for individuals with dementia (Farlow & Boustani, 2009).

Delusions and hallucinations can begin in the early stage of AD and are more common in the middle stage. Low-dose neuroleptics are sometimes used, and the atypical neuroleptics such as risperidone (Risperdal) and olanzapine (Zyprexa) are less likely to cause side effects (Peterson et al., 2001). However, the use of these medications is controversial due to the increased risk of stroke and death as well as only limited, if any, long-term improvements (Ballard, Corbett, Chitramohan, & Aarsland, 2009; Minati et al., 2009).

Disruptive behavior such as agitation and aggression is often a sign of a medical problem. Urinary tract infections or pneumonia can create delirium with agitation or aggression. Ruling out these and other concerns, such as environmental stress or pain, is the first step in reducing problem behaviors. If the behavior is truly caused by the underlying dementia, low-dose neuroleptics and mood stabilizers may be beneficial (Goldman et al., 2004). However, again, the use of neuroleptics in this situation may not be the best approach. Ballard et al. (2009) state that psychological interventions and caregiver training should be the first management strategies used, prior to pharmaceutical interventions.

Behavioral and Environmental Management

According to Hilgeman, Burgio, and Allen (2009), the environment surrounding a person with AD should be modified so as to restore the balance between the challenges presented and the person's current level of function. By creating an appropriate level of demand, the physical environment can serve to help maintain function and simultaneously provide stimulation and comfort to the individual with AD. Environmental considerations should be made for declining cognitive function as well as sensory loss and the potential for pain and discomfort. Some specific suggestions from Hilgeman et al. include

1. Reducing the size of space and number of individuals
2. Simplifying visual and auditory stimuli
3. Providing choices/options
4. Increasing the amount of familiar and meaningful stimuli
5. Providing redundant cues in multiple modalities
6. Increasing the sensory contrast of important stimuli

An appropriate environment is perhaps one of the most effective ways to manage problem behaviors of persons with AD. Hilgeman et al. (2009) point out that aggression is often a result of too much or too little stimulation, the anticipation or experience of pain, and frustration with one's inability to perform daily tasks or effectively communicate. They suggest breaking up long periods of low or high arousal activities with sensory stimulation or relaxation, providing orienting cues, emphasizing nonverbal communication, and working to relieve immediate discomforts. Addressing other underlying factors such as pain and depression may also help ameliorate agitated behavior. Neugroschl et al. (2004) add that infections, constipation, delirium, and medication or substance intoxication may also lead to agitated behavior in persons with AD. They suggest strategies such as promoting exercise, socialization, recreation, and predictable routines. Another way to address troublesome behavior, such as agitation, is to consider the "ABCs" (Xie et al., 2009; Neugroschl et al). This refers to the antecedents, the nature of the behavior itself, and the consequences. By considering factors that frequently lead up to the behavior, changes can be made to try to avoid the issue before it begins. Some changes may involve simplifying the task, providing different cues, or offering choices. The consequences of behavior should also be considered so that incooperative behavior, such as acting out in avoidance of a task, is not reinforced, and positive behavior is not punished or ignored.

Patients with AD may engage in a variety of problematic behaviors other than or in addition to aggression and agitation. Some examples include wandering, grabbing others, and swallowing inedible objects. A helpful guide for dealing with these behaviors based on Allen's 25 cognitive levels and modes is written by Pollard (2005) and listed as a recommended learning resource at the end of the chapter.

Impact of Condition on Client Factors

Early Stage

With the progressive loss of performance skills, AD affects increasing areas of occupation and performance patterns. Although this section outlines the expected impact of AD on client factors, it is important to remember that each individual will perform differently. Someone who has always been flexible and adaptive may compensate in ways that support function; another person who is prone to anxiety or has fewer coping skills might have more significant functional losses.

In the early stage, ADLs remain intact. The first signs of memory impairment manifest in IADLs. The person experiencing memory loss cannot adequately or safely fulfil the responsibilities of child rearing or caring for others. Memory impairment affects orientation to place, and so community mobility is impaired. The person easily becomes lost in a new environment. The person with early AD will be disoriented while vacationing or travelling away from home, and sometimes this is when family members begin to note the symptoms of AD. Financial management begins to deteriorate. The person may forget to pay a bill or may misplace it. Shopping becomes a problem when the person is disoriented, loses track of what he or she is trying to purchase, and has difficulty making the money transactions. Compensations can include shopping only in the neighborhood and using a credit or debit card.

Other IADLs may also be impacted. Meal preparation can be a problem if the person starts the task, gets distracted, and then forgets to finish preparing and even eating the meal. Health management can be a problem if the person forgets to make or keep appointments or forgets to take medication. Home management may not be a problem if there are well-established routines and no unexpected problems arise. However, routine car maintenance might be neglected, and response to problems and emergencies might be less organized.

The ability to drive is an IADL that deserves special attention. As a general rule, persons with early stage dementia who wish to continue to drive should have their driving skills evaluated. Many states offer driving assessments through their state departments. The Family Caregiver Alliance (2002) advises families to observe for behavioral signs that the person with dementia is no longer able to drive with safety. It is possible to determine a person is no longer safe to drive when he or she

1. Has become less coordinated
2. Has difficulty judging distance and space
3. Gets lost or feels disoriented in familiar places
4. Has difficulty engaging in multiple tasks

5. Has increased memory loss, especially for recent events
6. Is less alert to things happening around him or her
7. Has mood swings, confusion, or irritability
8. Needs prompting for personal care
9. Has difficulty processing information
10. Has difficulty with decision making and problem solving

Memory loss impacts performance in education. Learning becomes very difficult, if not impossible. Reading is problematic. The person is likely able to read, but will have difficulty retaining or remembering what is read. Work is also seriously impacted. Tasks that are routine may remain intact, but forgetfulness will impact the ability to get work started, attend to all details, and follow the task through to completion. As job performance deteriorates, relationships with coworkers and supervisors can become strained. Some employers make efforts to arrange workloads and expectations in order to maintain the worker in employment as long as possible. In other cases, the person in the early stage of AD may have to seek early or medical retirement. The person will likely need assistance in determining benefits and making plans for productive retirement. Volunteer exploration and participation will be difficult. New routines are difficult to establish, and the task demands, as with regular employment, may be too high for the person with memory and other cognitive impairments.

Leisure exploration will be difficult for the same reasons. Learning new tasks or routines, even for leisure, will be very difficult. The person might be able to maintain established leisure patterns that have little demand for problem solving. Other activities may be given up; attending the bridge club becomes stressful instead of relaxing when it is hard to remember your partner's name or what cards were just played.

The person with early stage AD will find social participation no longer easy nor enjoyable. The family begins to notice that the person avoids social contact, is rigid or irritable, and no longer spontaneous. He or she may drop out of community and family events or attend without actually participating. The changed behavior could be a result of depression, deteriorating language skills, or fear of embarrassment because of forgetfulness. For the same reasons, intimacy and sexual expression will be diminished.

In the early stage, performance skills will be unaffected. As cognition declines, the process skills of temporal organization are impacted. It is easy to be distracted in the middle of a task and then forget to continue, sequence, and properly terminate it. If the task is new or unfamiliar, adaptation may be too demanding. Communication and interaction skills are impaired as language problems develop, and the person may no longer be able to clearly articulate thoughts and needs.

Performance patterns begin to deteriorate. The person might rigidly cling to habits or routines as he or she becomes aware of, and attempts to compensate for, memory loss. Another person may begin to neglect habits and routines; the garbage is not taken out, or the person stops going to church. Roles begin to change: A grandmother can no longer baby-sit, but needs help to go shopping; a father can no longer help his family do the taxes, even though he worked all of his life as an accountant.

Cultural and spiritual contexts remain strong, but participation begins to decline as a result of memory impairment and communication difficulties. Family and friends need to provide ever-increasing support to ensure that the person is included in family, cultural, and spiritual events.

Client factors that are impacted in the early stage are the mental functions: memory, orientation, perception, higher-level cognition, mental functions of language, and calculation. Self concept will be impacted as the individual fears embarrassment or worries that his or her competence is declining.

Middle Stage

In the middle stage of AD, there is impairment in all areas of occupation, and the person can no longer live alone. ADLs are not always attended to, and, when attempted, performance may be poor or inadequate. The person may attempt to shower, but have difficulty setting the water temperature. Showering may consist of just getting wet, with no attention to the need for soap or shampoo. If shampoo is used, regulation is poor, with too much or too little used, using it on the top of the head only, or forgetting to rinse. Dressing requires decision making such as choosing attire based on weather and occasion and the sequence of donning each article. The person with AD might make mistakes in these decisions as well as in understanding the need to remove dirty clothing and replace with clean. Although the person begins misplacing glasses and dentures in the early stage, by now these articles might be lost as well as unnoticed. Toilet hygiene is no longer productive as the person may neglect to clean the body or properly refasten clothing. Eating difficulties and weight loss typically begin in the middle stage of AD (Neugroschl et al., 2004). The sleep-wake cycle is often disturbed, and wandering in the night can create a crisis for caregivers.

IADLs are neglected or performed without proper sequence and completion. Home management tasks that are repetitive, such as folding towels, can be performed after someone else has sorted, laundered, and dried them. The person is dependent in areas of community mobility, financial management, and shopping. Some cleaning and cooking tasks may be done with supervision and direction. Safety is a major concern for the person in the middle stage of AD. At first, he or she may be safe if left home alone for an hour. As the symptoms progress, there can be risk for wandering, letting a stranger in the house, or setting a fire while trying to cook.

There is no ability to perform in areas of work or education. Leisure participation is limited to activities that do not require problem solving or decision making such as singing or going out with a friend or family member to church or a restaurant. In fact, friends or family are needed for any social participation as the person will have difficulty initiating or organizing social interaction outside of his or her immediate environment.

Performance skills remain intact in the early stage. By the middle stage, some of these skills are affected. The decline in visuospatial skills leads to many problems. Positioning and reaching are not always effective. Poor judgment of distance, direction, and floor or ground surfaces creates fall risk. By the middle stage, all process skills are impacted. Attention is limited, and serious memory impairment compromises all aspects of knowledge, temporal organization, organizing space and objects, and adaptation.

In the early stage, the person begins to have problems with communication and interaction skills. By the middle stage, information exchange is limited because of memory impairment and aphasia. As a result, social interactions are affected, often becoming limited to caregivers. Communication may be driven by anxiety, and it is not unusual for the individual to perseverate, asking the same question or expressing the same worry over and over again.

Performance patterns are severely limited. The individual may attempt to engage in habits and may be successful in some such as brushing hair or teeth. Habits that require problem solving or adaptations, such as setting an alarm clock or sewing a button, will be less productive if attempted at all. While most people have established routines for workdays, weekends, and holidays, the person in the middle stage of AD can no longer differentiate days. This loss of routine can contribute to the person's anxiety and depression. Caregivers can help by maintaining structure in the day as well as creative use of meaningful occupations. Roles continue to be lost, and family and friends need to support the most significant roles by reminiscing and affirming the individual's importance.

Cultural contexts begin to diminish in middle-stage AD. Personal and temporal contexts may be confused, and some days the person may believe he or she is in an earlier stage of life. At first, cultural, social, and spiritual contexts may be intact. As the condition progresses, there is less attention given to beliefs and values that defined the individual.

Client factors of mental functions are seriously impaired. Orientation to person, place, and time is affected. Personality changes; instead of spontaneity, there is **disinhibition**; instead of motivation and goal direction, there is apathy or anxiety; instead of fluent verbal and nonverbal communication, there is disinter-est or perseveration. There is progressive impairment in all cognitive functions. The person may have hallucinations or delusional ideas. Emotions are not well regulated, and there can be outbursts of anger, fear of an imagined threat, or crying spells that come and go suddenly.

Late Stage

During the late stage of AD, all areas of occupation diminish and are lost. The person is fully dependent in all ADLs and can no longer ambulate with safety. All performance skills and patterns are impaired, and eventually the person loses all functional capacity. Speech is reduced to a few words, and then entirely lost. The person may moan or cry, and caregivers need to assess this as a possible response to pain, discomfort, or psychosis. There is no awareness or understanding of cultural, social, or spiritual contexts. Mental functions are completely impaired, and now there is serious impact on neuromusculoskeletal and movement-related functions. Nerve cell damage takes a toll on muscle strength and tone, and voluntary movement is limited. Once the ability to swallow is lost, the family must make the decision to provide artificial life support or allow the natural course of the illness to proceed to death.

It is important to note that individuals with AD will show a wide variance in the signs and symptoms within these stages. This is true for several reasons. An individual with a strong set of beliefs and values may maintain these ideas longer than expected; the woman who always took care and pride in her appearance will maintain grooming habits in the middle stage; someone who has always been organized may adapt for memory loss more productively; a formerly shy person may become very impulsive and disinhibited or become even more withdrawn. The course of the disease is also dependent upon the extent and the areas of neuronal damage.

Vascular Dementia

Etiology of Vascular Dementia

Vascular dementia is caused by one or more strokes that occur when blood cannot get to the brain. Blood clots or fat deposits can block a vessel from delivering oxygen and nutrients to part of the brain. A stroke can also occur when a blood vessel in the brain bursts. High blood pressure, diabetes, heart disease, and high blood cholesterol levels cause strokes.

Vascular dementia can be caused by large multi-infarcts, which are blockages in the large vessels of the brain. Lacunar strokes, in which the small arteries are affected, can also cause vascular dementia. Lacunar strokes affect very small areas of tissue, and people with a history of arrhythmias, or irregular heart beat rhythms, may be especially at risk for this problem (Cohen & Eisdorfer, 2001).

Incidence and Prevalence of Vascular Dementia

Szoeke et al. (2009) state that vascular dementia is second to AD as the most common type of dementia, accounting for approximately 10% to 20% of late-onset cases. However, some researchers suggest that "mixed" AD and vascular dementia may be the most common form, and in Japan, China, and Russia, vascular dementia is more common than AD. While there is a slightly greater risk of AD for women, vascular dementia is more likely to occur in men, although this gender difference becomes less prominent with age (Szoeke et al.).

Signs and Symptoms of Vascular Dementia

Signs and symptoms vary depending on the area and extent of damage to the brain. When damage in the deep brain areas leads to degeneration of the subcortical white matter, prominent symptoms are memory disturbance, changes in executive function, apathy, and amotivation. Thrombotic or embolic strokes in the large or small cerebral blood vessels produce a different pattern of symptoms. These symptoms include amnesia, receptive or expressive aphasia, constructional or other types of apraxia, and disturbance of executive function (Goldman et al., 2009).

The first two criteria that the *DSM-IV-TR* (American Psychiatric Association, 2000) gives for dementia are the same for all the dementia types. The criteria for vascular dementia are as follows:

1. There is development of multiple cognitive deficits manifested by memory impairment and at least one other cognitive disturbance (such as aphasia, apraxia, agnosia, and disturbance of executive function).
2. These cognitive deficits cause significant impairment in social or occupational function.
3. Signs and symptoms of cardiovascular disease are judged to be related to the cognitive deficits.

Although there are similarities between AD and vascular dementia, some symptoms are more prominent with vascular dementia. The person with vascular dementia tends to have more apraxia; moves with rapid, shuffling steps; and may have more falls. Emotional **lability** is also more common in vascular dementia, causing the person to laugh or cry inappropriately (Alzheimer's Disease Education & Referral Center, 2003b).

Course and Prognosis of Vascular Dementia

Because strokes occur quickly, symptoms will appear suddenly. The classic course of vascular dementia is a stepwise pattern of increased symptoms. This means that a small stroke can suddenly cause some memory impairment; then there may be no new symptoms arising for weeks or even months until another small stroke suddenly worsens memory or causes a new symptom. A slow, progressive course, much like that of AD, can also occur in vascular dementia (Goldman et al., 2004). Controlling the risk factors and treating cardiovascular disease can reduce the progression of vascular dementia.

Medical Management of Vascular Dementia

It is important for someone who may be having a stroke to get emergency treatment. The signs of a stroke are sudden numbness or weakness on one or both sides of the body and difficulty speaking, seeing, or walking. Immediate treatment can reopen a blocked blood vessel and reduce the severity of the stroke.

The diagnostic process for vascular dementia is similar to the process used to diagnose AD. The clinician will assess cardiovascular risk factors including high blood pressure, diabetes, high cholesterol, and heart disease. Assessment should also include diet, medications, sleep patterns, and stress factors. A CT scan or MRI test can identify signs of stroke as well as tumors or other sources of brain injury. Differentiating vascular dementia from AD can be difficult, and it is possible for an individual to have both diseases (Alzheimer's Disease Education & Referral Center, 2003b).

Treatment for cardiovascular risk factors may prevent further strokes and therefore halt the progression of the disease. High blood pressure is the primary risk factor, and this can be treated. Treatment needs to include strategies for managing diabetes, high cholesterol, and heart disease. The doctor may prescribe aspirin or other drugs to prevent clots from forming in small blood vessels. In some cases, the doctor may even recommend surgical procedures to improve blood flow or remove blockages in blood vessels (Alzheimer's Disease Education & Referral Center, 2003b).

Pharmaceuticals commonly used in the treatment of AD (cholinesterase inhibitors and Memantine) have also shown some usefulness in treating vascular dementia. This is reasonable considering that neurotransmitter deficits have been observed upon autopsy of vascular dementia patients, and neurotransmitters have a known role in modulating cerebral blood flow (Szoeke et al., 2009).

Frontotemporal Dementia

Memory impairment is considered the hallmark symptom of dementia. However, memory impairment is not the first symptom of FTD. This form of dementia was first identified by Pick in 1906 and was known as Pick's disease (Kertesz, 2004). Some researchers refer to this condition as Pick's complex and believe that it includes an overlapping of the following syndromes: primary progressive aphasia, corticobasal degeneration, progressive supranuclear palsy, and motor neuron disease (Kertesz, 2003).

Etiology of Frontotemporal Dementia

Findings on autopsy include bilateral atrophy of the frontal and anterior temporal lobes and degeneration of the
striatum (Snowden, Neary, & Mann, 2002). Researchers have discovered a link with chromosome 17 as well
as tau mutations (Kertesz, 2004). These genetic factors
continue to be the subject of research.

Incidence and Prevalence of Frontotemporal Dementia

FTD accounts for 5% of all dementias and up to 20% of
early-onset dementia. It occurs most commonly between
the ages of 45 and 65 years, though it can develop before
the age of 30 or after the age of 65. There is an equal incidence in men and women, and there is a family history of
dementia in about half of the cases (Snowden et al., 2002).

Signs and Symptoms of Frontotemporal Dementia

The most prominent feature of FTD is a change in character and social conduct. There is a decline in personal
grooming and hygiene. Mental rigidity and inflexibility
combined with distractibility can cause the person to
appear memory impaired, when, in fact, memory may
yet be intact. There may be perseverative and stereotyped
behavior, such as humming or hand rubbing. Utilization
behavior refers to touching or grasping anything within
sight and inappropriate use of objects such as trying to
drink from an empty cup. Speech is affected; there can be
aphasia, stereotyped speech, echolalia, perseveration, and
eventual mutism (Kertesz, 2004).

A striking feature of FTD is the combination of disinhibition with apathy, although, at various stages of the
disease, one or the other symptom may predominate. Disinhibited behaviors manifest as **hypersexuality**, **hyperorality**, and utilization behavior. For the middle-aged or
older person, hypersexuality may consist of verbalizations
or gestures. Hyperorality can be seen in excessive overeating or in developing a limiting food preference, such
as eating only milk and bananas. Some may grab food,
eat from other's plates, or eat inedibles. Another group
of behaviors are sometimes referred to as "negative
symptoms" because they represent a lack in behavior.
These include apathy, amotivation, indifference, and flat
affect. There may be striking disinterest in the affairs of
the family. The person may neglect to change clothing
or lack the ability to attend to any task to completion.
There is often decreased language and communication
(Mosimann & McKeith, 2003). However, episodic memory is generally less impaired in comparison with AD
(Xie et al., 2009).

FTD is often broken down into clinical subgroups
based on the configuration of symptoms. Borroni et al.
provide one such delineation by describing "behavioral
FTD," "semantic dementia," "progressive nonfluent aphasia," "corticobasal degeneration syndrome," and "progressive supranuclear palsy" as distinct phenotypes on the
FTD spectrum (Borroni et al., 2010).

Course and Prognosis of Frontotemporal Dementia

This disorder was often mistaken for AD, as its course is
progressive. There is a great variation in the symptom patterns of FTD, so the course will vary between individuals.

Medical Management

Treatments for FTD require further research. Since there
seems to be no abnormality in the cholinergic system,
the cognitive medications used for AD are not likely to
be effective. Some of the disinhibited behaviors may be
treated with an SSRI (Snowden et al., 2002).

Dementia with Lewy Bodies

DLB has often been misdiagnosed as AD, delirium, or
viewed as Parkinson's disease plus AD. Lewy bodies
are microscopic spherical neuronal inclusion bodies
within the cytoplasm of a cell. In DLB, Lewy bodies
are found in the cortical and subcortical structures of
the brain (distinguishing DLB from Parkinson's disease, in which Lewy bodies are found in the substantia
nigra) (Neugroschl et al., 2004).

Etiology of Dementia with Lewy Bodies

Just as with AD, the etiology of DLB is unknown. Examination at autopsy reveals, in addition to Lewy bodies, the
presence of senile plaques. Unlike the findings of AD,
there are sparse neurofibrillary tangles (Mosimann &
McKeith, 2003).

Incidence and Prevalence of Dementia with Lewy Bodies

DLB accounts for about 11% to 22% of dementia cases.
However, like vascular dementia, patients with both AD
and DLB complicate these statistics (Tarawneh & Galvin, 2009). The mean age of onset is between 75 and
80 years of age. There is a slightly higher risk for males
(Frank, 2003).

Signs and Symptoms of Dementia with Lewy Bodies

An international consortium established guidelines
for the diagnosis of DLB (Frank, 2003). According to
this guide, the central feature is progressive decline of
cognition, resulting in impaired social or occupational

function. Secondary features include fluctuation in cognition, alertness, and attention; recurrent visual hallucinations; and motor parkinsonism. In addition to these symptoms, there may be

1. Repeated falls
2. Syncope
3. Transient loss of consciousness
4. Neuroleptic sensitivity
5. Systematized delusions
6. Hallucinations in other sensory modalities
7. Rapid eye movement (REM) sleep behavior disorder

Course and Prognosis of Dementia with Lewy Bodies

The course of DLB is generally gradual and insidious. Early in the disease, frontal-subcortical structures are most severely affected, leading to problems in executive, visuospatial, attention, and memory function. Over time, the temporal and parietal lobes are affected, leading to aphasia, apraxia, and spatial disorientation. Parkinsonism, characterized by **bradykinesia**, facial masking, and rigidity, is a core feature of DLB. However, in contrast to Parkinson's disease with dementia, cognitive decline begins more than 12 months prior to motor impairment (Tarawneh & Galvin, 2009). Mean duration of the disease is 5 to 6 years with a range of 2 to 20 years (Mosimann & McKeith, 2003).

Medical Management of Dementia with Lewy Bodies

Clinical management is similar to that of AD, with a need for family involvement and assessment of safety. Medication management requires extreme care, as neuroleptics can result in serious side effects. Any medications with anticholinergic side effects should be avoided. The use of antiparkinsonian medication for motor symptoms is unproven. Research is beginning to show some effectiveness in the use of cholinesterase inhibitors for the treatment of neuropsychiatric and cognitive symptoms of DLB (Mosimann & McKeith, 2003).

Reversible Dementia

The idea that dementia may be reversible is a topic of debate. Most researchers today believe that reversible dementia is very uncommon (Knopman & Jankowiak,

2005). In many cases, what seemed to be a reversible dementia was simply some other cause of cognitive impairment that was misdiagnosed as dementia. Burke, Sengoz, and Schwartz (2000) refer to the term of reversible dementia as a misnomer and state that dementia should only be used to identify cognitive impairment in cases of irreversible degenerative brain disease.

It is a fact that cognitive impairment can be misdiagnosed as dementia. Having a potentially treatable impairment misidentified, and left untreated, could have drastic and dire consequences for the person's function and way of life. As a result, it is important to review what some may refer to as reversible dementia, and others see as reversible cognitive impairment.

Hejl, Hogh, and Waldemar (2002) state that the most frequently encountered potentially reversible conditions are depression, normal pressure hydrocephalus, alcohol-related conditions, space-occupying lesions, epilepsy, and metabolic conditions. Depression is sometimes known as pseudodementia when it presents with cognitive impairment in an elderly person. The National Institute of Aging (2003) also places depression high on its list of treatable causes of dementia. Its list is as follows:

1. Medication side effects
2. Depression
3. Vitamin B_{12} deficiency
4. Chronic alcoholism
5. Certain tumors or infections of the brain
6. Blood clots pressing on the brain
7. Metabolic imbalances, including thyroid, kidney, or liver disorders

Bear et al. (2001) also discussed reversible causes of dementia. Asymptomatic infections can cause a delirium that could be misdiagnosed as dementia. In addition to metabolic disorders, there may be nutritional disorders that lead to a false diagnosis of dementia. A disturbance in electrolytes or uncontrolled diabetes can cause impairment in cognition. Cardiovascular and pulmonary changes can reduce oxygen and nutrients needed by the brain for normal cognition. Medication-related problems may be the most common cause of cognitive impairment and yet are the most easily treated. Lastly, impaired vision or hearing can create the impression that the person's functional loss is a result of impaired cognition. It is for these reasons that any change in cognition must be treated as a serious, but possibly treatable, symptom of disease.

Case Illustrations

Case 1: Alzheimer's Disease

Mrs. L. was born in South America. She was bilingual, speaking her native Spanish as well as flawless English. In her early years, she had the luxury of maids and a cook. She was a widow before her two children were grown. At age 60, her adult daughter died, leaving Mrs. L. as the primary caregiver for her two young grandchildren. Soon after her daughter's death, Mrs. L. fled her native land for political reasons, bringing her orphaned grandchildren to live in New York. After raising them, she continued to live with her adult granddaughter G.

Early Stage

When Mrs. L. was 82, G. married and her new husband moved into their home. Mrs. L. had always told G. that "when you marry and no longer need me, it will be my time to die." She seemed angry at G. and showed her irritation by complaining. Nevertheless, she continued to prepare the family meals, make beds, and do some of the laundry. In spite of failing vision, she was aware of the need to dust. She continued to take impeccable care of her appearance, always setting her hair at night and never going out without wearing hose and high heels. Her social life was full, with friends and neighbors frequently visiting. She took pride in serving tea and dessert to her weekly women's support group who met at her apartment. There were times when Mrs. L. misplaced her dentures (in odd places such as in a plant pot) or forgot to use detergent when washing the dishes. She was often anxious and needy when G. came home from work, and she became defensive and easily upset when questioned about mistakes. Her granddaughter attributed these aberrations to Mrs. L.'s increased stress as a result of the marriage.

Middle Stage

At age 86, Mrs. L. broke her hip, her granddaughter had a new, colicky baby, and the family moved to a larger apartment in the same complex. As a result of these crises, Mrs. L. seemed to have slowed down and became more dependent on G. She began making more obvious mistakes, such as using the toilet brush to scrub the floor and neglecting to wash the dishes before putting them away. G. took over the housekeeping and cooking duties.

Mrs. L.'s hearing and sight continued to decline, and she complained about "nothing ever being right." G. got her books on tape, but Mrs. L. could not learn to operate the tape player. She continued to entertain her weekly women's group, basking in the compliments from her friends for the tasty desserts that they knew were now being made by G.

Mrs. L. became a picky eater, putting catsup on everything, including salads and fruit. She was still very particular about her appearance, but she began to need help doing her hair and became neglectful of her denture care. She could still fold laundry, make beds, and take her bath independently.

There were times when Mrs. L. became fearful of G.'s husband, accusing him of wanting to hurt her granddaughter.

At age 91, the family moved out of the apartment complex, where they had lived for many years, to a new home. Mrs. L. was no longer able to make impromptu visits to her neighbors, and her circle of friends now rarely visited. Mrs. L. was afraid to use anything in the new kitchen, especially the unfamiliar gas stove. Her appetite continued to be poor, and she was losing weight. Strategies to enable her to make her own tea and toast were unsuccessful, and she would forget to eat food left for her in the refrigerator when G. went to work.

Mrs. L. began to have incontinence of bowel and bladder, yet she would resist her granddaughter's suggestions that she needed to shower or bathe. Ironically, when Mrs. L. fell and broke her wrist, she became amenable to assistance. Insurance covered about 6 weeks of home health care, and Mrs. L. seemed to enjoy the attention.

Late Stage

At age 92, it was clear that Mrs. L. could not be left alone. She continued to be incontinent; she could not lift herself from the toilet and seemed afraid to use a bedside commode. When her granddaughter came home from work, she would follow her about, repeating the same question over and over. She was not eating lunch or dinner. Her granddaughter, pregnant with her second child, was having difficulty bathing Mrs. L. On one occasion they both ended up falling on the bathroom floor during a bathing session. In-home care proved unaffordable, and G. made the difficult decision to place Mrs. L. in a nursing home. The nursing home, known for its excellence, proved to be a positive move for Mrs. L. She regained some of her weight and seemed much less anxious. Mrs. L.'s deep-rooted social personality and gift for charming those around her made a reappearance. This served to ensure that a constant stream of staff and residents dropped by her room for brief chats. When G. and her family visited, Mrs. L. remained cool, as if to reprimand G. for sending her away.

Within a year, Mrs. L. was not always able to recognize G. when she came to visit. Sometimes she mistook G. for her daughter. Eventually she completely lost the ability to recognize G. Her granddaughter continued to visit with her own children, who delighted in playing word games with Mrs. L. The youngest child, himself learning to speak, would say a few words or phrases to Mrs. L., which she would mimic. This would set both children to giggling, in turn pleasing Mrs. L. to have had such an amusing effect on the children.

At age 94, Mrs. L. seemed no longer able to speak English. Her verbalizations in Spanish were limited to a few words, which were sometimes unintelligible. She was no longer able to ambulate and needed total care for feeding. Shortly after her 95th birthday, Mrs. L. died peacefully of heart failure.

Case 2: Vascular Dementia

Mr. B. is a 71-year-old African American who is cared for at home by his wife. Mrs. B. describes him as having been a quietly dignified person before the onset of his illness. He enjoyed spending time with his family, including his four children and other members of his extended family.

As a young college graduate, Mr. B. was unable to find work in his field of engineering but did get an unskilled job with the phone company. His supervisor recognized his talents and abilities, and, over time, he had a series of promotions that eventually took him to the position of personnel manager.

When Mr. B. was 60, his company was bought out and he was given an early retirement. Soon after this, he started taking classes in cabinet making and began working for an architect who was building a local church.

At age 64, Mr. B. began making errors in measurement in his work. He was aware of, and troubled by, this difficulty. He decided to cut back his hours at work. Mrs. B. noted at this time that he sometimes appeared confused. During family gatherings he was not only quieter than his usual self, but he would actually distance himself by sitting in another room. Although he was still driving, he began misplacing things. Mrs. B. had some concerns about these behaviors but attributed them to the stress of life changes.

It was when Mr. B. was no longer able to read a ruler that Mrs. B. began to realize something was seriously wrong. At about this time, Mr. B. had an episode in which he got lost on the way to the dentist. Mrs. B. turned to her family physician for help, and an 18-month period of medical and neurologic testing ensued.

At age 66, Mr. B. had a stroke. During hospitalization, the diagnosis of vascular dementia was finally made. When Mr. B. left the hospital, he was able to walk and perform his self-care activities independently.

At first, things went well at home. Both Mr. and Mrs. B. adjusted to a routine in which she would make sure that he was up, dressed, and had breakfast before she left for work. His lunch was prepared and left for him to retrieve from the refrigerator. One day Mrs. B. came home from work and found that the stove had been left on. At this point, she realized that Mr. B. was no longer safe when left alone, and she enrolled him in a daycare program.

About 8 months later, Mrs. B. made the decision to stop working. The day program cost almost as much as her pay. It was becoming more and more difficult to help Mr. B. get dressed and out of the house every morning. In fact, Mr. B. started choosing to undress himself several times a day. He began having problems speaking and understanding what others said to him. Mrs. B. felt he was losing his personality; he was not able to focus on conversation or show interest, even when his grandchildren visited. He was still ambulating with help. He began having difficulty swallowing, was losing weight, and was having bladder infections. He was no longer continent of bowel or bladder.

At age 69, Mr. B. had another stroke. Despite the efforts of the rehabilitation service, he could no longer ambulate. He returned home in a wheelchair. His home did not have a ground floor bedroom, so Mrs. B. converted the living room to his bedroom. For about 1 month, his insurance provided a home health aide who would give Mr. B. a weekly bed bath. Eventually Mrs. B. took over this responsibility, along with complete care for dressing and feeding him. Mr. B. often did not recognize Mrs. B. and no longer recognized his children.

During a recent visit to the outpatient clinic, Mrs. B. talked about the difficulty of getting through each day. "I rarely get out unless one of the family members can stay with my husband, and even then I'm just too tired. I think about the reality that someday I may need to put him in a nursing home. I'll do it when it gets to the point where I'm no longer able to take care of him or if my health goes bad. But if that happens, I'll lose our life savings—it's not much, but enough to help pay bills with my social security check." She also related an incident that illustrated the small daily frustrations of caring for her husband: "I was feeding him lunch, and he reached for the glass of milk with his left hand. I helped place the glass in his outstretched hand, but he began raising his right hand to his mouth as if to drink. Obviously that wasn't working, so I took the glass out of his left hand and put it in his right hand. This must have totally confused him, and he just looked at me as if to say 'what did you do that for?' I felt so helpless, and so bad that I couldn't even help him."

Mr. B., who at 71 is still handsome, sits straight and is tall in his wheelchair, appearing to emanate dignity and calm, faintly smiling and nodding as his wife tells their story.

RECOMMENDED LEARNING RESOURCES

Mace, N. L., & Rabins, P. V. (1999). *The 36-hour day: A family guide to caring for persons with Alzheimer's disease.* Baltimore, MA: Johns Hopkins University Press.

Peterson, R. (2002). *Mayo clinic on Alzheimer's disease.* Rochester, MN: Mayo Clinic Health Information.

Pollard, D. (2005). *A cognitive link: Managing problematic bodily behavior.* Monona, WI: SelectOne Rehab.

Robinson, A., Spencer, B., & White, L. (1996). *Understanding difficult behaviors: Some practical suggestions for coping with Alzheimer's disease and related illnesses.* Ypsilanti, MI: Eastern Michigan University Alzheimer's Education Program.

The National Institute on Aging. (2008). *Alzheimer's disease: Unraveling the mystery.* Silver Spring, MD: Author. Retrieved from www.nia.nih.gov/ Alzheimers

The National Institute on Aging. (2010). *Caring for a person with Alzheimer's disease: Your easy-to-use guide from the national institute on aging.* Silver Spring, MD: Author. Retrieved from www.nia.nih.gov/Alzheimers

REFERENCES

Alzheimer's Association. (2009). Alzheimer's disease facts and figures. *Alzheimer's and Dementia, 5*(3), 234–270.

Alzheimer's Disease Education & Referral Center. (2003a). *Alzheimer's disease genetics: Fact sheet.* U.S. Department of Health and Human Services. Washington, D.C.: National Institutes of Health.

Alzheimer's Disease Education & Referral Center. (2003b). *Multi-infarct dementia fact sheet.* (Publication no. 02–3433). National Institutes of Health. Washington, D.C.

American Psychiatric Association. (2000). *Diagnostic and statistical manual of mental disorders* (4th ed.). Washington, DC: Author.

Ballard, C., Corbett, A., Chitramohan, R., & Aarsland, D. (2009). Management of agitation and aggression associated with Alzheimer's disease: Controversies and possible solutions. *Current Opinion in Psychiatry, 22*(6), 532–540.

Beacher, F., Daly, E., Simmons, A., Prasher, V., Morris, R., Robison, C., et al. (2009). Alzheimer's disease and Down syndrome: An in vivo MRI study. *Psychological Medicine, 39*(4), 675–684.

Bear, M. F., Connors, B. W., & Paradiso, M. A. (2001). *Neuroscience: Exploring the brain* (2nd ed.). Baltimore, MA: Lippincott, Williams & Wilkins.

Blazer, D. G., Steffens, D. C., & Busse, E. W. (2004). *The American psychiatric publishing textbook of geriatric psychiatry* (3rd ed.). Washington, D.C.: American Psychiatric Publishing, Inc.

Borroni, B., Grassi, M., Agosti, C., Premi, E., Archetti, S., Alberici, A., Padovani, A. (2010). Establishing short-term prognosis in frontotemporal lobar degeneration spectrum: Role of genetic background and clinical phenotype. *Neurobiological Aging, 31*(2), 270–279.

Bouve, B. F. (2006). A review of the non-Alzheimer dementias. *Journal of Clinical Psychiatry, 67,* 1985–2001.

Breitner, J. C., & Albert, M. S. (2009). *The American*

Psychiatric Publishing textbook of Alzheimer disease and other dementias. Arlington, VA: American Psychiatric Publishing, Inc.

Burke, D., Sengoz, A., & Schwartz, R. (2000). Potentially reversible cognitive impairment in patients presenting to a memory disorders clinic. *Journal of Clinical Neuroscience, 7*(2), 120–123.

Cohen, D., & Eisdorfer, C. (2001). *The loss of self*. New York: W.W. Norton & Co.

Coppus, A., Evenhuis, H., Verberne, G. J., Visser, F., Van Gool, P., Eikelenboom, P., & Van Duijin, C. (2006). Dementia and mortality in persons with Down syndrome. *Journal of Intellectual Disability Research, 50*(10), 768–777.

DeCarli, C. (2001). The role of neuroimaging in dementia. *Clinical Geriatric Medicine, 17*(2), 255–279.

Family Caregiver Alliance. (2002). *Dementia & driving: Fact sheet*. Retrieved from National Center on Caregiving.

Farlow, M. R., & Boustani, M. (2009). *The American Psychiatric Publishing textbook of Alzheimer's disease and other dementias*. Arlington, VA: American Psychiatric Publishing.

Frank, C. (2003). Dementia with Lewy bodies. *Canadian Family Physician, 49*(10), 1304–1311.

Gauthier, S. (2002). Advances in the pharmacotherapy of Alzheimer's disease. *Canadian Medical Association Journal, 166*(5), 616–626.

Goldman, L. S., Wise, T. N., & Brody, D. S. (2004). *Psychiatry for primary care physicians* (2nd ed.). Atlanta, GA: AMA Press.

Hales, R. E., & Yudofsky, S. C. (2003). *The American psychiatric publishing textbook of clinical psychiatry* (4th ed). Washington, DC: American Psychiatric Publishing, Inc.

Hejl, A., Hogh, P., & Waldemar, G. (2002). Potentially reversible conditions in 1000 consecutive memory clinic patients. *Journal of Neurology, Neurosurgery, & Psychiatry, 73*(7), 390–394.

Hilgeman, M. M., Burgio, L. D., & Allen, R. S. (2009). *The American Psychiatric Publishing textbook of Alzheimer disease and other dementias* (4th ed.). Arlington, VA: American Psychiatric Publishing, Inc.

Hughes, C. P., Berg, L., & Danziger, W. L. (1993). A new clinical scale for the staging of dementia. *British Journal of Psychiatry, 140*, 566–572.

Josephs, K. A., Katsuse, O., Uitti, R. J., Lin, W. L., Fujino, Y. F., Boeve, B. F, et al. (2005). Clinicopathological features of multisystem tauopathy with corticospinal tract degeneration (MTCD). *Annals of Neurology, 58*, S12.

Kanehisa, M., Limviphuvadh, V., & Tanabe, M. (2010). *Neuroproteomics*. Boca Raton, FL: CRC Press.

Kawai, Y., Suenaga, M., Watanabe, H., & Sobue, G. (2009). Cognitive impairment in spinocerebellar degeneration. *European Neurology, 61*(5), 257–268.

Kawas, C. H., & Brookmeyer, R. (2001). Aging and the public health effects of dementia. *New England Journal of Medicine, 344*(15), 1160–1161.

Kertesz, A. (2003). Pick complex: An integrative approach to frontotemporal dementia: Primary progressive aphasia, corticobasal degeneration, and progressive supranuclear palsy. *Neurologist, 9*(6), 311–317.

Kertesz, A. (2004). Frontotemporal dementia/Pick disease. *Archives of Neurology, 61*(6), 969–971.

Knopman, D., & Jankowiak, J. Recovery from dementia: An interesting case. *Neurology, 64*(4), E18–E19.

Kovach, C. R. (1997). *Late-stage dementia care: A basic guide*. Milwaukee, WI: Taylor & Francis.

Kozoro, E., Hanley, J. G., Laptiva, L., & Filley, C. M. (2008). Cognitive dysfunction in systemic lupus erythmatosus: Past, present, and future. *Arthritis and Rheumatism, 58*(11), 3286–3298.

Lahiri, D. K., Zawia, N. H, Sambamurti, K., & Maloney, B. (2008). Early-life events may trigger biochemical pathways for Alzheimer's disease: The "LEARn" model. *Biogerontology, 9*(6), 375–379.

Liu, C., McDowd, J., & Lin, K. (2004). Visuospatial inattention and daily life performance in people with Alzheimer's disease. *American Journal of Occupational Therapy, 58*(2), 202–210.

Massoud, F., & Gauthier, S. (2010). Update on the pharmacological treatment of Alzheimer's disease. *Current Neuropharmacology, 8*(1), 69–80.

Mastrianni, J. A. (2004). Prion diseases. *Clinical Neuroscience Research, 3*(6), 469–480.

Minati, L., Edinton, T., Bruzzone, M. G., & Giaccone, G. (2009). Reviews: Current concepts in Alzheimer's disease: A multidisciplinary review. *American Journal of Alzheimer's Disease and Other Dementias, 24*(2), 95–121.

Miranda, E., & Lomas, D. A. (2006). Neuroserpin: A serpin to think about. *Cellular and Molecular Life Sciences, 63*(6), 709–722.

Mosimann, U. P., & McKeith, I. G. (2003). Dementia with Lewy bodies—diagnosis and treatment. *Swiss Medical Weekly, 133*(9–10), 131–142.

National Institute on Aging. (2003). *Alzheimer's disease: Unraveling the mystery*. Washington, DC: National Institutes of Health.

Neugroschl, J. A., Kolevzon, A. K., Samuels, S. C., & Marin, D. B. (2004). *Kaplan and Sadocks comprehensive textbook of psychiatry* (8th ed.). Philadelphia, PA: Lippincott Williams & Wilkins.

Peterson, R. C., Stevens, J. C., & Ganguli, M. (2001). Practice parameter: early detection of dementia: mild cognitive impairment (an evidence based review). *Neurology, 56*, 1133–1142.

Pollard, D. (2005). A cognitive link: Managing problematic bodily behavior. Monona, WI: SelectOne Rehab.

Reed, T. T., Sultana, R., & Butterfield, D. A. (2010). *Neuroproteomics.* Boca Raton, FL: CRC Press.

Reisberg, B., & Sclan, S. G. (1992). Functional assessment staging (FAST) in Alzheimer's disease; reliability, validity and ordinality. *International Psychogeriatric, 4,* 55–69.

Reitz, C., Tang, M. X., Schupf, N., Manly, J. J., Mayeux, R., & Luchsinger, J. A. (2010). A summary risk score for the prediction of Alzheimer's disease in elderly persons. *Archives of Neurology, 67*(7), 835–841.

Revesz, T., Holton, J. L., Lashley, T., Plant, G., Robstagno, A., Ghiso, J., et al. (2006). Sporadic and familial cerebral amyloid angiopathies. *Brain Pathology, 12*(3), 344–357.

Rocchi, A., Pellegrini, S., Siciliano, G., & Murri, L. (2003). Causative and susceptibility genes for Alzheimer's disease: A review. *Brain Research Bulletin, 61*(1), 1–24.

Samuels, S. C., & Neugroschl, J. A. (2004). *Kaplan & Sadock's comprehensive textbook of psychiatry* (8th ed.). Philadelphia, PA: Lippincott, Williams & Wilkins.

Schneider, R. K., & Levenson, J. L. (2008). *Psychiatry essentials for primary care.* Philadelphia, PA: The American College of Physicians.

Shah, K., Qureshi, S. U., Johnson, M., Parikh, N., Schulz, P. E., & Kunik, M. E. (2009). Does the use of antihypertensive drugs affect the incidence or progression of dementia? A systematic review. *American Journal of Geriatric Pharmacotherapy, 7*(5), 250–261.

Shenk, D. (2003). *The forgetting.* New York: Anchor Books.

Snowden, J. S., Neary, D., & Mann, D. M. (2002). Frontotemporal dementia. *British Journal of Psychiatry, 180,* 140–143.

Szoeke, C. E., Campbell, S., Chiu, E., & Ames, D. (2009). *The American Psychiatric Publishing textbook of Alzheimer disease and other dementias.* Arlington, VA: American Psychiatric Publishing, Inc.

Tanzi, R. E., & Bertram, L. (2001). New frontiers in Alzheimer's disease genetics. *Journal Neuron, 32*(2), 181–184.

Tarawneh, R., & Galvin, J. E. (2009). *The American Psychiatric Publishing textbook of Alzheimer disease and other dementias.* Arlington, VA: American Psychiatric Publishing, Inc.

Timmermans, M., & Carr, J. (2004). Neurosyphilis in the modern era. *Journal of Neurology, Neurosurgery and Psychiatry, 75*(12), 1727–1730.

Van Wynen, E. A. (2001). A key to successful aging: Learning-style patterns of older adults. *Gerontology Nurse, 27*(9), 6–15.

Varadarajan, S., Yatin, S., & Aksenova, M. (2000). Review: Alzheimer's amyloid beta-peptide associated free radical oxidative stress and neurotoxicity. *Structural Biology, 130*(2–3), 184–208.

Vickers, J. C., Dickson, T. C., & Adlard, P. A. (2000). The cause of neuronal degeneration in Alzheimer's disease. *Progress in Neurobiology, 60*(2), 139–165.

Wu, J., Basha, M.R., Brock, B., Cox, D. P., Cardozo-Palaez, F., McPherson, C. A., et al. (2008). Alzheimer's disease (AD)-like pathology in aged monkeys after infantile exposure to environmental metal lead (Pb): Evidence for a developmental origin and environmental link for AD. *Journal of Neuroscience, 28*(1), 3–9.

Xie, S. X., Libon, D. L., Wang, X., Massimo, L., Moore, P., Vesely, L., et al. (2009). Longitudinal patterns of semantic and episodic memory in frontotemporal lobar degeneration and Alzheimer's disease. *Journal of the International Neuropsychological Society, 15*(2), 1–9.

Zgola, J. M. (1999). *Care that works: A relationship approach to persons with dementia.* Baltimore, MA: The John Hopkins University Press.

Cerebrovascular Accident

- *David P. Orchanian*
- *Paula W. Jamison*

M.V. is a 68-year-old native New Yorker. She was born to Irish and Italian parents on the lower eastside of Manhattan. She attended private preparatory schools and readily was accepted at Columbia University, where she studied fashion marketing and design. She received a second undergraduate degree in business from Barnard College and immediately entered the hectic, high-energy world of finance, within the world of women's fashion and apparel. M.V. never married, finding her life fulfillment more in the glitter and glass world than in diapers and the seeming melancholia of suburbia. She worked ungodly hours, often never stopping for lunch, and sometimes missing dinner altogether. Timelines, deadlines, corporate demands, and constantly needing to exceed quotas in order to appease shareholders made her job monetarily rewarding, but extremely stressful in overt as well as insidious ways. M.V.'s weight was a constant stressor for her. She seemed to gain 2 to 3 lb each time she walked past a Baskin-Robbins ice cream store. She was always dieting or going to diet or thinking that she should be on a diet, but the Coke Zero did not make a discernable dent in her ever increasing midriff. In addition to her weight, she also had an ongoing relationship with cigarettes. She continued to be a pack-a-day smoker despite all of the Relays for Life, pink ribbons, and St. Jude's commercials that seemed to trumpet their anti-cancer messages directly at her, whenever she gave them a second glance. M.V. was 30 lb overweight and has had high blood pressure since she was a sophomore in college. M.V. was on her usual path from the subway station at 54th Street and Lexington Avenue to her office, when she began to sense that something was happening to her that she had never before experienced. The first sensation was one of a warm drape being pulled over her head; the air she was breathing became thick and difficult for her to draw into her chest. Then there was a bit of a tingle in her right hand, as though the pinky and ring fingers suddenly decided to fall asleep together;

the bag of bagels she was carrying to share with her coworkers slipped to the pavement unnoticed by M.V. As she attempted to make sense of what was happening to her, breathing became more challenging, like drawing thick soup through a too thin straw. She leaned on a nearby storefront and vomited. As she leaned there for a moment, a man came to her side and spoke in a language she seemingly had never heard before; she thought "was he speaking Russian, Latvian, certainly someone here speaks English?" Within a minute or two, M.V. was being guided to the pavement by two people who appeared to be wearing uniforms; possibly they worked for a Russian circus? She was now lying on the pavement feeling frightened, embarrassed, and very, very confused. There was no way she could move her right hand or arm, and her right lower body seemed to have floated away from her and onto another part of the universe. M.V. was taken to a hospital by ambulance, with much of that event lost to her memory. What is happening to M.V.? Is there enough evidence to suspect that a stroke may be evolving? This chapter will provide insight into M.V.'s condition and helps provide answers to these questions.

DESCRIPTION AND DEFINITIONS

A stroke, or **brain attack**, results from an interruption in the blood flow to the brain, either because a blood vessel is blocked or because of ruptures. The consequence is an inadequate supply of oxygen and nutrients to this vital organ. Even a brief disruption of this blood flow can lead to brain damage. Medical practitioners use the term "**cerebrovascular accident**," often abbreviated as CVA, for stroke. A stroke can occur in any part of the brain, the cerebral hemispheres, the cerebellum, or the brainstem. The site and extent of the affected area, or infarct, determines loss of function.

Strokes are divided into two main types: ischemic and hemorrhagic. Ischemic strokes are characterized by blockages (the term **ischemia** refers to the lack of blood supply) and include atherothrombotic, lacunar, and embolic infarctions, in that order of frequency. **Hemorrhagic strokes** include intracerebral and subarachnoid hemorrhages (Broderick et al., 2007). Both types of stroke lead to the death, or infarction, of brain tissue. These two groups of strokes can be differentiated further by the location of the insult and the precise causes of the

ischemia or hemorrhage (Kaspera, Majchrzak, Ladzinski, & Tomalski, 2005). In most cases, a loss of blood supply is the result of long-standing degeneration of the body's blood vessels. Less commonly, a CVA occurs because of an inborn abnormality or weakness of the brain's vascular supply. A brief review of cerebral circulation will help understand the impact of each type of stroke.

Cerebral Circulatory System

The blood supply of the brain is extremely important because the brain is one of the most metabolically active organs of the body. Although it comprises only 2% of the body's weight, the brain receives approximately 17% of the cardiac output and consumes about 20% of the oxygen used by the entire body (Lundy-Ekman, 2007).

In the brain, the arteries of the anterior circulation supply the front, top, and side portions of the cerebral hemispheres. The brainstem and cerebellum, as well as the back and undersurface of the cerebral hemispheres, are supplied by the posterior circulation. These two areas of circulation are further categorized into the extracranial portions (arising from outside the skull and traveling toward the brain) and the intracranial portions (arising from within the skull) (Lundy-Ekman, 2007).

Extracranial Vessels

Extracranial anterior circulation consists of the two carotid arteries, which travel in the front of the neck on each side of the trachea and esophagus (Lundy-Ekman, 2007). The word "carotid" is derived from the Greek word "karos" meaning "to stupefy" or render unconscious, indicating the significance of this main artery in maintaining consciousness and brain function (Qureshi et al, 2007). The right common carotid artery arises from the innominate artery. The left common carotid artery originates directly from the aortic arch. Around the fifth or sixth vertebra, these common carotid arteries divide into external carotid arteries, whose branches supply the face and its structures, and the internal carotid arteries, which supply the eyes and the cerebral hemispheres (Lundy-Ekman; Qureshi et al, 2007).

The vertebral arteries arise from the subclavian arteries and make up the extracranial posterior circulation. They remain within the vertebral column for part of their course from about C6 to C2. The vertebral arteries enter the cranium through the foramen magnum (Lundy-Ekman, 2007; Qureshi et al, 2007).

Intracranial Vessels

The internal carotid arteries enter the skull through the carotid canal and form an S-shaped curve called the carotid siphon (Qureshi et al., 2007). The artery then enters the subarachnoid space by piercing the dura mater. It gives rise to the ophthalmic arteries, which supply the eyes; the posterior communicating arteries, which join with the posterior circulation; and the anterior cerebral arteries, which supply the orbital and medial surfaces of the frontal lobes and part of the basal frontal lobe white matter and caudate nucleus. The internal carotid artery also gives off the middle cerebral arteries, which supply almost the entire lateral surface of the frontal, parietal, and temporal lobes as well as the underlying white matter and basal ganglia (Lundy-Ekman, 2007). The middle cerebral artery is the largest of the terminal branches of the internal carotid artery and is the direct continuation of this vessel.

The vertebral arteries enter the cranium within the posterior fossa and travel along the side of the medulla, where they give off their longest branch, the posterior inferior cerebellar artery. This artery supplies the lateral medulla and the back of the undersurface of the cerebellum (Zazulia, 2002). The two vertebral arteries then join at the junction between the medulla and pons to form the single midline basilar artery (Zazulia). The basilar artery gives off penetrating arteries to the base of the pons and two vessels (the anterior inferior and superior cerebellar arteries) that supply the upper and anterior undersurfaces of the cerebellum (Zazulia). At the level of the midbrain, the basilar artery bifurcates into the two posterior cerebral arteries (Zazulia). As they circle the brainstem, these two arteries give off penetrating branches to the midbrain and thalamus and then divide into branches that supply the occipital lobes as well as the medial and undersurfaces of the temporal lobes (Zazulia). One of the branches of the posterior cerebral artery, the calcarine artery, is of special significance because it is the main supplier of blood for the visual area of the cortex (Lundy-Ekman, 2007).

Communicating Arteries

The right and left carotid vessels connect with each other when they enter the brain, each sending out a small lateral branch that meets in the space between them. These are the anterior communicating arteries. They also branch backward to join with the right and left posterior cerebral arteries, called the posterior communicating arteries. This communicating vascular interchange is known as the circle of Willis, which is pictured in Figure 9.1. It protects the brain should one of the four major supplying arteries coming up through the neck be blocked (Zazulia, 2002). This important anatomical feature is named for Dr. Thomas Willis and was first described in the mid-17th century (Zazulia). Starting from the midline anteriorly, the circle consists of the anterior communicating, anterior cerebral, internal carotid, posterior communicating, and

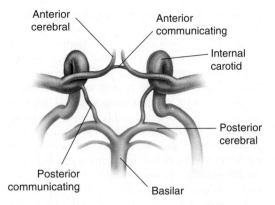

Figure 9.1 Circle of Willis.

posterior cerebral arteries, from which it continues to the starting point in reverse order (Zazulia). When one major vessel supplying the brain is slowly occluded, either within the circle of Willis or proximal to it, the normally small communicating arteries may slowly enlarge to compensate for the occlusion (Lundy-Ekman, 2007). This system is imperfect, however, and it often fails to prevent strokes. In many individuals, the same atherosclerotic processes that caused a stroke also may damage communicating arteries. In addition, only about one-fourth of strokes are caused by a blockage of the major neck vessels (Qureshi et al., 2007). For approximately one-third of the population, the communicating artery may be insufficient or even absent (Zazulia). Such anomalies are more common in those who have strokes than in the general population and may be linked to increased risk of stroke in persons who also have **atherosclerosis** (van Kooij, Hendrikse, Benders, de Vries, & Groenendaal, 2010).

ETIOLOGY

Ischemic Stroke

This is the most common type of stroke accounting for 80% of cases (Fulgham et al., 2004). Cerebral infarction, or brain tissue death, results when circulation to an area of the brain is obstructed, with the result being ischemia. Ischemic strokes are classified as thrombotic, embolic, or lacunar strokes. The damaged area has two components: the tissues that have died as a result of blood supply loss and the peripheral area in which there may be temporary dysfunction as a result of edema. Edematous brain tissue sometimes recovers slowly and gradually, resulting in a reappearance of function after a period of 4 to 5 months (Fulgham et al.). In the past, prognoses for functional recovery have been limited to this time frame. However, recent research offers promising evidence that recovery is possible months and even years post stroke

(Hankey et al., 2007). Explanations focus on the brain's ability to reroute neural pathways, a phenomenon known as neural plasticity (Johansson, 2000; Takatsuru et al., 2009).

The actual physiologic events that follow an ischemic stroke occur in characteristic steps. First, the membrane surrounding each affected neuron leaks potassium (a mineral necessary for producing electrical impulses) and adenosine triphosphate (ATP, an energy-producing biochemical found in the body). Fluid quickly accumulates between the blood vessel and neuron, making it difficult for oxygen and nutrients to pass from the bloodstream into the damaged neuron. The initial injury produces a vicious circle in which more cellular injury results. Irreversible cell death will occur in 5 to 10 minutes if oxygen and nutrients are unable to reach them from the bloodstream or in a slightly longer period if blood flow is only partially interrupted. These dead cells form a zone of infarction that will not regenerate (Zazulia, 2002).

Downstream from the infarct zone is a zone of injury (penumbra) (Gonzalez, 2006; Bose A, Henkes H, and Alfke, K. (2008). This area may be served by collateral blood vessels and is capable of returning to normal functioning. A third area that reacts differently to the stroke process may also exist. In this area of hyperemia, the blood vessels are congested and swollen and also may have the potential for recovery.

The presence of these two zones, the regions of penumbra and hyperemia, may serve to minimize the total area of infarction. However, they do present problems for treatment because interventions that benefit one region may not help the other (Gonzalez, 2006; Bose, 2008).

Thrombosis

Cerebral thrombosis occurs when a blood clot forms in one of the arteries supplying the brain, causing vascular obstruction at the point of its formation. The size and location of the infarct depends on which vessel is occluded and the amount of **collateral circulation**. Thrombosis occurs most frequently in blood vessels that have already been damaged by atherosclerosis (Ho, Huang, Khor, & Lin, 2008).

Atherosclerosis is a gradual degenerative disease of the blood vessel walls. It is a pathologic process rather than a normal effect of human aging (Ho et al.). Rough, irregular fatty deposits form within the intima and inner media of the arteries and often lead to the generation of a **thrombus** or blood clot. This is the most common cause of stroke, with stenosis or narrowing of the blood vessels, resulting in much fewer cases (Ho et al., 2008). Large-vessel atherosclerosis accounts for 60% of ischemic stroke (University of Medicine and Dentistry of New Jersey, 2010). Because the body's blood vessels have a

significant reserve capacity, ischemic strokes do not usually occur until the vessel is two-thirds blocked (University of Medicine and Dentistry of New Jersey, 2010). The impact of atherosclerosis on the vascular system is considerable; it is also a major risk factor for heart disease.

To understand the process that produces a mass of degenerated, thickened material (plaque) called **atheromas**, imagine a glue bottle that has been allowed to collect the residuals of dried glue. The more clogged the cap of the bottle becomes, the more difficult it is for the glue to flow through. Squeezing the glue through the opening can push already dried glue more firmly against the opening. The opening will become smaller and smaller until it closes completely or bursts from the increased pressure.

In the cerebral circulation, atherosclerosis and thrombus formation are most likely to occur in areas where blood vessels turn or divide, such as the origins of the internal carotid artery and the middle cerebral artery and the junction of the vertebral and basilar arteries (van Kooij et al., 2010).

Cerebral thrombosis often causes stuttering or progressive symptoms that occur over several hours or days. Onset during sleep is common. Often a patient notices mild arm numbness at night and then awakens the next morning with paralysis. **Transient ischemic attacks (TIAs)** precede actual infarction about half the time (van Kooij et al., 2010).

Lacunar Strokes/Penetrating Artery Disease

Lacunar strokes are small infarcts, usually lying in the deep brain structures, such as the basal ganglia, thalamus, pons, internal capsule, and deep white matter (Porter & Kaplan, 2004). Approximately 25% of ischemic strokes are the result of damage to these deep structures (Porter & Kaplan). Within a few months of onset of a lacunar stroke, a small cavity ("lacune" in French) is left (Porter & Kaplan).

Lacunar strokes result from an occlusion of small branches of larger cerebral arteries—middle cerebral, posterior cerebral, basilar, and, to a lesser extent, anterior cerebral and vertebral arteries (Jackson & Sudlow). Lacunar infarcts range in size from 2 to 15 mm (Porter & Kaplan, 2004; Jackson & Sudlow, 2005). Because of their small size, minimal neurologic symptoms are often present, and many such strokes go undetected. Recent findings indicate, however, that long-term prognosis is not good for lacunar strokes, and the recovery rate is similar to that for other types of stroke (Jackson & Sudlow). Typically, lacunar strokes produce purely motor deficits (weakness or **ataxia**), purely sensory deficits, or a combination of sensory and motor deficits (Jackson & Sudlow). Symptoms do not usually include aphasia, changes in cognition or personality, loss of consciousness, homonymous **hemianopsia**, or seizures (Jackson & Sudlow). The most consistently identified risk factor for lacunar infarction is hypertension, and treatment is aimed at controlling it (Jackson & Sudlow).

Embolism

Embolism occurs when a clot that has formed elsewhere (thrombus) breaks off (embolus), travels up the blood stream until it reaches an artery too small to pass through, and blocks the artery (Montaner et al., 2008). At this point, the effects of the embolus are similar to those produced by thrombosis. Embolic materials that travel to the arteries of the brain can originate from many sources, including the aortic arch and arteries arising from it, the extracranial carotid and vertebral arteries, and thrombi in the heart. Cardiac source emboli occur in approximately 20% of ischemic strokes and are referred to as cardiogenic (Cho et al., 2009). Many cardiac abnormalities can give rise to a cerebral embolism, including atrial fibrillation, coronary artery disease, valvular heart disease, and arrhythmias. Cardiac surgery is also a cause (Cho et al., 2009). The middle cerebral artery is by far the most common destination of cardiac emboli, followed by the posterior cerebral artery (Cho et al., 2009).

In contrast to thrombotic strokes, embolic strokes typically occur during daytime activity (Montaner, 2008). The embolism can be precipitated by a sudden movement, or even a sneeze, which raises blood pressure and dislodges the clot. Clinical symptoms are usually maximal at onset, but in some cases the neurologic symptoms improve or stabilize somewhat, then worsen as the embolus moves and blocks a more distal artery. A history of TIAs is rare. Seizures may be associated with embolic strokes.

Hemorrhagic Stroke

Approximately 20% of strokes are hemorrhagic (Amarenco, Bogousslavsky, Caplan, Donnan, & Hennerici, 2009). Hemorrhagic strokes are caused by a rupture in a blood vessel or an aneurysm, with resultant bleeding into or around cerebral tissue. An **aneurysm** is a bulging or outpouching of a wall of an artery as a result of weakness in the vessel wall; it is prone to rupture at any time (Mayo Clinic Staff, 2009). While fatality rates for hemorrhagic strokes are higher than for ischemic strokes, recent findings indicate that patients often make a better recovery after a hemorrhagic stroke (Amarenco et al., 2009). Hemorrhagic strokes are more common in young people than ischemic strokes as the vessel wall anomaly is often

congenital. There are two types of hemorrhagic strokes. An intracerebral hemorrhage refers to bleeding directly into brain substance, whereas a subarachnoid hemorrhage is bleeding occurring within the brain's surrounding membranes and cerebrospinal fluid (CSF) (Feigin, Lawes, Bennet, Barker-Collo, & Parag, 2009). These two types of hemorrhage differ in incidence, etiology, clinical signs, and treatment.

Intracerebral Hemorrhages

Intracerebral hemorrhage results in bleeding directly into the brain and accounts for a high percentage of deaths because of stroke (Feigin et al., 2009). It may occur in any part of the brain and is most commonly linked to hypertension. Other causes include blood vessel abnormalities, such as **arteriovenous** malformations (AVMs) or aneurysms, or trauma (Locksley, 2010). Release of blood into brain tissue and surrounding edema will then disrupt the function of that particular brain region (Locksley, 2010). Blood irritates the brain tissue and causes swelling, or it may form a mass called a **hematoma**. In either case the increased pressure on brain tissues can rapidly destroy them. Factors that increase the risk of intracerebral hemorrhage include blood and bleeding disorders such as hemophilia, sickle cell anemia, and leukemia; use of anticoagulants; and liver disease (Porter & Kaplan, 2004).

Clinical signs of intracerebral hemorrhage are usually focal; that is, unlike cerebral infarcts, hemorrhagic bleeds do not follow the anatomic distribution of blood vessels but move spherically through the tissue planes (Locksley, 2010). Typically they develop suddenly, often during activity (Amarenco et al., 2009). While extremely small hemorrhages may go undetected, a large hematoma causes headache, vomiting, convulsions, and decreased levels of alertness (Ohwaki et al., 2004).

Stupor and coma are common signs of very large hemorrhages and indicate a poor prognosis, especially among individuals over 85 (Ohwaki et al., 2004). Nevertheless, recovery is possible.

Cerebral injury caused by intracerebral bleeding is a result of the damaging effect that the abnormal presence of blood has on the neurons. In addition to the irritant of the blood, abnormal pressure on neurons distorts their normal architecture. It also prevents oxygen and nutrients from passing to the cells from the blood stream. Eventually, bleeding will stop and a hard clot will form. During a period of months, the clot slowly recedes, breaks down, and is absorbed by the body's white blood cells (Zhao, Grotta, Gonzales, & Aronowski, 2009). If not damaged by increased pressure, the tissues irritated by the blood may heal, leading to a positive outcome, perhaps even full recovery (Zhao et al., 2009).

Subarachnoid Hemorrhages

Subarachnoid hemorrhages account for about 5% to 10% of all strokes and are slightly more common in women (Ohwaki et al.). About 95% are caused by the leakage of blood from aneurysms (Ohwaki et al.). A combination of congenital and degenerative factors, usually at the points of origin or bifurcations of arteries, can precipitate formation of an aneurysm (Ohwaki et al., 2004). Blood may break through the weak point of the aneurysm at any time and, because of the force of arterial pressure, spread quickly into the CSF surrounding the brain. A subarachnoid hemorrhage also may be caused by bleeding from an AVM, which is an abnormal collection of vessels near the surface of the brain. Other less common causes of subarachnoid hemorrhages are hemophilia, excessive anticoagulation therapy, and trauma to the skull and brain (Amarenco et al., 2009). The extravasated, or escaped, blood irritates the meninges, and intracranial pressure is increased owing to extra fluid in the closed cranial cavity. This can lead to headache, vomiting, and an altered state of consciousness. Sleepiness, stupor, agitation, restlessness, and actual coma are various manifestations of reduced consciousness. Headaches are usually severe and are described as the worst in the patient's life (Stary, 2004). Because the bleeding takes place around the brain and not in the actual brain substance, motor, sensory, or visual abnormalities on one side of the body usually are not seen. Computed tomography (CT) scans (see later in this chapter) are the most reliable tool for detecting subarachnoid hemorrhage (Stary). If results are inconclusive, lumbar puncture with analysis of the CSF is the most reliable method of diagnosing subarachnoid hemorrhage (Stary).

INCIDENCE AND PREVALENCE

Stroke is the third leading cause of death in the United States, surpassed only by heart disease and cancer (Chiuve et al., 2008). Stroke, the most common cause of disability, is the most widespread diagnosis among clients seen by occupational therapists for the treatment of physically disabled adults (Legg et al., 2003). An estimated 600,000 to 730,000 people in the United States suffer an episode each year, and about 4.5 million stroke survivors are alive today (Xie et al., 2006). Approximately 50% to 70% of people regain functional independence after a stroke; however, 15% to 30% of those who survive an ischemic or hemorrhagic stroke suffer some permanent disability (Xie et al., 2007). Of the two main types, hemorrhagic strokes occur much less frequently (20% of all strokes) than ischemic strokes, which account for about 80% of all strokes (Xie et al., 2007). Depression affects approximately one-third of stroke survivors (Hackett et al., 2005;

Townend, Tinson, Kwan, & Sharpe, 2010). Impact on family and caregivers is also enormous. If adequate social services and support are not available, caregivers assume the burden for functional tasks that the patient is unable to perform (McCullagh, Brigstocke, Donaldson, & Kalra, 2005).

Despite these grim statistics, there is some good news. With the exception of subarachnoid hemorrhage, between 1950 and 1990 all types of strokes have shown a significantly decreased incidence (Chiuve et al., 2008). This may be partly the result of increased control of risk factors such as hypertension, diabetes mellitus, and heart disease (Chiuve et al.). Individuals who have had a stroke now live almost twice as long; interestingly, one study even reported that long-term survivors appeared to be less depressed than the comparison group (Patel, McKevitt, Lawrence, Rudd, & Wolfe, 2007). Fewer people now die of stroke, notwithstanding the continuing debate as to whether this decline is the result of the occurrence of fewer strokes or better medical treatment (Carandang et al., 2006). However, it should be noted that the absolute number of strokes occurring in the United States is rising, probably a result of the aging of the population (Carandang et al.). Moreover, dramatic increases in obesity, among children as well as adults, offer grave cause for concern, given the close links determined between obesity and vascular disease (Lawlor & Leon, 2005).

Stroke in young children occurs in about 2.5 cases per 100,000 children per year as compared to 100 cases per 100,000 in the adult population (Lawlor & Leon, 2005). It is more frequent in children younger than 2 years of age. The effects of stroke among children are similar to those described in adults. Although the etiology of pediatric stroke is often unknown, the most common known cause is a congenital defect affecting the structure of the heart (Lawlor & Leon). Sickle-cell disease, which affects blood-clotting mechanisms, and genetic disorders are the next most commonly known causes. Forty-five percent of pediatric stroke patients experience neurologic defects throughout their lives; however, one-third of children with strokes display no symptoms afterward (Steinlin, Roellin, & Schroth, 2004).

RISK FACTORS

A number of risk factors are associated with the likelihood of stroke and resemble those for heart disease. This is not surprising, considering that atherosclerosis is an underlying cause for both conditions. While some of these risk factors are inborn or otherwise unavoidable, many are related to lifestyle and behavioral choices. Adopting healthy eating and exercise patterns early in life is especially important for individuals who are genetically at risk, although everyone can benefit. Regular visits to a family physician are important.

- Ethnicity—although all minority groups are at risk, stroke death rates are much higher for African Americans than for whites: Data from 2005 indicated that out of 100,000 people there were 87 deaths from stroke for black males and 78 for black females, compared to 59 for white males and 58 for white females (Bravata et al., 2005). Recent data also indicate that blacks living in the South have a greater risk of dying from stroke than those who live in the northern states (Voeks et al., 2008).
- Age—risk for stroke increases with age, especially after age 65. People with high blood pressure and who exhibit the other risk factors listed in this chapter are increasingly vulnerable as they age. Younger people are not immune, either: Approximately 28% of strokes occur in individuals younger than age 65 (Bhat et al., 2008).
- Heredity—a family history of stroke, particularly on the father's side, increases one's risk (Bhat et al., 2008). Genetic factors account for 7% to 20% of cases of subarachnoid hemorrhage, and some researchers recommend that people with more than one close relative who suffered a hemorrhagic stroke be screened for aneurysms (Locksley, 2010).
- Obesity—being overweight is a known risk factor for hypertension and diabetes mellitus and also is associated with stroke. Weight that is centered in the abdomen (so-called apple shape) has a particularly high association with stroke as well as heart disease, while individuals whose weight is distributed around the hips are less at risk (Suk et al., 2003). A sedentary lifestyle is associated with rising levels of obesity and has been implicated in occurrence of strokes as well as hypertension (Bhat et al., 2008).
- Hypertension—called the "silent disease," hypertension has long been acknowledged as the most significant controllable risk factor for both stroke and heart attack (Bhat et al., 2008). Hypertension occurs in 25% to 40% of the U.S. population (Bhat et al., 2008). Symptoms of hypertension are not clearly identifiable: an occasional headache, dizziness, or light-headedness, which may indicate hypertension, can easily be attributed to other factors. Chronically elevated blood pressure exerts pressure on cerebral vessels, often resulting in lacunar infarctions or intracerebral hemorrhage (Jackson & Sudlow, 2005; Amarenco et al., 2009). Hypertension also has been implicated in the atherosclerotic process because it drives fatty substances into the arterial walls, making them brittle, narrowed, and hardened (Zazulia, 2002). The impact of hypertension increases with age (Bhat et al., 2008). For these reasons it is crucial to have regular blood pressure checks. Hypertension can be controlled through drug therapy, stress reduction, dietary control, and regular exercise—treatments that all require patient compliance for maximum effectiveness.

- Smoking—smoking doubles the risk of stroke (Bhat et al., 2008). Quitting smoking reduces the likelihood of stroke, and there is some evidence to suggest that 5 years after quitting smoking, individuals lower their risk of having a stroke to nearly that of people of who have never smoked (Zazulia, 2002).
- TIAs—a TIA is considered an important risk factor for an impending stroke. Approximately 30% of all patients who have had a TIA are at risk of having a stroke within 2 years. This risk is greatest in the first month, so it is important to seek medical intervention quickly (Fulgham et al., 2004).
- Geographic location—the highest death rates from strokes in the United States are in North and South Carolina, Georgia, northern Florida, Alabama, Mississippi, and Tennessee. Specific pockets of high death rates in Texas, Oklahoma, and all of the Hawaiian Islands have been noted (Voeks et al., 2008). This geographical strip, often termed the "stroke belt," is the source of numerous studies on environmental, cultural, or other geographically determined risk factors. A person who grows up in a high-risk area and then moves to a lower-risk area as an adult continues to carry the greater likelihood of having a stroke. This has led to the speculation that the causes may be diet related, cultural, or possibly even related to water supply or altitude (Glymour, Avendaño, & Berkman, 2007).
- Diabetes mellitus—this disease is more common in stroke patients than in a normal population of similar age (Lees & Walters, 2005). Having diabetes increases the risk of stroke by two to three times, as diabetics have a tendency to form blood clots (Lees & Walters). Men are more vulnerable than women (Lees & Walters).
- Oral contraceptives—women who have taken birth control pills, especially those with a high estrogen content, have an increased risk for stroke as they become older. Smoking while taking the pill further increases the risk (Slooter et al., 2005).
- Hyperlipidemia—including elevated triglycerides and "bad" cholesterol has long been suspected to be a risk factor for stroke (Milionis et al., 2005). Its role in CVA has been confirmed by several recent studies (Milionis et al.). Cholesterol levels should be monitored, and adults are encouraged to know their cholesterol counts. Dietary changes are effective in lowering cholesterol levels in some individuals; a class of drugs known as statins is also effective but may have side effects (Trubelja, Vaughan, & Coplan, 2005).

- Asymptomatic carotid bruits—bruit is an abnormal sound or murmur heard when a stethoscope is placed over the carotid artery. This slushing noise indicates turbulent blood, often caused by a significant degree of stenosis. Carotid bruit clearly indicates increased stroke risk. Complete occlusion of the carotid artery sometimes follows, resulting in stroke (Bhat et al., 2008).

- Prior stroke—risk of stroke for a person who has already suffered a stroke is increased four to eight times (Fang et al., 2005).

- Heart disease—diseased heart (whether it be chronic disease, acute heart attacks, or prosthetic heart valves) increases the risk of stroke. Independent of hypertension, people with heart disease have more than twice the risk of stroke than people with normally functioning hearts (Ohira et al., 2006). Atrial fibrillation, a condition in which the heart produces an irregular rhythm, is also a known risk factor for stroke (Fang et al., 2005).

- Infections and inflammation—inflammation occurring with various infections, often mild, has been associated with stroke. A study in 2005 indicated that periodontal (gum) disease is associated with a 20% high risk for ischemic stroke and heart disease and that the risk may be even greater in adults under the age of 65 (Beck & Offenbacher, 2005). Research is under way to determine whether other infections that produce arterial inflammation can lead to stroke or heart disease. For example, chronic infection with *Chlamydia pneumoniae*, which causes mild pneumonia in adults, has been linked with higher risk for stroke (Elkind et al., 2006b).

- Alcohol and drug abuse—numerous studies indicate that moderate consumption of alcohol decreases the risk of stroke and heart disease; however, excessive consumption and total abstinence are associated with higher risk (Elkind et al., 2006a). Cocaine and methamphetamine abuse are major factors in the incidence of stroke in young adults (Westover, McBride, & Haley, 2007). Use of anabolic steroids for bodybuilding is also associated with increased risk of stroke (Santamarina, Besocke, Romano, Loli, & Gonorazky, 2008).

- Sleep apnea—it is a common disorder in which the throat becomes obstructed during sleep, interfering with normal breathing and sleep. Sleep apnea is worsened by obesity and may contribute to the narrowing of the carotid artery. Sleep apnea is currently thought to increase the risk of stroke three- to sixfold (Arzt, Young, Finn, Skatrud, & Bradley, 2005).

Of these many risk factors, several can be controlled by changes in lifestyle, including elevated blood cholesterol and lipids, cigarette smoking, use of oral contraceptives, excessive drinking of alcohol, and obesity. Some, such as hypertension, heart disease, TIAs, carotid bruits, and polycythemia, can be controlled by medical intervention. Factors that cannot be changed are age, sex, race, family history, diabetes mellitus, and a prior stroke. The potential benefits of all medical and surgical interventions currently available for cerebrovascular disease pale in comparison to what can be achieved through risk factor control (Chiuve et al., 2008). Understanding and awareness of these risk factors for stroke is an important first step in reducing the likelihood of having stroke.

SIGNS AND SYMPTOMS

Neurologic Effects of Stroke

An occlusion that causes a serious stroke can occur anywhere in the extracranial or intracranial system, but the most common site is in the distribution of the middle cerebral artery and its branches in the cerebrum. The majority of cerebral strokes occur in one or the other cerebral hemisphere, but not both (Wintermark et al., 2002). It is important to note that even in individuals with the same neurologic deficit, the impact of disability is different, depending on the individual's life situation.

Stroke Warning Signs

To educate the public, the American Heart Association and National Stroke Association distribute pamphlets listing the warning signs of an impending serious stroke (American Heart Association [AHA], 2010). Many hospitals and community clinics also distribute this information. These include

- Sudden numbness or weakness of the face, arm, or leg, especially on one side of the body
- Sudden confusion, trouble speaking or understanding
- Sudden trouble seeing in one or both eyes
- Sudden trouble walking, dizziness, loss of balance, or coordination
- Sudden severe headache with no known cause

Some general medical symptoms related to type of stroke were discussed under Etiology. Signs and symptoms also depend on the size and location of the injury, and neurologists can often predict location by the symptoms the individual displays. However, it is important to remember that a stroke is complex, and each individual may experience a unique constellation of symptoms. Relying on stereotypical models of stroke leads to generalized and often inappropriate therapy.

In addition to the above list, it is important to be aware that symptoms resulting from a partial reduction or temporary change in the blood flow to the brain are extremely important warning signs for stroke (Fogle et al., 2008). Several of these conditions are discussed below.

Transient Ischemic Attacks

TIAs result from a temporary blockage of the blood supply to the brain. The symptoms occur rapidly and last for <24 hours. Seventy-five percent of TIAs last <5 minutes. The specific signs and symptoms depend on the portion of the brain affected but may include fleeting blindness in one eye, hemiparesis, **hemiplegia**, aphasia, dizziness, double vision, and staggering. Carotid artery disease and vertebral basilar artery disease may lead to TIAs (Mattace-Raso et al., 2006). The main distinction between TIAs and stroke is the short duration of the symptoms and the lack of permanent neurologic damage. People who have had TIAs are 9 1/2 times more likely to have a stroke than those of the same age and sex who have never had a TIA (Mattace-Raso et al., 2006). Without preventive treatment, a third of those who suffer TIAs will go on to have a stroke within 5 years (Mattace-Raso et al., 2006). Thus, it is crucial to detect the cause of a TIA and begin appropriate intervention promptly (Fogle et al., 2008).

Small Strokes (RINDs)

In some cases, the symptoms of a TIA may last longer than 24 hours. If they last a day or more and then completely resolve or if they leave only minor neurologic deficits, they are called small strokes or lengthy TIAs (Jackson & Sudlow, 2005). Often the remaining neurologic deficits are barely noticeable. Like TIAs, however, these small strokes are important warning signs that a more serious CVA may occur (Fogle et al., 2008). A small stroke that completely resolves is called a reversible ischemic neurologic deficit (RIND). An episode that lasts more than 72 hours and leaves some minor neurologic impairments is called a partially reversible ischemic neurologic deficit (PRIND). The mechanism of injury in RIND and PRIND is the same as that for a stroke or TIA. Like ischemic strokes, RINDs typically occur in the morning; since blood pressure is low during sleep, sudden increases in blood pressure upon arising may cause problems (Metoki et al., 2006).

Many small strokes are not reported to a medical practitioner, which makes the exact frequency of occurrence of these strokes difficult to determine. It is important to recognize the symptoms of a small stroke so that it can be treated early, reducing the risk of more permanent injury.

Subclavian Steal Syndrome

This is a rare condition caused by a narrowing of the subclavian artery that runs under the clavicle. Symptoms occur when the arm on the side of the narrowed vessel is exercised. Usually, movement of the arm produces light-headedness, numbness, and weakness. Other neurologic symptoms also may be present. In this syndrome, blood is "stolen" from the brain and instead is delivered to the exercised arm. It is a warning sign that advanced atherosclerosis may be present in the arteries throughout the body, including the cerebral arteries (Bicknell, Subramanian, & Wolfe, 2004).

DIAGNOSIS

The diagnosis of stroke requires knowledge of the incidence of the different types of stroke and awareness of the presence of the risk factors mentioned above. Symptoms must be carefully noted from the patient or, if the patient is too ill, frightened, or confused, from the family (Hand, Kwan, Lindley, Dennis, & Wardlaw, 2006). Neurologists, neurosurgeons, and some internists are the specialists usually involved in this acute diagnostic phase of treatment (Hand et al., 2006). A number of diagnostic techniques are utilized to distinguish stroke from other potential causes of observed symptoms and to assist in determining the location of lesions (Kidwell & Warach, 2003).

The physical examination of the patient with a suspected stroke or TIA includes a search for possible cardiac sources of emboli by listening to the heart and arteries of the neck. Also useful in the determination of cardiac-source emboli are electrocardiography, echocardiography, and monitoring for arrhythmias. In addition to cardiac testing, various neuroimaging techniques (see below) and analysis of blood and CSF may be performed (Feldmann et al., 2007). A neurologic examination assists in determining the neurologic disability and usually includes evaluation of higher cortical function (memory and language), level of alertness, reflexes, visual and oculomotor system, behavior, and gait (Feldmann et al.).

Other diagnostic methods include noninvasive studies of blood vessels and invasive techniques requiring injection of dye into the arterial system, for example.

COURSE AND PROGNOSIS

Strokes result in anoxic damage to nervous tissue that causes various neurologic deficits, depending on where the blood supply was lost. If neuronal cell death occurs, it is considered irreparable and permanent, as no way has yet been found to regenerate nerve cells (Yuan, Lipinski, & Degterev, 2009). However, the nervous system has a high level of plasticity, especially during early development, and individual differences in neural connections and learned behaviors play a major role in functional recovery. No two brains can be expected to be structurally or functionally identical (Carmichael, 2006). Spontaneous recovery may occur as edema subsides or viable neurons reactivate. Recovery also may occur with physiologic reorganization of neural connections or developmental strategies. Any injury brings different factors into play, affecting axonal and dendritic sprouting or collateral rearrangement, synaptic formation, the excitability of neurons, "substitution of parallel channels," and "mobilization of redundant capacity" (Huang, Shen, & Duong, 2010). Recovery from neurologic deficits thus depends on the etiology and size of the infarct (Carmichael). Approximately 90% of neurologic recovery occurs within 3 months, with the rest occurring over a more extended time (Rossini, Calautti, Pauri, & Baron, 2003). It should be noted that recovery from hemorrhagic strokes proceeds more slowly, however (Rossini et al., 2003).

Accuracy in the prediction of function or rate of return in a given stroke patient is difficult because of individual variability of anatomy and extent of brain damage as well as differences in types of CVA, learning ability, premorbid personality and intelligence, and motivation (Rossini et al., 2003). Generally, the prognosis for recovery of function is greater in young clients, possibly because the young brain is more plastic or because the young are generally in better physical condition.

Secondary complications are important to recovery and rehabilitation and may actually be more disabling than the stroke itself (McLean, 2004). These complications, are discussed in this chapter and include depression, seizures, infection, bowel/bladder incontinence, thromboembolism, shoulder subluxation, painful shoulder, shoulder-hand syndrome, abnormal muscle tone, and **associated reactions** and movements.

Individuals with good sensation, minimal **spasticity**, some selective motor control, and no fixed contractures seem to make the greatest improvements in functional abilities. If an individual has no concept of the affected side and cannot localize stimuli to the affected side or if he or she has fecal or urinary incontinence, the outlook for independence is generally poor. Some individuals may continue to have strokes, complicating recovery (McLean, 2004).

Left-Sided Cerebral Injuries: Middle Cerebral Artery

The left cerebral hemisphere controls most functions on the right side of the body because of the **decussation** of motor fibers (decussation of the pyramids) in the medulla. These fibers that cross, or decussate to the opposite side, form the lateral corticospinal tract. The rest of the fibers descend ipsilaterally, forming the anterior corticospinal tract (Wintermark et al., 2002). The proportion of crossing fibers varies from person to person, averaging about 85% (Wintermark et al.).

A CVA in the region of the middle cerebral artery in the left cerebral hemisphere may produce the following symptoms:

1. Loss of voluntary movement and coordination on the right side of the face, trunk, and extremities.
2. Impaired sensation, including temperature discrimination, pain, and proprioception on the right side (hemianesthesia).
3. Language deficits, called aphasia, in which the patient may be unable to speak or understand speech, writing, or gestures. The breakdown of language function is complex; the many types of aphasia will be discussed later in this chapter.
4. Problems with articulation of speech because of disturbances in muscle control of the lips, mouth, tongue, and vocal cords (**dysarthria**).
5. Blind spots in the visual field, usually on the right side.
6. Slow and cautious personality.
7. Memory deficits for recent or past events (Boyd & Winstein, 2003).

Right-Sided Cerebral Injuries: Middle Cerebral Artery

The right cerebral hemisphere controls most of the functions on the left side of the body and also is responsible for spatial sensation, perception, and judgment. Injury to the middle cerebral artery of the right cerebral hemisphere may produce a combination of the following deficits:

1. Weakness (hemiparesis) or paralysis (hemiplegia) on the left side of the body (face, arm, trunk, and leg)
2. Impairment of sensation (touch, pain, temperature, and proprioception) on the left side of the body
3. Spatial and perceptual deficits
4. **Unilateral neglect**, in which the patient neglects the left side of the body or the left side of the environment
5. Dressing **apraxia**, in which the patient is unable to relate the articles of clothes to the body (Walker, Walker, & Sunderland, 2003)
6. Defective vision in the left halves of visual fields or left homonymous hemianopsia in which there is defective vision in each eye (the temporal half of the left eye and the nasal half of the right eye)
7. Impulsive behavior, quick and imprecise movements, and errors of judgment (Boyd & Winstein, 2003)

Anterior Cerebral Artery Stroke

The territory of the anterior cerebral artery is rarely infarcted because of the side-to-side communication provided by the anterior communicating artery in the circle of Willis (Boyd & Winstein, 2003). Symptoms of an anterior cerebral artery stroke include

1. Paralysis of the lower extremity, usually more severe than that of the upper extremity, contralateral to the occluded vessel
2. Loss of sensation in the contralateral toes, foot, and leg
3. Loss of conscious control of bowel or bladder
4. Balance problems in sitting, standing, and walking
5. Lack of spontaneity of emotion, whispered speech, or loss of all communication
6. Memory impairment or loss (Boyd & Winstein, 2003)

Vertebrobasilar Stroke

The vertebrobasilar system of arteries supplies blood primarily to the posterior portions of the brain, including the brainstem, cerebellum, thalamus, and parts of the occipital and temporal lobes. This posterior circulation is not divided into right and left halves, as in the anterior circulation (Coward et al., 2007). An occlusion here might produce

1. A variety of visual disturbances, including impaired coordination of the eyes
2. Impaired temperature sensation
3. Impaired ability to read and/or name objects
4. Vertigo and dizziness
5. Disturbances in balance when standing or walking (ataxia)
6. Paralysis of the face, limbs, or tongue
7. Clumsy movements of the hands
8. Difficulty judging distance when trying to coordinate limb movements (dysmetria)
9. Drooling and difficulty swallowing (**dysphagia**)
10. Localized numbness
11. Loss of memory (Boyd & Winstein, 2003)
12. Drop attacks in which there is a sudden loss of motor and postural control resulting in collapse, but the individual remains conscious (Parry et al., 2009)

TIAs in this area are common in the elderly. The vertebral arteries travel up to the brainstem through a bony channel in the cervical vertebrae. In older adults, osteoarthritis may develop in the cervical bones, causing narrowing of the cervical canal, especially when the head is extended or rotated (Parry et al., 2009).

Wallenberg's Syndrome

Wallenberg's syndrome is a classic brainstem stroke that also is referred to as lateral medullary syndrome (Dietrich et al., 2005). It occurs as the result of an occlusion of a vertebral or cerebellar artery. Strokes in this

area may produce contralateral pain and temperature loss, ipsilateral Horner's syndrome (sinking of the eyeball, ptosis of the upper eyelid, and a dry, cool face on the affected side), ataxia, and facial sensory loss. Ischemia to ipsilateral cranial nerve fibers VIII, IX, and X results in palatal paralysis, hoarseness, dysphagia, and vertigo (Walton & Buono, 2003). There is no significant weakness in this syndrome (Dietrich et al.).

Brainstem strokes often result in coma because of damage to the centers involved with alertness and wakefulness (reticular system) (Parvizi & Damasio, 2003). A hemorrhage into the brainstem area is rare, quickly accompanied by loss of consciousness, and usually fatal. Among patients who survive brainstem stroke, however, recovery is often good (Parvizi & Damasio).

OTHER COMPLICATIONS OF STROKE

Secondary conditions may occur in addition to these deficits. These are important manifestations of the patient's recovery and rehabilitation and may actually be more disabling than the stroke itself (McLean, 2004). It is necessary to be aware of these complications so that they may be prevented.

Seizures

Brain scars that result from stroke may irritate the cortex and cause a spontaneous discharge of nerve impulses that may generalize to a full grand mal convulsion (Vespa et al., 2003). Seizures develop in up to 10% of stroke patients and are more common with embolic than thrombotic infarcts (Vespa et al., 2003). Anticonvulsant drugs are sometimes used in patients with early seizures, but their use is controversial (Camilo & Goldstein, 2004).

Infection

Alteration of swallowing function, aspiration, hypoventilation, and immobility in the stroke patient often lead to pneumonia (Prass, Braun, Dirnagl, Meisel, & Meisel, 2006). Changes in bladder function may lead to bladder distention and urinary tract infection (McLean, 2004). Impaired sensation and inadequate position changes may result in pressure sores (decubitus) and consequent infection of these areas (Turhan, Atalay, & Atabek, 2006).

Thromboembolism

Immobility of the legs and prolonged bed rest often lead to thrombosis of dependent leg veins (MacDougall,

Feliu, Boccuzzi, & Lin, 2006). In **deep vein thrombosis** (DVT), local pain and tenderness may develop in the calf, with some swelling and a slight increase in temperature. If the thrombosis is confined to the calf, it may not be serious. However, if the thrombosis spreads up toward the groin to involve the veins in the pelvis, there is a very real possibility of a clot breaking off into the blood stream. The clot will then travel through the right side of the heart and enter the lungs through the pulmonary arteries, resulting in sudden collapse and death owing to obstruction of the pulmonary arteries (MacDougall et al., 2006). Early mobilization of the patient is of utmost importance in preventing DVT and subsequent pulmonary embolism.

Medications and surgery may make a difference in the prognosis of an individual at risk for, or having had, a CVA.

NEUROIMAGING TECHNIQUES

CT and magnetic resonance imaging (MRI) are invaluable noninvasive tools that depict pathological changes in the brain in patients with stroke (Feldmann et al., 2007). One or the other of these is almost always used at some point for every patient with a suspected stroke. CT and MRI are also capable of showing zones of edema and the shifting of intracranial material (Feldmann et al.). Negative results of these tests may indicate that the ischemia is reversible (Feldmann et al.).

Computed Tomography

CT is a type of radiographic examination that is widely used for analysis of cerebral injury (Chalela et al., 2009). CT scans are employed to differentiate between a hemorrhagic stroke and an ischemic stroke (Chalela et al.). While they are useful in clarifying the location and the mechanism and severity of stroke, they are not particularly sensitive to subtle ischemic changes (Chalela et al.). It is most useful in the diagnosis of stroke caused by hemorrhage; CT findings may even be normal in patients with recent infarction. It is often not diagnostic in patients with TIAs and is not useful for imaging brainstem infarcts (Chalela et al.).

Magnetic Resonance Imaging

MRI is more sensitive than a CT scan and does not expose the patient to radiation. It provides detailed pictures of the brain by using a magnetic field. MRI is particularly helpful in revealing AVMs (Fiebach et al., 2004). It is superior to CT in imaging the cerebellum, brainstem, thalamus, and spinal cord. It also provides better anatomic definition of the injury, but it does not distinguish between hemorrhage, tumor, and infarction as well as a CT scan. (Fiebach et al.).

Positron Emission Tomography

Positron emission tomography (PET) scan is being used experimentally. This scan shows how the brain uses oxygen, glucose, and other nutrients and has increased understanding of the effects of stroke on the brain (De Reuck et al., 2006). Because these imaging techniques are not commonly available, PET scans are seldom used in the management of acute stroke (De Reuck et al.).

NONINVASIVE STUDY OF BLOOD VESSELS

Noninvasive procedures used to evaluate both extracranial and intracranial blood flow include duplex ultrasonography as well as color-flow and transcranial Doppler ultrasound. These techniques can localize and determine the approximate size of the lesions within the arteries (Aaslid, Huber, & Nornes, 2010).

Duplex ultrasonography is useful in detecting the presence and severity of the disease in the common and internal carotid arteries and in the subclavian and vertebral arteries in the neck. This scan can reliably differentiate between minor plaque disease, stenosis, and occlusive lesions. It is an excellent method of monitoring the progression or regression of atherosclerotic disease in the neck (Nederkoorn, van der Graaf, & Hunink, 2003).

Color-flow Doppler ultrasound is used because it is effective in showing lesions of the carotid and vertebral arteries (Aaslid et al., 2010).

Transcranial Doppler ultrasound gives information about pressure and flow in the intracranial arteries. This procedure is useful in monitoring changes in the arterial flow later in the course of the patient's disease (Aaslid et al., 2010).

INVASIVE TECHNIQUES

Cerebral angiography involves radiography of the vascular system of the brain after injecting a dye or other contrast medium into the arterial blood system. Computer-generated images are then produced that can show the entire visible length of cerebral arteries as well as the nature, location, and extent of pathological changes. This technique is now safer than before (<1% incidence of mortality and serious morbidity);

however, it is recommended when noninvasive techniques have failed to yield a conclusive diagnosis or when surgery is being planned or considered (Kaufmann et al., 2007).

Analysis of CSF is helpful in diagnosing subarachnoid hemorrhage. In a lumbar puncture, the subarachnoid space (usually between the third and fourth lumbar vertebrae) is tapped and CSF is withdrawn. Analysis of the pigments in the spinal fluid also can help in estimating the age of the hemorrhage and detecting rebleeding (Bykowski, Latour, & Warach, 2004).

OTHER TECHNIQUES

Other diagnostic techniques used for stroke include electroencephalography, single-photon emission tomography, and special cardiac and coagulation tests that are useful in detecting unusual heart and blood disorders that can bring on a stroke (Petrella, Coleman, & Doraiswamy, 2003). After this diagnostic phase of evaluation, a neurologist will evaluate the brain-damaged person's ability to function. Rehabilitation often will begin at that point to return the patient to the highest possible level of independent functioning (Duncan et al., 2005).

MEDICAL/SURGICAL MANAGEMENT

At present, the treatment of acute stroke is limited to management of the results of the primary event and preventive measures against further injury or occurrence (Zhao et al., 2009).

Much is still unclear about the effectiveness of the routine use of agents to reverse the cause or decrease the effects of stroke (Zhao et al., 2009).

Before the stroke can be treated, it must be accurately identified as either cerebral infarction or cerebral hemorrhage, since interventions that are beneficial with one type of stroke may be potentially dangerous to the other (Zhao et al., 2009).

Therefore, careful and exact diagnosis must be made first. Drug management of CVA is constantly evolving. Common categories of drugs used to minimize the damage of cerebral infarction are described in the following sections.

Antiplatelet Therapy

Aspirin is often prescribed to patients when the vascular lesion is not severely stenotic (Mant et al., 2007). Aspirin has been shown to reduce the risk of further stroke in patients who had suffered TIAs by 15% to 58%

(Mant et al.). It also benefits patients who have had a mild stroke but is not as effective in those with moderate or severe strokes (Sacco et al., 2006). Aspirin is clearly not suitable for patients with cerebral hemorrhage or those at risk of bleeding. It is less successful when used by women as compared with men. Aspirin is relatively safe and inexpensive. Recently published studies have recommended a lower dose of aspirin to reduce harmful side effects (Sacco et al.).

Anticoagulants

These drugs inhibit clotting by interfering with the activity of chemicals in the liquid portion of blood that are essential for the coagulation process (Mant et al., 2007). Short-term (2 to 3 weeks) heparin therapy is prescribed for patients with complete blockages of large arteries, as heparin is effective in preventing the formation of emboli (Diener et al., 2006). For longer-term treatment (1 to 3 months), the drug warfarin may be used to prevent blockages in areas that cannot be treated by surgery (Mant et al.).

Thrombolytics

Thrombolytic therapy (t-PA), used for dissolution of an occluding thrombus, is frequently applied in the acute treatment of myocardial infarction as well as in the treatment of stroke. It is effective before extensive brain infarction has occurred, so it is appropriate only in stroke patients whose arterial damage has been identified early (Thomalla et al., 2006). The potential benefit must be weighed against reperfusion damage, a bleeding tendency, and the possibility of reocclusion (Amarenco, G., Easton, J., Sacco, R., & Teal, P., 2008). The Food and Drug Administration has approved the use of t-PA for the treatment of acute stroke within 3 hours of onset (Gurm et al., 2008). One study reported that patients treated with t-PA were 30% to 50% more likely to have minimal or no disability 3 months after the onset of symptoms (Thomalla et al.).

Surgical Interventions

In some cases, surgical treatment may be the best choice for the patient. The neurosurgeon must carefully consider many factors before surgery is performed, including the patient's overall health and life expectancy. Carotid **endarterectomy** is among the most commonly performed vascular surgeries in the United States (Gurm et al., 2008).

During the procedure, the diseased vessel is opened, the clot is removed, and an artificial graft is put in place (Porter & Kaplan, 2004). Carotid endarterectomy is a treatment option for patients with more than 50% stenosis of the carotid artery ipsilateral to the affected hemisphere (Porter & Kaplan; Bhat, 2008).

Subarachnoid hemorrhages are often caused by ruptured aneurysms or AVMs. Surgical clipping or lesion removal is the most effective treatment of these anomalies. If the patient survives the initial bleeding, the goal of surgery is to correct the problem before bleeding recurs. In intracerebral hemorrhage, small hematomas usually resolve spontaneously (Zhao et al., 2009).

Large hematomas, however, often produce death. Some lesions may expand, causing gradually increasing neurologic signs. These expanding lesions can be drained surgically if they are near the surface of the brain, especially in the cerebral or cerebellar white matter. Generally, hemorrhages are evacuated only if they are large and life threatening or when surgery is necessary to treat an aneurysm, tumor, or AVM (Zhao et al., 2009).

Superficial temporal artery bypass is a new, more delicate surgical therapy for preventing future strokes (Charbel, Meglio, & Amin-Hanjani, 2005). The procedure begins with craniotomy to expose the brain; then a scalp artery is connected to an intracranial artery microsurgically. This operation is extremely challenging to perform and is thus performed less frequently than carotid endarterectomy. Surgeons who do the procedure, however, are enthusiastic about the results and claim that it revascularizes the brain better than endarterectomy (Pinar & Govsa, 2006).

Treatment of Secondary Effects

Specific pathophysiologic sequelae, or outcomes, follow the occurrence of any type of stroke. Treating these secondary effects is crucial to medical and functional recovery. Two of these are cerebral edema and ischemia. Oxygen therapy to reduce hypoxia, vasodilation to improve blood flow through ischemic areas, therapeutic hypertension, and hemodilution therapy are some of the treatments used for ischemia. Hemodilution results in a significant rise in cerebral blood flow and increased oxygen transfer (Vilea & Newell, 2008).

Edema often complicates ischemic strokes and must be controlled, because most deaths during the first week after a massive stroke are caused by extensive cerebral edema and increased intracranial pressure (Treggiari, Walder, Suter, & Romand, 2003). This pressure can displace the cerebrum downward and interfere with the functioning of the midbrain and lower brainstem, which control such basic vital functions as respiration and heart action (Treggiari et al., 2003).

Corticosteroid therapy can cause a significant reduction in interstitial cerebral edema, reducing swelling and improving outcomes after stroke (Thomas et al., 2007). However, a review of the literature indicates that there is no clear basis for evaluating the effect of corticosteroid treatment for people with acute ischemic strokes (Veltkamp et al., 2005).

IMPACT ON OCCUPATIONAL PERFORMANCE

The impact of stroke on an individual is unique and may affect any number of client factors. Deficits in motor, process, and communication skills as well as impaired sensory functions and problems with perceptual processing may be compounded by secondary complications such as infection or depression. Together, these profoundly affect an individual's performance in all areas of occupation: activities of daily living (both basic and instrumental), work, play, leisure, and social participation (Langhorne, 2007).

Sensory Functions

Sensory functions can be affected at the very basic level of awareness and at the point of processing and modulation of sensory input. Loss of protective tactile functions, such as diminished awareness of temperature and pain, is a common concern for those with a CVA. Loss of these functions poses a safety risk. Individuals with proprioceptive dysfunction may show asymmetrical posture, have difficulty maintaining balance, appear to forget affected body parts, be unable to describe position or movement of limbs, and be susceptible to joint damage (Davis & Donnan, 2004). Individuals with a loss of tactile sensation may demonstrate a lack of awareness of body parts simply because they forget what they cannot feel. They are also vulnerable to damage of affected body parts, particularly skin breakdown. Moreover, diminished tactile function hinders resumption of motor activities. Depending on the location of the infarct, individuals may experience diminished vestibular function, which will limit mobility efficiency and safety. Impaired balance may cause difficulties in assuming and maintaining a vertical posture and in automatic adjustments to changes of position and antigravity movement. As a result, individuals demonstrate an asymmetrical posture at rest, leaning or falling to the hemiplegic side during mobility, or fail to use normal protective reactions when falling (Ward, Brown, Thompson, & Frackowiak, 2006).

Defects in visual field functions may impair reading, even in the absence of language dysfunction. For example, patients with right cerebral lesions may find reading difficult or impossible, because visuospatial deficits hinder tracking or following the line of print across the page. Patients with homonymous hemianopsia on either side are unable to respond to people, objects, or the environment on the affected side. They may bump into objects or be startled by their sudden appearance. Individuals experiencing visual inattention have difficulty scanning and shifting their gaze, particularly toward the affected side (Tyson, Hanley, Chillala, Selley, & Tallis, 2008).

Perceptual deficits may be difficult to understand for patient and family alike, but their impact on the patient's ability to resume independent function may be profound. Depending on the location of the lesion, or infarct, such deficits include visual agnosia and visuospatial agnosia—difficulty in understanding the relationship between objects and between self and objects (Zhang, Kedar, Lynn, Newman, & Biousse, 2006). Individuals affected in this manner are unable to find their way in a familiar environment; they cannot trace a route on a map, pick out objects from a cluttered environment, copy drawings or simple construction, and may have difficulty in functional (spatial) tasks, such as dressing and reading a newspaper. **Agnosia** for sounds may also occur, so that the individual cannot understand or confuses nonverbal sounds (Lampinen, 2003; Vignolo, 2006). Another important loss is astereognosis, which affects functional use of the affected hand whenever vision is occluded: Tasks such as finding keys or coins in a pocket or a glass on a bedside table when it is dark may be difficult (Murray, Camen, Gonzalez, Bovet, & Clarke, 2006).

The location of the infarct determines which functions are lost and which remain intact. For example, somatagnosia, in which an individual has no awareness of his or her own body and its condition, is commonly seen in right parietal lobe lesions. Deficits that result from right cerebral injuries often cause unilateral perceptual problems of the left body side and space, such as unilateral inattention. Lesions in the left cerebral hemisphere, however, cause bilateral problems, such as right/left discrimination (Connell, 2008). Impairment of the left parietal lobe results in apraxia, whereby individuals are unable to adjust the movement of their own body parts. Yet impairment of the right parietal lobe causes an inability to adjust the position of external objects. Frontal lobe lesions may result in apraxia, in which sequencing of movement becomes difficult. Apraxic individuals may be unable to carry out a verbal request (for even a simple task such as combing the hair), although often they can perform such tasks automatically (Connell). They may perseverate, that is, persist in purposeless movement, or they may be unable to complete a required sequence of acts, copy gestures, drawings, or carry out simple spatial constructional tasks (Beis et al., 2004).

Motor Functions

Sensory loss seldom occurs in isolation but typically accompanies the loss of motor functions. Motor dysfunction because of stroke usually results in changes in muscle tone that render normal movement impossible. It has been commonly said that hypotonicity (flaccid hemiplegia) gives way to hypertonicity (spastic hemiplegia); occasionally there is progress into a final stage, in which normal movement patterns re-emerge (Kleinman et al., 2007; Formisano et al., 2005).

The muscle tone of individuals with an intact central nervous system operates within a range that permits effective voluntary movement. Normal muscle tone is high enough to stabilize and maintain a person through an activity, while at the same time low enough to allow ease of movement. This variability of tone allows mobility to be superimposed on stability (Formisano et al., 2005).

Abnormal tone may be termed either low or high. Hypotonus, or **flaccidity**, is felt as too little resistance or floppiness. When released, the extremity will drop. At the other extreme, when there is too much resistance, hypertonus, or spasticity, is felt. Spasticity is the result of hyperactive reflexes and loss of moderating or inhibiting influences from higher brain centers (Diserens, 2006; Sommerfeld et al., 2004). Spasticity may be aggravated by pain, emotional upset, or efforts to hurry. Spasticity is never isolated to one muscle group but is always a part of what is known as either an extensor or flexor synergy, that is, a grouping of stereotypical movements. These movement patterns usually consist of a flexion pattern in the arm (scapular retraction and depression, shoulder adduction and internal rotation, elbow flexion, forearm pronation, wrist flexion, finger and thumb flexion and adduction) and an extension pattern in the leg (pelvis rotated back and internal rotation, knee extension, foot plantar flexion and inversion, toe flexion and adduction).

Abnormal tone is not limited to the extremities, however, and is manifested in the head and trunk. The head is usually flexed toward the hemiplegic side and rotated so that the face is toward the unaffected side. The trunk is rotated back on the hemiplegic side with side flexion of the hemiplegic side (Lim, Koh, & Paik, 2008; Dipietro et al., 2007). These typical patterns of spasticity interfere with the normal, smooth, efficient, and coordinated movement necessary for locomotion in and manipulation of the environment. If untreated, spasticity may lead to contractures.

Addressing the return of motor function is an important part of rehabilitation, and a number of theories and treatment methods have been developed. In recent years, one approach that is being studied for its effectiveness is known as **constraint-induced therapy**, which is outlined in Table 9-1.

TABLE 9.1 An Overview of Constraint-Induced Movement Therapy

Upper-limb hemiparesis following stroke can make bathing, dressing, and feeding a challenge for patient and caregiver. Between 30% and 66% of stroke survivors have limited use of their affected arm (van der Lee et al., 1999), making the impairment one of the most commonly treated by rehabilitation clinicians (Page et al., 2001).

Forced use of the hemiplegic upper extremity and the subsequent emergence of constraint-induced movement therapy (CI therapy) have received considerable attention as a means of helping some stroke patients avoid or overcome learned nonuse and regain upper limb function.

Forced use refers to the restriction of a patient's stronger limb to encourage focused and frequent use of the impaired limb during daily activities.

The theory guiding forced use and CI therapy is based upon the principle of preventing or overcoming learned nonuse through intensive use of the affected limb.

Current health care trends have placed limitations on lengths of hospital and rehabilitation stays as well as curtailing the amount of therapy a stroke survivor can receive (Aycock et al., 2004).

Intensive training with CI therapy involves practicing functional task activities using repetitive task practice and shaping.

Overcoming learned nonuse and the improvements following CI therapy are thought to result from use-dependent cortical organization.

To be eligible for CI therapy, stroke patients must have adequate balance and remain safe while wearing the limb restraint. They also must be able to demonstrate active wrist extension of at least 10° from neutral, abduction/extension of the thumb of 10°, and movement in at least two additional digits in the affected extremity (Wolf et al., 2002).

The hemiplegic shoulder is also a common concern. Typical problems include shoulder subluxation, pain, and immobility. Because of the unstable nature of the glenohumeral joint, the anatomy of the shoulder is particularly vulnerable to problems. Normally this lack of stability is partly compensated for by a strong surrounding musculature. However, subluxation is inevitable once the surrounding musculature of the shoulder, especially the so-called rotator cuff muscles, has been damaged (Ward, 2006; Paci, Nannetti, & Rinaldi, 2005). A closer look at the biomechanics of the glenohumeral joint makes this clear.

Two-thirds of the humeral head is not covered by the glenoid fossa. In the normal orientation of the scapula, the glenoid fossa slopes upward. This orientation plays an important role in preventing downward dislocation of the humerus, as the humeral head would have to move laterally to move downward (Ward, 2006; Paci et al., 2005). When the arm is adducted, the superior part of the capsule and the coracohumeral ligament are taut, which prevents lateral movement of the humeral head and guards against downward displacement. The rotator cuff muscles play a crucial role: The supraspinatus muscle reinforces the horizontal tension of the capsule, while the infraspinatus and the posterior portion of the deltoid, because of their horizontal fibers, also play an important role in preventing subluxation. When the humerus is adducted sideways or flexed forward, the superior capsule becomes lax, eliminating support, and joint stability must then be provided by muscle contraction. Thus the integrity of the joint depends almost exclusively on the rotator cuff muscles (Paci et al., 2007).

After a stroke, changes in muscle tone and movement, the position of the scapula, and joint capsule stability allow the pull of gravity to draw the head of the humerus out of the glenoid fossa of the scapula, resulting in shoulder subluxation (Paci et al., 2007). Patients with hemiplegia have lost voluntary movement in muscles such as the supraspinatus, infraspinatus, and posterior fibers of the deltoid. In addition, the muscles that support the scapula in its normal alignment are affected, which leads to a change in the angulation of the glenoid fossa.

Another typical complication is "the painful shoulder." This condition may either develop quickly after a stroke or at a much later stage. It presents with flaccid or spastic muscle tone and with or without subluxation. In hemiplegia, the normal, coordinated, and timed movement of the scapula and humerus (scapulohumeral rhythm) has been disturbed by abnormal and unbalanced muscle tone. The typical hemiplegic postural components of depression and retraction of the scapula and internal rotation of the humerus are especially important to the mechanism of pain. Fear of pain during passive movement of the arm will further increase abnormal flexor tone, which can become a vicious circle (Dromerick, Edwards, & Kumar, 2008).

A chronically painful shoulder can lead to shoulder-hand syndrome, also known as reflex sympathetic dystrophy (RSD). This complex condition produces severe pain, edema of the hand, and limitations in range of motion on the involved side (Salisbury, Choy, & Nitz, 2003). These complications not only interfere with movement, they may have profound emotional consequences.

Another motor dysfunction caused by stroke is the presence of associated reactions. Associated reactions in hemiplegia are abnormal reflex movements of the affected side that duplicate the synergy patterns of the arm and leg (Poduri, 1993). These movements may be observed when the patient moves with effort, is trying to maintain balance, or is afraid of falling. A flexor pattern of involuntary movement in the arm is often observed when the individual yawns, coughs, or sneezes. Associated reactions also are seen when new activities, such as running or putting on socks, are attempted after a stroke. They are stereotyped reactions and may occur even if no active movement is present in the limb. The limb returns to its normal position only after cessation of the stimulus and usually does so gradually (Bhakta, O'Connor, & Cozens, 2008).

Unlike associated reactions, associated movements accompany voluntary movements and are normal, automatic postural adjustments. They reinforce precise movements of other parts of the body or occur when a great amount of strength is required. They are not pathological and can be stopped at will. Associated movements often can be observed in the unaffected extremities of stroke patients who are trying new activities (Bhakta et al., 2008).

Other motor dysfunctions include orofacial weakness, which may cause difficulties in expression, speech (dysarthria), mastication, and swallowing (dysphagia) (Honaga et al., 2007; Mackenzie & Lowit, 2007). Additionally, bladder or bowel incontinence may result from a communication disorder or from disruption of normal routine and diet, lack of awareness of body function, or emotional disorder (Daniels et al., 2009; Kovindha, Wyndaele, & Madersbacher, 2010).

Mental Functions

Severe strokes often result in cognitive deficits that affect global and specific mental functions (Hallevi et al., 2009). Milder strokes may have a more subtle impact on mental function, however. Commonly used psychometrics are not always sensitive to the wide range of mental functions and process skills that may permit effective occupational performance: initiation, recognition, attention, orientation, sequencing, categorization, concept formation, spatial operations, problem solving, and learning abilities (Nys et al., 2007). Moreover, basic visual deficits also have an impact on cognitive performance. For example, visual attending and scanning deficits lead to a decrease in the efficiency required for cognitive performance (Pendlebury et al., 2010; Hoffmann et al., 2010).

Emotional Functions

Stroke patients may experience a number of psychological changes, including depression, irritability, low tolerance for stressful situations, fear and anxiety, anger, frustration, swearing, emotional lability, and catastrophic reactions. Significant depression has been recorded in 30% to 50% of stroke survivors (Riggs et al., 2007; Berg et al., 2009). These changes often are a major cause of concern to relatives and the individual. While depression is often viewed as a natural and understandable consequence of reduced function caused by stroke, proper treatment can result in observable improvement. Depression is more frequent and severe with lesions in the left hemisphere, as compared with right hemisphere or brainstem strokes (Williams et al., 2007). Both organic and psychological factors are probably involved in poststroke depression (Williams et al., 2007).

Emotional lability, sudden and extreme shifts of mood, may be the result of a release of inhibition. The individual may switch from laughing to crying for no apparent reason. Excessive crying is the most common problem and is frequently the result of organic emotional lability rather than depression or sadness over perceived losses. Organic emotional lability is characterized by little or no obvious relation between the start of emotional expression and what is happening around the person (Provinciali et al., 2008).

Catastrophic reactions are outbursts in which frustration, anger, and depression are combined. When individuals cannot perform tasks that used to be very easy, they may be unable to inhibit emotional expression and may begin sobbing, expressing a sense of hopelessness (Carota & Bogousslavsky, 2008; Thompson & Ryan, 2009). Outbursts and emotional difficulties are to be expected after stroke. Relatives and families should be told that a tendency to cry easily or get upset will improve with time. Families and therapists need to develop a positive, understanding attitude if the individual is to overcome psychological sequelae. The psychosocial impact of stroke on patients and families can be lessened with increased social support and access to services once the patient has been discharged to home and community (Ferro, Caeiro, & Santos, 2009).

Case Illustrations

Case 1

Initial Presentation

Marilyn Purdue is a 72-year-old woman who has been a widow for several years since the sudden death of her second husband while they were vacationing on Sanibel Island in Florida. Marilyn has been treated consistently for the past 20 years for hypertension and hypercholesterolemia. She was told by a physician several years ago to watch her sugar, but she never thought she officially had diabetes. She had a stent placed in her right anterior descending artery in 2005 due to reported 90% blockage in one location. Marilyn has never done much in the way of organized or formal exercise; she has always chosen to keep active by tending her garden, doing mild yard work, and going out for coffee at least three times each week with her girlfriends. One of the gadgets that her two adult children were successful in convincing her to have is the "Life Line" emergency monitoring system. The "I've fallen, and I can't get up" button. Today is the first time she has ever even thought of using the button. It is 3:10 a.m., and Marilyn has gotten out of her bed to urinate, not an unusual event for her at all. On the journey back to bed from her bathroom she suddenly loses her sense of balance and stability and begins to list and lean to her right side. She makes it back to the edge of the bed, but misjudging the distance she is from the edge, she proceeds to slide from the bed edge to the carpeted floor. She thinks to herself that if her kids saw her they would say she had been drinking, but she has not touched even so much as a glass of wine since her husband died. Attempting to rise from the floor, Marilyn now senses that something more serious may be occurring, as she is unable to get herself off the floor and onto the bed. It is as though the entire right side of her body, her "strong side," is no longer actively supporting her in any way. She is sweating profusely and has become aware of her stomach feeling upset. She feels nauseous and will vomit if this feeling does not pass. She experiences no discernable pain, no headache, and no jaw pain radiating into her left arm. Good she thinks, "At least I am not having a damn heart attack." But the sensation in her right side is persistent, the feeling of disconnection to her environment pervasive. Marilyn makes the most important decision of her entire life in the next moment; she activates the emergency medical monitor button and within a minute's time she hears a voice. "Is it the operator?" She makes an utterance, which coming from her mouth sounds to her like a motor boat engine attempting to turn over, slow, sluggish, wet, and heavy. No response from the operator. Again the motorboat attempts to start and again the same gurgle with no clear acknowledgement from the dispatcher at the other end. What is going on? Fortunately the dispatcher has Marilyn's medical history accessible to him and realizes that she may be having a stroke. Her inability to articulate in a meaningful way to get her needs met causes the dispatcher to immediately activate the emergency medical services system. Within 3 or 4 minutes, the police and paramedics are at her door; they gain entrance to her ranch-style home through a back door that Marilyn inadvertently left unlocked earlier in the evening.

Hospital Course

After stabilization in the emergency department, Marilyn was admitted to a monitored bed in the intensive care unit (ICU). An intravenous solution of 5% dextrose in 0.45% normal saline was started. Laboratory tests were all normal except for a blood glucose level of 315 mg/dL and occasional unifocal premature ventricular contractions. CT scan of the brain, taken the day of admission, was positive for bleeding into the left temproparietal lobe. Nursing began regular turning and positioning and range of motion exercises. The physician ordered physical, occupational, and speech therapy consultations on the third day of hospital admission. On day 6 of her hospital admission, Marilyn continued to demonstrate dysphagia to all consistencies of food and fluid, and a videofluoroscopy study was ordered. A nasogastric tube remained in place for feeding and for the removal of gastric secretions. By day 8 Marilyn was medically cleared for transfer to the rehabilitation unit of the facility. It was determined by her treatment team including medicine, nursing, neurology, and physical medicine and rehabilitation that she would be well enough to benefit from the intensive therapy program provided.

Rehabilitation

At the end of her first week of stay in the rehabilitation unit, Marilyn began to demonstrate some active movement in her right hand and leg. None of the movement was yet considered purposeful or isolated, but it was active and somewhat volitional. Her bed mobility skills were improving, and she was able to roll from side to side with the use of the side rails, to relieve pressure on her back and buttocks when lying on the bed. She was able to wash her face with setup, and she was attempting more tasks each day using her nondominant left hand. The speech therapist was concerned about Marilyn's swallowing and the fact that she was at high risk for aspiration. She lost 4 lb since admission, and if not for the IV fluids being administered, she would likely have become dehydrated. The speech therapist recommended a second videofluoroscopic examination to observe Marilyn's functional swallow while ingesting a variety of consistencies of food and liquid. The outcome of the "cookie swallow" assessment should facilitate a decision regarding maintenance of the feeding tube. Physical therapy decided to hold program until Marilyn's nutritional status stabilized and her physical energy level improved. The rehabilitation stroke team was in close communication on a daily basis about this patient's status, to be able to grade the intensity of interventions as indicated. Occupational therapy continued on a twice per day basis, providing bedside passive range of motion, active assisted range of motion, and core strengthening exercises including rolling in bed and bridging in bed activities. Additionally, Marilyn indicated that she enjoyed listening to Country and Western music and that the noises of the ICU were distracting and disturbing her ability to rest. The OTR communicated with Marilyn's sister and had the sister bring in Marilyn's IPod on her next visit to the unit.

Marilyn's physical strength continued to improve over the next 2 weeks, and she began receiving all therapies bid for the remainder of her 4-week stay on the rehabilitation unit. She was subsequently discharged to her sister's home in a town approximately 20 miles from her own home in order to continue her recovery process. Upon discharge, Marilyn was able to stand independently from an armchair and ambulate with contact guard assist short distances. Although she regained minimal active movement in the right upper extremity, she was becoming adept with using her left hand for most of her self-care activities. Her speech abilities and cognitive-linguistic skills continue to progress steadily. Occupational therapist and speech therapist continue to see Marilyn two times a week as part of her home care program. A home health aide also comes to her sister's home to assist with bathing Marilyn two times a week. A skilled nurse continues to come to the home one time a week to tend to a stage 3 decubitus ulcer that unfortunately developed on her sacrum during her stay in the acute care setting.

Marilyn intends to eventually return to her own home, realizing that she may continue to require and benefit from the assistance of formal care providers, as well as some minor home adaptations and assistive equipment in the home to maximize her safety and function.

Case 2
Initial Presentation

Mrs. Stella Rojo is 66 years old, from Puerto Rico, and a retired housekeeper. She was brought into the emergency room (ER) by paramedics after complaining of a severe headache that began earlier in the day while she was cleaning the windows in her small apartment. She was on a step stool and reportedly fell to the ground and was unable to move her left arm or leg. She was able to pull herself to a coffee table in her living room and reach the telephone to dial 911. Initially in the ER she seemed confused about her surroundings, and it was reported that in the ambulance she had a generalized tonic-clonic seizure.

Hospital Course

Mrs. Rojo was intubated, and IV phenytoin sodium (Dilantin) was started for the seizures. An emergency CT scan of the head revealed an intracerebral hemorrhage in the internal capsule and thalamus. There was no evidence of intracranial pressure. Her blood pressure on admission to the ER was 190/110 mm Hg but decreased within the first hour to 170/95 mm Hg. She was admitted to the neuro-ICU of the facility. On day 2 she was extubated and began to open her eyes but still seemed confused.

Rehabilitation

Mrs. Rojo was much more alert by day 5. Her blood pressure was now 160/90 mm Hg. She started occupational therapy. When feeding, she demonstrated difficulty locating food items on the left side of her meal tray, and she called out for the nurses to find her drink container for her. When the nurses would tell her that it was on the left side of her tray she seemed to become irritated and think that they were belittling her. When visitors came to call on her Mrs. Rojo tended to become teary and even broke down into sudden crying spells. Her physician recommended transfer from the hospital to a skilled nursing facility.

At the time of discharge from the hospital the physician believed that Mrs. Rojo should be sent to a nursing facility because she was not thought to be a good candidate for inpatient rehabilitation. The rehabilitation therapy team in the hospital reached this decision because of her apparent cognitive deficits and severe left-sided neglect. Mrs. Rojo's daughter, Yvonne, was her patient advocate and durable power of attorney, and she also agreed with the team's decision.

The rehabilitation therapy team in the nursing facility received orders from the medical director for evaluation and treatment as indicated. All therapies initiated their respective assessments within 24 hours of her admission to the facility. These included occupational therapy, physical therapy, and speech-language pathology. Mrs. Rojo was assessed to be in need of skilled rehabilitative care and admitted to the rehabilitation wing of the facility. Her treatment would be covered by her Medicare part A. Her family and her physician were informed that her Medicare coverage under part A would continue as long as Mrs. Rojo continued to need skilled care and demonstrated functional progress and the care was reasonable and medically necessary.

Even though all these criteria were met, there were still limits to the length of care coverage, and these were also discussed with the client's health care advocate.

Mrs. Rojo made consistent functional gains in balance, mobility, self-care dressing, grooming, toileting, and feeding skills. After approximately 4 weeks of combined therapies she reached her maximum potential in functional performance and was recommended for discharge from the therapy programs. Prior to discharge from occupational therapy, a home safety assessment was done, equipment and adaptation recommendations were shared with the family, and preparatory plans were set in motion.

Thirty-six days postadmission to the nursing facility, Mrs. Rojo was discharged to her daughter's home. Home care services were arranged by the discharge planner and social services and included occupational therapy, physical therapy, and speech therapy. Home safety equipment was to include a wheelchair for trips to appointments, a quad-cane, overtoilet commode, transfer tub bench, wall safety grab bars, and a shower sprayer and flexible hose.

RECOMMENDED LEARNING RESOURCES

American Heart Association
www.americanheart.org
American Stroke Association
www.strokeassociation.org
Children's Hemiplegia and Stroke Association
www.chasa.org
Family Caregiver Alliance
www.caregiver.org
National Institute of Neurological Disorders and Stroke
www.ninds.nih.gov
National Stroke Association
www.stroke.org
Pediatric Stroke Network
www.pediatricstrokenetwork.com

Survivor and Family References
Gardner, R. (2008). *Take brave steps for stroke survivors and families.* Concord, MA: Infinity Publishing Co. ISBN 0-7414-4678-2.

Marler, J. R. (2005). *Stroke for dummies.* Hoboken, NJ: Wiley Publishing. ISBN-13:978-0-7645-7201-2.

Personal Stories
Berger, P. E., & Mensh, S. (2002). *How to conquer the world with one hand and an attitude* (2nd ed.). Merrifield, VA: Positive Power Publishing, 2002.

Bolte-Taylor, J. (2008). *My stroke of insight: A brain scientist's personal journey.* New York, NY: Penguin Group. ISBN 978-0-670-02074-4.

Brady, D. (2002). *When I learn ... surviving a stroke with pride.* Bloomington, IN: 1st Books Library.

Hutton, C., & Caplan, L. R. (2003). *Striking back at stroke: A doctor-patient journal.* New York, NY: Dana Press.

Robinson, R. (2005). *Peeling the onion: Reversing the ravages of stroke.* Key West, FL: SORA Publishing.

Simon, S. (2001). *A stroke of genius: Messages of hope and healing.* Cedars Group, 2001.

REFERENCES

Aaslid, R., Huber, P., & Nornes, H. (2010). Evaluation of cerebrovascular spasm with transcranial Doppler ultrasound. *Journal of Neurosurgery, 55*(2), 112–123.

Amarenco, G., Easton, J., Sacco, R., & Teal, P. (2008). Antithrombotic and thrombolytic therapy for ischemic stroke. American College of Chest Physicians Evidence-Based Clinical Practice Guidelines. *Chest, 133*(6), 1–5.

Amarenco, P., Bogousslavsky, J., Caplan, L., Donnan, G., & Hennerici, M. (2009). Classification of stroke subtypes. *Cerebrovascular Disease, 27*, 493–501.

American Heart Association. (2010). Retrieved August 17, 2010, from http://www.heart.org/HEARTORG/General/911—Warnings-Signs-of-a-Heart-Attack_UCM_305346_SubHomePage.jsp

Arzt, M., Young, T., Finn, L., Skatrud, J., & Bradley, T. (2005). Association of sleep disordered breathing and the occurrence of stroke. *American Journal of Respiratory and Critical Care Medicine, 172*, 1447–1451.

Aycock, D. M., Blanton, S., Clark, P. C., et al. (2004). What is constraint-induced therapy? *Rehabilitation Nursing, 29*(4), 114–116.

Beck, J., & Offenbacher, S. (2005). Systemic effects of periodontitis: Epidemiology of periodontal disease and cardiovascular disease. *Journal of Periodontology, 76*, 11, 2029–2030.

Beis, J., Keller, C., Morin, N., Bartolomeo, P., Bernati, T., Chokron, S., et al. (2004). Right spatial neglect after left hemisphere stroke. *Neurology, 63*, 1600–1605.

Berg, A., Lönnqvist, J., Palomäki, H., & Kaste, M. (2009). Assessment of depression after stroke. *Stroke, 40*, 523–529.

Bhakta, B., O'Connor, R., & Cozens, J. (2008). Associated reactions after stroke: A randomized controlled trial of the effect of botulinum toxin type a. *Journal of Rehabilitation Medicine, 40*, 36–40.

Bhat, M., Cole, J., Sorkin, J., Wozniak, M., Malarcher, A., Wozniak, A. (2008). Dose-response relationship between cigarette smoking and risk of ischemic stroke in young women. *Stroke, 39*, 2439–2443.

Bicknell, C. D., Subramanian, A., & Wolfe, J. (2004). Coronary subclavian steal syndrome. *European Journal of Vascular and Endovascular Surgery, 27*(2), 220–221.

Bose, A., Henkes, H., Alfke, K. (2008). The Penumbra System. *Catheter Cardiovascular Intervention, 72*, 705–709.

Boyd, L., & Winstein, C. (2003). Impact of explicit information on implicit motor-sequence learning following middle cerebral artery stroke. *Physical Therapy, 83*(11), 976–989.

Bravata, D., Wells, C., Gulanski, B., Kernan, W., Brass, L., Long, J., & Concato, J. (2005). Racial disparities in stroke risk factors: The impact of socioeconomic status. *Stroke, 36*, 1507–1511.

Broderick, J., Connolly, S., Feldmann, E., Hanley, D., Kase, C., Krieger, D., et al. (2007). Guidelines for the management of spontaneous intracerebral hemorrhage in adults: 2007 update: A guideline from the American Heart Association/American Stroke Association stroke council, high blood pressure research council, and the quality of care and outcomes in research interdisciplinary working group. *Circulation, 116*, 391–413.

Bykowski, J., Latour, L., & Warach, S. (2004). More accurate identification of reversible ischemic injury in human stroke by cerebrospinal fluid suppressed diffusion-weighted imaging. *Stroke, 35*. Retrieved from http://stroke.ahajournals.org/cgi/content/abstract/35/5/1100

Camilo, O., & Goldstein, L. (2004). Seizures and epilepsy after ischemic stroke. *Stroke, 35*, 1769–1775.

Carandang, R., Seshadri, S., Beiser, A., Kelly-Hayes, M., Kase, C., Kannel, W., & Carmichael, S. (2006). Cellular and molecular mechanisms of neural repair after stroke: Making waves. *Annals of Neurology, 59*(5), 735–742.

Carota, A., & Bogousslavsky, J. (2008). *Stroke related psychiatric disorders. Handbook of clinical neurology, stroke part II: Clinical manifestations and pathogenesis*, 623–651. Retrieved from: http://www.sciencedirect.com

Chalela, J., Kidwell, C., Nentwich, L., Luby, M., Butman, J., Demchuk, A., et al. (2009). Magnetic resonance imaging and computed tomography in emergency assessment of patients with suspected acute stroke: A prospective comparison. *Lancet, 369*(9558), 293–298.

Charbel, F., Meglio, G., & Amin-Hanjani, S. (2005). Superficial temporal artery to middle cerebral artery bypass. *Neurosurgery, 56*(1), 186–190.

Chiuve, S., Rexrode, K., Spiegelman, D., Logroscino, G., Manson, J., & Rimm, E. (2008). Primary prevention of stroke by healthy lifestyle. *Circulation, 118*, 947–954.

Cho, H. J., Cho, H. Y., Kim, Y., Nam, H., Han, S., Heo, J. (2009). Transesophageal echocardiography in patients with acute stroke with sinus rhythm and no cardiac disease history. *Journal of Neurosurgery and Psychiatry, 81*, 412–415.

Connell, L. (2008). Somatosensory impairment after stroke: Frequency of different deficits and their recovery. *Clinical Rehabilitation, 22*(8), 758–776.

Coward, L., McCabe, D., Ederle, J., Featherstone, R., Clifton, A., & Brown, M. (2007). Long-term outcome after angioplasty and stenting for symptomatic vertebral artery stenosis compared with medical treatment in the carotid and vertebral artery transluminal angioplasty study (CAVATAS): A randomized trial. *Stroke, 38*(5), 1526–1530.

Daniels, S., Schroeder, M., DeGeorge, P., Corey, D., Foundas, A., & Rosenbek, J. (2009). Defining and measuring dysphagia following stroke. *American Journal of Speech-Language Pathology, 18*, 74–81.

Davis, S., & Donnan, G. (2004). Steroids for stroke: Another potential therapy discarded prematurely? *Stroke, 35*, 230–231.

De Reuck, J., Claeys, I., Martens, S., Vanwalleghem, P., Van Maele, G., Phlypo, R., & Hallez, H. (2006). Computed tomographic changes of the brain and clinical outcome of patients with seizures and epilepsy after an ischemic hemispheric stroke. *European Journal of Neurology, 13*(4), 402–407.

Diener, H., Ringelstein, E., von Kummer, R., Landgraf, H., Koppenhagen, K., Harenberg, J., et al. (2006). Prophylaxis of thrombotic and embolic events in acute ischemic stroke with the low-molecular-weight heparin certoparin. *Stroke, 37,* 139–144.

Dietrich, M., Benses, S., Stephan, T., Brandt, T., Schwaiger, M., & Bartenstein, P. (2005). Medial vestibular nucleus lesions in wallenberg's syndrome cause decreased activity of the contralateral vestibular cortex. *Annals of the New York Academy of Sciences, 1039,* 368–383.

Dipietro, L., Krebs, H., Fasoli, S., Volpe, B., Stein, J., Bever, C., & Hogan, N. (2007). Changing motor synergies in chronic stroke. *Journal of Neurophysiology, 98,* 757–768.

Diserens, K., Vuadens, P., Michel, P., Reichhart, M., Herrmann, F., Arnold, P., Bogousslavsky, J., & Ghika, J. (2006). Acute autonomic dysfunction contralateral to acute strokes: a prospective study of 100 consecutive cases. *European Journal of Neurology, 13*(11), 1245–1250.

Dromerick, A., Edwards, D., & Kumar, A. (2008). Hemiplegic shoulder pain syndrome: Frequency and characteristics during inpatient stroke rehabilitation. *Archives of Physical Medicine and Rehabilitation, 89*(8), 1589–1593.

Duncan, P., Zorowitz, R., Bates, B., Choi, J., Glasberg, J., Graham, G., et al. (2005). Management of adult stroke rehabilitation care: A clinical practice guideline. *Stroke, 36.* Retrieved from http://stroke.ahajournals.org/cgi/content/full/strokeaha;36/9/e100

Elkind, M., Sciacca, R., Boden-Albala, B., Rundek, T., Paik, M., & Sacco, R. (2006a). Moderate alcohol consumption reduces risk of ischemic stroke: The northern Manhattan study. *Stroke, 37,* 13–19.

Elkind, M., Tondella, M., Feikin, D., Fields, B., Homma, S., & Di Tullio, M. (2006b). Seropositivity to *Chlamydia pneumoniae* is associated with risk of first ischemic stroke. *Stroke, 37,* 790–795.

Fang, M., Singer, D., Chang, Y., Hylek, E., Henault, L., & Jensvold, N. (2005). Gender differences in the risk of ischemic stroke and peripheral embolism in atrial fibrillation. *Circulation, 112,* 1687–1691.

Feigin, V., Lawes, C., Bennett, D., Barker-Collo, S., & Parag, V. (2009). Worldwide stroke incidence and early case fatality reported in 56 population-based studies: A systematic review. *The Lancet Neurology, 8*(4), 355–369.

Feldmann, E., Wilterdink, J., Kosinski, A., Lynn, M., Chimowitz, M., Sarafin, J., et al. (2007). The stroke outcomes and neuroimaging of intracranial atherosclerosis (SONIA) trial. *Neurology, 68,* 2099–2106.

Ferro, J., Caeiro, L., & Santos, C. (2009). Poststroke emotional and behavior impairment: A narrative review. *Cerebrovascular Disease, 27*(Suppl. 1), 197–203.

Fiebach, J., Schellinger, P., Gass, A., Kucinski, T., Siebler, M., Villringer, A., et al. (2004). Stroke magnetic resonance imaging is accurate in hyperacute intracerebral hemorrhage: A multicenter study on the validity of stroke imaging, *Stroke, 35,* 502–506.

Fogle, C., Oser, C., Troutman, T., McNamara, M., Williamson, A., Keller, M., et al. (2008). Public education strategies to increase awareness of stroke warning signs and the need to call 911. *Journal of Public Health Management & Practice, 14*(3), 17–22.

Formisano, R., Pantano, P., Buzzi, M., Vinicola, V., Penta, F., Barbanti, P., & Lenzi, G. (2005). Late motor recovery is influenced by muscle tone changes after stroke. *Archives of Physical Medicine and Rehabilitation, 86*(2), 308–311.

Fulgham, J. R., Ingall, T. J., Stead, L. G., Cloft, H. J., Wijdicks, E. F. M., & Flemming, K. D. (2004). Management of acute ischemic stroke. *Mayo Clinic Proceedings, 79*(11), 1459–1469.

Glymour, M., Avendaño, M., & Berkman, L. (2007). Is the 'stroke belt' worn from childhood? Risk of first stroke and state of residence in childhood and adulthood. *Stroke, 38,* 2415–2421.

Gonzalez, R. (2006). Imaging-guided acute ischemic stroke therapy: From "time is brain" to "physiology is brain." *American Journal of Neuroradiology, 27*(4), 728–735.

Hackett, M., Yapa, C., Parag, V., & Anderson, C. (2005). Frequency of depression after stroke: A systematic review of observational studies. *Stroke, 36*(10), 2296–2301.

Hallevi, H., Albright, K., Martin-Schild, S., Barreto, A., Morales, M., Bornstein, N. et al. (2009). Recovery after ischemic stroke: Criteria for good outcome by level of disability at day 7. *Cerebrovascular Disease, 28,* 341–348.

Hand, P., Kwan, J., Lindley, R., Dennis, M., & Wardlaw, J. (2006). Distinguishing between stroke and mimic at the bedside: The brain attack study. *Stroke, 37,* 769–775.

Hankey, G. J., Spiesser, J., Hakimi, Z., Bego, G., Carita, P., & Gabriel, S. (2007). Rate, degree, and predictors of recovery from disability following ischemic stroke. *Neurology, 68,* 1583–1587.

Ho, B. L., Huang, P., Khor, G. T., & Lin, R. T. (2008). The simultaneous thrombosis of cerebral artery and venous sinus. *Acta Neurologica Taiwan, 17,* 112–116.

Hoffmann, T., Bennett, S., Koh, C., & McKenna, K. (2010). A systematic review of cognitive interventions to improve functional ability in people who have cognitive impairment following stroke. *Topics in Stroke Rehabilitation, 17*(2), 398–412.

Honaga, K., Masakado, Y., Oki, T., Hirabara, Y., Fujiwara, T., Ota, T., et al. (2007). Associated reaction and spasticity among patients with stroke. *American Journal of Physical Medicine & Rehabilitation, 86*(8), 656–661.

Jackson, C., & Sudlow, C. (2005). Are lacunar strokes really different? A systematic review of differences in risk factor profiles between lacunar and nonlacunar infarcts. *Stroke, 36*, 891–901.

Johansson, B. (2000). Brain plasticity and stroke rehabilitation: The willis lecture. *Stroke, 31*, 223–230.

Kaspera, W., Majchrzak, H., Ladzinski, P., & Tomalski, W. (2005). Color doppler sonographic evaluation of collateral circulation in patients with cerebral aneurysms and the occlusion of the brachiocephalic vessels. *Neurosurgery, 57*(6), 1117–1126.

Kaufmann, T., Huston, J., Mandrekar, J., Schleck, C., Thielen, K., & Kallmes, D. (2007). Complications of diagnostic cerebral angiography: Evaluation of 19826 consecutive patients. *Radiology, 243*. Retrieved from http://radiology.rsna.org/content/243/3/812. abstract

Kidwell, C., & Warach, S. (2003). Acute ischemic cerebrovascular syndrome: Diagnostic criteria. *Stroke, 34*, 2995–2998.

Kleinman, J., Newhart, M., Davis, C., Heidler-Gary, J., Gottesman, R., & Hillis, A. (2007). Right hemispatial neglect: Frequency and characterization following acute left hemisphere stroke. *Brain and Cognition 64*(1), 50–59.

Kovindha, A., Wyndaele, J., & Madersbacher, H. (2010). Prevalence of incontinence during rehabilitation in patients following a stroke. *Current Bladder Dysfunction Report.*

Langhorne, P. (2007). Occupational therapy for patients with problems in personal activities of daily living after stroke: Systematic review of randomized trials. *British Medical Journal, 335*, 922.

Lawlor, D., & Leon, D. (2005). Association of body mass index and obesity measured in early childhood with risk of coronary heart disease and stroke in middle age. *Circulation, 111*, 1891–1896.

Lees, K., & Walters, M. (2005). Acute stroke and diabetes. *Cerebrovascular Disease, 20*(1), 9–14.

Legg, L., Drummond, A., Leonardi-Bee, J., Gladman JRF, Corr, S., Donkervoort, M., et al. (2003). Interaction with the physical environment in everyday occupation after stroke: A phenomenological study of persons with visuospatial agnosia. *Scandinavian Journal of Occupational Therapy, 10*(4), 147–146.

Lim, J., Koh, J., & Paik, N. (2008). Intramuscular botulinum toxin-a reduces hemiplegic shoulder pain. *Stroke, 39*, 126–131. Retrieved from http://stroke.ahajournals.org/cgi/content/abstract/39/1/126 accessed 8/21/10

Locksley, H. (2010). Natural history of subarachnoid hemorrhage, intracranial aneurysms and arteriovenous malformations: Based on 6368 cases in the cooperative study. *Journal of Neurosurgery, 112*, 2.

Lundy-Ekman, L. (2007). *Neuroscience: Fundamentals for rehabilitation* (3rd ed.). Philadelphia: WB Saunders.

MacDougall, D., Feliu, A., Boccuzzi, S., & Lin, J. (2006). Economic burden of deep-vein thrombosis, pulmonary embolism, and post-thrombotic syndrome. *American Journal of Health-System Pharmacy, 63*(20), 5–15.

Mackenzie, C., & Lowit, A. (2007). Behavioural intervention effects in dysarthria following stroke: Communication effectiveness, intelligibility and dysarthria impact. *International Journal of Language and Communication Disorders, 42*(2), 131–152.

Mayo Clinic Staff. (2009). *Brain aneurysm overview.* Retrieved August 16, 2010, from http://www.mayoclinic.com/health/brain-aneurysm/DS00582.

Mant, J., Hobbs, F., Fletcher, K., Roalfe, A., Fitzmaurice, D., Lip, G., & Murray, E. (2007). Warfarin versus aspirin for stroke prevention in an elderly community population with atrial fibrillation (the Birmingham Atrial Fibrillation Treatment of the Aged Study, BAFTA): A randomized controlled trial. *Lancet, 370*, 493–503.

Mattace-Raso, F., Van der Cammen, T., Hofman, A., van Popele, N., Bos, M., Schalekamp, M., et al. (2006). Arterial stiffness and risk of coronary heart disease and stroke. *The Rotterdam Study Circulation, 113*, 657–663.

McCullagh, E., Brigstocke, G., Donaldson, N., & Kalra, L. (2005). Determinants of caregiving burden and quality of life in caregivers of stroke patients. *Stroke, 36*, 2181–2186.

McLean, D. (2004). Medical complications experienced by a cohort of stroke survivors during inpatient, tertiary-level stroke rehabilitation. *Archives of Physical Medicine and Rehabilitation, 85*(3), 466–469.

Metoki, H., Ohkubo, T., Kikuya, M., Asayama, K., Obara, T., Hashimoto, J., et al. (2006). Prognostic significance for stroke of a morning pressor surge and a nocturnal blood pressure decline: The Ohasama study. *Hypertension, 47*(2), 149–154.

Montaner, J., Perea-Gainza, M., Delgado, P., Ribó, M., Chacón, P., Rosell, A., et al. (2008). Etiologic diagnosis of ischemic stroke subtypes with plasma biomarkers. *Stroke, 39*, 2280–2287.

Murray, M., Camen, C., Gonzalez, A., Bovet, P., & Clarke, S. (2006). Rapid brain discrimination of sounds of objects. *The Journal of Neuroscience, 26*(4), 1293–1302.

Nederkoorn, P., van der Graaf, Y., & Hunink, M. (2003). Ultrasound and magnetic resonance angiography compared with digital subtraction angiography in carotid artery stenosis. *Stroke, 34*:1324–1331.

Nys, G., van Zandvoort, M., de Kort, P., Jansen, B., de Haan, E., & Kappelle, L. (2007). Cognitive disorders in acute stroke: Prevalence and clinical determinants. *Cerebrovascular Disease, 23*, 408–416.

Ohira, T., Shahar, E., Chambless, L., Rosamond, W., Mosley, T., & Folsom, A. (2006). Risk factors for ischemic stroke subtypes: The atherosclerosis risk in communities study. *Stroke, 37,* 2493–2498.

Ohwaki, K., Yano, E., Nagashima, H., Hirata, M., Nakagomi, T., & Tamura, A. (2004). Blood pressure management in acute intracerebral hemorrhage relationship between elevated blood pressure and hematoma enlargement. *Stroke, 35,* 1364–1367.

Paci, M., Nannetti, L., & Rinaldi, L. (2005). Glenohumeral subluxation in hemiplegia: An overview. *Journal of Rehabilitation Research & Development, 42*(4), 557–568.

Paci, M., Nannetti, L., Taiti, P., Baccini, M., Pasquini, J., & Rinaldi, L. (2007). Shoulder subluxation after stroke: Relationships with pain and motor recovery. *Physiotherapy Research International, 12,* 95–104.

Parvizi, J., & Damasio, A. (2003). Neuroanatomical correlates of brainstem coma. *Brain, 126*(7), 1524–1536.

Patel, M., McKevitt, C., Lawrence, E., Rudd, A., & Wolfe, C. (2007). Clinical determinants of long-term quality of life after stroke. *Age and Aging, 36*(3), 316–322.

Pendlebury, S., Cuthbertson, F., Welch, S., Mehta, Z., & Rothwell, P. (2010).Underestimation of cognitive impairment by Mini-Mental State examination versus the montreal cognitive assessment in patients with transient ischemic attack and stroke: Population-based study. *Stroke, 41,* 1290–1293.

Petrella, J., Coleman, R., & Doraiswamy, P. (2003). Neuroimaging and early diagnosis of alzheimer disease: A look to the future. *Radiology, 226.* Retrieved from http://radiology.rsna.org/content/226/2/315.abstract

Pinar, Y., & Govsa, F. (2006). Anatomy of the superficial temporal artery and its branches: Its importance for surgery. *Surgical and Radiologic Anatomy, 28*(3), 248–253.

Poduri, K. (1993). Shoulder pain in stroke patients and its effects on rehabilitation. *Journal of Stroke and Cerebrovascular Diseases, 3*(4), 261–266.

Porter, R., & Kaplan, J. (Eds.). (2004). *Merck manual online.* Merck Sharp & Dohme. Neurologic Disorders Stroke. Retrieved from http://www.merck.com/mmpe/sec16/ch211/ch211b.html

Prass, K., Braun, J., Dirnagl, U., Meisel, C., & Meisel, A. (2006). Stroke propagates bacterial aspiration to pneumonia in a model of cerebral ischemia. *Stroke, 37,* 2607–2612.

Provinciali, L., Paolucci, S., Torta, R., Toso, V., Gobbi, B., & Gandolfo, C. (2008). Depression after first-ever ischemic stroke: The prognostic role of neuroanatomic subtypes in clinical practice. *Cerebrovascular Disease, 26,* 592–599. Accessed 8/12/10

Qureshi, A. I., Alexandrov, A. V., Tegeler, C. H., Hobson II, R. W., Baker, J. D., & Hopkins, L. N. (2007). MD guidelines for screening of extracranial carotid artery disease: A statement for healthcare professionals from the multidisciplinary practice guidelines committee of the American society of neuroimaging; cosponsored by the society of vascular and interventional neurology. *Journal of Neuroimaging, 17*(1), 19–47.

Page, S. J., Sisto, S. A., Levine, P., et al. (2001). Modified constraint induced therapy: A randomized feasibility and efficacy study. *Journal of Rehabilitation Research and Development, 38,* 583–590.

Parry, W., Reeve, L., Shaw, F., Davison, J., Norton, M., Frearson, R., et al. (2009). The Newcastle protocols 2008: An update on head-up tilt table testing and the management of vasovagal syncope and related disorders. *Heart, 95,* 416–420.

Riggs, R., Andrews, K., Roberts, P., & Gilewski, M. (2007). Visual deficit interventions in adult stroke and brain injury: A systematic review. *American Journal of Physical Medicine & Rehabilitation, 86*(10), 853–860.

Rossini, P., Calautti, C., Pauri, F., & Baron, J. (2003). Post-stroke plastic reorganization in the adult brain. *The Lancet Neurology, 2*(8), 493–508.

Sacco, R., Prabhakaran, S., Thompson, J., Murphy, A., Sciacca, R., Levin, B., & Mohr, J. (2006). Comparison of Warfarin versus Aspirin for the prevention of recurrent stroke or death: Subgroup analyses from the warfarin-aspirin recurrent stroke study. *Cerebrovascular Disease, 22,* 4–12.

Salisbury, S., Choy, N., & Nitz, J. (2003). Shoulder pain, range of motion, and functional motor skills after acute tetraplegia. *Archives of Physical Medicine and Rehabilitation, 84,* 1480–1485.

Santamarina, R., Besocke, A., Romano, L., Loli, P., & Gonorazky, S. (2008). Ischemic stroke related to anabolic abuse. *Clinical Neuropharmacology 31,* 2.

Slooter, A., Rosedaalo, F.,Tanis, B., Kemmeren, J., Vandergraaf, Y., & Algra, A. (2005). Prothrombotic conditions, oral contraceptives, and the risk of ischemic stroke. *Journal of Thrombosis and Haemostasis, 3*(6), 1213–1217.

Sommerfeld, D., Eek, E., Svensson, A., Holmqvist, L., & von Arbin, M. (2004). Spasticity after stroke: Its occurrence and association with motor impairments and activity limitations. *Stroke, 35.* Retrieved from http://stroke.ahajournals.org/cgi/content/abstract/35/1/134 accessed 8/21/10

Stary, H. (2004). *Atlas of atherosclerosis: Progression and regression* (2nd ed.) (p. 21:2). The Parthenon Publishing Group.

Steinlin, M., Roellin, K., & Schroth, G. (2004). Long-term follow-up after stroke in childhood. *European Journal of Pediatrics,163,* 245–250.

Suk, S., Sacco, R., Boden-Albala, B., Cheun, J., Pittman, J., Elkind, M., & Paik, M. (2003). Abdominal obesity and risk of ischemic stroke: The northern Manhattan stroke study. *Stroke, 34,* 1586–1592.

Takatsuru, D., Fukumoto, M., Yoshitomo, T., Nemoto, H., Tsukada, R., & Nabekurak, L. (2009). Neuronal circuit remodeling in the contralateral cortical hemisphere during functional recovery from cerebral infarction. *Journal of Neuroscience, 29*(32), 10081–10086.

Thomala, G., Schwark, C., Sobesky, J., Bluhmki, E., Fiebach, J., Fiehler, J., et al. (2006). Outcome and symptomatic bleeding complications of intravenous thrombolysis within 6 hours in MRI-selected stroke patients. *Stroke, 37,* 852–858.

Thomas, K., Gerlach, S., Jorn, H., Larson, J., Brott, T., & Files, J. (2007). Advances in the care of patients with intracerebral hemorrhage. *Mayo Clinic Proceedings, 82*(8), 987–990.

Thompson, H., & Ryan, A. (2009). The impact of stroke consequences on spousal relationships from the perspective of the person with stroke. *Journal of Clinical Nursing, 18*(12), 1803–1811.

Townend, E., Tinson, D., Kwan, J., & Sharpe, M. (2010). Feeling sad and useless': An investigation into personal acceptance of disability and its association with depression following stroke. *Clinical Rehabilitation, 24*(6), 555–564.

Treggiari, M., Walder, B., Suter, P., & Romand, J. (2003). A systematic review of the prevention of delayed ischemic neurological deficits with hypertension, hypervolemia, and hemodilution therapy following subarachnoid hemorrhage. *Journal of Neurosurgery, 98*(5), 978–984.

Trubelja, N., Vaughan, C., & Coplan, N. (2005). The role of statins in preventing stroke. *Preventive Cardiology, 8*(2), 98–101.

Turhan, N., Atalay, A., & Atabek, H. (2006). Impact of stroke etiology, lesion location and aging on post-stroke urinary incontinence as a predictor of functional recovery. *International Journal of Rehabilitation Research, 29*(4), 353–358.

Tyson, S., Hanley, M., Chillala, J., Selley, A., & Tallis, R. (2008). Sensory loss in hospital admitted people with stroke: characteristics, associated factors, and relationships with function. *Neurorehabilitation & Neural Repair, 22*(2), 166–172.

University of Medicine and Dentistry of New Jersey (2010). *Types of Stroke.* Retrieved May 20, 2011 from http://www.theuniversityhospital.com/stroke/types.htm

van Kooij, B., Hendrikse, J., Benders, M., de Vries, L., & Groenendaal, F. (2010). Anatomy of the circle of willis and blood flow in the brain-feeding vasculature in prematurely born infants. *Neonatology, 97,* 235–241.

van der Lee, J. H., Wagenaar, R. C., Lankhorst, G. J., et al. (1999). Forced use of the upper extremity in chronic stroke patients: Results from a single-blind randomized clinical trial. *Stroke, 30,* 2369–2375.

Veltkamp, R., Siebing, D., Sun, L., Heiland, S., Bieber, K., Marti, H., et al. (2005). Hyperbaric oxygen reduces blood–brain barrier damage and edema after transient focal cerebral ischemia. *Stroke, 36,* 1679–1683.

Vespa, P., O'Phelan, K., Shah, M., Mirabelli, J., Starkman, S., Kidwell, C., et al. (2003). Acute seizures after intracerebral hemorrhage: A factor in progressive midline shift and outcome. *Stroke, 60,* 1441–1446.

Vignolia, M. (2006). Agnosia and auditory agnosia: Dissociations in stroke patients. *Annals of the New York Academy of Sciences, 99,* 50–57.

Vilea, M., & Newell, D. (2008). Superficial temporal artery to middle cerebral artery bypass: Past, present, and future. *Neurosurgery, 24*(6), 566–579.

Voeks, J., McClure, L., Go, R., Prineas, R., Cushman, M., Kissela, B., & Roseman, J. (2008). Regional differences in diabetes as a possible contributor to the geographic disparity in stroke mortality: The reasons for geographic and racial differences in stroke study. *Stroke, 39,* 1675–1680.

Vuadens, P., Michel, P., Reichhart, M., Herrmann, F., Arnold, P., Bogousslavsky, J., & Ghika, J. (2006). Acute autonomic dysfunction contralateral to acute strokes: A prospective study of 100 consecutive cases. *European Journal of Neurology, 13*(11), 1245–125.

Walker, C., Walker, M., & Sunderland, A. (2003). Dressing after a stroke: A survey of current occupational therapy practice. *The British Journal of Occupational Therapy, 66*(1), 281–285.

Walton, K., & Buono, L. (2003). Horner syndrome. *Current Opinion in Ophthalmology, 14*(6), 357–363.

Ward, N. (2006). The neural substrates of motor recovery after focal damage to the central nervous system. *Archives of Physical Medicine and Rehabilitation, 87*(12), 30–35. Recovered from http://www.archives-pmr.org/article/S0003-9993(06)01282-2/abstract-article-footnote-1#article-footnote-1, http://www.archives-pmr.org/article/S0003-9993(06)01282-2/abstract-article-footnote-2#article-footnote-2

Ward, N., Brown, M., Thompson, A., & Frackowiak, R. (2006). Longitudinal changes in cerebral response to proprioceptive input in individual patients after stroke: An fMRI study. *Neurorehabitation Neural Repair, 20*(3), 398–405.

Westover, A., McBride, S., & Haley, R. (2007). Stroke in young adults who abuse amphetamines or cocaine: A population-based study of hospitalized patients. *Archives of General Psychiatry, 64*(4), 495–502.

Williams, L., Kroenke, K., Bakas, T., Plue, L., Brizendine, E., Tu, W., & Hendrie, H. (2007). Care management of post stroke depression. *Stroke, 38,* 998–1003.

Wintermark, M., Reichhart, M., Cuisenaire, O., Maeder, P., Thiran, J., Schnyder, P., et al. (2002). Comparison of admission perfusion computed tomography and qualitative diffusion and perfusion weighted magnetic resonance imaging in acute stroke patients. *Stroke, 33*(8), 2025–2032.

Wolf, S. L., Blanton, S., Baer, H., et al. (2002). Repetitive task practice: A critical review of constraint-induced movement therapy in stroke. *Neurologist, 8,* 325–338.

Xie, J., Wu, E., Zheng, Z., Croft, J., Greenlund, K., Mensah, G., & Labarthe, D. (2006). Impact of stroke on health-related quality of Life in the noninstitutionalized population in the United States. *Stroke, 37,* 2567–2572.

Yuan, J., Lipinski, M., & Degterev, A. (2009). Diversity in the mechanisms of neuronal cell death. *Neuron, 40*(2), 401–413.

Zazulia, A. R. (2002). Stroke. In V. S. Ramachandran (Ed.), *Encyclopedia of the human brain Vol. 4* (pp. 475–492). Boston, MA: Academic Press.

Zhang, X., Kedar, S., Lynn, M., Newman, N., & Biousse, V. (2006). Natural history of homonymous hemianopia. *Neurology, 66,* 901–905.

Zhao, X., Grotta, J., Gonzales, N., & Aronowski, M. (2009). Resolution as a therapeutic target: the role of microglia/microphages. *Stroke, 40,* 592–594.

10

Cardiopulmonary Disorders

■ *Carla Chase*

Nadine looked down at her feet and saw that they were really swollen today. She also felt more short of breath than she did a couple of days ago but assumed it was because she had been working hard to move some of her belongings into her daughter's home as she was going to help take care of her grandchildren for a few weeks. A couple of months ago, her doctor had told her that she had signs of **congestive heart failure** (CHF), and although she thought the name of the condition sounded serious, she was told she could control it. She had no time to think about it at the moment though, as she was focused on helping her daughter.

Over the next few days, her shortness of breath and fatigue worsened—and so did her swollen ankles. One night Nadine felt like she couldn't breathe if she lay flat in her bed, so she decided to sleep in her recliner. The next morning she decided to go see her doctor. While being weighed prior to her session, Nadine noticed that she had gained 4 pounds since last week, but also noted that she had been eating less. During their meeting, her doctor explained that her heart was not pumping hard enough to circulate her blood normally and that fluid was building up in her lungs and other parts of her body.

Occupational therapists often work with clients who have either a primary or secondary diagnosis that involves the cardiopulmonary system. This chapter reviews introductory anatomy and physiology information about the lungs and heart followed by descriptions of common conditions that negatively impact these important structures. **Hypertension** (HTN) and **coronary artery disease** (CAD) are presented together as these conditions are commonly involved in cardiopulmonary diagnoses. Major conditions of the lungs included are **pneumonia** and **chronic obstructive pulmonary disease** (COPD). Major conditions of the heart included are CHF and **myocardial infarction** (MI).

OVERVIEW OF THE CARDIOPULMONARY SYSTEM

The cardiopulmonary system includes the lungs, the heart, and their connections. In this section of the chapter, each component is discussed individually and then considered as a functional unit as the work of one impacts the other.

Lungs

Fast facts from the American Lung Association (2011):

- The surface area of the lungs is roughly the same size as a tennis court.
- The average adult takes 12 to 15 breaths a minute, which are over 6 million breaths per year.
- A sneeze can travel up to 100 miles per hour.

Lungs are a spongy, balloon-like part of the respiratory system where gas exchange occurs. The right side, with three lobes, is slightly larger than the left that has two lobes. Air moves into the nose or mouth, moves down through the pharynx, larynx, trachea, and bronchial tubes, and then into the lungs (Fig. 10.1) to complete the respiratory process.

To begin the inhalation process, the diaphragm muscle pulls down on the chest cavity, creating a vacuum for air to enter. Air moves through the lungs where small air sacs called **alveoli** perform the gas exchange. Oxygen is moved into the blood stream from the alveoli to be carried to cells throughout the body. Carbon dioxide, one of the body's waste products, is removed from the blood and exhaled during this exchange.

The respiratory system has several protective mechanisms. A thin flap of tissue called the **epiglottis** protects the lungs from foreign objects by covering the trachea during swallowing. This prevents food, drink, and other material from entering the air passages that lead to the lungs. Inhaled air is warmed and moistened within the nose and mouth and then cleaned by mucus that lines the remaining airway structures. This sticky substance is moved up and out of the system by **cilia** (hair-like structures). A cough is a forceful way of expelling material in order to keep airways clean (Lungs, 2011).

Heart

Fast facts from the Cleveland Clinic (2011):

- The adult heart pumps about 5 quarts of blood each minute.
- The heart beats about 100,000 times each day.
- The heart is more in the center of the chest than the left side, but the bottom is tilted left.

The heart is the main pumping station of the circulatory system, working to provide needed nutrients and oxygen to all organs of the body. The heart attempts to provide the right amount of blood at the proper rate to make sure oxygen gets where it is needed at all times. If the heart is not working properly, either pumping too quickly and thready (**tachycardia**) or otherwise inefficiently, circulation is impacted and oxygen may not be available to other body structures. The amount of oxygen needed throughout the body varies depending on the task being completed. More oxygen is needed in the gastrointestinal system after eating. More oxygen is needed by voluntary muscle groups while exercising. Heart rate changes to meet these needs.

The heart has muscular walls that surround four chambers with valves to keep the blood moving in one direction and to prevent back flow. The two upper chambers, called atria, collect blood, and the two lower chambers, called ventricles, pump blood out of the heart (Figs. 10.2 and 10.3). Starting with the upper chambers (atria), oxygen-poor blood enters the right atrium after circulating the body, and oxygen-rich blood enters the left atrium after leaving the lungs. The oxygen-poor blood continues to the right ventricle and then goes into the lungs to receive oxygen. The oxygen-rich blood from the lungs continues to the left ventricle and then goes out to the body.

There are two distinctive parts to a heartbeat that are measured when taking blood pressure readings. The **systolic** reading is taken during the constriction phase of blood flow through the heart and is the higher of the two numbers. The **diastolic** reading is taken during the resting part of the process and is the lower of the two (National Heart Lung and Blood Institute [NHLBI], 2011a).

The Heart and Lung Connection

The heart and lungs must work in tandem in order to efficiently and effectively transport oxygen and nutrients to all systems of the body. De-oxygenated blood is circulated through the alveoli (air sacs) of the lungs in order to gather oxygen from inhaled air, and remove carbon dioxide waste. The lungs then return the blood, which is now oxygenated, directly to the heart to be pumped back out to the body. Because of this direct connection between these two organs, conditions impacting one can cause impairments of the other. Barr et al. (2010) found a link between the extent of airflow obstruction and efficiency of the left ventricle of the heart in patients with emphysema. CHF, as described later in this chapter, also illustrates the partnership of the heart and lungs and the negative impact when this relationship is out of balance.

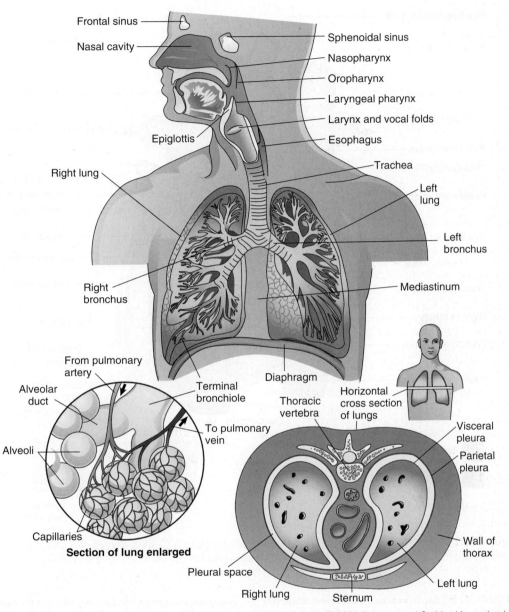

Figure 10.1 Respiratory system. (From Smeltzer, S. C. O., & Bare, B. G. [2002]. *Brunner and Suddarth's textbook of medical-surgical nursing* (9th ed.). Philadelphia, PA: Lippincott Williams & Wilkins.)

COMMON DISORDERS OF THE CARDIOPULMONARY SYSTEM

The conditions presented in this chapter may be present at the same time and may have overlapping symptoms. Some are curable while others are considered controllable or manageable. CAD and HTN are considered to be chronic diseases that can lead to further complications and are common preexisting conditions for many cardiopulmonary diagnoses.

Hypertension

HTN, commonly known as high blood pressure, is an increase in the amount of force that is pushing against the walls of the arteries as the heart pumps blood. It is usually asymptomatic, so it can go unnoticed and untreated for years, but it can be causing damage to the heart, kidneys, and other body structures during that time. NHLBI states that any reading between 120/80 and 139/89 is considered prehypertensive and treatment is recommended.

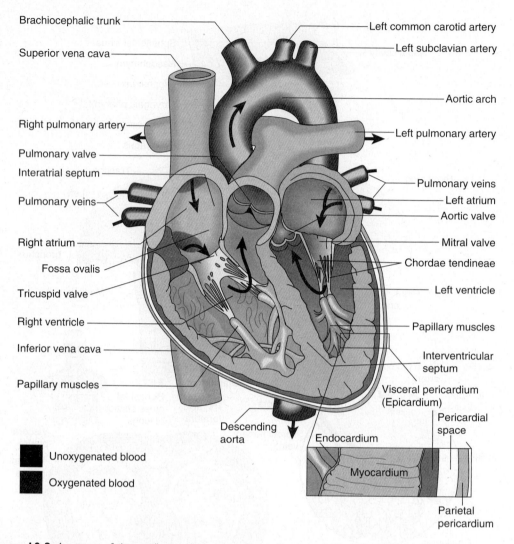

Figure 10.2 Anatomy of the cardiovascular system. (From Smeltzer, S. C. O., & Bare, B. G. [2002]. *Brunner and Suddarth's textbook of medical-surgical nursing* (9th ed.). Philadelphia, PA: Lippincott Williams & Wilkins.)

NHBLI (2011b) also reports that one in three adults has HTN. Prevention recommendations include healthy lifestyle choices such as getting regular exercise and eating a healthy diet. Treatment recommendations involve following a physician-recommended healthcare plan to include adhering to exercise and healthy eating plans, monitoring blood pressure levels, and taking medications.

Coronary Artery Disease

CAD, also known as coronary heart disease, is actually related to a larger condition called **atherosclerosis**, a condition where plaque made of cholesterol, fat, calcium, and other substances sticks to the inner lining of arteries that are taking oxygen-rich blood from the heart to the body.

Over time this plaque hardens and narrows the opening of the blood vessels, thus reducing the rate of oxygenated blood being delivered. When the arteries of the heart are affected, it is specifically called CAD. As with HTN, the causes are thought to be part lifestyle choices and part genetics. Smoking, obesity, diabetes, and high cholesterol are among the risk factors that may be controlled in some cases. Family history and age are risk factors that cannot be controlled.

Treatment for CAD is a physician-recommended plan of care that includes healthy lifestyle choices, medications, and, if severe enough, surgical procedures. Possible procedures are angioplasty, coronary artery bypass grafting, and carotid endarterectomy. **Angioplasty** is a procedure where a small mesh tube is inserted into the

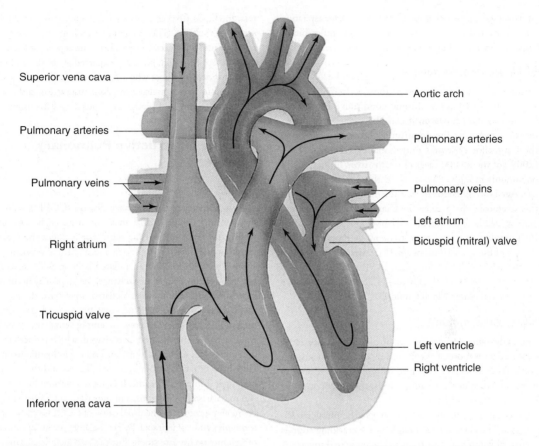

Figure 10.3 Blood flow through the heart. (From Anatomical Chart Co. [2004]. Baltimore, MA: Lippincott Williams & Wilkins.)

coronary artery to widen the opening, thus increasing the blood flow. If the blockage is more severe, arteries or veins from other parts of the body (often the legs) are "harvested" and then surgically attached to bypass the blocked arteries near the heart in a process called **coronary artery bypass grafting** (CABG). Last, **carotid endarterectomy** is a surgery where the carotid artery in the neck is opened in order to remove some of the plaque that has formed, thus allowing better blood flow to the brain. Each of these treatments has benefits and risks that must be considered in partnership with a physician.

Not all of the cardiopulmonary conditions seen by occupational therapists are included here as only the more common conditions were chosen. However, there are considerations for practice regardless of the cardiopulmonary condition the patient may have.

These include the following:

1. Know your patient's precautions.
2. Access appropriate, accurate, and updated Web sites or other sources for additional information about *any* condition when you are unsure.

3. Be comfortable using measurement devices (blood pressure cuff, stethoscope, pulse oximeter), taking a pulse, and assisting a patient with oxygen use such as placement and adjustment of the nasal cannula.
4. Communicate appropriately with your medical team, and know when to contact a doctor or nurse with status changes.

Pneumonia

Etiology

Pneumonia is an inflammation of the lung tissue caused by infection, usually from bacterial, viral, or fungal sources. The exposure to the bacteria or virus that can cause this condition most often occurs in the community and is called community-acquired pneumonia. Hospital-acquired pneumonia can happen following a surgery, especially if it was an abdominal or chest surgery or if the patient is in an intensive care unit or has a weakened immune system. Patients who have had a brain injury such as a cerebral vascular accident or traumatic brain injury that has impacted their swallowing sequence or gag reflex may be at risk for aspiration pneumonia, and it can occur when food or some other foreign substance enters the lungs and causes an infection.

Incidence and Prevalence

Pneumonia is most common in those over 65 years old and those who have a chronic condition or impaired immune system; however, it can also occur in younger, healthier people if the opportunity arises. According to the Center for Disease Control and Prevention (CDC) (2009), of the 60,000 cases of deaths from influenza and pneumonia in 2004, 85% involved those over 65 years of age. Age is a risk factor in that the older the person with this diagnosis, the greater the chance of hospitalization and/or death from pneumonia (Mayo Clinic, 2010a). Pneumonia as the cause of death increases drastically after the age of 85, with a jump from 37 deaths out of 100,000 for those 65 to 74 years of age to 137 per 100,000 deaths for those 75 to 84 and finally to 571.2 out of 100,000 for those 85 and older (Mayo Clinic, 2010a).

Signs and Symptoms

The early signs and symptoms of pneumonia are often confused with those of the flu and may start with a cough and a fever. Additional symptoms can include shortness of breath (**dyspnea**), sweating, chills, chest pain or tightness, headache, and fatigue.

Diagnosing pneumonia may involve the physician listening to the chest during breathing for crackling sounds (**rales**) or rumbling sounds caused by increased mucus. A chest x-ray may be necessary to further assess lung function. Blood and mucus tests may also be necessary to identify the infection-causing organism.

Course and Prognosis

The first signs may appear as if it is the onset of the flu, with coughing and a slight fever. The severity of the symptoms can vary widely depending on the infecting organism and the overall health and age of the patient. If caught early or if it is a mild case, hospitalization can be avoided. If hospitalization is deemed necessary, it typically lasts 3 to 4 days. Pneumonia can be serious for older adults, especially if they are over 85 years old or have additional health complications. If left untreated, pneumonia can lead to severe respiratory distress and death, as organs are no longer getting the oxygen they need and begin to fail (NHLBI, 2011b).

Medical/Surgical Management

Vaccines are important in the prevention of pneumonia. Getting an annual flu shot helps, as flu can turn into pneumonia. Pneumonia vaccines are helpful for older adults and those with a challenged immune system.

As the severity of symptoms varies, so do the treatments. The standard plan, however, includes antibiotics, rest, and fluids. Oxygen may be needed temporarily until the symptoms subside. Since coughing is an important mechanism for removing excess mucus from the airways, it should not be stopped totally, but can be quieted at times to allow for rest and sleep. Those who are more medically challenged may need to be hospitalized for close observation and may receive intravenous antibiotics and fluids as well as oxygen.

Chronic Obstructive Pulmonary Disease

Etiology

Chronic obstructive pulmonary disease (COPD), a progressive lung condition that makes it increasingly difficult to breathe, is an overarching term that includes the more specific conditions of emphysema and chronic bronchitis. Rather than resembling an inflated balloon with tension and pressure for proper air exchange, the lungs may become more floppy and somewhat deflated, may have damaged alveoli walls or thickened mucosal linings and therefore cannot support good airflow. In **emphysema**, the alveoli walls may become deflated or damaged, which reduces the amount of gas exchange that can occur. In **chronic bronchitis**, the bronchial tubes become inflamed and thickened making it difficult to breathe. It is not uncommon for a person to have both conditions, and thus the term COPD may be more appropriate. The usual cause of COPD is the long-term inhalation of irritants. By far the most common source of irritants is cigarette smoke but can also include air pollution, dust, or chemicals (American Lung Association, 2011).

Incidence and Prevalence

Over 12 million people are living with COPD, and it is the fourth leading cause of death in the United States (CDC, 2009). Because the condition worsens slowly and chronic exposure to an irritant may have occurred over several years, symptoms usually are not seen in people <40 years of age. Incidence is higher in areas of high pollution and from workers in high-risk areas (Mayo Clinic, 2010b).

Signs and Symptoms

Symptoms of COPD include persistent cough that produces a large amount of mucus (also called smoker's cough), wheezing or whistling while inhaling, chest tightness, and dyspnea with exertion. As the condition becomes more severe, swelling in the ankles and feet may be noticeable, and lips and fingernails may be bluish due to decreased oxygen levels.

In addition to listening to the lungs with a stethoscope and taking a thorough history related to smoking or other exposure to irritants, the physician may request a series of tests and labs to confirm the COPD diagnosis. Lung function tests such as spirometry, the main test of lung function for those with COPD, measures how much air is forcefully exhaled and how quickly.

Course and Prognosis

COPD is not curable and slowly worsens over time. Breathing becomes more difficult and less oxygen gets to the body. The heart may become enlarged from the strain and blood pressure increases. Eventually, lack of oxygen to body structures leads to cognitive deficits and organ failure, which then leads to death. The rate of decline can be modified and quality of life maintained longer by quitting smoking, organizing and simplifying daily life tasks, avoiding irritants, managing symptoms, getting annual flu shots, and preparing for emergencies by having medical information and medications conveniently located (NHBLI, 2011b).

Medical/Surgical Management

Medical management of COPD includes use of oxygen, inhaled medications, and oral medications such as steroids and antibiotics, which are all designed to ease breathing. Qualified patients with serious symptoms may have lung reduction surgery or lung transplants.

Congestive Heart Failure

Etiology

CHF, also known simply as heart failure, is a chronic, noncurable condition where the heart does not beat strongly enough to maintain adequate blood flow to all systems in the body, causing organs to be oxygen-deprived and the body to retain fluid. Because of the close connection to the lungs, when blood flow weakens, fluid can build up in the tissues around the lungs causing difficulties with breathing. CHF can be caused by infections or conditions such as a heart attack that damage the heart muscle, but the most common causes are CAD and HTN (American Heart Association, 2009).

Incidence and Prevalence

Currently, approximately 5.8 million people in the United States have CHF with about 670,000 people diagnosed each year (CDC, 2009). About 300,000 deaths each year are caused by CHF.

Signs and Symptoms

Symptoms may be subtle at first but will increase in intensity as the condition progresses. Shortness of breath, difficulty breathing while lying down, weight gain from fluid retention, and swelling of the feet and legs are common symptoms. Other symptoms that may be noticed include decreased urine output, general fatigue, decreased ability to focus, and occasional nausea and vomiting.

A physical examination by the physician provides information in order to make this diagnosis. Signs noted may be neck arteries that are distended, swollen liver noted during palpation, fluid sounds in the lungs, and swelling of the feet and legs. More formal diagnostic procedures include a chest x-ray, heart CT scan, echocardiogram, MRI, and various blood and urine analyses.

Course and Prognosis

Much like COPD, CHF is a condition that progresses slowly over time depriving the body of needed oxygen and eventually leading to death. Shortness of breath is one of the first signs of this condition and may be mistaken for a normal part of the aging early in the process. Decreasing endurance and increasing difficulty in breathing worsens as the condition progresses (American Heart Association, 2009).

As with all cardiopulmonary conditions presented in this chapter, eating right by taking smaller portions and avoiding salt, exercising regularly, avoiding smoking, and following a medical management plan can decrease the rate of progression and help minimize the symptoms as long as possible. A systematic review of research articles leads authors to report that although length of life was not significantly impacted, men with mild to moderate CHF who participated in regular exercise had a better quality of life and had better overall fitness than those who did not (Davies et al., 2010).

Medical/Surgical Management

Along with healthy lifestyle choices, medications and surgeries are also used to treat CHF and help minimize symptoms as they present. Medications may include angiotensin-converting enzyme (ACE) inhibitors that expand blood vessels and ease the heart's workload, diuretics that help the body get rid of fluid, and dioxin that helps the heart contract properly. Surgical procedures can provide some relief of symptoms. Insertion of a pacemaker to help maintain a consistent heartbeat, angioplasty to hold the arteries open, CABG and heart valve repair, or replacement to improve circulation are some of the more invasive treatment methods that are utilized when treating CHF.

Myocardial Infarction

Etiology

MI, more commonly known as a heart attack, occurs when a blood vessel to the heart is blocked, causing heart muscle tissue to be without oxygen and resulting in damage or death to that tissue. CAD, in which the artery walls have plaque formations that impair blood flow, diabetes, and high blood pressure all are known causes of MI. Other risk factors for this condition are increasing age, smoking, and family history.

Prevalence

According to the American Heart Association's 2009 statistics report, someone in the United States has a heart attack every 34 seconds, with approximately 16% of those dying from that event.

Signs and Symptoms

The major symptoms of a MI, particularly for men, are chest pain and tightness, feelings of indigestion, dizziness, shortness of breath, and excessive sweating. Women may be less likely than men to have the hallmark chest tightness symptom and tend to report shortness of breath, weakness, and fatigue (McSweeney et al., 2003).

A MI is a medical emergency that requires immediate attention. Once at the hospital, a physical exam will be completed, and tests such as a coronary angiography, CT scan, electrocardiogram, echocardiography, or MRI may be completed to make the final diagnosis.

Course and Prognosis

The prognosis for recovery depends on the amount of cardiac tissue that was damaged during the time of the blockage and the length of time it took to receive medical attention. If caught and treated early, full recovery and return to all activities of daily living (ADLs) may be possible. Sudden cardiac death can occur early in the process. During the early hospitalization stage of recovery, time in the intensive care unit may be necessary to monitor for irregular heart rhythms.

Cardiac rehabilitation that includes exercise, education, and counseling may be necessary to help patients ease back into their daily routine following strict precautions and progressing at a slow and steady pace. To help guide physical rehabilitation and determine safe recommended levels of activity, a **metabolic equivalent** (MET) chart is used. A MET is the amount of energy that an activity requires, with more sedentary tasks such as watching TV or doing computer work using 1.5 to 2 METS ranging up to some competitive sports requiring 11 or more METs. The physician and the team determines the maximum MET level for the patient until healing begins, and this will guide how much exercise can be completed or how much help the person needs with daily activities.

Medical/Surgical Management

In addition to the immediate emergency response that includes oxygen and stabilizing medications, surgeries to reestablish blood flow to the damaged area and additional medications are often necessary. One or more CABG procedures or angioplasty may be needed. Beta-blockers may be given to relieve chest pain and to treat heartbeat irregularities, ACE inhibitors reduce the workload and stress on the heart, and anticoagulants may help prevent blood clots from forming (PubMed Health, 2010).

TABLE 10.1 Common *Symptoms* and Their Impact on Occupational Performance

Dyspnea	Clients may need frequent breaks and may need chairs placed in various positions around their house to provide a place to sit.
Fatigue	Clients may need to have tasks broken down into smaller parts and to do them over a longer period of time. Work simplification and energy conservation techniques will be needed.
Depression	This is a multilayered symptom as many emotional issues, stressors, and life reviews are common with cardiopulmonary conditions. Encouraging participation, supporting successes, and being empathetic are important therapeutic skills for helping clients figure out ways to do what they need to do in their occupational areas.
Difficulty focusing	Visual reminders and verbal cues may be needed. Processing time may be lengthened, so a slower pace may be helpful when problem-solving more complex tasks.
Anxiety	Clients may have more fear when attempting tasks. More time, encouragement, and pleasant distractions can help them move forward with the small day-to-day tasks. This can, however, become a larger issue that keeps clients from doing what they need to do.
Light-headedness	Allow clients to sit whenever possible to complete a task. Have seats close, and encourage them to stand near a stable counter or table, or use a grab bar if standing is needed.

IMPACT ON OCCUPATIONAL PERFORMANCE

The primary focus of the field of occupational therapy (OT) is clients' occupations and how they perform them. *The OT Practice Framework*, 2nd ed. (American Occupational Therapy Association, 2008), has divided occupations into the following eight categories in an attempt to support a thorough analysis of our client's needs and to help organize our critical thinking process:

1. Activities of daily living (ADL)
2. Instrumental activities of daily living (IADL)
3. Work
4. Play
5. Leisure
6. Education
7. Sleep/rest
8. Social participation

Considering each of these areas of occupations and then further exploring the specific tasks within each area provides a good base for determining the best treatment for the client. After determining the occupational needs of the client, it is important to then determine the effects of his or her symptoms on occupational performance.

The symptoms listed in Table 10.1 are common to many of the conditions presented in this chapter.

Precautions

Precautions are determined by the diagnosis and general client health. Some are formally dictated and documented by the physician, whereas others are determined by anyone on the healthcare team that recognizes a safety or health concern. They will change as the client's health status changes. Not only is it important for the therapist to be familiar with all of the client's precautions in order to keep him or her safe during the treatment session, it is also important to consider how these precautions impact the client's ability to safely complete all areas of occupations (Table 10.2).

OT practitioners play a key role in helping people with cardiopulmonary diseases. Conditions such as CHF

TABLE 10.2 Common *Precautions* and Their Impact on Occupational Performance

No heavy lifting	Any task that would require lifting would need to be modified or completed by someone else. Lifting precautions also limit wheelchair self-propulsion as this, too, puts too much strain on the upper body.
Heart rate ≤ 110 beats/minute	Clients will need to be taught to take their own heart rate and be reminded to take it if more exertion is attempted. Written cues may be needed for reminders.
No activities at a MET rate higher than 6	Clients will be limited in the tasks they can complete until this precaution is lifted. In some cases, the activities that are of a higher MET value may not be permitted for many weeks.
Oxygen on at all times (liters determined by physician)	Clients will need to be connected to an oxygen source at all times. That usually involves a tank and a long hose that must be manipulated to ensure safety with mobility.
Maintain low-salt diet	Clients may need to modify cooking habits and seasoning habits and to explore alternatives.
Record daily weight	This is important for those with CHF. Clients may need a scale with large numbers and a system set up for recording their daily weight. Scale may need to be in a place where clients can hold on to a stable object while stepping up and down.
Follow recommended oral and inhaled medication schedule	Visual reminders and environmental set up may be needed. Having a dedicated site for the clients to go to when doing their breathing treatments can help.

and COPD are chronic conditions that require new self-management techniques to maintain health, and these new medical needs have to be integrated into daily routines. According to AOTA, OT practitioners work collaboratively with clients to identify needs and design strategies for independent health management, and helping clients take charge of their health care can improve their quality of life (as cited in Bondoc and Siebert, 2009).

Case Illustrations

Case Study 1

Wanda, an 87-year-old woman, was admitted to the intensive care unit in a hospital through the emergency room 2 days ago. Prior to being brought to the hospital by ambulance, she had been coughing and feeling ill for several days but had refused to go see her doctor. When she finally agreed to get medical help, she reported that she was short of breath and felt a weight on her chest. She was also weak and malnourished. Wanda was diagnosed with pneumonia. Antibiotics were started, a saline drip was inserted, and, due to her severe weakness, a catheter was inserted to limit transfers to the toilet. The occupational therapist evaluated her, according to doctor's orders, after she was transferred to a regular room.

Social History

Wanda's son moved into her single-story home with her following the death of her husband 10 years ago. She is particularly proud of her gardens and of the fact that she just retired a few years ago from seamstress work for an upholstery shop. Since retirement, she reports enjoying visits to the library to get stacks of romance novels and cooking for her family. She is no longer driving and reports feeling frustrated by the loss of independence but states that she is too nervous to drive now.

Current Activity Level

Wanda is currently much debilitated as she transitions from the intensive care unit to the regular hospital wing to continue her recovery. She is so weak that she is unable to move from supine to sit independently, but follows directions well and appears cognitively intact. Prior to coming into the hospital with pneumonia, she was doing her basic care and some light cooking independently using a wheeled walker. Her son reports that she appeared to be slowing down a bit and taking more rest breaks recently.

Case Study 2

William is a 63-year-old man who was diagnosed with emphysema 8 years ago. He had provided care for his mother as she struggled to breathe and had to be connected to her oxygen tank "like an umbilical cord" throughout the house until she had died of emphysema 2 years ago. He now has his own oxygen tank and takes breathing treatments throughout the day, but still he reports feeling little relief from the struggle. His activity level has steadily declined, and he has lost his appetite. The steroid medication he is taking to help his breathing has caused his face to look puffy and almost unrecognizable in the mirror. The homecare agency has received a referral to evaluate and treat William as he was recently discharged from the hospital following recovery from pneumonia.

Social History

William is divorced, and his only daughter has moved to another state and is no longer visiting or calling. He has numerous siblings and nieces and nephews that visit. However, they are more likely to ask for help than to provide it. He lives alone, with his dog, in a single-story home in a subdivision outside of town. He still drives, but becomes anxious when traveling more than 10 or 15 minutes from his home, which makes going to his doctor appointments 30 minutes away very stressful. He has many friends who involve him in social events and give him rides as often as he is willing, but he finds that his breathing becomes more labored after being out for more than a couple of hours. He admits to feelings of anxiety and depression.

Current Activity Level

Since his discharge from the hospital, William appears weak overall but is attempting to build his endurance as much as he is able. He is very active in online social media and spends hours each day online posting on social sites or playing games. He also reports having the television on "almost 24 hours a day." He is able to cook and do light housekeeping but finds that it is getting more and more difficult to keep it up as he has in the past. He also reports that taking a shower standing in the tub "takes a lot out of him." He appears eager to continue to maintain his independence and to take suggestions on best to do so.

REFERENCES

American Heart Association. (2009). Heart disease and stroke statistics 2009 update. *Circulation*. Retrieved from http://www.heart.org/HEARTORG/Conditions/HeartAttack/HeartAttackToolsResources/Patient-Information-Sheets-Heart-Attack_UCM_303950_Article.jsp

American Lung Association. (2011). *How lungs work*. Retrieved from http://www.lungusa.org/your-lungs/how-lungs-work

American Occupational Therapy Association. (2008). Occupational therapy practice framework: Domain and process (2nd ed.). *American Journal of Occupational Therapy, 62,* 625–683.

Barr, R. G., Bluemke, D. A., Ahmed, F. S., Carr, J. J., Enright, P. L., Hoffman, E. A., et al. (2010). Percent emphysema, airflow obstruction, and impaired left ventricular filling. *New England Journal of Medicine, 362,* 217–227.

Bondoc, S., & Siebert, C. (2009). The role of occupational therapy in chronic disease management. *American Occupational Therapy Association Fact Sheet*, Retrieved from http://www.aota.org

Center for Disease Control and Prevention. (2009). *FastStats A to Z*. Retrieved from www.cdc.gov/nchs/fastats

Cleveland Clinic. (2011). *Your heart and blood vessels*. Retrieved from http://my.clevelandclinic.org/heart/heartworks/heartfacts.aspx

Davies, E. J., Moxham, T., Rees, K., Singh, S., Coats, A. J. S., Ebrahim, S., et al. (2010). Exercise training for systolic heart failure: Cochrane systematic review and meta-analysis. *European Journal of Heart Failure, 12,* 706–715.

Lungs. (2011). In *Encyclopædia Britannica*. Retrieved from http://www.britannica.com/EBchecked/topic/351473/lung

Mayo Clinic Health Information. (2010a). *Pneumonia*. Retrieved from http://www.mayoclinic.com/health/pneumonia/DS00135

Mayo Clinic Health Information. (2010b). *Chronic obstructive pulmonary disease*. Retrieved from http://www.mayoclinic.com/health/copd/DS00916

McSweeney, J. C., Cody, M., O'Sullivan, P., Elberson, K., Moser, D. K., & Garvin, B. J. (2003). Women's early warning symptoms of acute myocardial infarction. *Circulation, 108,* 2619–2623.

National Heart Lung and Blood Institute (NHLBI). (2011a). *How the heart works*. Retrieved from http://www.nhlbi.nih.gov/health/dci/Diseases/hhw_anatomy.html

National Heart Lung and Blood Institute (NHLBI). (2011b). *Diseases and conditions index*. Retrieved from http://www.nhlbi.nih.gov/health/dci/Diseases/Hbp/HBP_WhatIs.html

PubMed Health. (2010). *Heart attack*. Retrieved from http://www.ncbi.nlm.nih.gov/pubmedhealth/PMH0001246/

11

Diabetes

■ *Joanne Estes*

Serena is a 12-year-old girl who lives in an urban Hispanic neighborhood of a large Midwestern city. She spends most of her time not in school watching television and playing video games with a couple of neighborhood friends or by herself. Serena has never been interested in playing sports, so her parents stopped encouraging her to do so. Serena's parents both hold full-time jobs, so she is often home alone and responsible for taking care of herself. Her meals and snacks consist of convenience and processed foods, and she also often eats at fast food restaurants. Serena is 5'5" tall, weighs 200 pounds, and has a body mass index (BMI) of 33.3 kg/m^2, placing her in a category of obese children/adolescents. Lately, her mother notices that Serena seems more tired than usual, drinks a lot of soda pop, and uses the bathroom frequently. Serena's mother takes her to the pediatrician where blood work results showed a random plasma glucose level of 225 mg/dL. She is diagnosed as having **type 2 diabetes**.

DESCRIPTION AND DEFINITION

Diabetes mellitus, more commonly known as diabetes, refers to a group of metabolic conditions characterized by a malfunction in the body's ability to either make or use insulin. Insulin is a hormone produced by the pancreas and functions to regulate glucose metabolism. Insulin transports glucose into the body's cells where it is used for growth and energy. Without insulin, glucose builds up in the bloodstream and is ultimately excreted in the urine (Fig. 11.1). Without insulin to transport it, organs and tissues do not receive glucose causing the body to break down its own fat or lipids to produce an energy source. Total lack of insulin is potentially lethal, and a chronic high blood glucose level has devastating effects on multiple tissues and organ systems.

Diabetes can be classified into five disease entities according to etiology. The two most common forms are type 1 and type 2. Type 1, formerly known as insulin-dependent or juvenile onset diabetes mellitus, typically occurs in children and accounts for 5% to 10% of all cases of diabetes (O'Keefe, Bell, & Wynne, 2009). **Type 1 diabetes** is a condition of complete insulin deficiency and requires insulin replacement for survival (O'Keefe et al., 2009). Onset of the disease is abrupt with the individual initially presenting in an acutely ill state and oftentimes with a life-threatening condition known as **diabetic ketoacidosis** (DKA) (Goodman, 2009).

In type 2 (formerly known as non–insulin-dependent or adult-onset) diabetes mellitus, insulin is secreted but insulin resistance is present and the amount of insulin may be insufficient (Goodman, 2009), producing a chronic

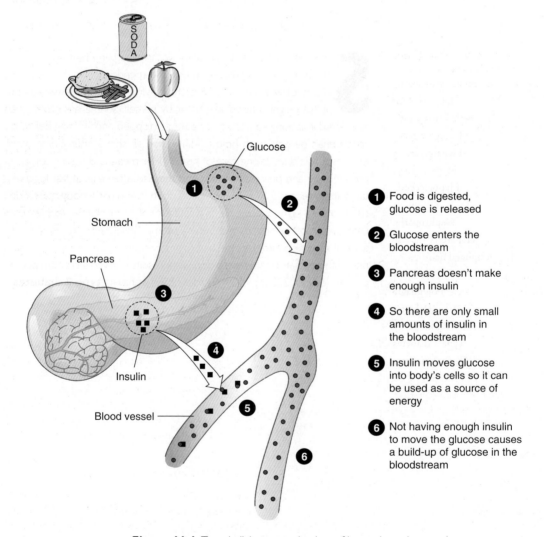

1 Food is digested, glucose is released

2 Glucose enters the bloodstream

3 Pancreas doesn't make enough insulin

4 So there are only small amounts of insulin in the bloodstream

5 Insulin moves glucose into body's cells so it can be used as a source of energy

6 Not having enough insulin to move the glucose causes a build-up of glucose in the bloodstream

Figure 11.1 Type 1 diabetes mechanism of hyperglycemia.

state of **hyperglycemia** (Surampudi, John-Kalarickal, & Fonseca, 2009). Type 2 accounts for 90% to 95% of all cases of diabetes and typically occurs with increasing age and in people who are obese (O'Keefe et al., 2009). A marked increase in prevalence of obesity in children and adolescents both in the United States and globally has resulted in increases in type 2 diabetes for these age groups (Lipton et al., 2005; Pinhas-Hamiel & Zeitler, 2004). Onset is gradual, and the disease may go undetected for years (O'Keefe et al.).

The third classification is gestational diabetes, a transient form of diabetes mellitus that occurs during pregnancy and typically requires no further treatment after delivery (Jovanovic, 2010). However, 35% of women with gestational diabetes will develop type 2 diabetes within 5 to 10 years (O'Keefe et al., 2009). Diabetes resulting from other causes forms the fourth classification. These include pathological conditions that damage the pancreas (e.g., chronic pancreatitis, cystic fibrosis) and certain genetic syndromes (e.g., Down's syndrome, Klinefelter's syndrome, Turner's syndrome, Freiderich's ataxia) (American Diabetes Association [ADA], 2007). Prediabetes is the fifth classification and occurs in individuals who have impaired glucose tolerance (IGT) or impaired fasting glucose (IFG). Approximately 25% of people with prediabetes eventually develop type 2 diabetes; however, some interventions (e.g., diet/exercise, medications, bariatric surgery) have been shown to slow the progression (O'Keefe et al.).

ETIOLOGY

Type 1

The exact cause of type 1 diabetes mellitus is not well understood. (Adeghate, Shattner, & Dunn, 2006). The disease process is precipitated by an autoimmune response whereby antibodies are produced that destroys pancreatic insulin-producing cells known as beta cells (Sherwin, 1996). It has a strong genetic predisposition with environmental factors thought to trigger the autoimmune process that destroys the beta cells (Daneman, 2006). Environmental factors can be divided into three categories: viral infections, infant diet, and exposure to toxins (Atkinson & Eisenbarth, 2001). While exposure to certain viruses (e.g., Enterovirus, Coxsackie B, Mumps) is thought to be a trigger (Daneman, 2006), research about their role is contradictory (Eisenbarth & McCulloch, 2010). Infant diet, specifically ingestion of cow's milk, early introduction of gluten-based cereals, and a short duration of breastfeeding are thought to be inciting factors (Akerblom, Vaarala, Hyoty, Ilonen, & Knip, 2002; Laron, 2002). Toxins in the form of ingested nitrates and nitrites in food (e.g., processed meat products) and water may also be a triggering factor (Akerblom et al., 2002; Devendra, Liu, & Eisenbarth, 2004).

Type 2

Genetic predisposition is stronger for type 2 diabetes than for type 1 as concurrence of the disease in monozygotic twins approaches 100% (Adeghate, Schattner, & Dunn, 2006; O'Keefe et al., 2009). Other factors include aging (Hseuh & Bryer-Ash, 2009), physical inactivity (Kriska et al., 2001), chronic stress (Adeghate et al., 2006), and being obese. Obesity is a strong contributing factor as 80% of people with type 2 diabetes are obese with the remaining 20% having a high percentage of abdominal body fat (Goodman, 2009). Finally, ethnicity is a risk factor in that African Americans, Hispanics, Native Americans, Asians, and Pacific Islanders are more likely to develop diabetes (O'Keefe et al., 2009; Pavkov et al, 2007).

INCIDENCE AND PREVALENCE

Children and Adolescence Incidence

The 2007 National Diabetes Fact Sheet provides statistics based on 2002 to 2003 data (Centers for Disease Control and Prevention [CDC], 2008a). According to this report, 15,000 youth (rate of 19 per 1,000) were newly diagnosed with type 1 diabetes, and 3,700 youth (rate of 5.3 per 100,000) with type 2 diabetes per year. Non-Hispanic white youth had the highest rate of newly diagnosed cases of type 1 diabetes (20 per 100,000), with type 2 being extremely rare in this group of youth under age 10. The highest rates of newly diagnosed type 2 cases occurred in American Indians (approximately 35 per 100,000); African Americans (approximately 20 per 100,000); Asian/Pacific Islanders (approximately 20 per 100,000); and Hispanics (approximately 10 per 100,000). For these groups, the incidence of type 2 diabetes was greater than that of type 1.

Adult Incidence

In 2007, about 1.6 million new cases of diabetes were diagnosed in people aged 20 or older in the United States, with the majority of cases in the 40 to 59 age group (CDC, 2008a). The age-adjusted incidence of diabetes was similar for men (8.4 per 1,000) and women (7.8 per 1,000) aged 18 to 79 in 2008 (CDC, 2008b). Incidence for Black, Native-American, Hispanic, and Asian Americans is 1.5 to 2 times that of Caucasian Americans (Goodman, 2009).

Prevalence of Diabetes

Nearly 24 million Americans or approximately 8% of the population now have diabetes (CDC, 2008a). This number tripled from 1980 to 2007 (CDC, 2008b). Prevalence is associated with race and ethnicity. For type 1 diabetes, African Americans and people of Asian descent have the lowest prevalence whereas Caucasians and people of Finnish, Scandinavian, Scottish, and Sardinian descent have the highest (Sherwin, 1996). Prevalence of type 2 diabetes is highest among American Indians and Alaskan natives (16.5%), followed by African Americans (11.8%), Hispanics (10.4%), Asian Americans (7.5%), and Caucasians (6.6%) (National Institute of Diabetes and Digestive and Kidney Diseases, 2008). Type 1 diabetes occurs equally among males and females (Dambro, 1995), with type 2 prevalence for males (9.3%) slightly higher than for females (7.2%) (Crawford et al., 2010).

SIGNS AND SYMPTOMS

Classic symptoms of diabetes are **polydipsia** (increased thirst), **polyuria** (frequent urination), **polyphagia** (increased hunger), blurred vision, weakness, fatigue, and dizziness (Goodman, 2009). Additional symptoms of type 1 are weight loss, muscle cramps, irritability, emotional lability, headaches, anxiety attacks, abdominal pain and discomfort, diarrhea or constipation, and altered school and work behaviors. The individual may also present with **ketonuria** (Goodman). Ketones are waste products from the body's breakdown of fat for energy, high concentrations of which leads to DKA (ADA, 2007). Symptoms of DKA include fruity odor breath, nausea and vomiting, confusion, difficulty breathing, and dry or flushed skin (ADA, 2007).

People with type 2 diabetes experience some of the same symptoms as type 1, including polyuria, polydipsia, polyphagia, unusual weight loss, extreme weakness and fatigue, and irritability. Additionally, frequent skin, gum, or bladder infections; cuts or bruises that are slow to heal; and numbness or tingling in the hands or feet are symptoms of type 2 diabetes (ADA, 2007). Symptoms related to hyperglycemia and complications can also occur (e.g., **nephropathy**, neuropathy, and **retinopathy**). These complications may be present upon diagnosis if preceded by long periods of hyperglycemia (Powers, 2001).

The clinical sign of diabetes is hyperglycemia or high plasma concentration of glucose measured following an 8-hour period of fasting. Normal fasting blood glucose level is <100 mg/dL. The range of fasting blood glucose level for IFG/IGT is 100 to 125 mg/dL (ADA, 2010). Diabetes is diagnosed if fasting blood glucose level is ≥126 mg/dL or random blood glucose level is >200 mg/dL with accompanying symptoms (ADA, 2010). **Hemoglobin A$_{1c}$** (HbA$_{1c}$) levels also diagnose the presence of diabetes. HbA$_{1c}$ level is the average concentration of glucose in the blood over a 6-week to 3-month time period, with levels ≥6.5% diagnostic of diabetes (ADA, 2010).

COURSE AND PROGNOSIS

After initial diagnosis of type 1 diabetes, a temporary remission period usually occurs for 3 to 6 months. During this time, overall control of the disease is easier and insulin needs are less. Insulin production gradually decreases until levels are insignificant and a state of total diabetes is reached (Dambro, 1995). Life expectancy is lower overall than for persons who do not have diabetes. One study showed a 7.5-year reduction for adult men and 8.5-year reduction for adult women with diabetes as compared to their nondiabetic counterparts (Franco, Steyerberg, Hu, Mackenbach, & Nusselder, 2007). Longevity and quality of life are currently better than in the past owing to improvements in insulin delivery regimens, medication treatment for hyperlipidemia, and lifestyle modifications (Miao, Brismar, Nyren, Ugarph-Morawski, & Ye, 2005). In 1993, the National Institute of Health completed a 9-year study called the "Diabetes Control and Complications Trial." Intensive insulin therapy was shown to slow the development of retinopathy and neuropathy (Sherwin, 1996). Prior to this landmark study it was unclear whether tight glucose control was beneficial.

People with diabetes experience periods of **hypoglycemia** or hyperglycemia. Hypoglycemia or insulin shock is a condition of too much insulin or oral hypoglycemic medication and not enough glucose in the blood stream (Dambro, 1995). Symptoms are vague: fatigue, headache, drowsiness, lassitude, tremulousness, shallow breathing, and nausea (Sherwin, 1996). It may produce seizures, accidental injury, catecholamine response, or arrhythmia or cardiac ischemia in patients with underlying cardiac disease (Sherwin). The patient needs to ingest some form of sugar, such as orange juice, cola, candy, or jelly, if able to swallow. On an emotional level, this could become a great fear of the patient's leading to less-than-optimal blood sugar control (Sherwin).

Hyperglycemia is a condition of too little insulin causing abnormally high blood glucose levels. Signs are thirst, heartburn, fast and deep breathing, excessive urination, headache, nausea, abdominal pain, blurred vision, and constipation (Dambro, 1995). If untreated, the patient is at risk for entering into a diabetic coma. Mortality from hyperglycemia increases with age and is usually caused by the presence of a comorbid condition (myocardial infarction, cerebral vascular accident, sepsis). Treatment depends on insulin to reverse metabolic abnormalities and on detection and successful treatment of the comorbid condition.

Hyperglycemia has a direct toxic effect on body tissues (Hsueh & Bryer-Ash, 2009). Few diseases have the same potential for damaging as many organ systems and producing impairments as diabetes (Fig. 11.2).

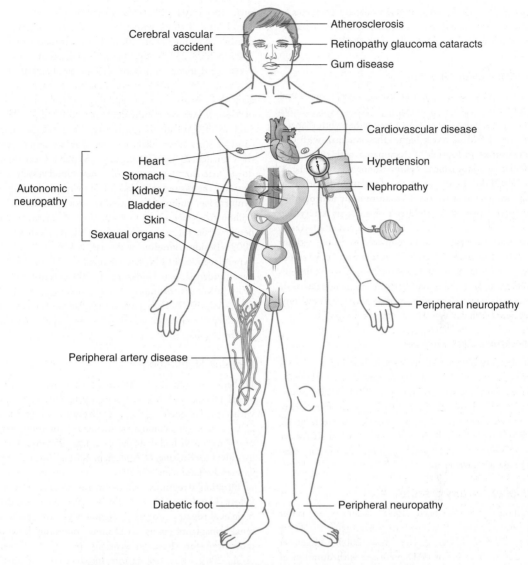

Figure 11.2 Impact of potential diabetes complications on body functions.

Damage occurs in macrovascular and microvascular structures as well as in autonomic and peripheral nerves. These complications are acute and chronic and impact the quality and duration of life for people with diabetes.

Macrovascular Complications

Hypertension

Essential **hypertension** (HTN) is defined as blood pressure >140/90 mm Hg (Bloomgarden, 2001). Although it varies across different racial and ethnic groups, HTN affects up to 70% of people with diabetes and is twice as common in people with diabetes as compared to those without (Klein, Klein, Lee, Cruickshanks, & Moss, 1996). In people with diabetes, incidence of HTN increases with longer duration of disease, older age, higher blood glucose levels, and being male (Klein et al., 1996). For people with type 1 diabetes, diabetic nephropathy is the most common cause of HTN (Lago, Singhy, & Nesto, 2007). Those with type 2 diabetes commonly develop HTN associated with central obesity (Lago et al., 2007). HTN combined with diabetes produces significant risk for cerebrovascular disease, retinopathy, and sexual dysfunction (Najarian et al., 2006). Each 10 mm Hg reduction in systolic blood pressure has been shown to reduce the risk of any complication by 12%, of death related to diabetes by 15%, of myocardial infarction by 11%, and of microvascular complications by 13% (Adler et al., 2000).

Cardiovascular Disease

Cardiovascular disease (CVD) is responsible for 75% of deaths for people with diabetes (O'Keefe et al., 2009). Risk of mortality due to CVD for women with diabetes (11- to 13-fold) is much higher than for men with diabetes (three- to fourfold) as compared with the general population (Juutilainen, Lehto, Ronnemaa, Pyorala, & Laakso, 2008). Predisposition to circulatory disturbances (e.g., accelerated atherosclerosis, **autonomic neuropathy**) produces a two- to fourfold risk of coronary artery disease and subsequent angina, acute myocardial infarction, and sudden cardiac death as compared to people without diabetes (Skyler et al., 2009; O'Keefe et al.). Active smoking doubles the risk of CVD in people with diabetes (O'Keefe et al.). The ADA (2010) recommends low-dose aspirin therapy (75 to 162 mg/day) for type 1 and type 2 patients with diabetes who are at risk for CVD.

Cerebrovascular Disease

Similarly, accelerated atherosclerosis leads to a 1.5 to 4 times greater risk of stroke as compared to people without diabetes (Hsueh & Bryer-Ash, 2009). Diabetes also doubles the risk of stroke recurrence, and patients have increased mortality following a stroke (O'Keefe et al., 2009). People with diabetes who have had a stroke are more likely to be discharged to a chronic care facility than to home (O'Keefe et al.).

Peripheral Artery Disease

Peripheral artery disease (PAD) occurs at an earlier age and at a rate of two to four times higher in people with diabetes (Hsueh & Bryer-Ash, 2009; O'Keefe et al., 2009). Severity of PAD increases with duration of diabetes (Beckman, Creager, & Libby, 2002). PAD predisposes people with diabetes to impaired wound healing (Falanga, 2005), tissue hypoxia, and decreased mobilization of white blood cells to infected tissues (Goodman, 2009), all of which contribute to diabetes being the leading cause of nontraumatic lower extremity amputation (O'Keefe et al.).

Microvascular Complications

Diabetic Retinopathy

Retinopathy is a key indicator of microvascular complications and as such of the impact of diabetes. Diabetic retinopathy is the leading cause of blindness in adults ages 18 to 74 (Mohamed, Gillies, & Wong, 2007). Duration of diabetes increases prevalence of retinopathy such that after 20 years most people with type 1 and 60% of those with type 2 will have some retinopathy (Mohamed et al., 2007). It was estimated that in 2005 to 2008, 28.5% of people with diabetes over age 40 years had diabetic retinopathy (Zhang et al., 2010). For this same group, 38.8% of non-Hispanic black individuals with diabetes had retinopathy as compared to 34.0% of Mexican American individuals and 26.4% of non-Hispanic white individuals (Zhang et al.). Similarly, males (38.1%) were more likely to have diabetic retinopathy than females (27.1%) (Zhang et al.). Vision loss can occur due to macular edema; rupture of new blood vessels that grow on the posterior surface of the vitreous leading to hemorrhage; pulling of new blood vessels on the retina leading to detachment; or formation of microvascular networks on the iris causing glaucoma (O'Keefe et al., 2009). Besides duration of disease, risk factors include hyperglecemia, HTN, use of insulin (Zhang et al.), hyperlipidemia (van Leiden et al., 2002), renal disease, heavy alcohol consumption, and smoking (Hseuh & Bryer-Ash, 2009). Tight glycemic control has been shown to reduce the incidence and progression of diabetic retinopathy (Mohamed et al.).

Diabetic Nephropathy

Diabetic nephropathy is the leading cause of End-Stage Renal Disease (ESRD), affecting up to 35% of people with type 1 diabetes (Hseuh & Bryer-Ash, 2009) and 25% to 40% (i.e., cumulative incidence) for those with type 2 who have had diabetes for at least 25 years (Parving, Hovind, Rossing, & Andersen, 2001). Thickening of glomerular basement membrane leads to the destruction of filtration structures and eventually to chronic renal failure (Goodman, 2009). Only 20% of people with diabetic nephropathy progress to hemodialysis treatment or renal transplantation as CVD more commonly leads to mortality before those interventions are needed (O'Keefe et al., 2009). Key risk factors for developing diabetic nephropathy include presence of obesity, hyperglycemia, and HTN; duration of diabetes; age of diabetes diagnosis (i.e., > age 50); gender (i.e., males > females); and race (i.e., Native Americans, Asians, Hispanics, and African Americans are at higher risk) (Hseuh & Bryer-Ash, 2009). Cigarette smoking also accelerates the rate of renal function loss (Hseuh & Bryer-Ash, 2009). Tight glycemic control and early treatment of HTN have been shown to slow progression of renal disease (Parving et al., 2001).

Neurologic Complications

Peripheral Neuropathy

Diabetic **peripheral neuropathy** (DPN) is the most common complication for patients with diabetes (Duby, Campbell, Setter, White, & Rasmussen, 2004) and the most common form of neuropathy in the Western world (Vinik, Park, Stansberry, & Pittinger, 2000). Prevalence estimates indicate that a range from 10% to 90% of people with diabetes have DPN (Hseuh & Bryer-Ash, 2009), with no difference based on the type of diabetes (Vinik et al., 2000). Most common symptoms include burning pain; stabbing, pricking, or tingling sensation; pathologic skin sensitivity; or deep aching pain (Boulton et al., 2000). Pain is worse at night, and symptoms are more common in lower extremities than in upper (Boulton et al., 2005). Proximal motor neuropathy (diabetic amyotrophy) is seen more in elderly people with diabetes, begins with pain in thighs and hips, and is followed by weakness of lower extremity proximal muscles (Vinik et al.).

Autonomic Neuropathy

Diabetic autonomic neuropathy (DAN) affects multiple systems in the body (Hsueh & Bryer-Ash, 2009), produces a wide spectrum of symptoms (Boulton et al., 2005), and can occur within 1 year of being diagnosed with type 2 diabetes (Hsueh & Bryer-Ash). Cardiac autonomic neuropathy occurs in 22% of patients with type 2 diabetes and can lead to sudden death, congestive heart failure, and silent myocardial infarction (Hseuh & Bryer-Ash). Symptoms include exercise intolerance, resting tachycardia (>100 bpm), and orthostasis (fall in systolic blood pressure >20 mm Hg upon standing) (Boulton et al., 2005). Autonomic neuropathy of the gastrointestinal system produces symptoms in 75% of people with diabetes (Hseuh & Bryer-Ash). Diabetes can cause an increase or decrease in gastric motility. The latter leads to delayed emptying and gastric retention (gastroparesis) (Duby et al., 2004). Patients may experience cramping, bloating, heartburn, loss of appetite, nausea, vomiting, constipation, and diarrhea (Boulton et al.; Duby et al., 2004; Hseuh & Bryer-Ash).

Genitourinary involvement produces bladder dysfunction in the form of decreased sensation that results in decreased voiding frequency, urinary retention, and subsequent increased risk of urinary tract infections (Hsueh & Bryer-Ash, 2009). Sexual dysfunction occurs in up to 50% of men over the age of 50 in the form of erectile dysfunction (Duby et al., 2004), the most common and typically the first sign of DAN for this group (Hseuh & Bryer-Ash).

Other Complications

Diabetic Foot

Several sequelae of diabetes combine to make the feet vulnerable to ulceration. **Diabetic foot** ulcers are caused by repetitive stress on the skin with body weight and activity level increasing the pressure (Goodman, 2009).

Autonomic neuropathy results in dry, cracked skin making it more prone to ulceration (O'Keefe et al., 2009) and allowing easier access for infection entry (Weintraub & Sexton, 2010). Sensory polyneuropathy diminishes pain and temperature perceptions causing lesions to go unnoticed (Weintraub & Sexton). PAD impairs blood supply needed for healing, and hyperglycemia reduces host defenses (O'Keefe et al.). Trauma to the foot combined with these risk factors results in lesions that can be slow to heal and subject to secondary infection (Weintraub & Sexton). Infections may extend to deeper soft tissues, bones, joints, and systemic circulation (Weintraub & Sexton). Mild infection is treated with antimicrobial therapy, with surgical intervention in the form of debridement, revascularization, and/or amputation indicated for more severe infection (Weintraub & Sexton). Diabetic foot ulcers are responsible for 50% to 75% of all nontraumatic amputations in the United States (Hseuh & Bryer-Ash, 2009). Mortality due to lower extremity amputation decreases with greater attention to glycemic control, blood pressure, and lipid management (Young, McCardle, Randall, & Barclay, 2008).

Periodontal Disease

Patients with type 1 and type 2 diabetes are more prone to gingivitis and periodontitis (Papapanouz, 1996). Research has shown a positive relationship between poor glycemic control and more severe periodontal disease in patients with type 2 diabetes (Campus, Salem, Uzzau, Baldoni, & Tonolo, 2005; Tsi, Hayes, & Taylor, 2002). It has been suggested that increased incidence of periodontal disease in this population is due to inhibition of cellular mechanisms that destroy bacteria in the mouth or to impaired functioning of reparative (i.e., wound healing) cells (Mealey, 2006).

MEDICAL/SURGICAL MANAGEMENT

Type 1

There is no known cure for diabetes, and until insulin was characterized and manufactured in 1921, diabetes was a death sentence. Medical management consists of glycemic control, insulin replacement, prevention of complications, and attention to lifestyle. The ADA recommends intense and ongoing patient/family education about the disease process and management along with prevention and screening for microvascular and macrovascular complications (ADA, 2010). Current standards for glycemic control for children vary with less stringent controls for younger children (i.e., <age 6 or 7) (ADA, 2010). Blood

glucose levels near normal are seldom attained after the initial remission period (ADA, 2010). Risk of hypoglycemia is a major limiting factor in glycemic control for individuals with type 1 diabetes (Atkinson & Eisenbarth, 2001; Bolli, 1999).

Insulin replacement uses combinations of rapid-acting (e.g., Humalog), short-acting (e.g., Humulin R), intermediate-acting (e.g., Humulin N), and long-acting insulin (e.g., Lantus) that can be delivered by syringe, subcutaneous insulin infusion (insulin pump), or inhalation (ADA, 2010; Plotnick, Clark, Brancati, & Erlinger, 2003; Skyler et al., 2005). Insulin schedule depends on the individual's age, compliance level, and severity of disease, with ADA recommendations of three to four injections per day (ADA, 2010). One regimen used to achieve tight (i.e., near normal) glycemic control is a basal/bolus insulin regimen (Skyler et al., 2005). This regimen attempts to mimic normal physiologic secretion of insulin by combining a long-acting insulin analog with a rapid-acting insulin analog that is given before meals and snacks. Basal/bolus therapy instituted at the time of diagnosis has been shown to result in better glycemic control as compared to a more conventional regimen (Adhikari, Adams-Huet, Wang, Marks, & White, 2009). Adherence to a basal/bolus injection regimen can be difficult for children to accept (Zgibor et al., 2000). Studies have shown delivery via insulin pumps (Plotnick et al., 2003) and inhaled insulin (Skyler et al., 2005) to be safe and effective alternatives to injected insulin.

In severe cases for people with type 1 diabetes and renal failure, surgical intervention in the form of a simultaneous pancreas-kidney (SPK) transplant is performed. Eligibility criteria include <55 years old, minimal cardiovascular risk, absence of amputations, history of adherence to medical regimes, willingness to adhere to posttransplant management, BMI <32, and presence of two or more potential type 1 diabetes end-organ complications (Becker et al., 2001). SPK transplant has been shown to improve HTN (Elliott et al., 2001), reduce coronary atherosclerosis (Jukema et al., 2002), and improve survival as compared to patients on hemodialysis (Witczak, Jenssen, Endresen, Roislien, & Hartmann, 2007).

Attention to lifestyle factors of diet and exercise are important to the management of type 1 diabetes. Nutritional requirements for children and adolescents with type 1 diabetes are the same as for those without the disease as there is no research addressing specific needs related to living with diabetes (ADA, 2010). Long delays between meals should be avoided, as not eating in a predictable pattern according to insulin regimen may cause hypoglycemia. Frequent, small snacks at the time of peak insulin action should also be taken to avoid hypoglycemia. Exercise has not been shown to influence glycemic control for people with type 1 diabetes (Goodman, 2009). However, regular exercise provides the same benefits to children and adolescents with diabetes as it does to the general population.

Type 2

Diet modification, exercise, glycemic control, and prevention and/or treatment of complications are the cornerstones for type 2 intervention (ADA, 2010). Medical nutritional therapy in the form of controlling the amount and types of fats, carbohydrates, and proteins is recommended for weight reduction and prevention of atherosclerotic vascular disease (O'Keefe et al., 2009). A Mediterranean-style diet (i.e., consumption of monosaturated and omega-3 fatty acids, fresh fruits and vegetables, high fiber, and vegetable protein) has been shown to reduce insulin resistance in people with type 2 diabetes (Ryan et al., 2000).

The health-promoting benefits of increased physical activity and regular exercise are well documented. The ADA recommends a minimum of 150 minutes of moderately intense physical activity (e.g., gardening, raking) and/or exercise per week (ADA, 2010). For patients with type 2 diabetes, regular exercise reduces insulin resistance, promotes cardiovascular health, and prevents/improves obesity, anxiety, and depression (Castaneda et al., 2002; O'Keefe et al., 2009).

The target for glycemic control is $HbA_{1c} < 7$ (ADA, 2010). When diet and exercise are ineffective in controlling blood glucose level, oral glucose-lowering agents are indicated. Several classes of these medications are used and individualized for each patient. Metformin (e.g., Glucophage) is typically the first line of intervention and is used to decrease liver output of glucose (Nathan). Glimepiride (e.g., Amaryl) and Repaglinide (e.g., Prandin) stimulate insulin secretion, and Pioglitazone (e.g., Actos) increases sensitivity of skeletal muscle tissues to insulin (Agency for Health Care Research and Quality, 2007; Nathan et al., 2006). Individuals with type 2 diabetes may initially respond to oral hypoglycemics but then not respond well after years of this therapy. This could be the result of decreased compliance with diet and exercise programs, progression of pancreatic failure to produce insulin, complications from comorbid medical conditions or medications, or development of tolerance to medications. Insulin therapy is indicated at this point.

Self-Monitoring of Blood Glucose Levels

Self-monitoring of blood glucose levels (SMBG) is crucial for both type 1 and type 2 diabetes.

Self-monitoring requires that individuals with diabetes take active control of their own health and well-being, allows for more rapid treatment adjustments, and reinforces dietary guidelines. Portable glucose meters are available that take blood for sampling, give a digital readout of glucose levels, and have a computerized memory for record keeping. People with type 1 diabetes should monitor glucose levels three to four times per day (ADA, 2010). People with type 2 who are insulin dependent should monitor before breakfast, dinner, and bedtime, with the goal of monitoring being to avoid hypoglycemia. People with type 2 who are non–insulin dependent should learn to do SMBG for urgent situations.

IMPACT OF CONDITION ON CLIENT FACTORS

Body Functions

Diabetes impacts specific mental functions in several ways due to both acute and chronic complications. Acutely, insulin and blood glucose levels influence the level of arousal. Symptoms of hypoglycemia include drowsiness and fatigue. Variations in blood glucose levels can also cause mood swings and irritability.

Chronic complications impact those with both type 1 and type 2 diabetes. Individuals with type 1 diabetes have intact learning and memory but slower mental speed and a lessening of mental flexibility (Brands, Biessels, deHaan, Kappelle, & Kessles, 2005). Type 2 diabetes has been shown to be a risk factor for Alzheimer's disease (Peila, Rodriguez, & Launer, 2002) and, especially when combined with HTN, for general cognitive decline in the elderly (Hassing et al., 2004). Adolescents (Kanner, Hamrin, & Grey, 2003) and young adults (Hislop, Fegan, Schlaeppi, Duck, & Yeap, 2008) with type 1 diabetes may be affected by depression. Anxiety is associated with type 2 diabetes (Li et al., 2008), while research about depression in this group is mixed. One study showed that type 2 diabetes does not increase the risk of depression (Brown, Majumdar, Newman, & Johnson, 2006), while another showed that younger females in this group may be at higher risk for being depressed (Lee et al., 2009). For elderly patients with type 2 diabetes, lower health-related quality of life and higher impairments in instrumental activities of daily living (IADL) have been shown to be predictors of depression (Pawaskar, Anderson, & Balkrishnan, 2007).

Sensory functions are also impacted. Diabetic retinopathy affects vision and may lead to blindness. Neuropathies result in diminished touch, temperature, and pressure sensations; a variety of painful sensations; and motor involvement in the form of muscle weakness and altered gait patterns in older adults (Brach, Talkowski, Strotmeyer, & Newman, 2008). Autonomic neuropathies lead to cracked and dry skin and to cardiac, gastrointestinal, and genitourinary dysfunction.

Occupational Performance

Performance in all areas of occupation may be affected by complications of diabetes. Common motor skill involvement includes impaired walking (leading to increased risk in falls), manipulation, and grip strength secondary to neuropathies. These impairments result in difficulty performing activities of daily living tasks such as dressing, grooming, and functional mobility. Effective personal hygiene and grooming care is critical in preventing diabetic foot complications. Sexual activity may also be impaired by fatigue, comorbid conditions, decreased sensation, and emotional issues (anxiety, fear, guilt, anger, or shame) (Tilton, 1997). Furthermore, sexual dysfunction leads to decreased quality of life for people with diabetes (DeBarardis, Franciosi, & Belfiglio, 2002; Enzlin et al., 2002).

Function in IADL tasks is also affected by diabetes. Meal preparation must meet dietary guidelines. Tasks that require cognitive functioning (e.g., managing medication routines, financial management) may be difficult due to fluctuations in blood glucose levels. Neuropathies can impact ability to use communication devices (e.g., writing) or perform home management tasks (e.g., meal preparation). Community mobility and shopping are also more difficult in the presence of neuropathies and gait abnormalities. Effective health management and maintenance related to SMBG levels and managing insulin regimen is vital to well-being and control of potential complications. Likewise, people with diabetes must demonstrate ability to respond to emergencies related to hyperglycemia or hypoglycemia.

Type 2 diabetes is associated with sleep disturbances, even in people who are not obese or have no other complications (Trento et al., 2008). Disturbances occur in the form of more movement in bed and less-efficient sleep and appear to be associated with glycemic control (Trento et al., 2008). Finally, social participation may be impacted by decreased mobility and fatigue (Schmader, 2002).

Case Illustrations

Case 1

Andrew is a 68-year-old Caucasian male diagnosed as having type 2 diabetes at age 52. His medical history includes a long-standing history of obesity with a BMI of 38 kg/m². He was diagnosed with HTN and hyperlipidemia (i.e., high cholesterol level) at age 52 and ESRD at age 62 that requires a three times per week regimen of hemodialysis. Andrew has decreased vision due to retinopathy and neuropathies in all four extremities.

Andrew's daily medication routine is extensive. He takes 5 mg Glipizide (oral hypoglycemic); 20 mg Lipitor (cholesterol-lowering medication); Catapres-TTS-3 change weekly (once per week blood pressure patch); one Nephrocap (multivitamin); 325 mg of ferrous sulfate twice a day for anemia; three 667 PhosLo tablets three times a day with meals (calcium binds phosphorus with foods eaten to prevent phosphorus from going into the body; normal kidneys eliminate extra phosphorus in body; secondary hyperparathyroidism can occur); Kayexalate 1T in diet soda pop by mouth daily (binds potassium so it can be eliminated with bowel movement); and 100 mg of Colace for constipation.

Andrew has been married to Jane for 48 years. They have six children and 15 grandchildren, all living within a 60-mile radius of Andrew and Jane. He retired 8 years ago from his job as a foreman in an auto factory. His hobbies include watching sports on television, attending his grandchildren's activities, and participating in family get-togethers.

Andrew is right-hand dominant and receives dialysis through his left upper extremity (LUE). He has pain and numbness in his LUE because of an ischemic neuropathy that is the result of decreased blood flow because blood is diverted to his dialysis access site. He has full bilateral upper extremity active range of motion but decreased peripheral sensation (tactile, pain, and temperature). A moderate decrease in bilateral grip and pinch strength has been noted, with his left side weaker than his right. Andrew recently stepped on a tack, did not feel it, and subsequently developed an infection that is not responding to antimicrobial medication. His physician has discussed the likelihood of a below the knee amputation. Dialysis nursing staff notes a chronic flat affect that may be an indication of mild depression. Andrew communicates little information to his physician during hemodialysis visits.

Transportation services bring him to and from dialysis, as his visual impairment prevents driving. He ambulates independently with guidance owing to his decreased vision. Andrew is independent in all transfers, feeding, dressing, bathing, and hygiene although his wife is noticing that it takes him longer to do these tasks and he tends to drop things. His laboratory results show poor compliance with fluid restriction (1,800 mL fluid/day) and noncompliance with dietary restrictions. Jane contacted his physician with concerns about his lack of interest in leaving their house, participating in family activities, and sexual activity. Jane seems supportive but notes recent marital tension.

Andrew is moderately disabled by the physical and emotional ramifications of diabetes, retinopathy, neuropathies, and renal failure. This affects his roles of husband, father, and grandfather. His physical environment must be adapted to accommodate his disabilities. Socially, he is becoming withdrawn and disinterested in participating in previously enjoyed activities. The context of his occupational performance further reflects the impact that diabetes has on decreasing his quality of life.

Case 2

Lisa is a 13-year-old girl who attends eighth grade at a local public school. She is an only child and lives with both parents. Lisa is an extremely bright and athletic child. She has several good friends and typically enjoys spending time with them, hanging out at the mall, having sleepovers, and attending school activities.

Lisa was in good health until 8 months ago when her parents found her in bed, lethargic, confused, weak, and complaining of being very thirsty and cold, and vomiting. They also noticed that her breath was "sweet-smelling." During ambulance transportation to the local emergency room, Lisa became unresponsive and had to be resuscitated. She was subsequently diagnosed as being in a state of DKA and having type 1 diabetes. Initially, management of her condition was easy. Her parents monitored blood glucose levels four times per day, and little insulin was needed for control. After this "honeymoon period" ended, Lisa's blood glucose levels became more difficult to manage.

Lisa says she is embarrassed and does not want her friends to know that she has diabetes. Consequently, she often does not follow dietary restrictions. She becomes irritable and combative with her parents regarding SMBG and insulin injections. She avoids socializing with friends, and her teachers report a significant decline in her academic performance. Lisa refuses to do homework and spends most of her time alone in her bedroom. She often says that she does not care what would happen to her if she does not follow dietary and medication requirements.

Sensorimotor and cognitive functioning is currently intact except for the level of arousal. As her glucose levels fluctuate, Lisa becomes drowsy and fatigue. This often occurs during school, where she lays her head on her desk and sleeps. These fluctuations subsequently impair her ability to learn.

At this point, psychosocial skills and psychological functioning are challenged. Lisa is having difficulty adjusting to the fact that she is different from her friends and often refuses to follow dietary restrictions in their presence. She quit playing soccer, no longer has

sleepovers with friends, and her mother has noticed increased arguing between Lisa and her friends.

Lisa's mother also is having difficulty coping with her daughter's diagnosis because her own father died of complications from diabetes when she was 14. She is distressed that Lisa is not enjoying her friends and school like a typical 13-year-old girl would. She is also concerned that Lisa's physical, social, emotional, and intellectual development will lag because of her diabetes. Lisa's father is spending more time at work than he used to. When he is home, he and Lisa often argue about her lack of interest in taking care of herself. These arguments escalate into screaming between Lisa and her father and end with Lisa running into her bedroom and slamming the door. Both parents are concerned about the increased tension in their marriage and home.

REFERENCES

Adeghate, E., Schattner, P., & Dunn, E. (2006). An update on the etiology and epidemiology of diabetes mellitus. *Annals of New York Academy of Science, 1084*, 1–29. doi: 10.1196/annals.1372.029.

Adhikari, S., Adams-Huet, B., Wang, Y. A., Marks, J. F., & White, P. C. (2009). Institution of basal-bolus therapy at diagnosis for children with type 1 diabetes mellitus. *Pediatrics, 123*, e673–e678. doi:10.1542/peds.2008–3027.

Adler, A. I., Stratton, I. M., Andrew, H., Neil, W., Yudkin, J. S., Matthews, D. R., et al. (2000). Association of systolic blood pressure with macrovascular and microvascular complications of type 2 diabetes (UKPDS 36): Prospective observational study. *British Medical Journal, 321*, 412–419.

Agency for Healthcare Research and Quality. (2007). Comparing oral medications for adults with type 2 diabetes (AHRQ Publication number 07(08)-EHC010-3). Retrieved from http://effectivehealthcare.ahrq.gov/ehc/products/6/29/OralHypo_Clin_07.02.08.pdf

Akerblom, H. K., Vaarala, O., Hyoty, H., Ilonen, J., & Knip, M. (2002). Environmental factors in the etiology of type 1 diabetes. *American Journal of Medical Genetics, 115*, 18–29. doi:10.1002/amjg.10340.

American Diabetes Association (ADA). (2007). Diagnosis and classification of diabetes mellitus. *Diabetes Care, 30*(Suppl. 1), S42–S47. doi:10.2337/dc07-S042.

American Diabetes Association (ADA). (2010). Standards of medical care in diabetes—2010. *Diabetes Care, 33*(Suppl. 1), S11–S61. doi:10.2337/dc10-S011.

Atkinson, M. A., & Eisenbarth, G. S. (2001). Type 1 diabetes: New perspectives on disease pathogenesis and treatment. *Lancet, 358*, 221–229.

Becker, B. N., Odorico, J. S., Becker, Y. T., Groshek, M., Werwinski, C., Pirsch, J. D., & Sollinger, H. W. (2001). Simultaneous pancreas-kidney and pancreas transplantation. *Journal of the American Society of Nephrology, 12*, 2517–2527.

Beckman, J. A., Creager, M. A., & Libby, P. (2002). Diabetes and atherosclerosis: Epidemiology, pathophysiology, and management. *JAMA, 287*(19), 2570–2581. doi:10.1001/jama.287.19.2570.

Bloomgarden, Z. T. (2001). Diabetes and hypertension. *Diabetes Care, 24*(9), 1679–1684.

Bolli, G. B. (1999). How to ameliorate the problem of hypoglycemia in intensive as well as nonintensive treatment of type 1 diabetes. *Diabetes Care, 22*(Suppl. 2), B43–B52.

Boulton, A. J. M., Vinik, A. I., Arezzo, J. C., Bril, V., Feldman, E. L., Freeman, R., et al. (2005). Diabetic neuropathies: A position statement by the American Diabetes Association. *Diabetes Care, 28*(4), 956–962.

Brach, J. S., Talkowski, J. B., Strotmeyer, E. S., & Newman, A. B. (2008). Diabetes mellitus and gait dysfunction: Possible explanatory factors. *Physical Therapy, 88*(11), 1365–1374.

Brands, A. M. A., Biessels, G. J., deHaan, E. H. F., Kappelle, L. J., & Kessles, R. P. C. (2005). The effects of type 1 diabetes on cognitive performance: A meta-analysis. *Diabetes Care, 28*(3), 726–735.

Brown, L. C., Majumdar, S. R., Newman, S. C., & Johnson, J. A. (2006). Type 2 diabetes does not increase the risk of depression. *CMAJ, 175*(1), 42–46. doi:10.1503/cmaj.051429.

Campus, G., Salem, A., Uzzau, S., Baldoni, E., & Tonolo, G. (2005). Diabetes and periodontal disease: A case-control study. *Journal of Periodontology, 76*(3), 418–425. doi:10.1902/jop.2005.76.3.418.

Castaneda, C., Layne, J. E., Munoz-Orians, L., Gordon, P. L., Walsmith, J., Foldvari, M., et al. (2002). A randomized controlled trial of resistance exercise training to improve glycemic control in older adults with type 2 diabetes. *Diabetes Care, 25*(12), 2335–2341.

Centers for Disease Control and Prevention. (2008a). *National Diabetes Fact Sheet: General information and national estimates on diabetes in the United States, 2007.* Atlanta, GA: U.S. Department of Health and Human Services, Centers for Disease Control and Prevention. Retrieved from http://www.cdc.gov/diabetes/pubs/pdf/ndfs_2007.pdf

Centers for Disease Control and Prevention. (2008b). *Diabetes data and trends.* Atlanta, GA: U.S. Department of Health and Human Services, Centers for Disease Control and Prevention. Retrieved from http://apps.nccd.cdc.gov/DDTSTRS/default.aspx

Crawford, A. G., Cote, C., Couto, J., Daskiran, M., Gunnarsson, C., Haas, K., et al. (2010). Prevalence of obesity, type II diabetes mellitus, hyperlipidemia, and hypertension in the United States: Findings from the GE Centricity Electronic Medical Record database. *Population Health Management, 13*(3), 151–161. doi:10.1089/pop.2009.0039.

Dambro, M. (1995). *Griffith's five minute clinical consult.* Baltimore, MD: Williams & Wilkins.

Daneman, D. (2006). Type 1 diabetes. *Lancet, 367,* 847–858.

DeBarardis, G., Franciosi, M., & Belfiglio, M. (2002). Erectile dysfunction and quality of life in type 2 diabetic patients. *Diabetes Care, 25,* 284–291.

Devendra, D., Liu, E., & Eisenbarth, G. S. (2004). Type 1 diabetes: Recent developments. *British Medical Journal, 328,* 750–754.

Duby, J. J., Campbell, R. K., Setter, S. M., White, J. R., & Rasmussen, K. A. (2004). Diabetic neuropathy: An intensive review. *American Journal of Health-System Pharmacy, 61,* 160–176.

Eisenbarth, G. S., & McCulloch, D. K. (2010). Pathogenesis of type 1 diabetes mellitus. *Up To Date.* Retrieved from http://www.uptodate.com/online/content/topic.do?topicKey=diabetes/5832&selectedTitle=4%7E150&source=search_result

Elliott, M. D., Kapoor, A., Parker, M. A., Kaufman, D. B., Bonow, R. O., & Gheorghiade, M. (2001). Improvement in hypertension in patients with diabetes mellitus after kidney/pancreas transplantation. *Circulation, 104,* 563–569. doi:10.1161/hc3001.093434.

Enzlin, P., Mathieu, C., Vanden Bruel, A., Bosteels, J., Vanderschueren, D., & Kemyttenaere, K. (2002). Sexual dysfunction in women with type 1 diabetes. *Diabetes Care, 25*(4), 672–677.

Falanga, V. (2005). Wound healing and its impairment in the diabetic foot. *Lancet, 366,* 1736–1743.

Franco, O. H., Steyerberg, E. W., Hu, F. B., Mackenbach, J., & Nusselder, W. (2007). Associations of diabetes mellitus with total life expectancy and life expectancy with and without cardiovascular disease. *Archives of Internal Medicine, 167,* 1145–1151.

Goodman, C. C. (2009). The endocrine and metabolic systems. In C. C. Goodman & K. S. Fuller (Eds.), *Pathology: Implications for the physical therapist* (3rd ed.) (pp. 453–518). Philadelphia, PA: Saunders.

Hassing, L. B., Hofer, S. M., Nilsson, S. E., Berg, S., Pedersen, N. L., McClearn, G., & Johansson, B. (2004). Comorbid type 2 diabetes mellitus and hypertension exacerbates cognitive decline: Evidence from a longitudinal study. *Age and Ageing, 33,* 355–361. doi:10.1093/ageing/afh100.

Hislop, A. L., Fegan, P. G., Schlaeppi, M. J., Duck, M., & Yeap, B. B. (2008). Prevalence and associations of psychological distress in young adults with type 1 diabetes. *Diabetic Medicine, 25,* 91–96. doi:10.1111/j.1464–5491.2007.02310.x.

Hsueh, W., & Bryer-Ash, M. (2009). *Contemporary diagnosis and management of type 2 diabetes* (3rd ed.). Newtown, PA: Handbooks in Health Care Company.

Jovanovic, L. (2010). Patient information: Gestational diabetes mellitus. *Up To Date.* Retrieved from http://www.uptodate.com/online/content/topic.do?topicKey=pregnan/8876&selectedTitle=4%7E56&source=search_result

Jukema, J. W., Smets, Y. F. C., van der Pijl, J. W., Zwinderman, A. H., Vliegen, H. W., Ringers, J., et al. (2002). Impact of simultaneous pancreas and kidney transplantation on progression of coronary atherosclerosis in patients with end-stage renal failure due to type 1 diabetes. *Diabetes Care, 25*(5), 906–911.

Juutilainen, A., Lehto, S., Ronnemaa, T., Pyorala, K., & Laakso, M. (2008). Similarity of the impact of type 1 and type 2 diabetes on cardiovascular mortality in middle-age subjects. *Diabetes Care, 31*(4), 714–719. doi:10.2337/dc07–2124.

Kanner, S., Hamrin, V., & Grey, M. (2003). Depression in adolescents with diabetes. *Journal of Child and Adolescent Psychiatric Nursing, 16*(1), 15–24.

Klein, R., Klein, B. E., Lee, K. E., Cruickshanks, K. J., & Moss, S. E. (1996). The incidence of hypertension in insulin-dependent diabetes. *Archives of Internal Medicine, 156*(6), 622–627.

Kriska, A. M., Pereira, M. A., Hanson, R. L., de Courten, M. P., Zimmet, P. Z., Alberti, K. G., et al. (2001). Association of physical activity and serum insulin concentrations in two populations at high risk for type 2 diabetes but differing BMI. *Diabetes Care, 24*(7), 1175–1180.

Lago, R. M., Singhy, P. P., & Nesto, R. W. (2007). Diabetes and hypertension. *Nature Clinical Practice, 3*(10), 667. doi:10.1038/ncpendme0638.

Laron, Z. (2002). Interplay between heredity and environment in the recent explosion of type 2 childhood diabetes mellitus. *American Journal of Medical Genetics, 115*, 4–7. doi:10.1002/ajmg.10338.

Lee, H., Chapa, D., Kao, C., Jones, D., Kapustin, J., Smith, J., et al. (2009). Depression, quality of life, and glycemic control in individuals with type 2 diabetes. *Journal of the American Academy of Nurse Practitioners 21*, 214–224. doi:10.1111/j.1745-7599.2009.00396x.

Li, C., Barker, L., Ford, E. S., Zhang, X., Strine, T. W., & Mokdad, A. H. (2008). Diabetes and anxiety in US adults: Findings from the 2006 behavioral risk factor surveillance system. *Diabetic Medicine, 25*, 878–881. doi:10.1111/j.1464–5491.2008.02477x.

Lipton, R. B., Drumm, M., Burnet, D., Rich, B., Cooper, A., Baumann, E., & Hagopian, W. (2005). Obesity at the onset of diabetes in an ethnically diverse population of children: What does it mean for epidemiologists and clinicians? *Pediatrics, 115*(5), e553–e560. doi:10.1542/peds.2004–1448.

Mealey, B. L. (2006). Periodontal disease and diabetes: A two-way street. *Journal of the American Dental Association, 137*, 26S–31S.

Miao, J., Brismar, K., Nyren, O., Ugarph-Morawski, A., & Ye, W. (2005). Elevated hip fracture risk in type 1 diabetic patients. *Diabetes Care, 28*(12), 2850–2855.

Mohamed, Q., Gillies, M. G., & Wong, T. Y. (2007). Management of diabetic retinopathy: A systematic review. *JAMA, 298*(8), 902–916. doi:10.1001/jama,298.8.902.

Najarian, R. M., Sullivan, L. M., Kannel, W. B., Wilson, P. W. F., D'Agostino, R. B., & Wolf, P. A. (2006). Metabolic syndrome compared with type 2 diabetes mellitus as a risk factor for stroke: The Framingham offspring study. *Archives of Internal Medicine, 166*, 106–111.

Nathan, D. M., Buse, J. B., Davidson, M. B., Heine, R. J., Holman, R. R., Sherwin, R., Zinman, B. (2006). Management of hyperglycemia in type 2 diabetes: A consensus algorithm for the initiation and adjustment of therapy. *Diabetes Care, 29*(8), 1963–1972. doi:10.2337/dc06-9912.

National Institute of Diabetes and Digestive and Kidney Diseases. (2008). *National Diabetes Statistics, 2007 fact sheet.* Bethesda, MD: U.S. Department of Health and Human Services, National Institutes of Health. Retrieved from http://diabetes.niddk.nih.gov/dm/pubs/statistics/index.htm

O'Keefe, J. H., Bell, D. S., & Wynne, K. L. (2009). *Diabetes essentials* (4th ed.). Sudbury, MA: Jones and Bartlett Publishers.

Papapanouz, P. N. (1996). Periodontal disease: Epidemiology. *Annals of Periodontology, 1*(1), 1–36.

Parving, H., Hovind, P., Rossing, K., & Andersen, S. (2001). Evolving strategies for renoprotection: Diabetic nephropathy. *Current Opinion in Nephrology and Hypertension, 10*, 515–522.

Pavkov, M. E., Hanson, R. L., Knowler, W. C., Bennett, P. H., Krakoff, J., & Nelson, R. G. (2007). Changing patterns of type 2 diabetes incidence among Pima Indians. *Diabetes Care, 30*(7), 1758–1763.

Pawaskar, M. D., Anderson, R. T., & Balkrishnan, R. (2007). Self-reported predictors of depressive symptomatology in an elderly population with type 2 diabetes mellitus: A prospective cohort study. *Health and Quality of Life Outcomes, 5*, 50–57. doi:10.1186/1477-7525-5-50.

Peila, R., Rodriguez, B. L., & Launer, L. J. (2002). Type 2 diabetes, APOE gene, and the risk for dementia and related pathologies: The Honolulu-Asia Aging Study. *Diabetes, 51*, 1256–1262.

Pinhas-Hamiel, O., & Zeitler, P. (2004). The global spread of type 2 diabetes mellitus in children and adolescents. *Journal of Pediatrics, 146*, 693–700. doi:10.1016/j.peds.2004.12.042.

Plotnick, L. P., Clark, L. M., Brancati, F. L., & Erlinger, T. (2003). Safety and effectiveness of insulin pump therapy in children and adolescents with type 1 diabetes. *Diabetes Care, 26*(4), 1142–1146.

Powers, A. C. (2001). Diabetes mellitus. In E. Braunwald, A. S. Fauci, & D. L. Kasper (Eds.), *Harrison's principles of internal medicine* (pp. 2109–2137). New York: McGraw-Hill.

Ryan, M., McInerney, D., Owens, D., Collins, P., Johnson, A., & Tomkin, G. H. (2000). Diabetes and the Mediterranean diet: A beneficial effect of oleic acid on insulin sensitivity, adipocyte glucose transport and endothelium-dependent vasoreactivity. *QJM: An International Journal of Medicine, 93*, 85–91.

Schmader, K. E. (2002). Epidemiology and impact on quality of life of postherpetic neuralgia and painful diabetic neuropathy. *The Clinical Journal of Pain, 18*, 350–353.

Sherwin, R. (1996). Endocrine and reproductive diseases. In J. Bennett & F. Plumb (Eds.), *Cecil textbook of medicine, Vol. 2* (20th ed.) (pp. 1258–1277). Philadelphia, PA: WB Saunders.

Skyler, J. S., Bergenstal, R., Bonow, R. O., Buse, J., Deedwania, P., Gale, E. A. M., et al. (2009). Intensive glycemic control and the prevention of cardiovascular events: Implications of the ACCORD, ADVANCE, and VA diabetes trials. *Diabetes Care, 32*(1), 187–192. doi:10.2337/dc08-9026.

Skyler, J. S., Weinstock, R. S., Raskin, P., Yale, J., Barrett, E., Gerich, J. E., & Getrstein, H. C. (2005). Use of inhaled insulin in a basal/bolus insulin regimen in type 1 diabetic subjects. *Diabetes Care, 28*(7), 1630–1635.

Surampudi, P. N., John-Kalarickal, J., & Fonseca, V. A. (2009). Emerging concepts in the pathophysiology of type 2 diabetes mellitus. *Mount Sinai Journal of Medicine, 76*, 216–226. doi:10.1002/msj.20113.

Tilton, M. (1997). Diabetes and amputation. In M. Sipski & C. Alexander (Eds.), *Sexual function in people with disability and chronic illness: A health professional's guide* (pp. 279–302). Gaithersbirg, MD: Aspen, Inc.

Trento, M., Broglio, F., Riganti, F., Basile, M., Borgo, E., Kucich, C., et al. (2008). Sleep abnormalities in type 2 diabetes may be associated with glycemic control. *Acta Diabetolgia, 45*, 225–229. doi:10.1007/x00592-008-0047-6.

Tsi, C., Hayes, C., & Taylor, G. W. (2002). Glycemic control of type 2 diabetes and severe periodontal disease in the US adult population. *Community Denistry and Oral Epidemiology, 30*, 182–192.

Van Leiden, H. A., Dekker, J. M., Moll, A. C., Nijpels, G., Heine, R. J., Bouter, L. M., et al. (2002). Blood pressure, lipids, and obesity are associated with retinopathy: The Hoon study. *Diabetes Care, 25*(8), 1320–1325.

Vinik, A. I., Park, T. S., Stansberry, K. B., & Pittenger, G. L. (2000). Diabetic neuropathies. *Diabetologia, 43*, 957–973.

Weintraub, A. C., & Sexton, D. J. (2010). Overview of diabetic infections of the lower extremities. *Up to Date*. Retrieved from http://www.uptodate.com/online/content/topic.do?topicKey=skin_inf/13375&selectedTitle=2%7E150&source=search_result

Witczak, B. J., Jenssen, T., Endresen, K., Roislien, J., & Hartmann, A. (2007). Risk factors for mortality in diabetic nephropathy patients accepted for transplantation. *Transplantation, 84*(3), 356–361. doi:10.1097/01.tp.0000276935.31584.4c.

Young, M. J., McCardle, J. E., Randall, L. E., & Barclay, J. I. (2008). Improved survival of diabetic foot ulcer patients 1995–2008. *Diabetes Care, 31*(11), 2143–2147. doi:10.2337/dc08-1242.

Zgibor, J. C., Songer, T. J., Kelsey, S. F., Weissfeld, J., Drash, A. L., Becker, D., & Orchard, T. J. (2000). *Diabetes Care, 23*, 472–476.

Zhang, X., Saaddine, J. B., Chou, C., Cotch, M. F., Cheng, Y. J., Geiss, L. S., et al. (2010). Prevalence of diabetic retinopathy in the United States, 2005–2008. *JAMA, 304*(6), 649–656. doi:10.1001/jama.2010.1111.

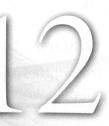

Acquired Brain Injury

■ *Gerry E. Conti*

It had been a hot summer day, and his construction job required every ounce of his strength and endurance. He had missed lunch and was roofing in the heat as the final part of his day, the tar radiating heat upward while the sun beat down on his back. At last, it was over. J.D. picked up Kathy, his girlfriend of 4 years, and headed for the beach. Five hours and many beers later, they sped home on familiar secondary roads. John negotiated the first part of an S-curve fine, but his reflexes were too slow to manage the second curve when a rabbit ran into the road. Overcompensating, he lost control of the car, slamming it up against a tree. In an instant, his life changed. Kathy was killed. J.D., age 20, survived. At the hospital, he was diagnosed with a moderate traumatic brain injury.

Acquired brain injury (ABI) is defined by the World Health Organization as "damage to the brain, which occurs after birth and is not related to a congenital or a degenerative disease. These impairments may be temporary or permanent and cause partial or functional disability or psychosocial maladjustment" (Bullock, Chestnut, & Clifton, 1995). ABI includes the conditions of traumatic brain injury (TBI), brain tumors, and stroke. This chapter will address TBI and brain tumors; stroke is discussed in a separate chapter.

TRAUMATIC BRAIN INJURY

Description and Definition

TBI, while it has been present throughout history, became a specialized area of rehabilitation only in the latter half of the 20th century. In 1973, only three major U.S. hospitals provided specialized care in rehabilitation for people with head injury, and it was not until 1995 that the first Guidelines for the Management of Severe Head Injury were established (Bullock et al., 1995). In the late 1990s, the term for the condition changed from head injury to traumatic brain injury, with the additional designation of open—cranium removed and dermis covering only the brain—or closed injury. Due to the short time that TBI has been studied, evidence-based knowledge is greatest concerning the medical assessment and management of TBI itself and its secondary sequelae, with less evidence available for the efficacy of interventions.

TBI involves a complex matrix of physical, cognitive, communicative, and neurobehavioral deficits that may have a lifetime effect on a person's ability to participate in work, leisure, and social occupations. The combination of these changes makes the total disability far greater than any single deficit (Jennett & Bond, 1975).

The extent of disability is typically identified within 48 hours of medical evaluation and is based on the length of amnesia and/or **coma**, using the Glasgow Coma Scale (GCS), where a greater score indicates more extensive brain damage. The following definitions will be used throughout this chapter.

> *Mild TBI:* clinically identified as a loss of consciousness, or amnesia, for <10 minutes, GCS rating of 13 to 15, no skull fracture on physical examination, and a nonfocal neurologic examination (Bazarian, McClung, & Shah, 2005).
>
> *Moderate TBI:* hospitalization of at least 48 hours, an initial GCS rating of 9 to 12 or more (Dawodu, 2005).
>
> *Severe TBI:* loss of consciousness and/or postacquired amnesia >24 hours, and a GCS rating of 1 to 8 (Dawodu, 2005).

Mild TBI represents 80% of all brain injury, and about 85% of these people will recover without intervention over a 3-month period (Greenwald & Rigg, 2009). Persons with mild TBI typically report symptoms such as headaches, dizziness, fatigue, visual disturbance, and memory and executive-thinking difficulties during the first week following injury. However, for some individuals, these difficulties persist from 3 months to a lifetime, causing significant distress and disruption of daily activities (Ponsford, Willmott, & Rothwell, 2000).

Intensive assessment and intervention is not beneficial for people with mild TBI, a meta-analysis from the Cochrane Collection suggests. Rather, early and structured education is recommended, with recommendations for symptom amelioration as needed (Turner-Stokes, Nair, Sedki, Disler, & Wade, 2005). Therefore, issues addressed in this chapter will pertain to moderate and severe TBI and to the 15% of people with mild TBI who experience primary deficits.

Etiology

The onset of TBI is sudden, following a single-incident neurologic insult, and results in both primary and secondary brain damage. Primary brain damage may be focal (localized) or diffuse and is created by acceleration, deceleration, and rotation or by the intrusion into the brain of a penetrating object. Focal lesions are limited in scope and are associated with direct impact of short duration such as occurs with a bullet. Diffuse lesions occur throughout multiple brain areas and may result from shrapnel, motor vehicle accidents, or sports. Diffuse axonal injuries (DAIs) occur as a result of collisions with the head at a velocity of approximately 15 miles per hour or greater (Meythaler, Peduzzi, & Eleftheriou, 2001). DAI therefore can occur with high-speed running collisions with others, as in football, soccer, or hockey, as well as with higher-speed motor vehicle accidents. Motor vehicle accidents typically result in both coup and **contrecoup injuries**. With these injuries, direct damage is incurred as the cerebrum rotates on the more stable brainstem while accelerating from the force of impact. The cerebrum strikes the skull (coup), and then accelerates in the opposite direction to strike the skull at an opposite location (contrecoup). This continues until the force of impact has been absorbed (Adams, Graham, & Murray, 1982; Strich, 1970).

The mechanism for DAI is stretching and shearing of brain cell axons and is associated with immediate coma following brain injury. Injury to the tracts leading from the hypothalamus and/or pituitary results in medical complications of hyperventilation, hormonal changes, electrolyte disturbances of salt and water, altered temperature regulation, and dysfunctional control of hunger (Meythaler et al., 2001). Structures sensitive to diffuse axonal injury (DAI) include the parasagittal white matter of the cerebral hemisphere, including the sensory and motor cortices and the frontal lobe, corpus callosum, brainstem, and the cerebellum (Adams et al., 1982; Dawodu, 2005; Meythaler et al., 2001; Strich, 1970). Common cognitive deficits associated with these structures include difficulty remembering new information, decreased ability to process information, and limited **executive functions** (Meythaler et al.). A common motor deficit is difficulty with bilateral integration due to callosal damage.

Secondary damage occurs shortly after impact and is mainly a result of limited oxygenation of the brain or

DAI. Factors causing secondary damage include increased intracranial pressure, ischemia or cerebral hypoxia, and intracranial hemorrhage. Increased intracranial pressure results in swelling, which cannot be accommodated within the rigid structure of the skull. Swelling, in turn, may lead to herniation of brain tissue (Jennett, 1990). Ischemia occurs when blood vessels can no longer provide sufficient blood to the brain. Intracranial hemorrhage is an additional source of hypoxia, leading to cell death within minutes after injury.

Medical complications are frequent and impair recovery following TBI. Following a high-impact TBI, such as occurs with a motor vehicle accident, victims may have single or multiple seizures (Frey, 2003), **hydrocephalus** (Beyerl & Black, 1984), extremity injuries including lacerations and fractures (Rimel & Jane, 1983), and/or cardiovascular complications (Bontke, 1989). Respiratory function is often impaired, requiring nasal intubation or tracheostomy, and pneumonia may occur. Neurogenic bowel and bladder disorders require catheterization and close monitoring to avoid the development of decubiti.

Incidence and Prevalence

The great incidence of TBI around the world has led the World Health Organization to refer to TBI as a "silent epidemic" (Binder, Corrigan, & Langlois, 2005). An estimated 1.4 million Americans sustain a TBI each year; of these 235,000 require hospitalization and 50,000 die (Langlois, Rutland-Brown, & Thomas, 2006). Included in the numbers of hospitalized people are about 60,000 children and adolescents (Ragnarsson, 2006). Of this 1.4 million people, approximately 70,000 to 90,000 live with a significant TBI-related disability (National Institutes of Health, 1998). The incidence of disability increases with the severity of brain injury. Permanent disability occurs in about 10% of those with mild TBI, 66% of those with moderate TBI, and 100% of those with severe TBI (Jallo & Narayan, 2000). Additionally, age, gender, and ethnicity may affect the incidence rate. At greatest risk for injury are young men between the ages of 15 and 24, who are twice as likely as women of the same age to sustain a head injury (Centers for Disease Control and Prevention [CDC], 2001). However, it is not known whether gender affects the severity of TBI and the outcome from TBI (Ragnarsson, 2006). Age groups that show an increased incidence of ABI include adults older than 75 years and children below the age of 5 years. A review of current evidence suggests that injury in older adults may result in greater impairment and more limited recovery (Ragnarsson, 2006). Inner-city environments have higher incidence rates (Bruns, 2003), with persons of African American ethnicity having the highest death rates from TBI of all races (CDC, 2001; Whitman & Coonley-Hoganson, 1984). It is currently uncertain whether this incidence is due to issues of ethnicity or to lack of medical and rehabilitation outcomes (Ragnarsson, 2006).

The three leading causes of TBI are falls, motor vehicle accidents, and violence. Falls are the most common cause of TBI, but motor vehicle accidents are the most common cause of severe TBI. Children below the age of 5 and elderly adults over 85 years are the most commonly seen groups with brain injury in hospital emergency departments (Gordon et al., 2006). According to a major statewide study of 2003 to 2006, males accounted for approximately 61% of all motor vehicle accidents, both with and without the presence of alcohol or substance use (Rochette, Conner, & Smith, 2009). In addition, young adults between 16 and 30 years were also at increased risk for motor vehicle accidents. Among children involved in vehicular crashes resulting in moderate to severe injury, half were unrestrained at the time of the accident (Department of Transportation, National Highway Traffic Safety Administration [NHTSA], 2006). In the United States, survivors of violence, the second major cause of TBI, are more likely to be men, single, unemployed, and from a minority background (Bogner, Corrigan, & Mysiw, 2001; Bushnik, Hanks, Kreutzer, & Rosenthal, 2003). A history of previous arrests in survivors of violence also has been shown (Bushnik et al., 2003).

Severity of injury is related to cause. Surviving vehicle crash victims tend to be injured more severely than survivors of either falls or violence, and to have additional injuries such as long bone fractures and plexopathies; falls are more often associated with mild injury. Intoxication, which is present in one-third to one-half of individuals at the time of injury (Corrigan, 1995), is significantly negatively correlated with outcome. Persons who were intoxicated when injured tend to be hospitalized longer and have greater severity of injury, greater incidence of death, and a lower cognitive status at the time of discharge, as well as greater periods of postacquired amnesia (Bogner et al., 2001; Corrigan, 1995; Cummings, Rivara, Olson, & Smith, 2006; Cunningham, Maio, Hill, & Zink, 2002). People injured by violence tend to have more severe injuries and poorer community reintegration (Gordon et al., 2006).

The costs of TBI, both individually and for society, are staggering. In 1996, approximately $5.4 billion were spent on TBI hospitalizations (Schootman, Buchman, & Lewis, 2003). Between 1997 and 1999, the individual cost of hospitalization varied from $15,860 for falls and $20,522 for motor vehicle accidents (McGarry et al., 2002). A study completed in Missouri between 2001 and 2005 also found that $1.1 billion for lost productivity accrued due to TBI-related deaths in the state. Severity of injury also affects cost. Examining a multiregional database, McGarry et al. (2002) found that costs of individual hospitalization averaged $8,189 for moderate and $14,603 for severe TBI.

The average lifetime cost of health care for each person with severe TBI is between $600,000 and $1,875,000 (Johnstone, Mount, & Schopp, 2003). As only 20% to 50% of TBI survivors are employed ("NIH Consensus Development Panel on Rehabilitation of persons with traumatic brain injury. Rehabilitation of persons with Traumatic Brain Injury," 1999), an additional $1 billion annually may be incurred due to lost wages, lost income taxes, and increased public assistance (Johnstone et al., 2003).

Signs and Symptoms

People with TBI experience a wide range of deficits, depending on the location and severity of their injuries.

Medical Complications

Seizures

Seizures are a frequent complication of moderate or severe TBI (Ragnarsson, 2006) and are typically classified as immediate, delayed, or postraumatic, depending on whether they occur within 24 hours, 1 week, or after 1 week, respectively (Elvidge, 1939). Risk factors for seizures include a depressed skull fracture and intracranial hematoma (Jennett, 1975). Additional risk factors include the type and site of the lesion, loss of consciousness, amnesia for more than 1 day, and being older than 65 years.

The risk of seizure varies for different groups, however. For example, seizure rates for adults of up to 53% have been identified after military injuries, while a 4% seizure incidence may occur with a small intracranial injury (Frey, 2003). Children tend to be more prone to early seizures than adults (Asikainen, Kaste, & Sarna, 1999; Jennett, 1975). The overall incidence of seizures in children is <10%, with the greatest risk for those under the age of 7 (Strich, 1970). The risk of a first seizure for people of any age continues to be elevated for more than 10 years after brain injury (Annegers, Hauser, & Coan, 1999).

Hydrocephalus

Posttraumatic hydrocephalus is the most common neurosurgical complication of people with TBI, with rates of incidence varying from approximately 2% to 45% (Gordon et al., 2006). Those with more severe injuries and those who have undergone decompressive craniotomies are at more risk to develop posttraumatic hydrocephalus.

Dysautonomia

Dysautonomia is frequently seen after severe TBI and is characterized by hypertension, tachycardia, increased body temperature and blood pressure, profuse sweating and decerebrate, or decorticate posturing (Gordon et al.,

2006; Hendricks, Heeren, & Vos, 2010). People experiencing dysautonomia have been shown to have longer rehabilitation lengths of stay, longer periods of posttraumatic amnesia, and lower Glasgow Outcome Scale scores (Baguley, Nicholls, & Felmingham, 1999; Gordon et al., 2006).

Deep Venous Thrombosis

It has been estimated that up to 20% of people with TBI have deep venous thrombosis (DVT) on admission to the hospital (Carlile et al., 2010). DVT results from prolonged immobilization. DVT can give rise to pulmonary emboli, which is the most common preventable cause of hospital death in TBI (Anderson, Wheeler, & Goldberg, 1991; Gordon et al., 2006).

Depressed Level of Consciousness

Brain injury involves associated cerebral and brainstem depression or destruction that, in turn, affects the person's level of consciousness. Mild brain injury may result in a relatively short loss of consciousness. Coma, defined as an alteration of consciousness associated with decreased arousal and awareness of all stimuli (*Plum and Posner's diagnosis of stupor and coma*, 2007), is typically present following moderate to severe brain injury.

Either diffuse cerebral hypoxia or extensive cortical damage, with minimal to no impairment of the brainstem, may result in a vegetative state. In this state, the individual's eyes may be open and follow a moving object, and the limbs may move but without apparent purpose. However, there is no response to pain or simple verbal requests, and there is no evidence of cortical function related to voluntary movement (Bazarian et al., 2005). Persons in such a vegetative state may live briefly or for years.

Motor Deficits

Damage to the brainstem between the vestibular nuclei and the red nucleus produces **decerebrate rigidity**, defined as an extensor posture of all limbs and/or the trunk. When the brainstem is intact despite severe cortical damage, **decorticate rigidity** is present, with flexion of the upper and extension of the lower limbs. Abnormal reflexes complicate movement patterns. During deep coma, brainstem reflexes may result in grimacing to noxious stimuli, which may be accompanied by a change in postural tone in the extremities.

These deficits decline as coma lightens, and motor disturbances reflecting neural damage become apparent. These deficits may include quadriparesis, hemiplegia, or monoplegia, with or without fluctuating muscle tone or spasticity as well as disorders of coordination.

Spasticity is characterized by velocity-dependent increase in muscle tone resulting from hyperexcitability of the stretch reflex (Kandel, Schwartz, & Jessell, 2000). Spasticity is common in adults after moderate and severe TBI, interfering with limb mobility and performance capabilities (Burnett, Watanabe, & Greenwald, 2003; Gordon et al., 2006), and 65% of children also have spasticity following TBI (Dumas, Haley, Carey, Ludlow, & Rabin, 2003). With immobility, **heterotopic ossification** may form at synovial joints surrounded by spastic musculature, particularly the hips, knees, and elbows (Gordon et al., 2006).

Coordination deficits include tremor and ataxia. Tremor types include cerebellar, resting, essential, and physiologic. Cerebellar tremors are associated with ataxia, hypotonia, and balance disorders. They tend to occur in trunk and proximal muscles with intentional movement, at a frequency of approximately 4 to 6 per second. Resting tremors are correlated with striatal damage and involve pill-rolling movement at rest, occurring at a similar rate. Essential tremors affect more distal musculature, occur at a frequency of 8 to 12 per second, and increase with anxiety and maintained positions. Physiologic tremor, commonly seen with aging, occurs at the same rate and is exacerbated by fatigue and stress. Postacquired ataxia is a result of damage to the sensory, equilibrium, or cerebellar systems and has been shown in 20% to 30% of persons sustaining DAI (Weintrab & Opal, 1989).

Cranial Nerve Dysfunction

As the cranial nerves originate from the brainstem, TBI typically results in damage to both the sensory and motor functions of these nerves. Lower levels of coma may permit only assessment of cranial nerves III, VI, and VII (Keane & Baloh, 1992). Pupillary reflexes are important early indicators of brain damage. The absence of a pupillary reflex in response to light by an unconscious patient is an indication of damage to the midbrain, from which the oculomotor nerve (III) originates. A fixed dilated pupil, indicative of pressure on the oculomotor nerve, is frequently seen following moderate to severe ABI (Kandel et al., 2000).

As coma lightens, significant visual deficits typically become apparent, because of damage to the oculomotor (III), trochlear (IV), and abducens (VI) nerves. These deficits include binocular, oculomotor, accommodative, refractive, visual field, and eyelid movement dysfunction, as well as nystagmus, ptosis, and diplopia (Burnett et al., 2003; Freed & Hellerstein, 1997). Indeed, the composite signs of diplopia, blurred vision, visual-field loss, decreased oculomotor skills, and seeing movement in the stable external environment has been termed posttrauma vision syndrome (Hellerstein, Freed, & Maples, 1995). Double vision has been called the hallmark of visual deficits for persons with TBI and often results in the individual closing one eye for greater clarity. In addition to sensory deficits, visual perceptual disorders may infrequently occur, including unilateral neglect or inattention. However, visual rather than perceptual deficits are more common in the person with TBI.

Loss of the sense of smell (cranial nerve I) occurs in up to 40% of the brain-injured population, as a result of damage to the olfactory nerve (Costanzo & Becker, 1990). It is often the only cranial nerve damaged in mild brain injury (Burnett et al., 2003; Costanzo & Becker, 1990). Anosmia, or the absence of smell, is especially common following frontal or occipital blows, as nerve endings cross through the thin and easily fractured cribriform plate of the ethmoid bone in the nose. Recovery of smell is not universal and is often incomplete. A study of persons with TBI by Costanzo and Becker found that only 33% of TBI victims improved in smell function. If recovery occurs, it typically occurs between 6 and 12 months postinjury (Burnett et al.; Costanzo & Becker).

The external ear is the most commonly damaged sensory organ following trauma, which may impact hearing (Sakai & Mateer, 1984). Eighty to ninety percent of individuals with TBI who receive a longitudinal fracture of the temporal bone will experience a conductive hearing loss as a result of damage to the vestibulocochlear nerve (VIII). Positional vertigo also has been found in about 50% of people with temporal bone fractures as well as in approximately 20% of people with severe brain injury without a skull fracture (Keane & Baloh, 1992).

As oral feeding is attempted, damage to the glossopharyngeal (IX) and vagus (X) nerves in the medulla may become apparent. Dysfunction results in an absent or depressed gag reflex and decreased movement of the palate and uvula. This limited oral-motor movement makes swallowing hazardous and may necessitate continued use of nasogastric or gastrostomy feeding tubes. In a study of swallowing disorders in brain-injured patients, Lazarus and Logemann (1987) found that 81% of patients had a delayed or absent swallowing reflex, 50% demonstrated limited tongue control, and 33% had slowed peristalsis. **Aspiration**, or pathologic inhalation of food or mucus into the respiratory tract, was found in one-third of all persons with TBI. The presence of aspiration is highly correlated with the development of pneumonia, which may be life threatening. In later stages of recovery, there may be hypotonia of the oral musculature, resulting in drooling, limited lip closure and tongue control, pocketing of food in the cheek, and a delayed swallow trigger (Logemann, Pepe, & Mackey, 1994; Mackay, Morgan, & Bernstein, 1999).

Course and Prognosis

Response to and recovery from TBI tends to be highly individual, due to the variety of neuropathologic effects that may be present as well as individual factors of age, gender, and preinjury history.

Significant functional, emotional, behavioral, and social difficulties remain for many years following injury. Useful factors in determining a person's prognosis are the trauma score, the GCS, presence of certain biomarkers such as S-100-B, and the presence or absence of hypoxia. In addition, consideration of neuroimaging studies and electrodiagnostic findings, length of coma, and duration of posttraumatic amnesia help determine general psychosocial and functional outcomes (Gordon et al., 2006).

The GCS was the first scale developed to predict both mortality and outcome for the comatose patient and remains the best-known and widely accepted scale of coma (Kornbluth & Bhardwaj, 2010). The Disability Rating Scale (DRS) (Fig. 12.1) has expanded on this information to provide a quantitative assessment of the disability of patients with severe brain injury. The DRS includes eight categories, including assessments of the cognitive components of self-care activities, the general level of functioning/dependence on others, and psychosocial skill/employability (Rappaport, Hall, & Hopkins, 1982). The DRS has demonstrated high interrater and test-retest reliability as well as concurrent and predictive validity (Hall, Cope, & Rappaport, 1985; Hall, Hamilton, & Gordon, 1993).

The Levels of Cognitive Functioning Scale (LCFS) (Hagan, 1997) (Fig. 12.2) is used in many rehabilitation programs. This scale classifies the admitted patient into one of eight levels of cognitive functioning and has been shown to have good interrater and test-retest reliability (Gouvier, Blanton, & LaPorte, 1987). Limitations for the scale are that it does not adequately reflect small changes in recovery, may not accurately place a patient with characteristics of two or more categories, and is less accurate at higher levels (Gouvier et al., 1987).

Level I of the LCFS is a period of dense unresponsiveness to all external stimuli. In level II, an inconsistent, nonpurposeful, and often delayed response to external stimuli is seen. Responses may be gross body movements, vocalizations, or physiologic changes such as sweating. Visual tracking of large objects is present, but the eyes may not appear focused. In level III, the level of localized response, there is an inconsistent but specific response to a strong stimulus such as pain or a bright object. An inconsistent response to simple verbal commands may be present. The person may respond to discomfort by pulling at nasogastric or catheter tubing. At level III, observations of deficits of vision and/or visual perception, somatosensation, and movement may be present.

Level IV is a highly variable stage, which may last for shorter or longer periods of time for the individual person. In level IV, the confused-agitated level, the person is confused and agitated, primarily responsive to internal stimuli and unable to cooperate with treatment. Behavior may be aggressive, explosive, and nonpurposeful, with incoherent verbalization. As this behavior may be out of character for the person, it can upset family and friends and provide challenges for the treatment team. No short-term memory is present. Attention is severely limited and is frequently driven by visual stimuli. In the absence of motor deficits, sitting, standing, reaching, and ambulating are possible but do not occur purposefully or consistently on request (Hagan, 1997).

Level V is the confused, inappropriate, nonagitated level; more consistent motor response to requests becomes possible. Agitated and exaggerated behavior may still occur, especially in response to external stimuli. An inability to maintain selective attention is present, and frequent redirection is needed for any task completion. Simple social and automatic communication is possible but only for short periods of time. Memory is severely impaired, and initiation is often limited. While the person may be physically able to complete simple self-care and feeding, verbal supervision is needed to accomplish tasks. The use of selected formal or standardized assessments may become possible at level V.

In stages VI through VIII, the injured person becomes increasingly more aware of his or her person, the external environment, and other persons and is able to intentionally plan movement sequences. Responses to request become consistently more appropriate, and the supervision level decreases for previously learned tasks. New academic learning is generally impaired until level VIII (Hagan, 1997).

Other factors such as memory loss, age, and intracranial pressure are also associated with outcome. Postinjury amnesia of <1 day suggests a mild injury, whereas amnesia lasting more than 1 day is indicative of a more severe injury. A younger age at injury improves both the chance of survival and overall outcome in adults. In children, higher death rates are associated with younger ages, and mortality below the age of 1 is great, with abuse common as the primary cause (Craig, Campbell, Richards, Ventureyra, & Hutchison, 2004).

Cognitive, Behavioral, and Psychological Deficits

Cognitive and behavioral problems are among the most common, difficult, and long-lasting consequences of all levels of TBI in both adults and children. Limited memory, especially, is typically present from coma through the person's life span. **Retrograde amnesia** and **anterograde amnesia** inhibit learning and cognitive rehabilitation. Retrograde amnesia, or memory loss prior to the accident, may gradually but incompletely improve. Anterograde amnesia, defined as the inability to learn new long-term declarative information, is typically the last to improve.

Other effects of cognitive dysfunction are apparent in delayed and inconsistent cognitive function, impairment in routine activities of daily living (ADL), difficulty

TBI NATIONAL DATABASE COLLECTION FORM

Patient Name: _____ Date of Rating:_____

Name of Person Completing Form: _____

DISABILITY RATING SCALE:
Disability Rating Scale ratings to be completed within 72 hours after Rehab. Admission. And within 72 hours before Rehab. Discharge.

A. EYE OPENING:

☐ (0) Spontaneous
☐ (1) To Speech
☐ (2) To Pain
☐ (3) None

0-SPONTANEOUS: eyes open with sleep/wake rhythms indicating active arousal mechanisms, does not assume awareness.
1-TO SPEECH AND/OR SENSORY STIMULATION: a response to any verbal approach, whether spoken or shouted, not necessarily the command to open the eyes. Also, response to touch, mild pressure.
2-TO PAIN: tested by a painful stimulus.
3-NONE: no eye opening even to painful stimulation.

B. COMMUNICATION ABILITY:

☐ (0) Oriented
☐ (1) Confused
☐ (2) Inappropriate
☐ (3) Incomprehensible
☐ (4) None

0-ORIENTED: implies awareness of self and the environment. Patient able to tell you a) who he is; b) where he is; c) why he is there; d) year; e) season; f) month; g) day; h) time of day.
1-CONFUSED: attention can be held and patient responds to questions but responses are delayed and/or indicate varying degrees of disorientation and confusion.
2-INAPPROPRIATE: intelligible articulation but speech is used only in an exclamatory or random way (such as shouting and swearing); no sustained communication exchange is possible.
3-INCOMPREHENSIBLE: moaning, groaning or sounds without recognizable words, no consistent communication signs.
4-NONE: no sounds or communications signs from patient.

C. MOTOR RESPONSE:

☐ (0) Obeying
☐ (1) Localizing
☐ (2) Withdrawing
☐ (3) Flexing
☐ (4) Extending
☐ (5) None

0-OBEYING: obeying command to move finger on best side. If no response or not suitable try another command such as "move lips", "blink eyes", etc. Do not include grasp or other reflex responses.
1-LOCALIZING: a painful stimulus at more than one site causes limb to move (even slightly) in an attempt to remove it. It is a deliberate motor act to move away from or remove the source of noxious stimulation. If there is doubt as to whether withdrawal or localization has occurred after 3 or 4 painful stimulations, rate as localization.
2-WITHDRAWING: any generalized movement away from a noxious stimulus that is more than a simple reflex response
3-FLEXING: painful stimulation results in either flexion at the elbow, rapid withdrawal with abduction of the shoulder or a slow withdrawal with adduction of the shoulder. If there is confusion between flexing and withdrawing, then use pinprick on hands.
4-EXTENDING: painful stimulation results in extension of the limb.
5-NONE: no response can be elicited. Usually associated with hypotonia. Exclude spinal transection as an explanation of lack of response; be satisfied that an adequate stimulus has been applied.

D. FEEDING (COGNITIVE ABILITY ONLY)

☐ (0.0) Complete
☐ (1.0) Partial
☐ (2.0) Minimal
☐ (3.0) None

Does the patient show awareness of how and when to perform this activity? Ignore motor disabilities that interfere with carrying out this function. (This is rated under Level of Functioning described below.)
0-COMPLETE: continuously shows awareness that he knows how to feed and can convey unambiguous information that he knows when this activity should occur.
1-PARTIAL: intermittently shows awareness that he knows how to feed and/or can intermittently convey reasonably clearly information that he knows when the activity should occur.
2-MINIMAL: shows questionable or infrequent awareness that he knows in a primitive way how to feed and/or shows infrequently by certain signs, sounds, or activities that he is vaguely aware when the activity should occur.
3-NONE: shows virtually no awareness at anytime that he knows how to feed and cannot convey information by signs, sounds, or activity that he knows when the activity should occur.

E. TOILETING (COGNITIVE ABILITY ONLY)

☐ (0.0) Complete
☐ (1.0) Partial
☐ (2.0) Minimal
☐ (3.0) None

Does the patient show awareness of how and when to perform this activity? Ignore motor disabilities that interfere with carrying out this function. (This is rated under Level of Functioning described below.) Rate best response for toileting based on bowel and bladder behavior
0-COMPLETE: continuously shows awareness that he knows how to toilet and can convey unambiguous information that he knows when this activity should occur.
1-PARTIAL: intermittently shows awareness that he knows how to toilet and/or can intermittently convey reasonably clearly information that he knows when the activity should occur.
2-MINIMAL: shows questionable or infrequent awareness that he knows in a primitive way how to toilet and/or shows infrequently by certain signs, sounds, or activities that he knows when the activity should occur.
3-NONE: shows virtually no awareness at anytime that he knows how to toilet and cannot convey information by signs, sounds, or activity that he knows when the activity should occur.

Figure 12.1 Disability Rating Scale (DRS). (From Wright, J. (2000). The Disability Rating Scale. *The Center for Outcome Measurement in Brain Injury.* http://www.tbims.org/combi/drs. Accessed August 31, 2010.)

F.GROOMING (COGNITIVE ABILITY ONLY)

☐ (0.0) Complete
☐ (1.0) Partial
☐ (2.0) Minimal
☐ (3.0) None

Does the patient show awareness of how and when to perform this activity? Ignore motor disabilities that interfere with carrying out this function. (This is rated under Level of Functioning described below.) Grooming refers to bathing, washing, brushing of teeth, shaving, combing or brushing of hair and dressing.
0-COMPLETE: continuously shows awareness that he knows how to groom self and can convey unambiguous information that he knows when this activity should occur.
1-PARTIAL: intermittently shows awareness that he knows how to groom self and/or can intermittently convey reasonably clearly information that he knows when the activity should occur.
2-MINIMAL: shows questionable or infrequent awareness that he knows in a primitive way how to groom self and/or shows infrequently by certain signs, sounds, or activities that he is vaguely aware when the activity should occur.
3-NONE: shows virtually no awareness at any time that he knows how to groom self and cannot convey information by signs, sounds, or activity that he knows when the activity should occur.

G.LEVEL OF FUNCTIONING (PHYSICAL, MENTAL, EMOTIONAL OR SOCIAL FUNCTION)

☐ (0.0)   Completely Independent
☐ (1.0)   Independent in special environment
☐ (2.0)   Mildly Dependent-Limited assistance (non-resid - helper)
☐ (3.0)   Moderately Dependent-moderate assist (person in home)
☐ (4.0)   markedly Dependent-assist all major activities, all times
☐ (5.0)   Totally Dependent-24 hour nursing care.

0-COMPLETELY INDEPENDENT: able to live as he wishes, requiring no restriction due to physical, mental, emotional or social problems.
1-INDEPENDENT IN SPECIAL ENVIRONMENT: capable of functioning independently when needed requirements are met (mechanical aids)
2-MILDLY DEPENDENT: able to care for most of own needs but requires limited assistance due to physical, cognitive and/or emotional problems (e.g., needs non-resident helper).
3-MODERATELY DEPENDENT: able to care for self partially but needs another person at all times. (person in home)
4-MARKEDLY DEPENDENT: needs help with all major activities and the assistance of another person at all times.
5-TOTALLY DEPENDENT: not able to assist in own care and requires 24-hour nursing care.

H."EMPLOYABILITY"(AS A FULL TIME WORKER, HOMEMAKER, OR STUDENT)

☐ (0.0) Not Restricted
☐ (1.0) Selected jobs, competitive
☐ (2.0) Sheltered workshop, Non-competitive
☐ (3.0) Not Employable

0-NOT RESTRICTED: can compete in the open market for a relatively wide range of jobs commensurate with existing skills; or can initiate, plan execute and assume responsibilities associated with homemaking; or can understand and carry out most age relevant school assignments.
1-SELECTED JOBS, COMPETITIVE: can compete in a limited job market for a relatively narrow range of jobs because of limitations of the type described above and/or because of some physical limitations; or can initiate, plan, execute and assume many but not all responsibilities associated with homemaking; or can understand and carry out many but not all school assignments.
2-SHELTERED WORKSHOP, NON-COMPETITIVE: cannot compete successfully in a job market because of limitations described above and/or because of moderate or severe physical limitations; or cannot without major assistance initiate, plan, execute and assume responsibilities for homemaking; or cannot understand and carry out even relatively simple school assignments without assistance.
3-NOT EMPLOYABLE: completely unemployable because of extreme psychosocial limitations of the type described above, or completely unable to initiate, plan, execute and assume any responsibilities associated with homemaking; or cannot understand or carry out any school assignments.

The psychosocial adaptability or "employability" item takes into account overall cognitive and physical ability to be an employee, homemaker or student.
This determination should take into account considerations such as the following:
1.   Able to understand, remember and follow instructions.
2.   Can plan and carry out tasks at least at the level of an office clerk or in simple routine, repetitive industrial situation or can do school assignments.
3.   Ability to remain oriented, relevant and appropriate in work and other psychosocial situations.
4.   Ability to get to and from work or shopping centers using private or public transportation effectively.
5.   Ability to deal with number concepts.
6.   Ability to make purchases and handle simple money exchange problems
7.   Ability to keep track of time and appointments

Revised 03/2010

Figure 12.1 (*Continued*)

RANCHO LOS AMIGOS SCALE
AKA level of cognitive functioning scale (LCFS)

____(1) **Level I** - *No response.*

Patient does not respond to external stimuli and appears asleep.

____(2) **Level II** - *Generalized response.*

Patient reacts to external stimuli in nonspecific, inconsistent, and nonpurposeful manner with stereotypic and limited responses.

____(3) **Level III** - *Localized response.*

Patient responds specifically and inconsistently with delays to stimuli, but may follow simple commands for motor action.

____(4) **Level IV** - *Confused, agitated response.*

Patient exhibits bizarre, nonpurposeful, incoherent or inappropriate behaviors, has no short-term recall, attention is short and nonselective.

____(5) **Level V** - *Confused, inappropriate, nonagitated response.*

Patient gives random, fragmented, and nonpurposeful responses to complex or unstructured stimuli - simple commands are followed consistently, memory and selective attention are impaired, and new information is not retained.

____(6) **Level VI** - *Confused, appropriate, response.*

Patient gives context appropriate, goal-directed responses, dependent upon external input for direction. There is carry-over for relearned, but not for new tasks, and recent memory problems persist.

____(7) **Level VII** - *Automatic, appropriate response.*

Patient behaves appropriately in familiar settings, performs daily routines automatically, and shows carry-over for new learning at lower than normal rates. Patient initiates social interactions, but judgment remains impaired.

____(8) **Level VIII** - *Purposeful, appropriate response.*

Patient oriented and responds to the environment but abstract reasoning abilities are decreased relative to premorbid levels.

Figure 12.2 Rancho Los Amigos AKA Level of Cognitive Functioning Scale (LCFS). (From Sander, A. (2002). The Level of Cognitive Functioning Scale. *The Center for Outcome Measurement in Brain Injury.* http://www.tbims.org/combi/lcfs. Accessed August 31, 2010.)

learning new motor routines, and adapting to new or cognitively demanding situations (Cicerone, Dahlberg, & Kalmar, 2000). Motor learning, or the ability to relearn previously well-known or learn anew adaptive motor skills, is often functional during the rehabilitation process despite memory loss.

As coma subsides, cognitive deficits become apparent. These may include difficulties with sustained attention, concentration, memory, comprehension, reasoning, self-monitoring and impulse control, other-awareness, and executive function. Executive functions involve the ability to formulate context-appropriate goals and to initiate, plan and organize, sequence, and adapt behavior based on anticipated or actual consequences of actions (Cicerone et al., 2000; Hawley, 2004).

Neurobehavioral deficits occur as a result of cognitive deficits interacting with brain dysfunction. These deficits are typically seen whether the TBI is mild, moderate, or severe (Cicerone et al., 2000; Hawley, 2004) and include impulsivity, perseveration, irritability, poor control of temper, aggression, disinhibition, and apathy (Noggle & Pierson, 2010; Ylvisaker et al., 2007). Limited self-awareness or a lack of insight may slow rehabilitation progress as well as the ability to participate successfully in academic, vocational, and/or social roles.

Depression and loss of self-esteem may be particularly prevalent in children with TBI as they age. An increasing awareness of their deficits coupled with decreased academic achievement (Fay et al., 1994) may lead to depression in children.

Onset of an Axis 1 or Axis 2 psychiatric disorder may occur following a TBI. In one large sample of 722 outpatients with TBI, major depressive disorder was found in 42% of the sample (Kreutzer, Seel, & Gourley, 2001); another large study of 666 people found the incidence to be 27% (Seel, Kreutzer, & Rosenthal, 2003). Neither time since injury nor severity of injury is correlated with depression (Gordon et al., 2006). With depression comes the potential for suicide. Suicide rates for people with TBI vary between 2.7 and 4.1 times that of the general population when matched for age and sex (Engberg & Teasdale, 2004; Teasdale & Engberg, 2001). A diagnosis of TBI and evidence of aggression and hostility are predictive of suicide attempts (Gordon et al., 2006).

Posttraumatic stress disorder is also seen in people with TBI. Studies have found that symptoms of posttraumatic stress disorder were related to the person's level of insight, but not severity of injury, years of education, intelligence, or memory impairment (Gordon et al., 2006). Additional Axis I diagnoses correlated with TBI include substance abuse and aggressive behavior and agitation. Aggressive behavior has been shown to be three times greater in people with TBI compared to people with multiple trauma (Baguley et al., 1999). Axis II diagnoses associated with TBI include borderline, avoidant, paranoid, obsessive-compulsive, and narcissistic personality. The onset of an Axis II disorder is independent of severity of injury, age at injury, and time since injury (Gordon et al.).

Medical/Surgical Management

Medical Intervention in the Acute Phase

Physicians from neurology, neurosurgery, nternal medicine, or orthopaedics may direct overall medical management in the acute phase. The focus of acute medical management is preservation of life, management of secondary complications, and the prevention of secondary damage. Maintaining an effective airway and circulatory function are critical life-preserving steps immediately after injury. An endotracheal tube is typically placed to support breathing. After arrival at the hospital, diagnostic tests are begun to identify the location and severity of all injuries. The patient typically receives a computerized axial tomography scan. If this reveals an intracranial hematoma, immediate surgical decompression is performed. Constant monitoring of consciousness occurs, as the duration and depth of coma are significant indicators of both mortality and morbidity (Carlile et al., 2010).

Diagnosis and management of secondary diagnoses also occurs upon arrival at the hospital. More than 50% of persons with severe head injury have associated injuries. A common secondary complication from the brain injury is hydrocephalus, which is a serious complication for up to 75% of individuals with TBI. Fractures are common as well, as 82% of those with TBI have one or more extracranial fractures, with 10% of these cervical spinal cord injuries. In the latter case, immediate medical management is needed for both a brain injury and a high-level spinal cord injury (Hanscom, 1987).

Intensive-care medical management is constant. An indwelling urinary catheter is placed and closely monitored. About one-third of those hospitalized with TBI aspirate food into their lungs, resulting in aspiration pneumonia. These persons usually have a delayed or absent swallowing reflex (Lazarus & Logemann, 1987; Logemann et al., 1994; Mackay et al., 1999). A nasogastric tube is positioned and used for high caloric feeding for people with swallowing dysfunction. Close attention to skin integrity is essential, and the person's total body position is changed frequently. Suctioning of the endotracheal tube and vigorous respiratory therapy are implemented to prevent additional pulmonary problems (Costanzo & Becker, 1990).

Ongoing management of common medical complications occurs in the acute phase. Prophylactic medication for seizures is provided typically for only the first 7 days following injury and then discontinued unless the person has recurring seizures. As a result of rigid abnormal posturing and other motor disturbances, many persons with TBI develop contractures of the neck, trunk, and/or extremities. The longer the duration of coma, the greater is the potential for the development of contractures, heterotopic ossification, and DVTs. Treatment to prevent these complications commonly includes range of motion in the acute phase. Medical intervention for spasticity in the acute phase includes physical and pharmacologic interventions. Acute physical interventions include range of motion and splinting. Commonly prescribed medications include baclofen, tizanidine, dantrolene, and botulinum toxin (Greenwald & Rigg, 2009).

Rehabilitation interventions in the acute phase may begin as soon as neurologic stability is achieved. The focus of acute rehabilitation is to prevent joint deformity and to provide graded and specific sensory stimulation, with the assumption that selective sensory input may speed or improve neurologic recovery.

Medical Intervention in Rehabilitation

Admission to an inpatient rehabilitation unit is needed for people with moderate to severe TBI. Criteria for transfer to the rehabilitation phase include medical stability, potential for improvement, and tolerance for therapy. Inpatient rehabilitation requires tolerance for at least 3 hours of two or more therapies 5 to 7 days per week; subacute rehabilitation requires the ability to participate for 0.5 to 2 hours each day. Intensive rehabilitation is usually directed by a physiatrist, a physician specializing in rehabilitation medicine. Goals of the rehabilitation program are to maximize the person's function, minimize additional physical or psychosocial impairments, and prevent complications (Greenwald & Rigg, 2009). Along with the primary physician, core rehabilitation members include specialists in occupational therapy, physical therapy, speech/language pathology, nursing, neuropsychology, and social work. In 2005, a major review of multidisciplinary rehabilitation of adults with TBI found "strong evidence of benefit from formal intervention," with earlier functional gains from more intensive programs (Turner-Stokes et al., 2005).

The long-term rehabilitation goals in occupational therapy are to reestablish occupational performance skill, sensorimotor integration and control, and the integration of perceptual, cognitive, and communication skills with daily tasks. Where remediation is not possible or when maximal neurologic recovery is assumed to be complete, the use of compensation strategies may be appropriate. As basic goals are accomplished, discharge from the hospital may occur, with more advanced skills learned on an outpatient basis. Outpatient occupational therapy goals include instrumental ADL, further community reintegration, and work reentry.

Impact of TBI on Client Factors

All areas identified in the Occupational Therapy Practice Framework are affected with TBI. The deeply comatose person, with cognitive levels I through III, shows depressed function in all function. With further recovery, improvement in performance skills and patterns, as well as client factors, may occur and enable the performance of preferred or required occupations. In a study of 1,170 records from the Traumatic Brain Injury Model Systems database, Bushnik et al. (2003) found that individuals with TBI as a result of a vehicular accident were initially admitted with significantly lower functional independence measure motor scores than those who were admitted because of violence, falls, or other causes. However, at discharge from rehabilitation, no significant differences were found among patients in the four etiology groups for most psychosocial and functional outcome measures. In fact, 85% to 96% of all patients demonstrated sufficient basic ADL skills to live in a private residence upon discharge.

Despite basic ADL skills, independence in community living is difficult for many people after TBI. A study of 175 survivors of moderate to severe TBI 2 years after acute rehabilitation found that over 75% of these survivors reported ongoing cognitive, emotional, and behavioral problems. Of those with remaining problems, between 60% and 75% reported difficulty with memory, fatigue, word-finding difficulties, irritability, decreased speed of thinking, and impaired concentration (Ponsford, Olver, & Curran, 1995).

Effect of TBI on Productivity

Most persons with TBI have major difficulties returning to a productive life after injury whether the injury is mild or severe. Ruffolo, Friedland, and Dawson (1999) reported that while 42% of people with mild brain injury returned to work, only 12% returned to their premorbid level of employment. Cognitive and behavioral issues were cited for this decreased function.

For those with moderate to severe injuries, the ability to return to work has been inconsistently correlated with self-awareness. Sherer, Bergloff, and Levin (1998), in a multicenter TBI Model System study, found that limited self-awareness accounted for a substantial proportion (0.31) of the variance in positive vocational outcomes, while Coetzer and du Toit (2002) found no comparable correlation in their study of 40 people with TBI of varying levels of severity. In the absence of definitive findings to date, the difficulty of people with TBI to be aware of the effect of their statements and physical actions on others should be considered in planning for return to productivity. Indeed, psychosocial skills that affect social integration show a stronger correlation with successful return to work than either cognitive or sensorimotor skills, or any combination of the three factors (Conti, 1992).

Bushnik et al. (2003) found the unemployment rate for persons with TBI because of violence to be 70%, significantly greater than the rate of approximately 50% for those with TBI from all other causes. An additional factor independently predicting poorer productivity outcomes was preinjury substance abuse (Sherer, Bergloff, & High, 1999).

Neither gender nor race has been consistently linked to productivity outcomes. A review by van Reekum (2001) found conflicting evidence that females had poorer outcomes, partly based on varying definitions of productivity. A major study of race (Sherer, Nick, & Sander, 2003) and productivity found that African Americans and others from minority backgrounds had less productive outcomes than whites, but race alone accounted for little of the variance in productivity. Race and productivity had confounding associations with preinjury productivity, educational level, and cause of injury.

The DRS has been found to predict employment. In a study of 145 persons with TBI, Cope, Cole, and Hall (1999) found that 62% of those with scores of 1 to 3 on rehabilitation admission were employed or in school at 1 year after discharge, while 39% of those with scores of 4 to 6 and only 11% of those with a DRS score of 7 to 20 were similarly employed. For those returning to work, supported part-time employment has been shown to be a viable and cost-effective option (Cope et al., 1999). However, limited employment opportunities with typically lower wages and decreased work hours often result in the need for public assistance (Johnstone et al., 2003; Wehman et al., 2003).

Factors Affecting Driving

Physical disabilities, as well as cognitive, visual, or perceptual, and self-awareness deficits can significantly impair driving function. A number of studies have attempted to identify factors that predict those persons with TBI who may successfully return to driving, with inconclusive results (Coleman, Rapport, & Ergh, 2002; Novack et al., 2010; Pietrapiana et al., 2005; Rapport, Coleman, & Hanks, 2008). Severity of injury and duration of coma have not shown clear predictive value (Coleman et al., 2002; Rapport, Hanks, & Bryer, 2006). One study found that persons more likely to return to driving included those discharged from rehabilitation with independence or modified independence in scores on the Functional Independence Measure (Fisk, Schneider, & Novack, 1998). Neuropsychologic testing may provide insight into driving potential, but these findings may be limited by the person's level of self-awareness (Novack et al., 2010).

Nevertheless, about 50% of people with moderate to severe TBI have resumed driving within 5 years, with most driving within the first year of injury (Novack et al., 2010; Rapport et al., 2006). Tamietto et al. (2006) note, however, that as many as two-thirds of these may resume driving without any formal examination. In a study comparing nondrivers to drivers with TBI, Rapport found that nondrivers who wanted to drive rated themselves as physically and cognitively fit to drive, despite cognitive skills that were significantly worse than drivers with TBI (Rapport et al., 2006). In discussing this finding, Rapport et al. stated that

> even nondrivers rate their current driving abilities as better than average (which) may reflect unawareness of deficit, denial, resistance to role change or accurate self-perception.

TUMORS OF THE CENTRAL NERVOUS SYSTEM

Descriptions and Definitions

Brain tumors have increased in the past few decades. Fortunately, this appears to be due to enhanced neuroimaging techniques and improved medical treatment options (Fisher, Schwartzbaum, Wrensch, & Berger, 2006), rather than a rise in natural incidence. Tumors are classified as primary or secondary, and malignant or benign. The site of origin for the tumor is considered its primary site, even when the tumor has spread to other parts of body or brain. **Malignant tumors** are composed of abnormal cells that multiply rapidly, with the ability to invade, or **metastasize**, into other tissues. Brain tumors, conversely, rarely metastasize beyond the brain. There are four general categories of malignant brain tumors: gliomas, meningiomas, germ cell tumors, and sellar region tumors (Bondy et al., 2008; Fisher et al., 2006). **Benign tumors**, on the other hand, are not cancerous, and they do not invade other body tissues or spread to other body parts. Benign tumors may become life threatening as they cause increasing deficits with cell growth, because they press upon nearby structures and tissues (Fisher, Schwartzbaum, Wrensch, & Wiemels, 2007). This chapter will discuss malignant primary brain tumors. However, the signs and symptoms of, and diagnosis, and treatment for a secondary brain tumor are similar.

Etiology

Chemical changes in brain cells lead to the formation of brain tumors. However, why these changes occur is not fully understood. Most brain tumors develop for no apparent reason and are not associated with anything the person did or did not do.

A few risk factors are known. A small number of genetic factors are associated with brain tumor risk; however, in a study of 500 patients with tumors, <1% had a known hereditary genetic syndrome (Wrensch, Lee, & Miike, 1997).

Gender appears to be associated with the risk for certain types of tumors. Men are more susceptible to glioma and germ cell tumors, while women are twice as likely as men to have meningiomas. In addition, relatively consistent research results show that being premenopausal confers a greater meningioma risk than being postmenopausal (Fisher et al., 2007).

High levels of ionizing radiation are strongly associated with tumor development, as was found following the atomic bombing of Hiroshima in World War II (Fisher et al., 2007). Types of tumors associated with radiation include glioma, schwannoma, and pituitary tumors. In the past infants and children have been treated with radiation in the treatment of tinea capitis and skin hemangioma and have shown increased risk for nerve sheath tumors, meningioma, and pituitary adenoma. Taken as a whole, however, exposure to high levels of radiation is rare.

Many studies suggest that the risk for glioma is reduced as a result of allergies and immune-related conditions. This may arise from the anti-inflammatory effects of cytokines present in allergic and autoimmune diseases (Fisher et al., 2007).

Inconsistent results have been found for exposure to other environmental factors. Early studies of cell phone use and glioma risk have been generally inconclusive. However, long-term studies are needed to determine definitively any risk factor between cell phone use and glioma. Inconsistent, minimal or no evidence is present to suggest any relationship with increased brain tumor risk and head trauma, certain dietary supplements, alcohol consumption, tobacco smoking, and exposure to electromagnetic fields (Fisher et al., 2006, 2007). Inconclusive evidence is also present for many occupational risk factors.

Incidence and Prevalence

About 22,070 persons were diagnosed with primary malignant brain tumors in 2009, including 12,060 men and 10,060 women (CBTRUS, 2010). An estimated 2,300 new cases of primary brain tumors were expected to occur in children (American Cancer Society, 2010a). Incidence differs according to gender, age, race and ethnicity, and geography. Adult men tend to have higher rates than women of primary malignant brain tumors while nonmalignant meningioma is more common in women (Bondy et al., 2008).

Age affects the survival rate for both the youngest and oldest people. Childhood cancer is rare; <1% of all new cancer diagnoses occur in children. Nevertheless, it is the second leading cause of death (after accidents) in children between 1 and 14 years (American Cancer Society, 2010a). It is also the third leading cause of death in young adults ages 20 to 39 (Jemal, Siegel, Xu, & Ward, 2010). In general, and for most tumors, the 5-year survival rate increases with age (Bondy et al., 2008) through the 50s and early 60s.

Studies of race and ethnicity are confounded by issues related to low socioeconomic status. African Americans are more likely to develop tumors than any other racial or ethnic group, and death rates from cancer are 34% higher for African American men and 17% higher for African American women than their Caucasian counterparts. Hispanic people tend to have lower incidence rates for cancer. These figures must be placed in context with concerns of poverty. According to the U.S. Census Bureau, one in four African Americans and Hispanic people lived below the poverty line in 2008. By comparison, only one in 10 non-Hispanic Caucasian people lived below the poverty line. Furthermore, one in five African Americans and one in three Hispanic persons were uninsured and therefore less able to receive needed treatment. Finally, discrimination may play a role in the provision of health care. According to the American Cancer Society (American Cancer Society, 2010a),

> racial and ethnic minorities tend to receive lower quality health care than whites even when insurance status, income, age, and severity of conditions are comparable.

Cancer rates tend to be higher in more developed countries, partly due to greater technology resources for evaluation and treatment. In the United States, the lowest average annual rate of all central nervous system (CNS) tumors in 2004 was reported in Virginia, and the highest rate was found in Colorado (Fisher et al., 2007).

Signs and Symptoms

Signs and symptoms of brain tumors include fatigue, sleep disturbance, pain, mood disorders, and cognitive dysfunction. Fatigue may be the single most significant problem with brain tumors, resulting in increased daytime sleep and decreased or interrupted nighttime sleep. Nightly sleep disturbance is reported by up to 50% of people with brain tumors (Liu, Page, Solheim, Fox, & Chang, 2009). One study of people with recurrent malignant gliomas found that as many as 94% reported severe fatigue (Osoba, Brada, Prados, & Yung, 2000).

Headache is the most common type of pain experienced, with up to 50% of people with gliomas reporting severe pain. Mood disorders accompanying brain tumors include, not surprisingly, anxiety and depression. Depression particularly has been linked to survival, and yet one study found that only 60% of people who reported this to their physician received antidepressants (Litofsky et al., 2004). Problems with memory and executive functions are found in almost half of all people with glioma tumors (Liu et al., 2009).

Diagnosis, Course, and Prognosis

Diagnosis begins with the onset of unexplained symptoms. As tumor cells multiply in the brain, they create pressure on and irritate normal brain tissue. As a result, two-thirds of those with primary brain tumors report symptoms as just described. Amazingly, about one-third of all people with brain tumors have no symptoms initially.

The presence of symptoms is typically assessed by a neurologist, with the use of such diagnostic procedures as magnetic resonance imaging (MRI), computerized tomography (CT), positron emission tomography (PET), or biopsy. The MRI uses an extremely strong magnet and radio waves to produce brain images. It may or may not be used with angiography, in which a dye is inserted into the bloodstream to differentiate between healthy and tumor tissues. People receiving an MRI may not have pacemakers or metal implants or be allergic to the dye used in angiography.

CT scans involve multiple x-rays of the brain from different angles. From this, a computerized three-dimensional model of the brain can be displayed. Iodine is commonly used as a contrast agent to enhance the image. As a result, this may not be the best diagnostic procedure for people with allergies, diabetes, or a heart, kidney, or thyroid condition.

PET scans are typically an ancillary diagnostic tool to either the MRI or PET scan. Finally, a biopsy of the suspected brain tissue may be made. Following the biopsy surgery, histologic analysis of brain cell tissue occurs (Family Caregiver Alliance, 2010).

In most cancer, an important next step is to determine the stage of the tumor. However, brain tumors rarely spread to other organs, although they may spread within the brain. Therefore there is no formal staging system for the prognosis of brain tumor. Instead the oncologist will use the following information to determine the outlook: the type of tumor, the grade of the tumor (how quickly it can be expected to spread), the person's age, the person's functional status (whether symptoms are present or not), the size and location of the tumor, the feasibility of surgical removal of the tumor, and whether there is evidence of spread to other parts of the brain and/or spinal cord (American Cancer Society, 2010a).

The course following diagnosis involves immediate medical management, described below, followed by ongoing medical checkups for years.

In general, survival from any tumor is lowest in the oldest age groups. When types of tumors are examined, the relative survival probability of those with glioblastomas is the lowest, with a 37.7% 2-year survival rate and a 30.2% 5-year survival rate. The survival rates for benign meningioma are much less well known, but appear to be significantly better. One estimate is that the 5-year survival rate for meningioma may be 81% for people ages 21 to 64 years and 56% for those 65 or older at diagnosis (McCarthy, Davis, & Freels, 1998).

Medical/Surgical Management

Management of brain tumors may involve surgery, radiation therapy, and/or chemotherapy. Surgery is now more sophisticated than in the past. It can now be guided at least partially by the use of MRI, to determine locations of important brain areas and their distance from a tumor. Surgery also may be directly aided by image guidance, which provides better visualization of the brain area (American Cancer Society, 2010a).

Radiation therapy uses x-rays, gamma rays, electron beams, or protons to destroy cancer cells. Because radiation can be localized, it affects only the body part being treated. It may be used alone or in combination with surgery or chemotherapy, where some drugs may actually make cancer cells more sensitive to radiation. Radiation may be given externally, using a linear accelerator, or internally, where a radioactive source in an implant is surgically placed near the tumor (American Cancer Society, 2010d).

Significant improvements have occurred to radiation therapy recently, allowing smaller doses of radiation and more precise placement of the radiation. Stereotactic radiosurgery is not really surgery, but the delivery of precise radiation to a brain site is guided by MRI or CT scans. Nearby tissue is affected as little as possible. Types of stereotactic radiosurgery include using a moving linear accelerator, the Gamma Knife, or accelerator-delivered proton and helium ions. Stereotactic radiosurgery typically uses just one treatment session to deliver the full radiation dose (American Cancer Society, 2010d).

Common side effects of radiation therapy, requiring medical management, include fatigue, fever/chills, and a sore or dry mouth. Because radiation therapy to the brain may increase the chance of tooth cavities, ongoing dental consultations are advised. Hair loss also is a common side effect (American Cancer Society, 2010c). While this is not a dangerous side effect, it is often distressing to the person.

Newer approaches to chemotherapy are also available. Traditionally, chemotherapy drugs have had difficulty crossing the blood-brain barrier. Research is currently under way to modify these drugs to successfully cross the barrier, so that they can reach more easily the bloodstream in the brain. Some targeted drug treatments have been developed that focus on specific abnormalities within cancer cells. These treatments are very new and are still undergoing rigorous study in clinical trials. One targeted drug used to treat brain tumors is bevacizumab (Avastin). This drug, given intravenously, stops the formation of new blood cells, which cuts off the blood supply to a tumor and results in the death of the tumor cells (Mayo Clinic, 2010).

The schedule for chemotherapy is dependent on a number of factors and may be provided daily, weekly, or even monthly. After each treatment cycle, a break is provided to allow the body time to rebuild healthy new cells and recuperate from the strong chemicals used. Common side effects of chemotherapy include fatigue, nausea, vomiting, sore mouth, diarrhea or constipation, loss of appetite, pain or difficulty swallowing, swelling in hands or feet, itching or rash, shortness of breath, cough, muscle or joint pain, or numbness in hands or feet (American Cancer Society, 2010b).

In addition to chemotherapy, the medications most commonly prescribed for brain tumors are steroids and antiepileptic drugs. Steroids are used to reduce brain edema and ameliorate the person's symptoms. They may be prescribed at diagnosis or before or after surgery. Common steroids include dexamethasone, Decadron, prednisone, or methylprednisone. Short-term side effects include insomnia, weight gain and increased appetite, mood swings, and irritability. Side effects from long-term use include cataracts, osteoporosis, muscle weakness, and diabetes (National Brain Tumor Society, 2010).

Antiepileptic medications may be used as a precautionary measure or in response to seizure activity. Common anticonvulsant drugs include Dilantin, Tegretol, Depakote, Keppra, Neurontin, Topomax, Phenobarbital, and Lamictal. Side effects from these medications include fatigue, weakness, nausea and vomiting, and incoordination.

Complementary and alternative therapies may also be used, not to replace medical treatment, but to lessen symptoms. Complementary therapies may include stress management, relaxation and imagery training, meditation, acupuncture, herbal medicine, and massage.

Education and support is critical throughout the course of treatment. Support groups may be helpful to both the person with cancer and his or her caregivers. Additionally, individual or family counseling may provide additional support and individual-specific information.

Impact of a CNS Tumor on Client Factors

Cancer of any type, located anywhere in the body, is terrifying. While rates of survival have improved for some types of cancer, most people consider a tumor to be deadly. Values and beliefs may be in conflict. For example, a highly valued commitment to honesty may conflict with the desire not to cause others distress. A basic belief in fairness may be shaken by the timing of the diagnosis. Spiritual beliefs may be overturned, or spirituality may grow.

Mental functions are likely to decline, as well as movement-related skills, vision, and/or communication, depending on the site of the tumor. Pain is likely to increase. Fatigue and side effect from medical treatment may make participation in all daily activities and preferred occupations difficult. While ADL may or may not remain intact for a considerable amount of time, instrumental activities such as work and leisure pursuits are likely to suffer fairly quickly from both physical dysfunction and cognitive deficits. Rest may be disrupted and daytime sleep ineffective in decreasing perceptions of fatigue. In a study comparing people with malignant glioma to age- and gender-matched people with lung cancer, greater problems with vision, motor function, communication, headaches, and seizures were identified by the people with glioma (Klein, Taphoorn, & Heimans, 2001).

Both TBI and brain tumors result in physical, cognitive, and social-emotional deficits affecting all areas of occupation. For the occupational therapist, assessment and intervention is challenging, at times frustrating, and ultimately rewarding.

Case Illustration

Case 1

J.D., age 20, survived an automobile accident with a moderate TBI. After 2 weeks each in intensive care and an acute medical unit, he is to begin intensive rehabilitation. His occupational therapist cannot get reliable information from him, so she relies on a medical record review for his medical history and a discussion with his mother to identify his previous occupations.

His mother does not seem to be very aware of his activities. She states that he has had three jobs as a garage mechanic in the last 2 years. She says he seemed to get tired of routine and did not get along well with his bosses. He moved into her two-bedroom apartment about 6 months ago, so he could start saving money for a new car. He does not participate in any home-care tasks but does help with the rent. Leisure activities included fixing up his old car and "hot-rodding" around. J.D.'s mother does not care for many of his friends, but becomes tearful when asked about his relationship with Kathy. She says they were planning to be married in the fall.

The medical record review reveals that J.D. sustained a right tibia-fibula fracture with the TBI. After 3 days of general unresponsiveness, he began to obey simple commands (LCFS level III). In a few days, he became agitated and confused. A few words could be understood, including swear words. He persis-

tently pulled out both his urinary catheter and his nasogastric tube.

The agitation has lessened somewhat, but he continues to be intermittently disoriented, as when he calls his occupational therapist "Kathy." There is a 1- to 2-second delay before any requested movement. His gaze appears divergent, and he performs best when closing one eye. When fatigued or perhaps frustrated, he is irritable and the therapist has used protective measures she was taught to both protect herself and J.D. from injury as he jabs his fist out toward her.

Motor deficits include poor sitting balance and right hemiplegia, with moderate to severe spasticity. The left upper extremity is within functional limits in range of motion and strength. Transfers require moderate assistance.

J.D. is independent in eating but requires assistance for all other tasks. He requires moderate assistance and verbal cuing for showering using a shower chair, donning and removing a T-shirt, and transferring to and from the bed and wheelchair. Wheelchair mobility is slow, but he can wheel himself from one area to another with verbal cuing for the route. J.D. is unable to read, and perseveration is apparent when writing his name. J.D. has come a long way, but there is still a longer way to go to achieve maximal possible independence.

Case 2

As a part of routine fourth-grade vision screening, the school nurse noticed that Jesus appeared to have some vision problems that were not present last year. Jesus said things seemed fuzzy. She sent a note home with Jesus to his mother, but never received a response. Six weeks later, his teacher sent Jesus to see the school nurse again, this time because of ongoing complaints of a headache. While with the nurse, Jesus vomited, and said that he had been routinely vomiting for the last few weeks. He had no fever. Alarmed, the school nurse drove Jesus home to the trailer in which he and his mother, brother, and two sisters lived.

She spoke to the mother and stressed the need for immediate evaluation by a physician. Maria, the mother, stated she had no physician and no insurance and that the only medical care she and her family received was at the free clinic, open only on Tuesday afternoons and evenings. The school nurse wrote out information for the doctor there, and Maria promised to take Jesus to the next clinic.

The physician at the clinic examined Jesus and immediately set Jesus up for an evaluation by a pediatric oncologist. Social workers at the clinic assisted in finding transportation and assured Maria that medical care would be provided despite her inability to pay. The visit to the pediatric oncologist provided a diagnosis of glioma. This message was sent to the social worker at the clinic, where there was a telephone. The social worker drove to Maria's to give Maria this information and to plan how to achieve the medical care Jesus needed. School was put on the back burner. Jesus entered a regional children's cancer center. Maria arranged for the other children to stay with an aunt and stays nearby the center.

It was a confusing and fun and sad time for Jesus. He missed his friends and his family, but he enjoyed the activities of the center. He did not like how he felt after radiation therapy, and it was hard to understand that something that made him feel so bad could make him better. He was glad that his mother is around, and, for the first time in years, spent time sitting on her lap.

Jesus came home, to a great family celebration. Maria ended the celebration after an hour, seeing that Jesus was tired. But Jesus was happy to be home. He did not care that he had no hair, because he was beginning to feel better, even though he tired easily. He missed his friends at school and hoped to go back soon, but he knew he still could not see well. Maria feared for the future of Jesus and her family and worried about bills that would certainly come.

RECOMMENDED LEARNING RESOURCES

Consumer and Professional Resources

Brain Injury Association of America, Inc.
1608 Spring Hill Rd.
Suite 110
Vienna, VA 22182
Brain Trauma Foundation
415 Madison Ave.
14th floor
New York, NY 10017
education@braintrauma.org
http://braintrauma.org
Tel: 212-772-0608
Fax: 212-772-0357
Centers for Disease Control and Prevention
1600 Clifton Rd.
Atlanta, GA 30333
Public Inquiries
Tel: (800) 311-3435
www.cdc.gov

Family Caregiver Alliance/National Center on Caregiving
180 Montgomery Street
Suite 1100
San Francisco, CA 94104
info@caregiver.org
Tel: 800-445-8106
Fax: 415-434-3508
National Rehabilitation Information Center (NARIC)
8201 Corporate Drive
Suite 600
Landover, MD 20785
naricinfo@heitechservices.com
www.naric.com
Tel: 301-459-5900
Fax: 301-562-2401

SUGGESTED READINGS

Umphred, D. A. (2001). *Neurological rehabilitation* **(4th ed.). St. Louis, MO: Mosby, Inc..**

REFERENCES

Adams, J. H., Graham, D. I., & Murray, L. S. (1982). Diffuse axonal injury due to non-missile head injury in humans. An analysis of 45 cases. *Annals of Neurology, 12,* 557–563.

American Cancer Society. (2010a). *Cancer facts and figures 2010.* Retrieved from http://www.cancer.org/acs/groups/content/@epidemiologysurveilance/documents/document/acspc-026238.pdf

American Cancer Society (Producer). (2010b, August 30, 2010). *Chemotherapy side effects worksheet.* Retrieved from http://www.cancer.org/acs/groups/content/@nho/documents/document/acsq-009502.pdf

American Cancer Society (Producer). (2010c, August 30, 2010). *External radiation side effects worksheet.* Retrieved from http://www.cancer.org/acs/groups/content/@nho/documents/document/acsq-009503.pdf

American Cancer Society. (2010d). *Understanding radiation therapy: A guide for patients and families.* Retrieved from http://www.cancer.org/Treatment/TreatmentsandSideEffects/TreatmentTypes/Radiation/UnderstandingRadiationTherapy-AGuideforPatientsandFamilies/understanding-radiation-therapy-intro

Anderson, F. A., Jr., Wheeler, H. B., & Goldberg, R. J. (1991). A population-based perspective of the hospital incidence and case-fatality rates of deep vein thrombosis and pulmonary embolism. The Worcester DVT Study. *Archives of Internal Medicine, 151,* 933–938.

Annegers, J. F., Hauser, W. A., & Coan, S. P. (1998) A population-based study of seizures after traumatic brain injuries, New England Journal of Medicine, 338(1), 20-24.

Asikainen, H., Kaste, M., & Sarna, S. (1999). Early and late posttraumatic seizures in traumatic brain injury rehabilitation patients: Brain injury factors causing late seizures and influence of seizures on long-term outcome. *Epilepsia, 40*(5), 584–589.

Baguley, I. J., Nicholls, J. L., & Felmingham, K. L. (1999). Dysautonomia after traumatic brain injury: A forgotten syndrome? *Journal of Neurology, Neurosurgery, and Psychiatry, 67,* 39–43.

Bazarian, J. J., McClung, J., & Shah, M. N. (2005). Mild acquired brain injury in the United States, 1998–2000. *Brain Injury, 19,* 85–91.

Beyerl, B., & Black, P. M. (1984). Postacquired hydrocephalus. *Neurosurgery, 15,* 257.

Binder, S., Corrigan, J. D., & Langlois, J. A. (2005). The public health approach to traumatic brain injury: An overview of CDC's research and programs. *Journal of Head Trauma Rehabilitation, 20,* 189–195.

Bogner, J. A., Corrigan, J. D., & Mysiw, J. (2001). A comparison of substance abuse and violence in the prediction of long-term rehabilitation outcomes after acquired brain injury. *Archives of Physical Medicine and Rehabilitation, 82,* 571–577.

Bondy, M. L., Scheurer, M. E., Malmer, B., Barnholtz-Sloan, J. S., Davis, F. G., Il'yasova, D., et al. (2008). Brain tumor epidemiology: Consensus from the Brain Tumor Epidemiology Consortium. *Cancer, 113*(7 Suppl.), 1953–1968.

Bontke, C. F. (1989). Medical complications related to acquired brain injury. In L. J. Horn & D. N. Cope (Eds.), *Physical medicine and rehabilitation: State of the art reviews. Traumatic brain injury* (pp. 43–58). Philadelphia, PA: Hanley & Belfus.

Bruns, J. J. (2003). The epidemiology of acquired brain injury: A review. *Epilepsia, 44,* 2–10.

Bullock, R., Chestnut, R. M., & Clifton, G. (1995). Guidelines for the management of severe head injury: A joint initiative of the Brain Trauma Foundation, the American Association of Neurological Surgeons, the Joint Section on Neurotrauma and Critical Care: Brain Trauma Foundation.

Burnett, D. M., Watanabe, T. K., & Greenwald, B. D. (2003). Congenital and acquired brain injury. 2. Brain injury rehabilitation: Medical management. *Archives of Physical Medicine and Rehabilitation, 84*(Suppl 1), S8–S11.

Bushnik, T., Hanks, R. A., & Kreutzer, J., & Rosenthal, M. (2003). Etiology of brain injury: Characterization of different outcomes up to 1 year postinjury. *Archives of Physical Medicine and Rehabilitation, 84,* 255–262.

Carlile, M., Nicewander, D., Yablon, S. A., Brown, A., Brunner, R., Burke, D., et al. (2010). Prophylaxis for venous thromboembolism during rehabilitation for traumatic brain injury: A multicenter observational study. *The Journal of Trauma, Injury, Infection, and Critical Care, 68,* 916–923.

CBTRUS. (2010). *Primary brain and central nervous system tumors diagnosed in the United States in 2004–2006.*

Retrieved from http://www.cbtrus.org/2010-NPCR-SEER/CBTRUS-WEBREPORT-Final-3-2-10.pdf

Centers for Disease Control and Prevention (CDC). (2001). Acquired brain injury in the United States: A report to congress. Retrieved July 4, 2006, from http://www.cdc.gov/ncipc/TBI/TBI–congress/index.htm

Cicerone, K., Dahlberg, C., & Kalmar, K. (2000). Evidence-based cognitive rehabilitation: Recommendations for clinical practice. *Archives of Physical Medicine and Rehabilitation, 81,* 1596–1615.

Coetzer, B. R., & Du Toit, P. L. (2002). Impaired awareness following brain injury and its relationship to placement and employment outcomes. *Journal of Cognitive Rehabilitation, 20,* 20–24.

Coleman, R. D., Rapport, L. J., & Ergh, T. C. (2002). Predictors of driving outcome after traumatic brain injury. *Archives of Physical Medicine and Rehabilitation, 83,* 1415–1422.

Conti, G. E. (1992). *Factors affecting return to work for persons with Traumatic Brain Injury.* Unpublished thesis. Eastern Michigan University.

Cope, D. N., Cole, J. R., & Hall, K. M. (1999). Brain injury: Analysis of outcome in a post-acute rehabilitation system. Part I: General analysis. *Brain Injury, 5,* 111–125.

Corrigan, J. D. (1995). Substance abuse as a mediating factor in outcome from acquired brain injury. *Archives of Physical Medicine and Rehabilitation, 76,* 302–309.

Costanzo, R. M., & Becker, D. P. (1990). Smell and taste disorders in head injury and neurosurgery patients. In R. L. Meiselman & R. S. Rivlin (Eds.), *Clinical measurement of taste and smell* (pp. 565–578). New York, NY: Macmillan.

Craig, G. N., Campbell, S. M. K., Richards, P. M. P., Ventureyra, E., & Hutchison, J. S. (2004). Medical and cognitive outcome in children with traumatic brain injury. *The Canadian Journal of Neurological Sciences, 31,* 213–219.

Cummings, P., Rivara, F. P., Olson, E. M., & Smith, K. M. (2006). Changes in traffic crash mortality rates attributed to use of alcohol, or lack of a seat belt, air bag, motorcycle helmet, or bicycle helment. *Injury Prevention, 12,* 148–154.

Cunningham, R. M., Maio, R. F., Hill, E. M., & Zink, B. J. (2002). The effects of alcohol on head injury in the motor vehicle crash victim. *Alcohol, 37,* 236–240.

Dawodu, S. T. (2005). *Acquired brain injury: Definition, epidemiology, pathophysiology. eMedicine.* Retrieved July 4, 2006.

Department of Transportation, National Highway Traffic Safety Administration (NHTSA). (2006). Traffic safety facts 2006. Retrieved July 4, 2006, from http://www.nhtsa.gov/portal/site/

Dumas, H. M., Haley, S. M., Carey, T. M., Ludlow, L. H., & Rabin, J. P. (2003). Lower extremity spasticity as an early marker of ambulatory recovery following traumatic brain injury. *Childs Nervous System, 19,* 114–118.

Elvidge, A. R. (1939). Remarks on post-traumatic convulsive state. *Transactions of the American Neurological Association, 65,* 125–129.

Engberg, A. W., & Teasdale, T. W. (2004). Psychosocial outcome following traumatic injury in adults: A long-term population-based follow-up. *Brain Injury, 18,* 533–545.

Family Caregiver Alliance. (2010). *Fact sheet: Brain tumor.* Retrieved October 2, 2010, from http://www.caregiver.org/caregiver/jsp/content_node.jsp?nodeid=568#

Fay, G. C., Jaffe, K. M., Polissar, M. L., Liao, S., Rivara, J. B., & Martin, K. M. (1994). Outcome of pediatric traumatic brain injury at 3 years: A cohort study. *Archives of Physical Medicine and Rehabilitation, 75,* 733–741.

Fisher, J. L., Schwartzbaum, J. A., Wrensch, M., & Berger, M. S. (2006). Evaluation of epidemiological evidence for primary adult brain tumor risk factors using evidence-based medicine. *Progressive Neurological Surgery, 19,* 54–79.

Fisher, J. L., Schwartzbaum, J. A., Wrensch, M., & Wiemels, J. L. (2007). Epidemiology of brain tumors. *Neurologic Clinics, 25,* 867–890.

Fisk, G., Schneider, J., & Novack, T. (1998). Driving following Traumatic Brain Injury: Prevalence, exposure, advice, and evaluations. *Brain Injury, 12,* 683–695.

Freed, S., & Hellerstein, L. F. (1997). Visual electrodiagnostic findings in mild traumatic brain injury. *Brain Injury, 11,* 25–36.

Frey, L. C. (2003). Epidemiology of posttraumatic epilepsy: A critical review. *Epilepsia, 44*(Suppl. 10), 11–17.

Gordon, W. A., Zafonte, R., Cicerone, K., Cantor, J., Brown, M., Lombard, L., et al. (2006). Traumatic brain injury rehabilitation. State of the science. *American Journal of Physical Medicine and Rehabilitation, 85,* 343–382.

Gouvier, W. D., Blanton, P. D., & LaPorte, K. K. (1987). Reliability and validity of the Disability Rating Scale and the Levels of Cognitive Functioning Scale in monitoring recovery from severe head injury. *Archives of Physical Medicine and Rehabilitation, 68,* 94–97.

Greenwald, B. D., & Rigg, J. L. (2009). Neurorehabilitation in traumatic brain injury: Does it make a difference? *Mount Sinai Journal of Medicine, 76,* 182–189.

Hagan, C. (1997). *Levels of cognitive functioning.* Retrieved from http://www.neuroskillls.com/rancho.shtml

Hall, K. M., Cope, D. N., & Rappaport, M. (1985). Glasgow Outcome Scale and Disability Rating Scale: Comparative usefulness in following recovery in traumatic head injury. *Archives of Physical Medicine and Rehabilitation, 66,* 35–37.

Hall, K. M., Hamilton, B., & Gordon, W. A. (1993). Characteristics and comparisons of functional assessment indices: Disability Rating Scale, Functional Independence Measure, and Functional Assessment Measure. *Journal of Head Trauma Rehabilitation, 8,* 60–74.

Hanscom, D. A. (1987). Acute management of the multiply injured head trauma patient. *Journal of Head Trauma Rehabilitation, 2,* 1–12.

Hawley, C. A. (2004). Behavior and school performance after head injury. *Brain Injury, 18,* 645–659.

Hellerstein, L. F., Freed, S., & Maples, W. C. (1995). Vision profile of patients with mild brain injuries. *Journal of the American Optometric Association, 66,* 634–639.

Hendricks, H. T., Heeren, A. H., & Vos, P. E. (2010). Dysautonomia after severe traumatic brain injury. *European Journal of Neurology, 17,* 1172–1177.

Jallo, J. I., & Narayan, R. K. (2000). Craniocerebral trauma. In W. G. Bradley, R. B. Daroff, & G. M. Fenichel (Eds.), *Neurology in clinical practice* (pp. 1055–1087). Boston: Butterworth-Heinemann.

Jemal, A., Siegel, R., Xu, J., & Ward, E. (2010). Cancer statistics 2010. *CA: A Cancer Journal for Clinicians, 60,* 277–300.

Jennett, B. (1975). *Epilepsy after non-missile injuries* (2nd ed.). Chicago, IL: Year Book Medical Publishers.

Jennett, B. (1990). Scale and scope of the problem. In M. Rosenthal, E. R. Griffith, & M. Bond (Eds.), *Rehabilitation of the adult and child with traumatic brain injury* (pp. 59–74). Philadelphia, PA: F. A. Davis.

Jennett, B., & Bond, M. (1975). Assessment or outcome after severe brain damage. *Lancet, 1,* 480–484.

Johnstone, B., Mount, D., & Schopp, L. H. (2003). Financial and vocational outcomes 1 year after acquired brain injury. *Archives of Physical Medicine and Rehabilitation, 84,* 238–241.

Kandel, E., Schwartz, J., & Jessell, T. (2000). *Principles of neural science.* New York, NY: McGraw-Hill.

Keane, J. R., & Baloh, R. W. (1992). Posttraumatic cranial neuropathies. *The Neurology of Trauma, 10*(4), 849–867.

Klein, M., Taphoorn, M. J., & Heimans, J. J. (2001). Neurobehavioral status and health-related quality of life in newly diagnosed high-grade glioma patients. *Journal of Clinical Oncology, 19,* 4037–4047.

Kornbluth, J., & Bhardwaj, A. (2010). Evaluation of coma: A critical appraisal of popular scoring systems. *Neurocritical Care.* doi:10.1007/?s12028-010-9409-3

Kreutzer, J. S., Seel, R. T., & Gourley, E. (2001). The prevalence and symptom rates of depression after traumatic brain injury: A comprehensive examination. *Brain Injury, 15,* 563–576.

Langlois, J. A., Rutland-Brown, W., & Thomas, K. E. (2006). *Traumatic brain injury in the United States: Emergency department visits, hospitalizations, and death.* Atlanta, GA: Centers for Disease Control and Prevention, National Center for Injury Prevention and Control.

Lazarus, C., & Logemann, J. (1987). Swallowing disorders in closed head trauma patients. *Archives of Physical Medicine and Rehabilitation, 68,* 79–84.

Litofsky, N. S., Farace, E., Anderson, F., Jr., Meyers, C. A., Huang, W., & Laws, E. R., Jr. (2004). Depression in patients with high-grade glioma: Results of the Glioma Outcome Project. *Neurosurgery, 54,* 358–367.

Liu, R., Page, M., Solheim, K., Fox, S., & Chang, S. M. (2009). Quality of life in adults with brain tumors: Current knowledge and future directions. *Neuro-Oncology, 11,* 330–339.

Logemann, J. A., Pepe, J., & Mackey, L. E. (1994). Disorders of nutrition and swallowing: Intervention strategies in the trauma center. *Journal of Head Trauma Rehabilitation, 9,* 43–56.

Mackay, L. E., Morgan, A. S., & Bernstein, B. A. (1999). Swallowing disorders in severe brain injury: Risk factors affecting return to oral intake. *Archives of Physical Medicine and Rehabilitation, 80,* 365–371.

Mayo Clinic. (2010). *Brain tumor. Treatments and drugs.* Retrieved October 2, 2010, from http://www.mayoclinic.com/health/brain-tumor/DS00281/DSECTION=treatments-and-drugs

McCarthy, B. J., Davis, F. G., & Freels, S. (1998). Factors associated with survival in patients with meningioma. *Journal of Neurosurgery, 88*(5), 831–839.

McGarry, L. J., Thompson, D., Millham, F. H., Cowell, L., Snyder, P. J., & Lenderking, W. R. (2002). Outcomes and costs of acute treatment of treatment of traumatic brain injury. *Journal of Trauma, 53,* 1152–1159.

Meythaler, J. M., Peduzzi, J. D., & Eleftheriou, E. (2001). Current concepts: Diffuse axonal injury—Associated acquired brain injury. *Archives of Physical Medicine and Rehabilitation, 82,* 1461–1471.

National Brain Tumor Society. (2010). Treatment FAQ. Retrieved October 2, 2010: http://www.caregiver.org/caregiver/jsp/content_node.jsp?nodeid=568#

National Institutes of Health. (1998). Rehabilitation of persons with acquired brain injury. *NIH Consensus Statement, 16,* 1–41.

NIH Consensus Development Panel on Rehabilitation of persons with traumatic brain injury. Rehabilitation of persons with Traumatic Brain Injury. (1999). *Journal of the American Medical Association, 282,* 974–983.

Noggle, C. A., & Pierson, E. E. (2010). Psychosocial and behavioral functioning following pediatric TBI: Presentation, assessment, and intervention. *Applied Neuropsychology, 17*(2), 110–115.

Novack, T. A., Labbe, D., Grote, M., Carlson, N., Sherer, M., Arango-Lasprilla, J. C., et al. (2010). Return to driving within 5 years of moderate-severe traumatic brain injury. *Brain Injury, 24*(3), 464–471.

Osoba, D., Brada, M., Prados, M. D., & Yung, W. K. (2000). Effect of disease burden on health-related quality of life in patients with malignant gliomas. *Neuro-Oncology, 2,* 221–228.

Pietrapiana, P., Tamietto, M., Torrini, G., Mezzanato, T., Rago, R., & Perino, C. (2005). Role of premorbid factors in predicting safe return to driving after severe TBI. *Brain Injury, 19*, 197–211.

Plum and Posner's diagnosis of stupor and coma. (2007). (4th ed.). New York, NY: Oxford University Press.

Ponsford, J., Olver, J. H., & Curran, C. (1995). A profile of outcome: 2 years after traumatic brain injury. *Brain Injury, 9*, 1–10.

Ponsford, J., Willmott, C., & Rothwell, A. (2000). Factors influencing outcome following mild traumatic brain injury in adults. *Journal of the International Neuropsychological Society, 6*, 568–579.

Ragnarsson, K. T. (2006). Traumatic brain injury research since the 1998 NIH Consensus Conference. Accomplishments and unmet goals. *Journal of Head Trauma Rehabilitation, 21*(5), 379–387.

Rappaport, M., Hall, K. M., & Hopkins, H. K. (1982). Disability rating scale for severe head trauma: Coma to community. *Archives of Physical Medicine and Rehabilitation, 63*, 118–123.

Rapport, L. J., Coleman, B. R., & Hanks, R. A. (2008). Driving and community integration after traumatic brain injury. *Archives of Physical Medicine and Rehabilitation, 89*, 922–930.

Rapport, L. J., Hanks, R. A., & Bryer, R. C. (2006). Barriers to driving and community integration after traumatic brain injury. *Journal of Head Trauma Rehabilitation, 21*(1), 34–44.

Rimel, R. M., & Jane, J. A. (1983). Characteristics of the head injured patient. In M. Rosenthal & E. R. Griffith (Eds.), *Rehabilitation of the head injured adult.* Philadelphia, PA: F.A. Davis.

Rochette, L. M., Conner, K. A., & Smith, G. A. (2009). The contribution of traumatic brain injury to the medical and economic outcomes motor vehicle-related injuries in Ohio. *Journal of Safety Research, 40*, 353–358.

Ruffolo, C. F., Friedland, J. F., & Dawson, D. R. (1999). Mild traumatic brain injury from motor vehicle accidents: Factors associated with return to work. *Archives of Physical Medicine and Rehabilitation, 80*, 392–398.

Sakai, C. S., & Mateer, C. A. (1984). Otological and audiological sequelae of closed head trauma. *Seminar of Hearing, 5*, 157–173.

Schootman, M., Buchman, T. G., & Lewis, L. M. (2003). National estimates of hospitalization charges for the acute care of traumatic brain injuries. *Brain Injury, 17*, 983–990.

Seel, R. T., Kreutzer, J. S., & Rosenthal, M. (2003). Depression after traumatic brain injury: A National Institute on Disability and Rehabilitation Research Model Systems multicenter investigation. *Archives of Physical Medicine and Rehabilitation, 84*, 177–184.

Sherer, M., Bergloff, P., & High, W., Jr. (1999). Contribution of functional ratings to prediction of longterm employment outcome after traumatic brain injury. *Brain Injury, 13*, 973–981.

Sherer, M., Bergloff, P., & Levin, E. (1998). Impaired awareness and employment outcome after traumatic brain injury. *Journal of Head Trauma Rehabilitation, 13*, 52–61.

Sherer, M., Nick, T. G., & Sander, A. M. (2003). Race and productivity outcome after traumatic brain injury: Influence of confounding factors. *Journal of Head Trauma Rehabilitation, 18*, 408–424.

Strich, S. J. (1970). Lesions in the cerebral hemispheres after blunt head injury. *Journal of Clinical Pathology, 23*, 154.

Tamietto, M., Torrini, G., Adenzato, M., Pietrapiana, P., Rago, R., & Perino, C. (2006). To drive or not to drive (after TBI)? A review of the literature and its implications for rehabilitation and future research. *NeuroRehabilitation, 21*, 81–92.

Teasdale, T. W., & Engberg, A. W. (2001). Suicide after traumatic brain injury: A population study. *Journal of Neurology, Neurosurgery, and Psychiatry, 71*, 436–440.

Turner-Stokes, L., Nair, A., Sedki, I., Disler, P. B., & Wade, D. T. (2005). Multi-disciplinary rehabilitation for acquired brain injury in adults of working age. *Cochrane Database of Systematic Reviews* (3), CD004170.

van Reekum, R. (2001). Review: Women have worse outcomes than men after traumatic brain injury. *Evidence Based Mental Health, 4*, 58.

Wehman, P., Kregel, J., Keyser-Marcus, L., Sherron-Targett, P., Campbell, L., West, M., & Cifu, D.X. (2003). Supported employment for persons with acquired brain injury: a preliminary investigation of long-term follow-up costs and program efficiency. *Archives of Physical Medicine and Rehabilitation, 84*, 192–196.

Weintrab, A. H., & Opal, C. A. (1989). Motor and sensory dysfunction in the brain-injured adult. In L. J. Horn & D. N. Cope (Eds.), *Physical medicine and rehabilitation: State of the art reviews. Traumatic brain injury* (pp. 59–84). Philadelphia: Hanley & Belfus.

Whitman, S., & Coonley-Hoganson, R. T. (1984). Comparative head trauma experiences in two socioeconomically different area communities: Chicago—a population study. *American Journal of Epidemiology, 119*, 570–580.

Wrensch, M., Lee, M., & Miike, R. (1997). Familial and family history of cancer and nervous system conditions among adults with glioma and controls. *American Journal of Epidemiology, 145*(7), 581–593.

Ylvisaker, M., Turkstra, L., Coehlo, C., Yorkston, K., Kennedy, M., & Sohlberg, M. M. (2007). Behavioral interventions for children and adults with behavior disorders after TBI: A systematic review of the evidence. *Brain Injury, 21*(8), 769–805.

13

Burns

■ *Elizabeth L. Phillips*

Sam, age 15, is scheduled for a burn dressing change at the outpatient burn clinic. Sam suffered 46% mixed partial- and **full-thickness burns** to his face, neck, chest, and bilateral arms 4 months ago when he added gasoline to a brush fire. The resulting explosion set Sam's clothes on fire. Sam panicked and started running. A neighbor who heard the explosion from inside his house tackled Sam and smothered the flames with a blanket. Sam spent 2 months as an inpatient on the burn unit where he received extensive grafting to his face, neck, arms, and chest. He was discharged 2 months ago but continues to have scattered small open areas. Sam arrives at the clinic, accompanied by his mother, and immediately requests assistance to remove his coat. When he is asked to try to remove his coat himself, he is able to complete the task but is noted to have extremely limited range of motion (ROM) and severe bilateral axillary contractures. It is noted that both his clothing and temporary **compression garment** have been cut apart at the arms and shoulder and duct-taped together. When asked why this was done he replies that it is easier to remove his clothes this way. His mother states, "I told him he shouldn't do that."

DESCRIPTION AND DEFINITIONS

Anatomy and Physiology of the Skin

An understanding of burn injury must begin with a review of the anatomy and physiology of the skin. The skin is the largest organ of the body. The thin nonvascular outer layer, called the epidermis, consists of layers of epithelial cells. Beneath the epidermis is the thicker dermis, which makes up the bulk of the skin. Housed within the dermis are hair follicles, blood vessels, sweat glands, nerve ending, and sebaceous glands, which play an integral part in the functions of the skin (Fig. 13.1). The functions of the skin include (McGrath & Uitto, 2010):

■ Protection against infection
■ Prevention of loss of body fluid
■ Control of body temperature

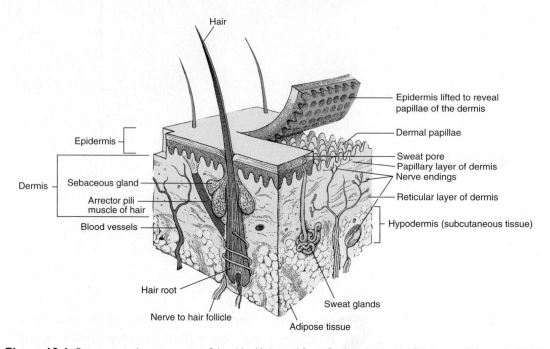

Figure 13.1 Structure and components of the skin. (Adapted from *Stedman's Medical Dictionary.* (27th ed.). (2000). Baltimore, MD: Lippincott Williams & Wilkins.)

- Functioning as an excretory organ
- Production of Vitamin D
- Helping to determine personal identity

Pathophysiology of Burns

The two primary factors that influence the amount of tissue destruction that occurs following a burn injury are temperature and duration of exposure (McGrath & Uitto, 2010). The tissue damage that occurs following a burn injury can be divided into three zones. The zone of coagulation is the area of irreversible tissue destruction. Surrounding this is the zone of stasis, where damage results in decreased perfusion. The outer zone is referred to as the *zone of hyperemia* (Kao & Garner, 2000). The tissues in the outer zones are damaged and considered at risk but with proper care should recover and heal. Without proper care of these at-risk tissues, further damage will result and increased tissue loss can occur (Kao & Garner, 2000). The aim of care after a burn injury is to reduce or prevent dermal ischemia, therefore avoiding further tissue death. The residual necrotic layers of skin destroyed by direct heat damage or the injury occurring secondary to heat damage is referred to as **eschar**.

SIGNS AND SYMPTOMS

Depth of Burn

The depth of a burn injury reflects how deep into the skin layers a burn extends and influences survival rates,

healing time, treatment, and scar formation. The depth of the burn wound is not always clear on admission, and burn depth is often underestimated at initial examination (Sheridan, 2002). The old terminology used to categorize burn depth *first degree*, *second degree*, and *third degree* have been replaced by the terms *superficial, superficial partial thickness versus deep partial thickness*, and *full thickness*.

Superficial Burn Injury

A **superficial burn** injury involves only the epidermal layers of the skin (Kao & Garner, 2000). This burn is characterized by redness and pain. The wound is dry and does not form blisters. The wound blanches readily and is exquisitely sensitive to air and/or light touch. A superficial burn injury can result from a variety of causes such as a sunburn or flash from an explosion. This wound will generally heal within 3 to 6 days and does not produce any residual scarring (Morgan, Bledsoe, & Barker, 2000).

Partial-Thickness Burn Injury (Superficial versus Deep)

A partial-thickness injury destroys the epidermal layer and extends down into the dermal layer of the skin. Some portion of the dermis remains in a partial-thickness injury, which allows this wound to eventually regenerate skin cells (Lewis, Flint, Meredith, Schwab, Trunkey, Rue, L & Taheri, P. (2008). Meredith, Schwab, Truniey,

& Rue, 2008). The differentiation between superficial partial thickness and deep partial thickness is dependent upon how deep the burn extends into the dermal layer. A **partial-thickness burn** is characterized by large thick-walled blisters, which will increase in size, and is deep red to waxy white in color. This wound leaks body fluid, is moist to the touch and blanches readily. The wound is soft and elastic in texture and is sensitive to pressure. This wound will generally heal in 7 to 20 days if it is properly managed (Lewis et al., 2008). This wound does leave a residual scar, which ranges from pigment changes in superficial partial thickness to hypertrophy and has the potential for contracture formation in deep partial thickness Kao & Garner, 2000).

Full-Thickness Burn Injury

A full-thickness burn injury destroys the entire epidermal and dermal layers of the skin and extends down into subcutaneous fat. Because both layers of the skin are destroyed, this wound will not heal spontaneously. Some very small full-thickness injuries can regenerate from the margins of the wound, but this delays healing time and is associated with significant scarring (Kao & Garner). A full-thickness injury may be in a variety of colors. The wound can be charred black, cherry red, tan, or pearly white in color. This wound may present with small fragile, thin-walled blisters that break easily and do not increase in size. Overall, the wound is dry and leathery hard in texture (Kao & Garner, 2000). Since nerve endings are destroyed, the wound is initially anesthetic but remains sensitive to deep pressure. Because burn wounds often have a mixture of differing depths, pain is never a good indicator of depth of wound. Healing time is dependent upon the availability of donor sites. This wound will leave a residual scar and is at severe risk for contracture formation (Morgan, Bledsoe, & Barker, 2000).

Extent of Burn

It is important to accurately estimate the total body surface area (TBSA) involved in the burn injury, as this will guide management. There are two common methods utilized to estimate extent of burn. The Rule of Nine (Fig. 13.2) is a convenient and rapid method that may be effectively used at the scene of accident to estimate extent of burn (Kao & Garner, 2000). It divides the body surface into areas, representing 9% or multiples of 9%. This method has limited accuracy when used with children. The Lund and Browder scale should be used when calculating the extent of burns in children (Fig. 13.3). This scale modifies the percentages of areas according to age thus reflecting the fact that the head and neck of the child make up a greater percentage of the body surface area than that of an adult (Migliore, 2008). In the presence of scattered, spotty burns, one helpful rule of thumb is that the surface of the patient's palm is roughly 1% of their TBSA (Migliore).

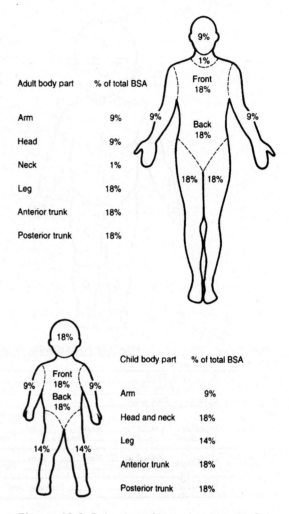

Figure 13.2 Estimation of burn size using the Rule of Nines.

INCIDENT AND PREVALENCE

Each year approximately 1 million Americans seek treatment for burn injuries, with 45,000 requiring hospitalization. About half of those hospitalizations are admitted to the 125 specialized burn treatment centers and the other half to the nation's 5,000 hospitals. It is estimated that one third of these injuries are children. (American Burn Association, 2010). Of those admitted for burn injuries, the survival rate is 94.8% with 70% being male and 30% female. Caucasians are the largest ethnic group affected (63%) followed by African American (17%), Hispanic (14%), and other (6%). Causes of burns include fire/flame inury (42%) followed by scalding (31%), contact burns (9%), electrical (4%), chemical (3%), and other (11%). Most burns occur in the home (66%) followed by occupational (10%), street/highway (8%) and other mechanisms (16%). (American Burn Association, 2010). Advancements in the

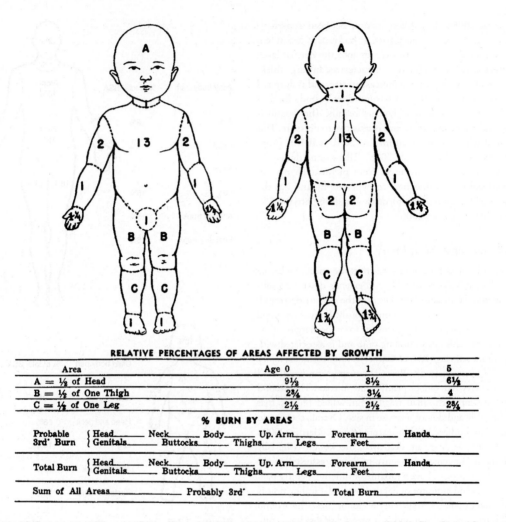

RELATIVE PERCENTAGES OF AREAS AFFECTED BY GROWTH

Area	Age 0	1	5
A = ½ of Head	9½	8½	6½
B = ½ of One Thigh	2¾	3¼	4
C = ½ of One Leg	2½	2½	2¾

% BURN BY AREAS

| Probable 3rd° Burn | { Head_____ Neck_____ Body_____ Up. Arm_____ Forearm_____ Hands_____ |
| | { Genitals_____ Buttocks_____ Thighs_____ Legs_____ Feet_____ |

| Total Burn | { Head_____ Neck_____ Body_____ Up. Arm_____ Forearm_____ Hands_____ |
| | { Genitals_____ Buttocks_____ Thighs_____ Legs_____ Feet_____ |

Sum of All Areas_____ Probably 3rd°_____ Total Burn_____

Figure 13.3 Lund and Browder Scale. (From Harwood-Nuss, A., Wolfson, A. B., et al. (2001). *The Clinical Practice of Emergency Medicine.* (3rd ed.). Philadelphia, PA: Lippincott Williams & Wilkins.)

treatment of burn injuries, such as early excision and skin grafting, improved antibiotic treatment, and the use of cultured epithelium, have decreased morbidity and mortality rates. Factors that increase the risk of death following a burn injury include increasing burn size, age of the patient, and the presence of an inhalation (pulmonary) injury (American Burn Association, 2010).

MEDICAL AND SURGICAL MANAGEMENT

Burn injuries require specialized care not available at all hospitals. The American Burn Association has identified criteria (Table 13.1) for burn injuries that should be transferred to a hospital with a designated burn/trauma unit, capable of providing the specialized care required by

significant burn injuries (Herndon & Spies, 2001). A burn injury has the potential to affect all body systems. The two major systems affected are the cardiac and pulmonary systems. Immediately following a burn injury, during the emergency phase of treatment, pulmonary and/or cardiac complications are the most common cause of death (Muller, Pegg, & Rule, 2001).

The most common pulmonary complications that can occur are carbon monoxide poisoning, upper-airway obstruction, and restrictive defects. Almost all products release carbon monoxide during combustion. It is an odorless, colorless gas that has a greater affinity for binding hemoglobin than oxygen, thus displacing oxygen and leading to asphyxia (Kao & Garner, 2000). Upper-airway obstruction occurs because toxic byproducts of combustion, such as various gases, are released during the burning process and are inhaled. These gases are highly

TABLE 13.1 American Burn Association Criteria for Burn Center Referral

Partial-thickness burns >10% TBSA.

Burns involving face, hands, feet, genitalia, perineum, and major joints.

Full-thickness burns in any age group.

Electrical burns, including lightning.

Chemical burns.

Inhalation injury.

Burn injuries in patients with complicating preexisting medical conditions.

Burns with concomitant additional trauma in which burn injury poses the greatest risk of morbidity or mortality.

Burned children in hospitals without qualified personnel or equipment.

Burn injury in patients requiring special social, emotional, or long-term intervention.

irritating to the respiratory mucosa causing upper-airway edema (Yowler & Fratianne, 2000). Restrictive defects can lead to respiratory distress when the presence of a tight, circumferential, restrictive eschar on the chest, neck, or abdomen causes difficulty with inspiration and expiration (Sheridan, 2002).

It is essential to assess for the presence of respiratory difficulty, as this may indicate pulmonary complications. Signs and symptoms that may indicate the potential for respiratory complications include the presence of facial burns, singed nasal hair and/or darkened oral mucosa, hoarse voice, cough, drooling, stridor, tachypnea, and hypoxia (Yowler & Frataianne, 2000). Those patients whose injuries occurred in an enclosed space, such as a house fire, are at a much greater risk for developing pulmonary complications. Treatment is aimed at maintaining adequate oxygenation through the administration of humidified 100% oxygen by mask. Intubation and ventilator support may be indicated in the presence of severe respiratory obstruction or restrictive defects. In the presence of restrictive eschar on the chest or abdomen, the patient may require escharotomies. Escharotomies are incisions through the eschar down to viable tissue to release the restriction and allow for expansion of the chest wall during inspiration and expiration (Sheridan, 2002). The primary cardiac complication that occurs after a burn injury is referred to as *burn shock* (Yowler & Fratianne, 2000). Unlike other causes of shock, the problem is not a loss of blood but rather the fluid or plasma portion of the circulating blood volume. Immediately following a burn injury an increase in capillary permeability allows fluid in the intravascular space to shift into the interstitial space producing burn wound edema. The effect on the cardiovascular system is a marked increase in peripheral

vascular resistance accompanied by a decrease in cardiac output. This shift is greatest in the first 8 hours postinjury but continues for 24 hours postinjury (Sheridan). After the first 24 hours, capillary wall function returns and gradually burn wound edema will shift back into the intravascular volume and be excreted by the kidneys. In the presence of a burn wound greater than 25%, this fluid shift occurs throughout the body and edema develops in areas that have not been burned (Yowler & Fratianne). In burns less than 25% the fluid shift is usually confined to the burn area.

When hypovolemia from this fluid shift is untreated, shock, organ failure (most commonly renal), and tissue hypoxia occur (Herndon & Spies, 2001). The treatment for burn shock is **fluid resuscitation**, which is the administration of intravenous fluid. The fluid replacement of choice is crystalloid, or lactated Ringer's solution (Yowler & Fratianne). The goal of fluid resuscitation is to maintain the intravascular volume in sufficient amounts to ensure adequate perfusion and oxygenation to all tissues and organs. Once fluid resuscitation is initiated, burn wound edema increases. If circumferential burn wounds are present on the extremities, distal areas should be checked frequently for compromised blood supply. If compromised perfusion is detected, escharotomies will need to be performed to improve circulation (Sheridan).

The Baxter (also called Parkland) formula is commonly utilized to calculate the amount of fluid required (Abston et al., 2010). This formula calculates fluid requirements based on the patient's weight and TBSA burned. According to the Baxter (Parkland) formula, the patient should receive 4 mL/kg body weight/% burn, as a volume of fluid needed for the initial 24-hour fluid resuscitation. One half of this amount is given in the first 8 hours postinjury.

The remaining half is given over the next 16 hours. Adequate assessment of the effectiveness of fluid resuscitation is important, as excessive fluids can cause increased burn wound edema and compromised local blood supply. Inadequate fluid resuscitation can lead to hypovolemia and renal failure. Monitoring hourly urine output is a reliable guide to evaluate the effectiveness of fluid resuscitation. The use of the Baxter (Parkland) formula as a guide to predict fluid requirements has been proven effective but continuous monitoring of the patient is needed to insure adequate treatment of burn shock (Abston et al., 2010; Cartotto et al., 2002; Inoue, Okabayashi, & Ohtani, 2002).

A large burn injury triggers a significant and prolonged stress response in the body and initiates the release of stress hormones such as catecholamines, prostaglandins, glucagon, and cortisol (Murphy, Lee, & Herndon, 2003). The release of these hormones initiates and mediates a hypermetabolic response in the body. This hypermetabolic state will result in increased energy catabolism, skeletal muscle catabolism, immune deficiencies, peripheral lipolysis, and reduced bone mineralization and growth. Nutritional support is needed to meet the resulting increase in basal energy expenditure. Most patients cannot consume enough calories through eating and require nutritional support via the enteral route (nasogastric feedings). Early initiation of nutritional support via enteral feedings will help reduce the risk of bacterial translocation from the gut and the development of sepsis (Kao & Garner, 2000).

Burn Wound Management

Eschar facilitates bacterial access and acts as the common denominator for burn sepsis. After the emergency phase of burn treatment, the patient enters the acute phase. In the acute phase of treatment, the most common cause of death is sepsis. Until the burn wound is healed, the patient remains vulnerable to invasive infection. **Debridement** is the cleansing and removal of nonadherent and nonviable tissue (Palmieri & Greenhalgh, 2002). Daily cleansing and debridement of the burn wound is necessary to decrease the potential for burn wound sepsis, to facilitate healing, and to prepare the wound for grafting if this procedure is needed to achieve wound closure.

Debridement is a painful procedure, and it is important to make sure the patient has been premedicated with analgesics and sedative medication prior to starting the dressing change. Commonly used analgesics include morphine, fentanyl, or codeine. A common drug given to sedate the patient is ketamine. Anxiolytics, such as diazepam or midazolam, are drugs given to control anxiety. Anxiety influences pain perception. The use of anxiolytics is beneficial in reducing anticipatory anxiety regarding future dressing changes (Murphy, Lee, & Herndon, 2003). The use of alternative therapies such as guided imagery, relaxation techniques, and music along with pharmaceuticals may further decrease the pain response during burn wound dressing changes.

Hydrotherapy (tub bath) is the optimal place for burn wound cleansing as the jets help loosen nonviable tissue and facilitate ROM exercises. If a patient's condition is unstable, burn wound dressing changes are done in bed. A mild soap, soft washcloth, tweezers, and scissors are utilized to aid in debridement. To decrease the potential for hypothermia, time in the bath is limited and the temperature of the room should be kept at 82.4°F to 87.8°F (28°C to 31°C) (Herndon & Spies, 2001). Once the wound has been cleansed, an antimicrobial agent and outer bandages are applied. The burn dressings act as a barrier to the environment, decrease temperature loss through the wound and promote comfort (Konigova, Matouskova, & Broz, 2000). Dressing changes are usually only done once a day. If outer bandages become saturated with drainage, however, it is necessary to replace them with dry outer bandages to prevent the wicking of bacteria down to the surface of the wound.

Topical antimicrobial agents are used to delay and/or minimize burn wound colonization (Murphy, Lee, & Herndon, 2003). The topical antimicrobial agent of choice is silver sulfadiazine 1% (Silvadene). Silvadene is a broad-spectrum antimicrobial agent effective against gram-positive and gram-negative bacteria with some antifungal activity. Silvadene does not penetrate burn eschar. It controls bacterial growth only on the surface of the wound, has few side effects, and is usually well tolerated by the patient. When there is a need to penetrate the eschar, such as on the ears to prevent chondritis, 10% mafenide (Sulfamylon) is used (Palmieri & Greenhalgh, 2002). Sulfamylon is effective against a broad range of microorganisms but does not treat yeasts. This drug may produce metabolic acidosis and application is painful, so the use of Sulfamylon is limited to small areas (Murphy, Lee, & Herndon). The use of intravenous antibiotic therapy is reserved for documented wound infections and is not given prophylactically (Palmeiri & Greenhalgh).

In full-thickness injuries, the risk of bacterial entrance and fluid/heat loss through the wound continues until the wound is closed either temporarily or permanently through the application of synthetic dressings (Biobrane; Integra) or biologic coverage (Konigova, Matouskova, & Broz, 2000). Grafting priorities are influenced by the location and size of the burn. If the patient requires long-term intravenous fluid administration, skin grafting may be needed on the chest to allow for insertion of a central line. Hands, because of their functional importance, are given grafting priority. Faces and ears have a dense cross section of dermal appendages and are given additional time to ascertain if healing will occur without surgical intervention (Kao & Garner, 2000).

If the patient does not have available donor sites, the burn wound can be excised down to viable tissue and temporarily closed through the application of a synthetic dressing such as Biobrane or a biologic coverage such as an **allograft**. An allograft (also referred to as a *homograft* or *cadaver skin*) is donor skin taken from another person. The body, through cell-mediated immunity, will reject an allograft usually within 10 to 14 days after application (eMedicine, 2006; Kao & Garner, 2000). These temporary means of wound closure provide the time needed to achieve a permanent method for closing the wound.

The only way to achieve permanent wound closure in large full-thickness burn injuries is through surgical intervention and the application of either an **autograft** or cultured epithelium. An autograft is the surgical transplantation of the patient's own skin from one area to another. A split-thickness skin autograft is the standard method of achieving wound closure (Shakespeare, 2001). Donor skin is taken from areas of unburned skin. The harvested skin is 0.008 to 0.012 inches in thickness. This leaves a wound, referred to as a *donor site*, that takes about 7 to 10 days to heal. Once healed, donor sites can be reharvested but will take longer to heal. Burn eschar is excised down to viable tissue, and bleeding is controlled prior to placement of the skin graft. A split-thickness skin autograft can be applied as a mesh graft or a sheet graft. A mesh graft is a graft that has small holes placed evenly throughout the graft, which allows it to be expanded (eMedicine, 2006). Use of a mesh graft allows more area to be covered than the actual size of the donor skin taken. Unfortunately this results in an unsightly "cobblestone" appearance in the scar (eMedicine). Because of this, mesh grafts are avoided in areas where there are concerns about the appearance of the scar, such as on the face or hands. Split-thickness grafts can be applied as a sheet graft in areas with aesthetic concerns. A sheet graft is a graft in which the donor skin has been laid intact over the area to be grafted. While sheet grafts are preferred because of cosmetic reasons, limited availability of donor sites in large burn injuries limits their use.

In large burns with limited availability of donor sites, cultured epithelium can be used to achieve wound closure. A biopsy of unburned skin is taken and sent to a laboratory that can grow cultured epithelium. It takes 3 to 4 weeks for cultured epithelium to be available for grafting. The resulting grafts are extremely fragile and sensitive to infection. Because of the expense of this form of treatment and the fragile nature of the graft, the use of cultured epithelium is controversial and is reserved for patients with massive burn injury (Kao & Garner, 2000).

Immediately after grafting, with either an autograft or cultured epithelium, the graft is fragile and susceptible to loss. Factors that can cause graft failure include shearing/motion, hematoma formation, and infection (Kao & Garner, 2000). To prevent loss of graft, the grafted area is immobilized in a functional position and remains in that position until the first dressing change. If grafts are placed on the chest or back, the bandages are sutured to the body to decrease the risk of shearing when repositioning the patient. Extremities are elevated to prevent/minimize edema formation. The timing of the first dressing change is controversial, and each physician will have his or her own preference. ROM to the grafted area is avoided until the graft is stable which is usually about 4 to 5 days after surgery.

Healing begins immediately after the burn injury so it is important to consider and initiate rehabilitation activities upon admission. While the scope of this book is not focused on specific rehabilitation approaches and methods, an overview is provided here with the expectation that the reader will be studying specific procedures in a course designed for that purpose. Rehabilitation needs are influenced by the phase of treatment the patient is experiencing. During the emergency phase and fluid resuscitation, edema formation is to be expected and may be profound. The emphasis should be placed on preservation of joint function and maintaining appropriate positioning of the affected area (Jordan, Daher, & Wasil, 2000). ROM exercises help to reduce edema and maintain joint mobility. ROM exercises should be preformed during the dressing change and throughout the day when the patient is awake (Celis, et al., 2003). Timing ROM exercises to occur when the patient has been medicated for pain will help patients tolerate the discomfort associated with this activity (Sheridan, 2002).

Splints are constructed to prevent the formation of contracture deformities and should be worn when the patient is asleep or resting (Jordan, Daher, & Wasil, 2000). In the acute phase of treatment, reconditioning exercises are started and ROM exercises and splinting are continued. Once the patient's condition is stable, ambulation is initiated and patients are encouraged to participate in activities of daily living (ADL). Assistive devices may be needed to help patients participate in ADL.

When burn wounds have been grafted/healed, the patient enters the rehabilitation phase of treatment. The focus of rehabilitation includes reconditioning, ROM, scar revision, contracture release, and reconstruction. Healed burn scars are initially fragile, dry, itchy, and susceptible to sunburns (Endorf & Arbabi, 2008). Destruction of sebaceous glands in partial- and full-thickness injuries cause dry skin and itching. It is important that patients receive proper education regarding how to care for their burn scars. Use of an unscented soap and application of a moisturizing lotion several times a day will help lubricate the skin and reduce itching. Antihistamines (such as Benadryl) can be taken orally to control itching and promote comfort. Application of a sunscreen is important if burn scars are exposed to the sun.

Burn scars are prone to **hypertrophic scar** formation. Hypertrophic scars are scars in which the tissues are enlarged above the surrounding skin and typically present as red, raised, and rigid (Puzey, 2001). Hypertrophic scars are differentiated from keloid scar formation by the fact that they remain within the boundary of the original wound and will eventually fade in color, flatten, and become more pliable as they mature. Hypertrophic scar formation is more common in children, people of color, and over areas involved in stretch or motion (Kao & Garner, 2000). Hypertrophic scar formation is frequently seen in deep dermal wounds that heal spontaneously but take a longer time to heal (Sheridan, 2002). The exact mechanism of hypertrophic scar formation is unclear. Excessive deposition of tissue **collagen** appears to play a significant role, leading to a thickening of the scar (Atiyeh, Ioannovich, & Al-Amm, 2002). Collagen is a basic structural fibrous protein found in all tissue. There is no single effective method to prevent hypertrophic scar formation.

Methods that may help control hypertrophic scar formation include the use of compression garments, scar massage, topical silicone, steroid injection, and surgery (Sheridan, 2002). Compression garments are the preferred conservative method to treat hypertrophic scars and have been in use since the early 1970s. Compression garments are thought to reduce oxygen flow to the scar thereby decreasing collagen production (Engrav et al., 2010). Shortly after the burn wound is healed, measurements are taken and compression garments are custommade for each patient. Compression garments are fit for all areas of partial- and full-thickness injuries and apply a pressure of 25 mm Hg to the scar. The garments need to be worn 23 hours a day; they should be removed only for bathing and the application of a moisturizing lotion.

It is important to verify that compression garments fit properly as excessive pressure may contribute to skin breakdown. Children who are growing and adults who have a significant weight gain after discharge from the hospital may need to be refitted for new compression garments. Compression garments will need to be worn until burn scars are mature which can take from 1 to 2 years depending upon the individual. Mature burn scars are softer, more pliable, and are no longer hyperemic in color; their color is similar to the surrounding unburned skin. Once burn scars are mature, nothing can be gained by the continued use of compression garments.

Wound healing involves three processes: epithelialization, connective tissue deposition, and contraction. Wound contraction is an active process generated by fibroblasts and myofibroblasts and is one of the most powerful mechanical forces in the body. **Burn scar contracture** is the shortening and tightening of the burn scar. Burn scar contracture deformities are most problematic over large joints. They can severely limit ROM and interfere with the ability to perform ADLs. Mature burn scars do not have the capacity to stretch that is found in normal skin. Children with large full-thickness injuries may develop burn scar contractures years after their initial burn injury as they literally grow out of their scar.

Immature burn scars have a greater capacity to stretch but are prone to the development of contracture deformities. Prevention of burn scar contracture through exercise, positioning, and splinting is important until the burn scar is mature. It is essential for practitioners, patients, and family members to realize that position of comfort often results in contracture formation. A prime example of this is the use of a pillow during sleep; while more comfortable, this action may facilitate the development of neck contractures. Simple acts such as having the bed flat when sleeping or avoiding the use of straws when drinking cause the patient to have to assume a position that provides a stress tension on the scar and help to prevent contracture deformities. ROM exercises help reduce the risk of contracture formation. An individualized exercise plan should be developed that meets the needs of the patient. It is important to involve both the patient and his or her family members in the development and execution of this plan to increase the likelihood that it will be followed. Incorporating exercises into activities that a patient likes to do may increase the likelihood that the patient will adhere to an exercise regimen. Engaging a child in play that involves large and/or fine motor groups is a great way for a child to perform ROM exercises. The use of splints at night will aid in maintaining the stretch achieved during the day through ROM exercises. Even with a patient's best efforts, contracture deformities may develop that will require surgical intervention to release.

IMPACT ON OCCUPATIONAL PERFORMANCE

A burn injury is a devastating injury that has far-reaching consequences that continue even after the wound is healed. The impact of a burn injury on an individual's occupational performance is influenced by the size, location, and depth of the burn injury. A burn injury may impact an individual's ability to perform basic ADLs, work activities, or play/leisure activities. Burn injuries that have the greatest potential to impact occupational performance include deep partial-thickness or full-thickness burns, burns involving major joints, and larger burn injuries. It is critical to follow up with the patient on a routine basis after discharge to identify and initiate early intervention if significant hypertrophic scar formation and contracture deformities are detected that are impacting the patient's occupational performance.

It is important to recognize and assist patients and families in dealing with the psychological and psychosocial impact of a major burn injury. Burn support groups can be helpful in assisting patients and families in dealing with the lifelong disfigurement and dysfunction that may result from a major burn injury. Having patients meet with a burn survivor can help them realize what challenges they may face and ways to overcome these challenges. Family members may experience many emotions such as fear, guilt, or sadness. If these emotions are not addressed, family members may feel the need to "take care of their loved one" and to do things for the patient that they need to do for themselves. Having family members meet with

another burn survivor and their families will help prepare them for the challenges ahead and assist them to deal with their emotions. This preparation will enable the family to provide the patient both the support and independence they will need to achieve the best outcome.

Additionally, children can benefit from school reentry and summer burn camp programs. School reentry programs prepare classmates on what to expect and help in the transition back to school. Summer camp for burn children can also help to improve self-esteem and allow them to realize that they can overcome the difficulties they face.

Case Illustrations

Case 1

L.S., a 5-year-old, is playing outside when her father arrives home. He is having difficulty with his car, which is overheating. Unaware that L.S. has come over to watch him work on the car he removes the radiator cap. Hot radiator fluid and steam strikes L.S. and she sustains a 32% mixed partial- and full-thickness burn injury to her face, neck, chest, and scattered area on bilateral arms.

During the emergency phase she required fluid resuscitation and intubation to maintain her airway during the initial fluid shift and resulting swelling. She was extubated on postburn day 3 and has had no further problems with her airway. Three weeks have passed and L.S. has been to surgery twice. During the first surgery, mesh grafts were placed on her chest and arms. During the last surgical procedure, a sheet graft was placed on her neck. Her grafts are intact and healing well, but scattered open areas remain at the margins of the grafts. L.S. has donor sites on her bilateral thighs and buttock, which are healing without difficulty.

Neuromuscular components of ROM, strength, and soft-tissue integrity have all been affected by the burn injury L.S. sustained. She has participated in ROM exercises since she was extubated. ROM exercises were halted for a few days, after the grafting procedures, to facilitate adherence of the graft. Currently, L.S.

has some restriction of ROM to bilateral axillary areas and has been fitted with an airplane splint to be worn when sleeping. This splint will maintain a 90-degree abduction to the axillary area. While she currently does not demonstrate any restriction of neck ROM, she is at great risk for developing contractures in this area. Her parents have been instructed to not allow L.S. to sleep with a pillow and to avoid the use of straws when drinking to promote adequate stretch on the neck. L.S. has been fitted for her compression garments, which should arrive in the next 2 weeks.

ADLs and play or leisure activities are the occupational performance areas that have been affected. Currently, L.S. has few limitations on ROM to most joints, but because of the discomfort experienced during ROM she is hesitant to move. Her parents have been instructed to apply lotion twice daily to facilitate stretching of the scar during ROM activities. Both parents express a great deal of difficulty with the discomfort that L.S. has experienced during her treatment and are hesitant to make her do things that may cause discomfort. L.S.'s father expresses a lot of guilt surrounding the circumstances that caused the burn injury. Arrangements are made for parents to meet with another burn survivor and the survivor's family prior to discharge.

RECOMMENDED LEARNING RESOURCES

American Burn Association
625 North Michigan Ave, Suite 2550
Chicago, IL 60611
Tel: 312-642-9260
Toll free: 800-548-2876
Fax: 312-642-9130
www.ameriburn.org

Shriners Burn Institutes
2900 Rocky Point Dr
Tampa, FL 33607-1460
Tel: 813-281-0300
www.shrinershq.org/Hospitals/BurnInst/
The Phoenix Society for Burn Survivors, Inc.
1835 R W Berends Dr SW

Grand Rapids, MI 49519-4955
Tel: 800-888-2876
Fax: 616-458-2831
www.phoenix-society.org
Burn Summer Camps for Kids
(Information available at Kids Camps)
2500 N. Military Trail Suite 450

Boca Raton, FL 33431
Tel: 877-242-9330
Fax: 866-665-2904
www.kidscamps.com/special_needs/burn.html
Total Burn Care
www.Totalburncare.com Associated online support at:
www.totalburncare.com

REFERENCES

Abston S., Blakeney P., Desai M., Edgar P., Heggers, J., Herndon, D., Hildreth M., Nichols R.J. (2010). *Burn care: Resident orientation manual.* Galvesoton Shriners Burn Hospital and University of Texas Medical Branch Blocker Burn Unit.

American Burn Association. (2010). *National Burn Repository: report of data from 2000–2009.*

Atiyehm, B., Ioannovich, J., Al-Amm, C., El-Musa K., & Dham, R. (2002). Improving scar quality: A prospective clinical study. *Aesthetic Plastic Surgery, 26,* 470–476.

Cartotto, R., Innes, M., Musgrave, M., Gomez, M., & Coope, A. (2002). How well does the Parkland formula estimate actual fluid resuscitation volumes. *Journal of Burn Care Rehabilitation, 23,* 258–265.

Celis, M., Suman, O., Huang, T., Yen P., & Herndon, D. (2003). Effect of a supervised exercise and physiotherapy program on surgical interventions in children with thermal injury. *Journal of Burn Care Rehabilitation, 24,* 57–61.

Endorf, F., & Arbabi, S. (2008). Burn Injury. In L. Flint, J. Meredith, C. Schwab, D. Trunkey & L. Rue, (Eds.) Trauma: Contemporary Principles and Therapy. Lippincott Williams & Wilkins: Phildadelphia.

eMedicine "Skin, Grafts," (February 2006) [Online]. Available http://www.emedicine.com/plastic/topic 392.htm [Retreived January 13, 2011]

Engrav, L., Heimbach, D., Rivara, F., Moore, M., Wang, J., Carrougher, G., Costa, B., Numhom, S., Calderon, J., Gibran, N. (2010). 12-year within-wound study of custom pressure garment efficacy. *Burns* 36(7): 975–983, 2010.

Engrav, L. H., Colescott P. L., Kemalyan, N., et al. (2001). A biopsy of the use of the Baxter formula to resuscitate burns or do we do it like Charlie did it. *Journal of Burn Care Rehabilliltation, 21,* 91–95.

Flint, L., Meredith, W., Schwab, W., Trunkey, D., Rue, L & Taheri, P.(Eds). (2008). Trauma: Contemporary principles and therapy.Baltimore: Lippincott, Williams & Wilkins.

Herndon, D. & Spies, M. (2001). Modern burn care. *Seminars in Pediatric Surgery, 10,* 28–31.

Inoue, T., Okabayashi, K., & Ohtani, M. (2002). Circulating blood volume in burn resuscitation. *Hiroshima Journal of Medical Science, 51,* 7–13.

Jordan, R., Daher, J., & Wasil, K. (2000). Splints and scar management for acute and reconstructive burn care. *Clinical Plastic Surgery, 27,* 71–85.

Kao, C., & Garner, W. (2000). Acute burns. *Plastic Reconstruction Surgery, 101,* 2482–2492.

Konigova, R., Matouskova, E., & Broz, L. (2000). Burn wound coverage and burn wound closure. *Acta Chirurgiae Plasticae, 42,* 64–68.

McGrath, J. & Uitto, J. (2010). Anatomy and organization of human skin. In T. Burns, C. Breathnac, N. Cox, & C. Griffiths (Eds.), *Rooks textbook of dermatology* (8th ed., Vol. 1). Oxford, UK: Wiley-Blackwell.

Migliore, S. (2008). Rehabilitation of the child with burns. In J. S. Tacklin (Ed.) *Pediatric physical therapy* (4th ed.). Baltimore, MD: Lippincott Williams & Wilkins.

Morgan, E., Bledsoe, S., & Barker, J. (2000). Ambulatory management of burns. *American Family Physician, 62,* 2015–2026.

Muller, M., Pegg, S., & Rule, M. (2001). Determinants of death following burn injury. *British Journal of Surgery, 88,* 583–587.

Murphy, K., Lee, J., & Herndon, D. (2003). Current pharmacotherapy for the treatment of severe burns. *Expert Opinion on Pharmacotherapy, 4,* 369–384.

Palmieri, T., & Greenhalgh, D. (2002). Topical treatment of pediatric patients with burns. *American Journal of Clinical Dermatology, 3,* 529–534.

Puzey, G. (2001). The use of pressure garments on hypertrophic scars. *Journal of Tissue Viability, 12,* 11–15.

Shakespeare, P. (2001). Burn wound healing and skin substitutes. *Burns, 27,* 517–522.

Sheridan, R. (2002). Burns. *Critical Care Medicine, 30,* S500–S514.

Yowler, C., & Fratianne, R. (2000). Current status of burn resuscitation. *Clinical Plastic Surgery, 27,* 1–10.

Progressive Neurological Disorders

■ *Diane K. Dirette*

Shortly after the birth of her second child, Joan started getting the sensation of pins and needles in her hands and feet. Within a couple of months, she noticed some numbness and weakness in her arms and legs. She was having difficulty walking for long distances and began to worry that she might drop her 2-year-old son or even her newborn. When the children napped in the afternoon, she found herself slumped on the couch for a much-needed rest. Convinced that this was just part of her postpartum recovery, Joan did not inform her doctor of this difficulty. However, when she found herself struggling 1 day to focus on the words of her son's bedtime story, she decided to seek medical advice.

Over time, Joan found out she had a progressive neurologic disorder (PND) called multiple sclerosis (MS). PNDs are a group of diseases that affect various areas of the central nervous system (CNS), are chronic in nature, and cause a deterioration of function over time. This chapter discusses three of the most common PNDs: MS, Parkinson's disease (PD), and amyotrophic lateral sclerosis (ALS).

There is little known about the underlying etiology and there is no known cause of any of these three PNDs, but research indicates that the etiology is a combination of interrelated factors (Armon, Kurland, Beard, O'Brien, & Mulder, 1991; Kenealy, Pericak-Vance, & Haines, 2003). These include genetic predisposition, viruses, and environmental influences. A genetic predisposition is suspected because these diseases are more prevalent among families and certain racial groups. Viruses and their resulting autoimmune response also may be involved as an external cause of these PNDs. Specific viruses have not been isolated, but particular interest has focused on a viral subgroup called retroviruses. What causes them is unknown, and they can remain silent for years before the onset of a disease. Environmental factors, including exposure to such toxins as lead or pesticides, have also been associated with a higher incidence of PND (Armon et al., 1991; Kamel et al., 2006; Lieberman & Williams, 1993). None of these factors, however, have been isolated as the single cause of any of the PNDs.

MULTIPLE SCLEROSIS

Description and Definitions

MS is a debilitating immunologic and neurodegenerative disease in which the person's own body attacks the **myelin** sheath that surrounds the brain and spinal cord neurons (Kalb, 1996; Kenealy et al., 2003; Matthews, 1993). MS is characterized by chronic inflammation and diffuse **demyelination** not only in the white matter, but also in the grey matter and the axons (Compston & Coles, 2002). Demyelination of the neurons in the CNS results in scar tissue formation or plaques that reduce the axons' ability to conduct impulses (Kenealy et al.). The location of demyelination varies from person to person. The visual, motor, sensory, cognitive, psychological, and bowel and bladder systems can be affected (Fig. 14.1).

Etiology

Why the attack on the myelin sheath begins is unknown because the exact cause of MS is unknown. It is hypothesized to be a combination of genetic and environmental factors, such as a virus or infection (Murray, 2002). The latest evidence regarding MS suggests that a viral infection triggers the immune system to wage an attack on the nerve cells of people who are genetically susceptible (Hanson & Cafruny, 2002). The specific gene or genes have not been isolated, but the genetic factor is suggested by an increased risk among family members (Neilsen et al., 2005). Other factors that have been suggested that may contribute to the cause of MS include smoking (Hernan, Olek, & Ascherio, 2001), a lack of ultraviolet

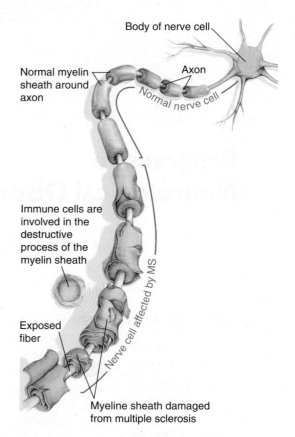

Figure 14.1 Nerve cell in multiple sclerosis.

light exposure, and heavy metal toxins in the environment (Noonan et al., 2010).

Incidence and Prevalence

MS affects approximately 1% of the population of the United States, and there is evidence that those numbers are increasing (Kalb, 1996; Kenealy et al., 2003; Noonan, Kathman, & White, 2002). Currently, an estimated 300,000 to 400,000 people in the United States have MS (Kenealy et al., 2003), and the distribution of these individuals varies geographically. The closer a person lives to the equator, the less likely he or she is to have MS (Matthews, 1993; Noonan et al., 2010). For example, in the southern United States, the rate of incidence is 20 to 39 for every 100,000 persons. In the northern United States and Canada, the rate is more than 40 out of every 100,000 persons (Matthews, 1993). If a person migrates from a location near the equator prior to age 15, the incidence of MS is reduced, which contributes to the theory of a possible childhood infection having a role in the onset (Hanson & Cafruny, 2002) or of the influence of limited exposure to ultraviolet light (Noonan et al., 2010).

The incidence of MS also varies according to gender. MS affects females more often than males at a ratio of between 2 and 3 females for every 1 male with the disease (Hanson & Cafruny, 2002). The current trend supports an increasing prevalence among women, with approximately 125 per 100,000 women and 40 per 100,000 men in the United States reporting MS as a cause for limitation in activity (Noonan, Kathman, & White, 2002).

Population prevalence studies and family aggregation studies provide evidence of a genetic contribution to the disease (Kenealy et al., 2003). MS occurs more frequently among people of European ancestry than other white racial groups. People of Scandinavian and Scottish descent are most susceptible to MS. It is twice as common among Caucasians as other races, and it is rare among people of Mongolian, Japanese, Chinese, Native American, Eskimo, African Black, and Aborigine descent (Hanson & Cafruny, 2002; Matthews, 1993). Studies of offspring, twins, siblings and adopted children demonstrate that the closer a relation genetically, the more likely a person is to have MS (Neilsen et al., 2005). The incidence of MS decreases as biological relationship decreases. If a person has MS, the identical twin, full siblings, half siblings, and offspring have increased risk of also having MS in that order (Kenealy et al., 2003). In adoption studies, increased risk was only noted in biological relatives. Immediate relatives of a person who has MS are 12 to 20 times more likely than an unrelated person of the same ethnicity living in the same climate to develop the disease (Matthews, 1993).

Signs and Symptoms

Some of the more common signs of MS include visual deficits such as diplopia or unilateral **optic neuritis**, sensory disturbances such as **dysesthesia** or paresthesia, urinary incontinence or retention, muscle weakness, gross and fine motor incoordination, fatigue, ataxia, dysphagia,

dysarthria, vestibular dysfunction, and cognitive or emotional disturbances. Each person with MS has symptoms that result from lesions in specific areas of the CNS. The types of symptoms, their intensity, and their effects on the person's functional status are highly individualized (Delisa, Hammond, Mikulic, & Miller, 1985). Table 14-1 includes a summary of common signs and symptoms.

Visual disturbances often are among the earliest signs of MS. They usually appear as a partial loss of vision (scotoma), double or blurred vision, or ocular pain. Sudden loss of vision with pain in or behind the eye is caused by optic neuritis. These early signs may subside after 3 to 6 weeks without any residual deficit. For others, visual loss may be insidious and painless. Nonetheless, nearly 80% of all persons who have MS have some loss of visual acuity. Oculomotor control may also be affected due to lesions of the supranuclear connection to the oculomotor nuclei in the brainstem. As a result, the person loses horizontal eye movement either unilaterally or bilaterally.

The individual with MS can experience a variety of other sensory disturbances such as numbness; impairment of vibratory, proprioceptive, pain, touch, and temperature sensation; and distortion of superficial sensation. Because of these sensory losses, the person also may lose various perceptual skills such as stereognosis, kinesthesia, and body scheme (Umphred, 1990).

Fatigue is the most common complaint and is often identified as the most debilitating symptom (Delisa et al., 1985; Filippi et al., 2002). Increased energy is required for nerves to conduct their impulses in a demyelinated nervous system, making it difficult for the individual to initiate movement and perform sustained activities. The individual also may experience muscle weakness. As the disease progresses, the person requires more frequent rest periods between activities, and decreased levels of activity lead to further debilitation.

Approximately 50% of individuals with MS experience some change in their cognitive ability. Short-term memory,

TABLE 14.1 Common Signs and Symptoms of Multiple Sclerosis

Tactile Awareness	Motor	Visual	Cognitive	Psychological
Numbness	Spasticity	Double vision	Memory loss or	Depression
Disturbance in	Limitations in	Pain behind the eyes	disturbance	or euphoria
pain sensation	tolerance/low energy	Blurred vision	Difficulty with	Impulsivity
Hypersensitivity	Weakness	Partial blindness/	complex ideas	Lability
	Ataxic-like symptoms	scotoma	Decreased	
	Intention tremor	Nystagmus	attention span	

Adapted from Umphred, D. A. (Ed.). (1985). *Rehabilitation* (1st ed.) (p. 401). St. Louis, MO: CV Mosby.

attention, processing speed, visuospatial abilities, verbal fluency, and executive functions have all been identified as deficit areas related to MS (Bobholz & Rao, 2003; Lyros, Messinis, Papageorgiou, & Papathanosopoulos, 2010). As with all aspects of MS, there is considerable variability among individuals with the disease depending on the area of the brain affected (Bobholz & Rao, 2003). An emotional component to this disease results in some individuals having bouts of depression, euphoria, or lability caused by lesions in the frontal lobes of the brain (Feinstein, 2006).

Course and Prognosis

MS is the most common PND found in young adults. MS is usually diagnosed between the ages of 20 and 40 years (Matthews, 1993). It is rarely seen in children or diagnosed in adults older than age 50. No two people with MS follow the same course, and each person experiences variation in symptoms over time (Kalb, 1996). The clinical course of this disease can be roughly organized into four types or patterns including benign, relapsing-remitting-nonprogressive, relapsing-remitting-progressive, and progressive.

The first type of MS is benign, in which the person experiences one or two episodes of neurologic deficits with no residual impairments. This person's chance of remaining symptom free increases with each nonsymptomatic year. The next pattern of progression is relapsing-remitting-nonprogressive. In this pattern the person returns to the previous level of function after each exacerbation. With the third type, relapsing-remitting-progressive, however, the person has some residual impairment with each remission. The course of this type is unpredictable with varied patterns of exacerbation and remission. Finally, there is the progressive pattern, which involves a steady decline in function without remissions and exacerbations. Individuals with MS may shift from one pattern to another, with no reliable predictors of these shifts (Delisa et al., 1985). Approximately 80% of people have one of the relapsing-remitting forms of MS in which they experience neurologic symptoms followed by complete or partial recovery (Hanson & Cafruny, 2002). Approximately 15% experience the progressive pattern of decline in function, without periods of remission of symptoms (Noonan et al., 2010).

Overall, about 60% of individuals with MS remain fully functional up to 10 years after their first exacerbation, and about 30% remain functional 30 years after their first attack (Andreoli, Carpenter, Plum, & Smith, 1986). In spite of the seriousness of this disease, it does not significantly decrease the person's life expectancy. A few people, however, do become severely disabled and die prematurely because of recurring infections or complications resulting from inactivity (Andreoli et al., 1986; Umphred, 1990).

Diagnosis

The diagnosis of MS involves excluding other conditions that share the symptomatology of MS such as B_{12} deficiency, AIDS, rheumatoid arthritis, lupus, Sjogrens syndrome, and Lyme disease (Kenealy et al., 2003). To make a definitive diagnosis of MS, the physician examines the person's medical history, symptoms reported by the person, and signs detected by various tests (Kalb, 1996). These tests include magnetic resonance imaging (MRI) to detect plaques or lesions in two distinct areas of the CNS, neurologic examination, evoked potentials (visual, brainstem auditory, and somatosensory), and spinal tap to assess cerebral spinal fluid proteins.

The results of these diagnostic procedures help contribute to a diagnosis of MS, but they do not determine the diagnosis independently. Many other conditions can elicit positive results. The physician and the individual must work together to rule out other causes before a diagnosis can be made. A definitive diagnosis of MS is made when the person has episodes of exacerbation and remission and slow or step-by-step progression over 6 months. There also must be evidence of lesions in more than one site in the white matter (as determined by MRI) and no other neurologic explanation for the clinical picture (Umphred, 1990).

Medical/Surgical Management

For each of the PNDs discussed in this chapter, surgical intervention is not part of the routine care given. Several medications are used to alleviate the myriad signs caused by each of these diseases. The medications most often prescribed to treat the signs of MS include antispasmodics, muscle relaxants, and anticonvulsants. Some current medications include methylprednisolone for functional skills and Prokarin, amantadine, pemoline, and 4-aminopyridene for fatigue (Bobholz & Rao, 2003; Lyros et al., 2010). Acetylocholinesterase inhibitors such as donepexil, rivastigmine, and galantamine, which were developed for the treatment of Alzheimer's disease, have shown some promise for alleviating cognitive symptoms such as attention, information processing, and memory/learning (Bobholz & Rao, 2003; Lyros et al., 2010). Immunomodulating drugs such as Interferon A-1b, Interferon B-1b, glatiramer acetate, mitoxantrone, and natalizumab show some potential to provide a reduction in lesions for relapsing-remitting MS via anti-inflammatory effects (Noseworthy, 2003; Lyros et al., 2010). Possible future treatments include antiviral medications, vaccinations, transplantation of schwann cells, cell lines or stem cells, and/or gene therapy (Noseworthy, 2003).

Nonpharmacologic interventions that have been found to alleviate some symptoms of MS include cognitive rehabilitation, occupational therapy, psychotherapy, and early nursing education (Bobholz & Rao, 2003; Lyros et al., 2010; Wassem & Dudley, 2003). Low impact exercise with a gradual increase in intensity, duration, and frequency was also found to be effective for reducing fatigue in adults with MS (Neill, Belan, & Reid, 2006).

PARKINSON'S DISEASE

Description and Definitions

PD is a PND identified by depigmentation of the substantia nigra and the presence of Lewy bodies (Hutton & Dippel, 1989; Zhang, Dawson, & Dawson, 2000). The substantia nigra, which is located in the basil ganglia, produces dopamine, a neurotransmitter, and transports it to the striatum (Fig. 14.2). The decrease in dopamine leads to deficits in the speed and quality of motor movements, postural stability, cognitive skills, and affective expression (DeLong, 2000; Duvoisin & Sage, 1996; Lieberman & Williams, 1993). Neuronal degeneration progresses beyond the substantia nigra and the brainstem and can affect other neurotransmitter systems (Zhang et al., 2000). There are variations in the clinical and pathological presentation of PD, and there is overlap with other parkinsonian disorders (Albanese, 2003). The differentiation of PD from other parkinsonian disorders does not have definitive, validated tests.

Etiology

The underlying cause of PD is unknown although there is some evidence that implicates both genetic and environmental factors (Kamel et al., 2007). Two types of PD include familial PD in which there is a genetic association and the more common type called sporadic PD. Several genetic factors, such as linkages to chromosomes 2P and 4P, have been identified in familial PD (Zhang et al., 2000). As many as 50% of people with familial PD have an affected relative. The involvement of genetic factors in sporadic PD has not been fully established (Kamel et al., 2007).

The environmental factors that have been associated with PD are dietary intake and exposure to environmental elements. Several studies have found that living in rural areas, drinking well water, farming, and exposure to certain pesticides increase a person's risk for PD (Kamel et al., 2007; McCormack et al., 2002; Priyadarshi, Khuder, Schaub, & Priyadarshi, 2001). Diet may not be a primary cause of PD, but many studies have found an association between diet and the risk for PD, suggesting a role in the susceptibility to the disease (Gao et al., 2008). Some examples include exposure to iron sources and intake of too much iron supplement were associated

with increased risk of PD (Logroscino, Gao, Chen, Wing, & Ascherio, 2008), increased dairy consumption was associated with increased risk of PD in men (Chen et al., 2007), and higher total blood cholesterol levels was associated with decreased risk of PD in women (de Lau, Koudstaal, Hofman, & Breteler, 2006).

Incidence and Prevalence

PD is the second most common neurodegenerative disease (Zhang, Dawson, & Dawson, 2000). Worldwide the prevalence of PD is estimated at 1% of the population above the age of 65, with estimates as high as 1 million cases in the United States (Kamel et al., 2007). These cases appear to be evenly distributed throughout the world, based on available diagnoses. Diagnostic data, however, vary from one medical care system to another.

PD has been reported to affect males slightly more than females, but recent studies report an equal distribution among the genders (Duvoisin & Sage, 1996). PD occurs in all races worldwide (Duvoisin & Sage, 1996). However, in the United States, there is a lower incidence among African Americans compared to Caucasians (Lieberman & Williams, 1993).

Signs and Symptoms

The major symptoms of PD are resting tremor, muscle rigidity, bradykinesia, and postural instability (Albanese, 2003; Duvoisin & Sage, 1996) (Table 14-2). The most obvious and familiar of these symptoms is tremor, which is usually noted initially in the hand on one side and sometimes in the foot. In the hand, the movement is frequently described as "pill-rolling." The tremors are usually variable. They disappear when the person is asleep or calmly resting, and they increase under stress or intense mental activity (Duvoisin & Sage, 1996). Infrequent eye blinking is often an early sign of PD followed by progressive loss of facial expression.

Secondary symptoms of PD include gait disturbances referred to as a "festinating gait" (short stepped or shuffling with reduced arm swing), dexterity and coordination difficulties, involuntary immobilization, micrographia (small handwriting), cognitive impairments (visuospatial, memory, and frontal lobe functions), sensory loss, muffled speech, frequent swallowing, poor balance, oculomotor impairments, reduced perception of and expression of emotions, sleep disturbances, reduced bowel and bladder function, painful cramping, sexual dysfunction, low blood pressure, seborrhea, depression or anxiety, and fatigue (Breitenstein, Van Lancker, Daum, & Waters, 2001; Carbon & Marie, 2003; Chen, Schernhammer, Schwarzschild, & Ascherio, 2006; Hutton & Dippel, 1989;

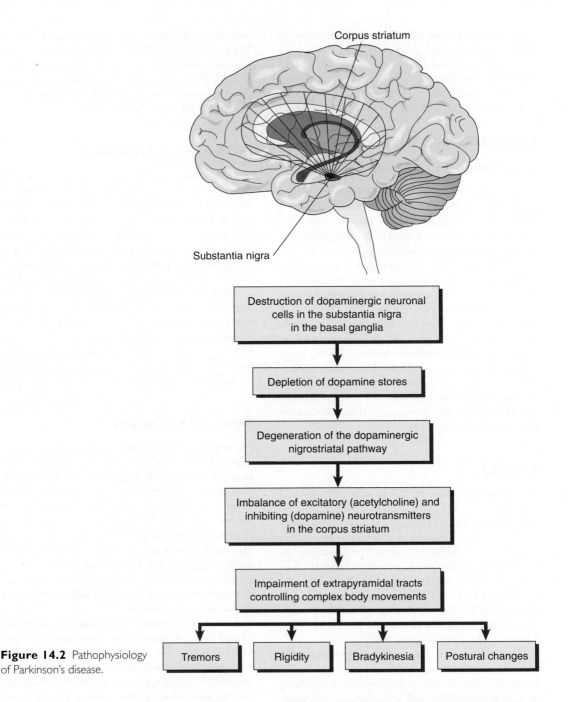

Corpus striatum

Substantia nigra

Destruction of dopaminergic neuronal cells in the substantia nigra in the basal ganglia

Depletion of dopamine stores

Degeneration of the dopaminergic nigrostriatal pathway

Imbalance of excitatory (acetylcholine) and inhibiting (dopamine) neurotransmitters in the corpus striatum

Impairment of extrapyramidal tracts controlling complex body movements

Tremors | Rigidity | Bradykinesia | Postural changes

Figure 14.2 Pathophysiology of Parkinson's disease.

Rearick, Stelmach, Leis, & Santello, 2002). This array of symptoms varies among people with PD. It is highly unlikely that any person with PD would develop all of the symptoms listed above. Some people may not experience a specific symptom, whereas for another person, that symptom might be a major complaint. For example, some people may experience cognitive deficits, such as executive functions impairment, as the initial symptoms, while others may never demonstrate any cognitive decline.

Course and Prognosis

PD is usually first diagnosed when a person is older than 50 years, with the average onset age at about 60. It rarely affects people younger than age 40 (Duvoisin & Sage, 1996). As with MS, the progression of PD differs with each person. In general, PD is a slow, progressive disorder (Hutton & Dippel, 1989). The three phases of the disease include the preclinical period when neurons have

TABLE 14.2 Primary and Secondary Signs and Symptoms of Parkinson's Disease

Primary Signs and Symptoms	Tremor (resting, pill-rolling)
	Rigidity (cogwheel)
	Bradykinesia (slowness of movement)
	Postural changes (stooped, unsteady)
Secondary Signs and Symptoms	Gait disturbances (shuffle, reduced reflexes, falling)
	Impaired dexterity and coordination
	Involuntary immobilization (freezing)
	Speech difficulties (soft, monotone, rapid)
	Swallowing difficulties (drooling)
	Poor balance
	Oculomotor impairments (deficits in fixation, scanning, tracking)
	Reduced facial expression
	Sleep disturbances
	Reduced bowel and bladder function
	Painful cramping of muscles
	Sexual dysfunction
	Low blood pressure
	Sensory disturbances (numbness, tingling, burning sensations)
	Seborrhea (oily skin, dandruff)
	Fatigue

begun to degenerate, but no symptoms are yet evident (Albanese, 2003). In this first phase, there may be some peripheral neuroinflammation that can be found with medical testing, but the implications of this are still being researched (Chen, O'Reilly, Schwarzschild, & Ascherio, 2008). The second phase of PD is the prodromal period that can last months or even years. During this phase generalized symptoms such as depression, anxiety, fibromyalgia, or shoulder pain may appear. The third phase is the symptomatic period when the PD symptoms are evident (Albanese). According to a clinical scale by Hoehn and Yahr, the third phase can be divided into five stages, as follows.

Stage I: Signs of PD are strictly one sided, affecting only one side of the body.

Stage II: Signs of PD are bilateral and balance is not impaired.

Stage III: Signs of PD are bilateral and balance is impaired.

Stage IV: PD is functionally disabling.

Stage V: Person is confined to bed or a wheelchair.

Progression through these stages is variable for each person. Usually, a person will have PD for 15 to 20 years before entering the most severe stages. Some people may be in the first asymptomatic, preclinical phase and remain there until death (Albanese, 2003). There are also fluctuations within each stage. The loss of function is not a linear progression. Each person experiences some periods of improvement scattered throughout the progressive loss of function. Because of advances in medical treatment, life expectancy is not significantly affected by a diagnosis of PD.

Diagnosis

Historically, a definitive diagnosis of PD could only be made by autopsy (Albanese, 2003). Therefore, a person was given a diagnosis of probable PD. To determine this diagnosis, the physician observed the current symptoms, eliminated other diseases as the cause of those symptoms, and evaluated the person's response to medications used to treat PD (Lieberman & Williams, 1993). Recent advancements in the medical community's ability to diagnose PD include positron emission topography to detect metabolic changes, such as a loss of dopamine, and genetic testing to determine familial PD (Merims & Freedman, 2008). At least one of the primary symptoms (resting tremor, rigidity, bradykinesia, or postural instability) must be present. Several tests, such as computerized axial tomography scan, MRI, or **electroencephalogram**, are also used to eliminate the possibility of other neurologic disorders.

Medical/Surgical Management

The medications usually prescribed to treat the symptoms of PD include dopamine replacement medications, acetylcholine inhibitors, and antiviral compounds. Some of the dopamine replacement medications include carbidopa/levodopa, pergolide, bromocriptine, ropinirole, and pramipexole. Some possible side effects of these medications include nausea, loss of appetite, dyskinesias, dry mouth, sleepiness, confusion, hallucinations, and neurotoxicity.

Many surgical procedures have also been developed to treat the symptoms of PD. These procedures include thalamotomy, pallidotomy, and deep brain stimulation (neurostimulation) (DeLong, 2000; Merims & Freedman, 2008). Thalamotomy is a surgical procedure in which heat via an electrode or gamma-knife radiosurgery is used to destroy part of the thalamus. The thalamus is an area of the brain involved in movement. A thalamotomy can reduce tremors associated with PD and may sustain the improvement for over 10 years. A pallidotomy is a surgical procedure in which heat via an electrode or gamma-knife radiosurgery is used to destroy part of the globus pallidus. The globus pallidus is also an area of the brain involved in movement. A pallidotomy can reduce tremors, shuffling gait, flat affect, rigidity, and slowness of movement. These symptoms may be dramatically reduced following this procedure, and the effects may last for at least 5 years. Deep brain stimulation (neurostimulation) is the implantation of a type of "brain pacemaker" that delivers electrical impulses to the subthalamic nucleus, the internal globus pallidus, or the thalamus to reduce tremors associated with PD. The potential side effects of this procedure include depression, slurred speech, tingling in the head and hands, and problems with balance. The generator usually needs to be replaced every 3 to 5 years.

Other medical management techniques that are being explored are gene therapy to replace enzymes involved in dopamine synthesis or to enhance the survival of dopamine neurons (Bohn, 2000), the use of growth factors pumped directly into dopamine-deficient areas of the brain (Mayor, 2002), and stem cell transplantation to generate dopamine-producing cells in the substantia nigra (Merims & Freedman, 2008).

AMYOTROPHIC LATERAL SCLEROSIS

Description and Definitions

ALS, also known as Lou Gehrig's disease, is a fatal, progressive, degenerative motor neuron disease in which scars form on the neurons in the corticospinal pathways, the motor nuclei of the brainstem, and the anterior horn cells of the spinal cord (Beresford; Przedborski, Mitsumoto, & Rowland, 2003; Weydt, Weiss, Moller, & Carter, 2002). Degeneration of motor neurons leads to progressive atrophy of muscles, usually beginning with the loss of strength in the small muscles of the hands or feet (Beresford; Maloney, Burks, & Ringel, 1985). When the motor neurons are affected, the reflexes can become hyperactive. Progressive loss of muscle movement, spasticity, difficulty speaking and swallowing, loss of emotional control, and reduced body temperature regulation are common (Beresford, 1995; Maloney et al., 1985). The actual mechanism of neurodegeneration remains a mystery. There is speculation that cytostolic and mitochondrial pathway dysfunction results in the buildup of proteins that lead to motor neuron death (Shaw, Al-Chalabi, & Neigh, 2001). There is also evidence of an inflammatory component in the mechanisms of the disease process (Weydt et al., 2002) (Fig. 14.3).

Etiology

There is no known cause of ALS, but it is speculated that several disorders with several causes lead to this motor neuron disease (Weydt et al., 2002). The two types of ALS, familial and sporadic, may have different causes. Only 5% to 10% of cases are familial (Zoccolella, Santamato, & Lamberti, 2009). Recent advances have discovered a genetic mutation as one cause for familial ALS (Shaw et al., 2001). There is also evidence of genetic causes using familial patterns of susceptibility. Family history of a first- or second-degree relative with ALS is a significant risk factor for the disease.

In most cases, however, ALS occurs sporadically and is presumed to be acquired. There is no known cause of sporadic ALS, but there is some speculation regarding viral, retroviral, and environmental causes (Shaw et al., 2001). Recent research has identified several risk factors associated with sporadic ALS, including occupational exposure such as chemicals or electromagnetic fields (Weisskopf et al., 2005), lead exposure (Kamel et al., 2003), cigarette smoking (Nelson, McGuire, Longstreth, & Matkin, 2000; Weisskopf et al., 2004), and dietary consumption with increased fat and glutamate intake associated with increased risk and fiber intake with reduced risk (Nelson, Matkin, Longstreth, & McGuire, 2000). Some of these risk factors may also be involved in the familial type of ALS with an environmental exposure combined with genetic susceptibility (Kamel et al., 2003).

Incidence and Prevalence

The prevalence rate of people with ALS is estimated to be 4 to 7 out of every 100,000 people uniformly worldwide (Przedborski et al., 2003; Weydt et al., 2002), with

Normal nerve cell and muscle   **ALS-affected nerve cell and muscle**

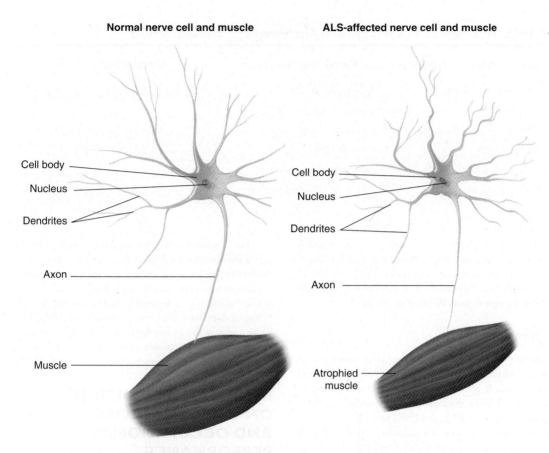

Figure 14.3 Motor neuron changes in amyotrophic lateral sclerosis.

approximately 30,000 Americans diagnosed annually (Weisskopf et al., 2004). It is the most common motor neuron disease in adults. ALS affects males more often than females with a ratio of 1.7:1 (Shaw et al., 2001), but there is evidence that this gender difference is decreasing over time (Noonan, Hildsdon, White, Wong, & Zack, 2002). Ongoing investigation indicates the possibility of increasing prevalence of ALS in the United States (Noonan, Hildsdon, et al., 2002) and worldwide (Durrleman & Alperovitch, 1989; Przedborski et al., 2003). Approximately 5% to 10% of cases are the familial type, with approximately 90% of cases the sporadic type (Kamel et al., 2003; Weisskopf et al., 2004).

Signs and Symptoms

The most common initial signs of ALS is weakness of the small muscles of the hand or an asymmetrical foot drop (Beresford, 1995). Night cramps, particularly in the calf muscles, also may be present. The signs and symptoms of ALS are progressive, most commonly in a distal to proximal pattern. The symptoms can be divided into three areas, including lower motor neuron, corticospinal tract, and corticobulbar tract dysfunction (Table 14-3). The lower motor neuron dysfunction symptoms include focal and multifocal weakness, atrophy, cramps, and muscle twitching. Spasticity and hyperresponsive reflexes are associated with corticospinal tract dysfunction (Nelson et al., 2000). Dysphagia and dysarthria are associated with corticobulbar dysfunction (Beresford; Mitsumoto, Hanson, & Chad, 1988).

Course and Prognosis

The onset of ALS occurs between 16 and 77 years, but it is usually diagnosed when a person is between the ages of 55 and 75 (Noonan Hilsdon, White, Wong & Zack, 2002). The course of ALS is usually progressive and rapid. The duration of survival after diagnosis is usually 1 to 5 years, with a mean survival of 3 years (Beresford, 1995; Weisskopf et al., 2004). The younger a person is and the more mild the symptoms at the time of diagnosis, the longer the course.

TABLE 14.3 Signs and Symptoms of Amyotrophic Lateral Sclerosis

Lower Motor Neuron	Corticospinal Tract	Corticobulbar Tract
Focal and multifocal weakness	Spasticity Hyperreactive reflexes	Dysphagia (difficulty swallowing)
Atrophy (progressive, distal to proximal)	Dysphagia (difficulty swallowing)	Dysarthria (impaired quality of speech production)
Muscle cramping Muscle twitching	Dysarthria (impaired quality of speech production)	

There is some evidence of a "resistance in ALS," in which a person may demonstrate improvements and live longer than 10 years. This is seen in approximately 10% to 16% of people with ALS (Mitsumoto et al., 1988). Death is usually from respiratory failure (Weydt et al., 2002).

Diagnosis

As with the other PNDs, the physician pieces together clinical symptoms, electromyogram (EMG) results, and tests to exclude other causes of the clinical presentation to make a definite diagnosis of ALS (Beresford, 1995; Mitsumoto et al., 1988). The EMG findings will include motor denervation and fasciculation (twitching) with intact sensory responses. A CT scan or MRI of the CNS may be used to rule out other causes of the symptoms. Blood tests are usually normal. Cerebrospinal fluid is often normal but may show raised protein levels.

Medical/Surgical Management

The medical treatments that are currently available do little to alter the fatal course of ALS (Weydt et al., 2002). The medications prescribed to treat the symptoms of ALS include antispasmodic medications, nonsteroidal anti-inflammatory medications, and antibiotics. There is evidence that Riluzole helps people stay in the milder stages for a longer time, and it is the only medication that increases survival, although for only a modest amount of time (Zoccolella et al., 2009). Experimental medications that have been in clinical trials include celecoxib (Celebrex) and minocycline, which are anti-inflammatory drugs, and topiramate, gabapentin, and riluzole (Rilutek), which are antiglutamatergic drugs (Weydt et al.).

Gastrostomy and noninvasive positive-pressure ventilation have been shown to increase both quality and possibly length of life (Przedborski et al., 2003). Low-dose radiation and botulinum toxin injections into the salivary glands are sometimes used to treat drooling.

There is some evidence that attending a clinic staffed by a multidisciplinary team (including neurologists; specialist nurses; physical, occupational, and speech therapists; a pulmonologist; a nutritionist; a psychologist; and a social worker) is effective for improving quality and length of life (Traynor, Alexander, Corr, Frost, & Hardiman, 2003). Palliative care may also be very important for people with ALS and their families. It has been estimated that 62.4% die in a hospice-supported environment (Przedborski et al., 2003).

IMPACT OF CONDITIONS ON CLIENT FACTORS AND OCCUPATIONAL PERFORMANCE

Each of these PNDs is progressive and can affect all client factors, performance patterns, performance skills, and areas of occupation. The extent of this effect depends on the stage and severity of the disease. In each case, a person may have any combination of the deficits listed.

Activities of Daily Living

Self-care skills are affected by changes in the person's sensorimotor skills. Changes are usually noted in gross and fine motor coordination, postural control, muscle tone, endurance, and sensation (except in ALS). Loss of independence in bathing, dressing, personal device care, and toilet hygiene may occur. Toileting can become problematic for persons with MS or PD because of the loss of bladder and bowel control. The individual may experience any combination of the complications noted earlier in this chapter.

Eating may be difficult, either because the person loses the strength and coordination to self-feed or because of chewing or swallowing difficulties (dysphagia). The latter is caused by weakness or incoordination of the pharyngeal musculature, which also can make it difficult for an individual to ingest oral medications.

Functional mobility is another critical concern. Neuromuscular and motor problems make ambulation difficult or impossible, either independently or with assistive devices, even in an electrically propelled wheelchair. Acquiring alternate methods of mobility requires the ability to adapt. The person must be able to change motor patterns, requiring concurrent new and varied perceptual and cognitive strategies. At the same time, the individual is challenged psychologically to make the necessary adjustments to new and different types of mobility. As the person's function decreases, issues of home and work accessibility must be considered, and the necessary adaptations must be made to maintain performance in activities of daily living.

Instrumental Activities of Daily Living

Deficits in neuromusculoskeletal, movement-related functions and motor skills due to PNDs usually lead to reduced ability to perform all instrumental activities of daily living. In addition to neuromusculoskeletal losses, reduced sensory, cognitive, and perceptual functions may also interfere with independence in this area. In the early stages of these diseases adaptations need to be made to afford the person the opportunity to maintain function for as long as possible. Most of these tasks, however, eventually need to be delegated to other members of the household, creating further issues of dependence and loss of role function.

A normal activity for many persons, including those with PND, is the care of others, including a spouse or significant other; children; or older, dependent adults. The individual with a PND may have increasing difficulty fulfilling this role. In fact, he or she may have to rely on these care receivers to provide support and care, creating a major role reversal. These changes in responsibilities can be very stressful for all concerned; they challenge everyone's ability to maintain the integrity of relationships.

Education

Because of the age of onset for these PNDs, many people will not be involved in formal educational activities. Those who are may gradually experience a reduced ability to physically participate due to decline in underlying neuromusculoskeletal and movement-related functions and motor skills. Deficits in cognitive and perceptual functions may further limit learning ability. Adaptations such as computer-based courses for formal and informal education may be a viable option.

Work

All client factors have the potential to affect work activities. Work is a crucial area of occupational performance and, for many adults, is an important part of self-identity.

As motor skills decline, the ability to perform specific work tasks also declines. "Invisible symptoms" such as fatigue, weak or blurred vision, and difficulties with bladder control often confound the issue. Coworkers may not understand why someone who does not look ill cannot work. Again, this affects the person psychologically, with changes in societal roles and self-concept. This is particularly true for an individual whose job requires a high degree of physical stamina and skill. For example, assembly workers or truck drivers may lose their jobs fairly early in the course of these diseases. An individual who has been the breadwinner of the family and whose identity is closely tied to physical strength and endurance may have serious adjustment problems. Cognitive deficits also may make it difficult for the person to function and continue to find satisfaction in work.

Play and Leisure

Many leisure activities can be affected by the changes that result from PNDs. Alternative leisure activities must be explored as more and more performance deficits occur. A balance between work and play should be maintained as long as possible. However, if the person can no longer engage in usual work and daily living activities, it is even more critical to have meaningful and fulfilling leisure pursuits. These activities will grow in importance as a means of self-actualization and satisfaction.

Social Participation

Communication, mobility, sexual dysfunction, and eating problems may all affect the person's normal socialization with individuals or groups. Dysarthria or imperfect articulation is caused by a lack of control of the tongue and other oral muscles essential to speech. This problem can affect the person's ability to communicate thoughts, needs, and desires and can limit social interaction. The individual may lose upper extremity function, making it difficult to compensate for speaking problems with written communication

Sexual dysfunction may also be present. Because of depression and diminished self-concept, the person may no longer feel attractive, which causes problems in sexual expression. Also, loss of specific motor and sensory function can affect physical performance.

Because of the unpredictable nature of the course of each PND, potential dependency issues are ongoing problems. This may lead to secondary psychosocial issues caused by these lifestyle changes. PNDs require an initial social-psychological adjustment as well as continual readjustment because of erratic progression of symptoms. A person who was active and outgoing may have a diminished self-concept because of the inability to engage in activities that were once of interest and value. The result is a variety of role changes in the family or society.

Role expectations, which exist in every social situation, are ways of behaving or reacting that fit with one's self-image and the expectations of others. These include attitudes, activities, and patterns of decision making, expressing feelings, and meeting the needs of significant others. Some individuals with loss of bladder control may avoid going out in public. Mothers may be unable to care for their children. Some may come to see themselves as no longer useful or attractive to others. Marriages may break up under the strain of living with PNDs. Occasionally, individuals with PNDs threaten suicide. An individual with a PND must think seriously about current role expectations and how these might be threatened by the PND.

Case Illustrations

Case 1: Multiple Sclerosis

M. A. is a 28-year-old woman who was diagnosed with MS 5 years before this hospital admission. She was admitted because she noticed a progressive deterioration of function during the past 6 months. The main problems she identifies are an increase in fatigue, difficulty with bowel and bladder function, and several falls. She complains of feeling moody and forgetting information.

She is married and has two children, an 11-year-old girl and a 5-year-old boy. She is self-employed as a paralegal, which requires her to spend many hours typing on the computer. Her husband works full-time and has been very supportive. At the time of admission, he seemed overwhelmed.

M. A. tries to do her morning self-care but is finding it more difficult and frustrating. Getting dressed is particularly fatiguing, and she admits that at times she goes to bed fully dressed to avoid having to get dressed in the morning. She has been using a manual wheelchair off and on for the past 2 years.

Her daughter is currently helping with the laundry, cooking, and simple cleaning. M. A. states that she has problems doing household tasks because she must hold onto something stable before reaching for, or lifting, an object.

She currently enjoys no leisure activities. At one time, she liked to knit, but it has become too frustrating to be pleasurable.

She complains of bladder urgency but often cannot void. She also has a mild dysarthria, spasticity of the lower extremities, weakness of the upper extremities (able to move against gravity withstanding minimal resistance), poor sitting balance, poor fine and gross motor coordination, blurred vision, and loss of stereognosis and light touch.

When the occupational therapist spoke with her, it became apparent that she did not comprehend the nature and course of MS. She is feeling frustrated and depressed about her recent decline of function.

She is currently taking Tylenol, Senokot, Metamucil, Colace, heparin, and multivitamins and is using Dulcolax suppositories.

Case 2: Parkinson's Disease

C. R. is a 72-year-old man with stage III PD. He has recently experienced a severe loss of balance and functional mobility. He reports difficulty moving quickly and gracefully. He also complains of poor handwriting, problems sleeping, and numbness in both hands.

C. R. is a single, retired accountant who lives independently in a two-story home. His bedroom and bathroom are on the second floor. There are four steps to enter the home. He has no children. He has one sister who lives within walking distance of his home. She, however, is suffering from arthritis and has difficulty offering much assistance.

C. R. has been caring for himself thus far, but his sister reports she is concerned about his safety, especially with activities such as cooking and bathing. She reports that he has fallen on several occasions recently and spends most of his time sitting in his chair in his living room.

His sister brings him meals as often as possible but is unable to bring meals in the morning or during bad weather. Her children live out of state and are only able to offer assistance to him during occasional visits when they try to do some of the major household chores such as painting, repairs, and cleaning.

C. R. was once interested in music and art. He played the piano and painted with watercolors. He reports that he has not participated in these leisure activities for "a long time." He also played tennis on a regular basis at the local club. He is still a member of the club but has not been there in more than a year.

C. R. is reportedly self-conscious of his illness and, therefore, does not like to go out in public very much. His sister, who has always been very close to her brother, expresses concern about his "depression and lack of motivation." She states that she has tried on several occasions to get him to go to local musical concerts or museums, but she feels he is just too depressed.

He is currently taking Sinemet CR and Artane. His sister, however, reports that he does not consistently take his medications because they "make him feel sick."

Case 3: Amyotrophic Lateral Sclerosis

T. M. is a 48-year-old man who has recently been diagnosed with ALS. Six months before being referred to O.T. services, he began to experience some weakness in his hands and he began dropping objects, such as tools. He reports loss of strength in his arms and legs. The weakness in his legs has become so severe that he now uses a borrowed wheelchair part of the time. He complains of difficulty sleeping due to cramps in his legs. He also reports that he has lost almost 20 lb in the last 6 or 8 months.

T. M. is married and has two sons, ages 6 and 4. He independently owns and operates a lawnmower shop at which he sells and repairs lawnmowers. He reports significant difficulty performing the repair parts of his job because of weakness in his hands and arms. Most of the repairs have become backed up in the shop, and he is considering hiring assistance or sending the work to another shop.

His wife is employed full-time as a legal secretary. She has helped with the business as much as possible by completing some of the bookkeeping after hours. She is very busy caring for their boys and trying to maintain the household. She appears to be very supportive of T. M. but also seems very burdened by her responsibilities.

T. M. has many interests in sports and outdoor activities. He has been racing in "Iron Man" triathlons and marathons for the last several years. He was a high school track and cross country star. He enjoys biking and camping. Every summer, he and his family take a 2-week trip to a remote location where they hike and camp.

He is also supportive of his sons' sports events and enjoys teaching them various sports. Last year, he was a soccer coach for his oldest boy's team.

The course and prognosis of ALS has been explained to T. M. and his wife, and they have reportedly been discussing future plans. They are, however, "hoping for a miracle." At this time, he is taking pain relievers to reduce the pain from the cramping in his legs.

RECOMMENDED LEARNING RESOURCES

Multiple Sclerosis

National Multiple Sclerosis Society
http://www.nmss.org/
The Multiple Sclerosis Association of America
http://www.msaa.com/
The Multiple Sclerosis Foundation
http://www.msfacts.org/

Parkinson's Disease

National Parkinson Foundation
http://parkinson.org/
Parkinson's Disease Foundation, Inc.

http://pdf.org/
The American Parkinson Disease Association, Inc.
http://www.apdaparkinson.com/

Amyotrophic Lateral Sclerosis

The ALS Association
http://www.alsa.org/
World Federation of Neurology Amyotrophic Lateral Sclerosis
http://www.wfnals.org/

REFERENCES

Albanese, A. (2003). Diagnostic criteria for Parkinson's disease. *Neurological Sciences, 24*, S23–S26.

Andreoli, T. E., Carpenter, C. C. J., Plum, F., & Smith, L. H. (1986). *Cecil essentials of medicine.* Philadelphia, PA: WB Saunders.

Armon, C., Kurland, L. T., Beard, C. M., O'Brien, P. C., & Mulder, D. W. (1991). Psychologic and adaptational difficulties anteceding amyotrophic lateral sclerosis: Rochester, Minnesota, 1925–1987. *Neuroepidemiology, 10*(3), 132–137.

Beresford, S. (1995). *Motor neurone disease (amyotrophic lateral sclerosis).* London, UK: Chapman & Hall.

Bobholz, J. A., & Rao, S. M. (2003). Cognitive dysfunction in multiple sclerosis: A review of recent developments. *Current Opinions in Neurology, 16,* 283–288.

Bohn, M. C. (2000). Parkinson's Disease: A neurodegenerative disease particularly amenable to gene therapy. *Molecular Therapy, 1*(6), 494–496.

Breitenstein, C., Van Lancker, D., Daum, I., & Waters, C. H. (2001). Impaired perception of vocal emotions in Parkinson's Disease: Influence of speech time processing and executive functioning. *Brain and Cognition, 45,* 277–314.

Carbon, M., & Marie, R. (2003). Functional imaging of cognition in Parkinson's disease. *Current Opinions in Neurology, 16,* 475–480.

Chen, H., O'Reilly, E., McCullough, M. L., Rodriguez, C., Schwarzschild, M. A., Calle, E. E., & Ascherio, A. (2007). Consumption of dairy products and risk of Parkinson's Disease. *American Journal of Epidemiology, 165*(9), 998–1006.

Chen, H., O'Reilly, E., Schwarzschild, M. A., & Ascherio, A. (2008). Peripheral inflammatory biomarkers and risk of Parkinson's Disease. *American Journal of Epidemiology, 167*(1), 90–95.

Chen, H., Schernhammer, E., Schwarzschild, M. A., & Ascherio, A. (2006). A prospective study of night shift work, sleep duration and risk of Parkinson's Disease. *American Journal of Epidemiology, 163*(8), 726–730.

Compston, A., & Coles, A. (2002). Multiple sclerosis. *Lancet, 359,* 1221–1231.

de Lau, L. M. L., Koudstaal, P. J., Hofman, A., & Breteler, M. B. (2006). Serum cholesterol levels and the risk of Parkinson's Disease. *American Journal of Epidemiology, 164*(10), 998–1002.

Delisa, J. A., Hammond, M. C., Mikulic, M. A., & Miller, R. M. (1985). Multiple sclerosis: Part 1. Common physical disabilities and rehabilitation. *American Family Physician, 32*(4), 157–163.

Delisa, J. A., Miller, R. M., Mikulic, M. A., & Hammond, M. C. (1985). Multiple sclerosis: Part 2. Common functional problems and rehabilitation. *American Family Physician, 32*(5), 127–132.

DeLong, M. (2000). Parkinson's Disease. *Neurobiology of Disease, 7,* 559–560.

Durrleman, S., & Alperovitch, A. (1989). Increasing trend of ALS in France and elsewhere: Are the changes real? *Neurology, 39,* 768–773.

Duvoisin, R. C., & Sage, J. (1996). *Parkinson's Disease: A guide for patient and family.* Philadelphia, PA: Lippincott-Raven.

Feinstein, A. (2006). Mood disorders in multiple sclerosis and the effects on cognition. *Journal of the Neurological Sciences, 245,* 63–66.

Filippi, M., Rocca, M. A., Colombo, B., Falini, A., Codella, M., Scotti, G., & Comi, G. (2002). Functional magnetic resonance imaging correlates of fatigue in multiple sclerosis. *NeuroImage, 15,* 559–567.

Gao, X., Chen, H., Choi, H. K., Curhan, G., Schwarzschild, M. A., & Ascherio, A. (2008). Diet, urate, and Parkinson's Disease in men. *American Journal of Epidemiology, 167*(7), 831–838.

Hanson, L. J., & Cafruny, W. A. (2002). Current concepts in multiple sclerosis: Part 1. *South Dakota Journal of Medicine, 55*(10), 433–436.

Hernan, M. A., Olek, M. J., & Ascherio, A. (2001). Cigarette smoking and incidence of multiple sclerosis. *American Journal of Epidemiology, 154*(1), 69–74.

Hutton, T., & Dippel, R. L. (1989). *Caring for the Parkinson patient.* New York, NY: Prometheus Books.

Kalb, R. C. (1996). *Multiple sclerosis: The questions you have, the answers you need.* New York, NY: Demos Vermande.

Kamel, F., Tanner, C. M., Umbach, D. M., Hoppin, J. A., Alavanja, M. C. R., Blair, A.,... & Sandler, D. P. (2007). Pesticide exposure and self-reported Parkinson's Disease in the agricultural health study. *American Journal of Epidemiology, 165,* 364–374.

Kamel, F., Umbach, D. M., Lehman, T. A., Park, L. P., Munsat, T. L., Shefner, J. M., et al. (2003). Amyotrophic lateral sclerosis, lead and genetic susceptibility: Polymorphisms in the aminolevulinic acid dehydratase and vitamin D receptor genes. *Environmental Health Perspectives, 111*(10), 1335–1339.

Kenealy, S. J., Pericak-Vance, M. S., & Haines, J. L. (2003). The genetic epidemiology of multiple sclerosis. *Journal of Neuroimmunology, 143,* 7–12.

Lieberman, A. N., & Williams, F. L. (1993). *Parkinson's disease.* New York, NY: Simon and Schuster.

Logroscino, G., Gao, X., Chen, H., Wing, A., & Ascherio, A. (2008). Dietary iron intake and risk of Parkinson's Disease. *American Journal of Epidemiology, 168*(12), 1381–1388.

Lyros, E., Messinis, L., Papageorgiou, S. G., & Papathanosopoulos, P. (2010). Cognitive dysfunction in multiple sclerosis: The effects of pharmacological interventions. *International Review of Psychiatry, 22*(1), 35–42.

Maloney, F.P., Burks, J.S., & Ringel, S.P. (1985). *Interdisciplinary Rehabilitation of Multiple Sclerosis and Neuromuscular Disorders,* New York, NY: Lippincott.

Matthews, B. (1993). *Multiple sclerosis: The facts* (3rd ed.). Oxford, UK: Oxford University Press.

Mayor, S. (2002). New treatment improves symptoms of Parkinson's Disease. *British Medical Journal, 324*(7344), 997.

McCormack, A. L., Thiruchelvam, M., Mannig-Bog, A. B., Thiffault, C., Langston, J. W., Cory-Slechta, D. A., & Di Monte, D. A. (2002). Environmental risk factors and Parkinson's Disease: Selective degeneration of nigral dopaminergic neurons caused by the herbicide paraquat. *Neurobiology of Disease, 10,* 119–127.

Merims, D., & Freedman, M. (2008). Cognitive and behavioural impairment in Parkinson's Disease. *International review of Psychiatry, 20*(4), 364–373.

Mitsumoto, H., Hanson, M. R., & Chad, D. A. (1988). Amyotrophic lateral sclerosis: Recent advances in pathogenesis and therapeutic trials. *Archives of Neurology, 45,* 189–202.

Murray, J. (2002). Infection as a cause of multiple sclerosis. *British Medical Journal, 325*(7373), 1128.

Neill, J., Belan, I., & Reid, K. (2006). Effectiveness of non-pharmacological interventions for fatigue in adults with multiple sclerosis, rheumatoid arthritis, or systemic lupus erythematosus: A systemic review. *Integrative Literature Reviews and Meta-analyses,* 617–635.

Neilsen, N. M., Westergaard, T., Rostgaard, K., Frisck, M., Hjalgrim, H., Wohlfahrt, J., Koch-Henriksen, N., & Melbye, M. (2005). Familial risk of multiple sclerosis: A nationwide cohort study. *American Journal of Epidemiology, 162*(8), 774–778.

Nelson, L. M., Matkin, C., Longstreth, Jr., W. T., & McGuire, V. (2000). Population-based case-control study of amyotrophic lateral sclerosis in western Washington state. II. Diet. *American Journal of Epidemiology, 151*(2), 164–173.

Nelson, L. M., McGuire, V., Longstreth, Jr., W. T., & Matkin, C. (2000). Population-based case-control study of amyotrophic lateral sclerosis in western Washington state. I. Cigarette smoking and alcohol consumption. *American Journal of Epidemiology, 151*(2), 156–163.

Noonan, C. W., Hilsdon, R., White, M. C., Wong, L. -Y., & Zack, M. (2002). Continuing trend of increased motor neuron disease mortality in the United States. *Epidemiology, 13,* S202.

Noonan, C. W., Kathman, S. J., & White, M. C. (2002). Prevalence estimates for MS in the United States and evidence for an increasing trend for women. *Neurology, 58,* 136–138.

Noonan, C. W., Williamson, D. M., Henry, J. P., Indian, R., Lynch, S. G., Neuberger, J. S., et al. (2010). The prevalence of multiple sclerosis in 3 US communities. *Preventing Chronic Disease, 7*(1). Retrieved from http://www.cdc.gov/pcd/Issues/2010

Noseworthy, J. H. (2003). Management of multiple sclerosis: Current trials and future options. *Current Opinion in Neurology, 16,* 289–297.

Priyadarshi, A., Khuder, S. A., Schaub, E. A., & Priyadarshi, S. S. (2001). Environmental risk factors and Parkinson's Disease: A metaanalysis. *Environmental Research Section A, 86,* 122–127.

Przedborski, S., Mitsumoto, H., & Rowland, L. P. (2003). Recent advances in amyotrophic lateral sclerosis research. *Current Neurology and Neuroscience Reports, 3,* 70–77.

Rearick, M. P., Stelmach, G. E., Leis, B., & Santello, M. (2002). Coordination and control of forces during multifingered grasping in Parkinson's Disease. *Experimental Neurology, 177,* 428–442.

Shaw, C. E., Al-Chalabi, A., & Neigh, N. (2001). Progress in pathogenesis of amyotrophic lateral sclerosis. *Current Neurology and Neuroscience Reports, 1,* 69–76.

Traynor, B. J., Alexander, M., Corr, B., Frost, E., & Hardiman, O. (2003). Effect of a multidisciplinary amyotrophic lateral sclerosis (ALS) clinic on ALS survival: A population based study, 1996–2000. *Journal of Neurology, Neurosurgery & Psychiatry, 74,* 1258–1261.

Umphred, D. A. (1990). *Neurological rehabilitation* (2nd ed.). St Louis, MO: CV Mosby.

Wassem, R., & Dudley, W. (2003). Symptom management and adjustment of patients with multiple sclerosis: A 4-year longitudinal intervention study. *Clinical Nursing Research, 12*(1), 102–117.

Weisskopf, M. G., McCullough, M. L., Calle, E. E., Thun, M. J., Cudkowicz, M., & Ascherio, A. (2004). Prospective study of cigarette smoking and amyotrophic lateral sclerosis. *American Journal of Epidemiology, 160*(1), 26–33.

Weisskopf, M. G., McCullough, M. L., Morozova, N., Calle, E. E., Thun, M. J., & Ascherio, A. (2005). Prospective study of occupation and amyotrophic lateral sclerosis mortality. *American Journal of Epidemiology, 162*(12), 1146–1152.

Weydt, P., Weiss, M. D., Moller, T., & Carter, G. T. (2002). Neuro-inflammation as a therapeutic target in amyotrophic lateral sclerosis. *Current Opinion in Investigative Drugs, 3*(12), 1720–1724.

Zhang, Y., Dawson, V. L., & Dawson, T. M. (2000). Oxidative stress and genetics in the pathogenesis of Parkinson's Disease. *Neurobiology of Disease, 7,* 240–250.

Zoccolella, S., Santamato, A., & Lamberti, P. (2009). Current and emerging treatments for amyotrophic lateral sclerosis. *Neuropsychiatric Disease and Treatment, 5,* 577–595.

15

Rheumatic Diseases

■ *David P. Orchanian*

Vincent O'Malley is a pleasant, energetic 11-year-old sixth-grade student at West Middle School. He enjoys riding his minibike in the fields around his neighborhood, playing street hockey, and playing video games with his Xbox 360. He has a variety of friends in school and is never one to be without something to do on most days. There are two other children in his family, a younger brother, Jimmy, age 8, and an older sister Carrie, age 16. His mother is a paraprofessional working in an elementary school with special needs children. His dad is a regional manager for Wal-Mart, and he works long hours, sometimes up to 50 to 60 hours per week. Approximately 4 months ago, Vincent was diagnosed with **juvenile rheumatoid arthritis** (JRA) of the pauciarticular type (four or fewer joints involved). The diagnosis was quite a while in coming from their pediatrician, and was made after a series of laboratory tests, radiographs, and physical examinations. Vincent's mother remembers him complaining of mild, intermittent pain and stiffness in his lower back and hips for almost 3 months prior to the diagnosis. Performance areas affected include play, self-care, and education. Involved neuromuscular components include hip and trunk range of motion (ROM), lower extremity muscle strength, endurance, and at times postural control. His hip musculature is stiff at the end of range in the early morning and after sitting for periods of time >1 hour. Muscle strength is measured as 3/5 for hip extension and flexion and 3+/5 for trunk extension. On days when he is experiencing significant "stiffness" in his trunk and hips, his postural control is compromised and he cannot react quickly during play. His musculoskeletal endurance diminishes in the afternoon, particularly after a busy day at school. He has limited his street hockey play to weekends when he tends to have more energy. Vincent's parents feel it best to share as much information about his condition with his teachers each school year as is practical in an effort to optimize Vincent's learning experience. His teachers have appreciated this input and guidance and have a clear and compassionate perspective on what they may be confronted with on a day-to-day basis in their classrooms. One accommodation that they all have agreed to is to allow Vincent the opportunity to stand and walk around the classroom periodically in order to relieve the stiffness that might be developing from extended static positioning at his desk. Regarding self-care, Vincent prefers showers to baths. This is actually better for him as there is only a 4-inch step over into the shower stall, and there is also a small bench built into the shower wall in case he needs to sit and rest. The bench seat is positioned approximately 17 inches above the floor, and there is a wall safety grab bar positioned on a 45-degree diagonal to the plane of the seat rest. He uses a squeeze bottle for shampoo and enjoys liquid soap, also administered from a lightweight squeeze bottle. His dad just installed a small shelf in the stall shower to hold these items. Dressing, grooming, feeding, and use of the toilet do not present any problems at this time for Vincent. He tends to avoid wearing tight clothing and generally wears T-shirts and loose-fitting cargo jeans or shorts on most days. He has just been fitted with braces for his teeth, and he is a little concerned about being able to maintain the high level of oral hygiene that his dentist is stressing. Vincent has never been one to floss his teeth, but now he must, and his parents will assist him in finding the right tools and technique to accomplish this task. Vincent is blessed with a very understanding and supportive family. His parents have chosen to not treat him as a "special child." He is required to participate in the routine activities of the family, including some yard work and other household chores. Generally, Vincent has been adjusting well to the limitations imposed by this disease, although there are some occasions when he is severely limited by stiffness and painful movement, and these occasions upset and anger him. He is at an age and stage of life where he is trying many new things and experiencing many opportunities in school and leisure. His friends know of his condition, but they have been accepting as a whole, and Vincent is fortunate that his positive attitude and warm family atmosphere help him to attract and retain friendships with his peers.

DESCRIPTION AND DEFINITION

Augustin-Jacob Landre-Beauvais is given credit for the earliest description of **rheumatoid arthritis** (RA) in his thesis of 1800. It was not until 1858 that A.B. Garrod coined the actual term rheumatoid arthritis, and it was in 1941 that the American Rheumatism Association (ARA) adopted the terminology. The appearance and distribution of lesions in ancient skeletons suggests that RA may have existed in North America 3,000 years ago (Rothchild & Woods, 1990). More than 100 different forms of **arthritis** are documented. Arthritis is divided into eight major categories, with RA included under the synovitis category. Though less common than other forms of the disease, such as **osteoarthritis**, it is considered to be more serious. Annual excess health care costs of RA patients were $8.4 billion, and costs of other RA consequences were $10.9 billion (Centers for Disease Control and Prevention, 2003). These costs translate to a total annual cost of $19.3 billion. From a stakeholder perspective, 33% of the total cost was allocated to employers, 28% to patients, 20% to the government, and 19% to caregivers. Adding intangible costs of quality-of-life deterioration ($10.3 billion) and premature mortality ($9.6 billion), total annual societal costs of RA (direct, indirect, and intangible) increased to $39.2 billion (Birnbaum et al., 2010). In one study done in the United States in 2009, of 10,298 patients, 8,916 had RA alone (86.6%), 608 had RA + cardiovascular disease (CVD) (5.9%), 716 had RA + depression (7.0%), and 58 had RA + CVD + depression (0.5%). All patients with CVD and/or depression incurred significantly higher follow-up costs compared with patients with RA alone. Adjusted annual mean health care costs were highest for RA + CVD (US$14,145), followed by RA + CVD + depression ($13,513), RA + depression ($12,225), and RA alone ($11,404). Although patients with CVD and/or depression had a greater rate of RA-related hospitalization, adjusted RA-related health care costs did not reflect any statistically significant differences as compared to the RA-alone cohort (Joyce, Smith, Khandker, Melin, & Singh, 2009). A significant proportion (13.4%) of patients with prevalent RA have comorbid CVD and/or depression. The presence of these conditions significantly affects annual health care costs as well as specific RA-related utilization patterns.

ETIOLOGY

It is essential to have a full awareness of the joint anatomy and related structures (Fig. 15.1) as a preamble to discussing the etiology, signs and symptoms, and course of RA. The word "arthritis" derives from the Greek words "athron" (meaning joint) and "itis" (meaning inflammation or infection). Therefore, the word is defined as "**inflammation** or infection of the joint"

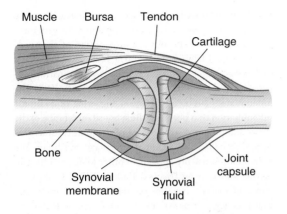

Figure 15.1 Anatomy of a joint. Arthritis can affect different parts of a joint.

(Arnett, 1996). The base "rheum" in rheumatoid refers to the stiffness, general aching, weakness, and fatigue that is experienced throughout the body. The basic anatomy of a healthy joint as shown in Figure 15.1 should be referred to when, later in the chapter, the disease process and its effects on the joint are discussed. RA results from interplay among immunogenetic risk factors, environmental insults, and random modulations of the musculoskeletal and immune systems (Sen & Carson, 2003). RA develops when the synovium changes into disorganized lymphoid granulation tissue. Multiple factors involving both resident and infiltrating cells contribute to **synovial** lining hyperplasia

and cartilage or bone erosion. Deposition of infectious agents and immune complexes into the synovial layer triggers complement activation and inflammation in joint tissue (Baecklund, Askling, Rosenquist, Ekbom, & Klareskog, 2004). Some recent studies report increased lymphoma risks linked to RA disease activity. The hypothesis that disease-modifying drugs, in particular methotrexate, increase the lymphoma risk receives little support. Observation times for the tumor necrosis factor (TNF)-blocking therapies are still short, but so far no clear increased risk for lymphoma has been observed. Presence of **Epstein-Barr virus** (EBV), as analyzed with Epstein-Barr virus–encoded ribonucleic acid in situ hybridization, appears to be uncommon in RA-related lymphomas. Hypothetically, an increased proliferative drive caused by self- or nonself-antigens may play a role in lymphoma development in RA patients, but this has to be further studied. **Rheumatologists** need to be aware of the increased lymphoma risk in their RA patients. The reason for the increased lymphoma risk in RA patients is still unclear, but available studies support the hypothesis of a link between RA disease severity and the risk of lymphoma rather than increased risks associated with specific treatment regimens (Baecklund et al., 2004). RA is a chronic, inflammatory, systemic disease that produces most prominent manifestations in the diarthrodial joints (Fig. 15.2). **Diarthroses** are the most mobile joints and are by far the most common articular pattern (Simkin, 1997). Because these joints possess a synovial

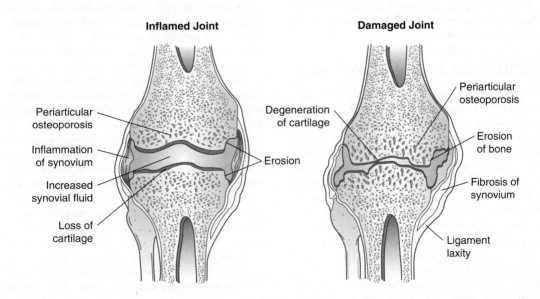

Figure 15.2 The postinflammatory response to joint inflammation is fibrosis, not unlike the scarring (fibrosis) that results from a surgical incision. The function of the postinflammatory joint depends on the degree of fibrosis and the destruction that occurred during the inflammatory stage. The damage influences the alignment, angle of tendon pull (joint integrity), ROM, and stability. (Reprinted with permission from the Arthritis Foundation. [1988]. *The AHPA Arthritis Teaching Slide Collection.* [2nd ed.].)

membrane and contain synovial fluid, diarthrodial joints are more commonly referred to as synovial joints. Synovial joints are subclassified according to shape: ball and socket (hip), hinge (interphalangeal), saddle (first carpometacarpal [CMC]), and plane (patellofemoral) joints. These widely varying configurations demonstrate the fact that form parallels function in the design of diarthrodial joints (Simkin, 1997). In all cases noted, a well-lubricated bearing develops from essentially congruent cartilaginous surfaces that slide freely against each other. The shape and the size of the opposing surfaces define the direction and extent of the available motion. Within the limits of each joint, a wide variety of designs permit motion in flexion (bending), extension (straightening), abduction (movement away from the midline of the body), adduction (moving toward the midline of the body), and rotation. It is seen that individual joints can act in one (humeroulnar joint), two (wrist), or up to three (shoulder) axes of movement (Simkin). Persistent and progressive synovitis develops in peripheral joints. The initial event inciting the inflammatory response is unknown. An infectious etiology of RA has been vigorously pursued without yielding convincing evidence (Goronzy & Weyand, 1997). Genetic and environmental factors control the progression, extent, and pattern of the inflammatory response and are, as such, responsible for the heterogenous clinical features. Genetic factors have been identified as potentially influential in the disease. RA is not inherited; it is not passed directly from parents to children. A susceptibility or tendency to develop RA can be inherited, but not everyone who inherits this susceptibility will have the disease develop (Goronzy & Weyand).

INCIDENCE AND PREVALENCE

Nearly 47 million Americans in 2008 reported that a doctor told them they have arthritis or other rheumatic conditions. Another 23 million people have chronic joint symptoms, but have not been diagnosed with arthritis. Arthritis is the leading cause of disability in the United States, limiting the activities of more than 16 million adults (Bolen et al.). Approximately one in seven people in the general population is affected, and women are affected three times more than men (Bolen et al., 2010). RA has a worldwide distribution and involves all ethnic groups (Escalante & dle Ricon, 2001). Though the disease can occur at any age, the prevalence increases with age, and the peak incidence is between the fourth and sixth decades. Data from population-based prevalence and incidence studies have to be interpreted cautiously because there is no unique feature to establish the diagnosis of RA. Studies of incidence and prevalence have not had a major impact on the understanding of the disease

pathogenesis. Insignificant differences in prevalence rates among ethnic groups are likely explained by variations in disease assessment and age distribution of the study populations (Helmick et al., 2007). It is speculated that a high proportion of individuals with RA demonstrate circulating antibodies to an antigen present in the EBV. The inflammatory problem involves a triggering of a chronic inflammation that begins in the synovial membrane of the joints and progresses to erosion of the joint capsule, tendons, ligaments, and eventually cartilage and bone. The inflammation usually spreads to other joints, resulting in further joint damage (Beers & Berkow, 1999). Leukocytes (white blood cells) have been studied for hereditary factors that predispose a person to RA. One type of leukocyte, the T cell, matures under the influence of the thymus and mediates cellular immunity. This cell-mediated immunity provides the body's main defense against intracellular organisms and involves the identification and removal of foreign substances (antigens) from the body. The entire process depends on the interaction of the antigen with receptors on the surface of the T cell; therefore, T cells are further classified into genetic classes containing human leukocyte antigen (HLA) receptors. A large accumulation of data links specific HLA antigens with particular disease states in the human (Goronzy & Weyand, 1997). The T cell has a binding cleft (receptor site) with specific sensitivity to certain antigens and is complimentary to the structures found in **antibodies**. One particular class, the HLA-DR4 type, does not distinguish between antigens and healthy tissue and is associated with a susceptibility to RA. As a result, substances that facilitate inflammation of the synovial lining are released. The following description helps to provide an understanding of the molecular process. Initially, an antigen such as EBV comes in contact with the T-cell receptor; the T-cell membrane becomes activated and is transformed into a large blast cell that then proliferates. The sensitized T cells indirectly stimulate macrophage-like cells of the synovial lining of the joints. During this inflammatory phase the affected joint demonstrates increased heat, swelling, pain, redness, and decreased ROM (Beers & Berkow, 1997). Later there is a proliferation of connective tissue and a heavy infiltration by more lymphocytes as well as plasma cells. The activated synovial cells grow out as a malignant pannus (Fig. 15.3) over the cartilage, leading to cartilage breakdown. This granulation tissue continues to spread, the joint space is slowly effaced by fibrous adhesions, and eventually fibrous ankylosis appears. The by-product of the synovial lining destruction further stimulates the inflammation process, leading to more tissue damage than tissue repair (Goronzy & Weyand) as shown in Figure 15.4. Additional research has demonstrated that individuals who have inherited a specific gene sequence from both parents have a higher risk of developing much

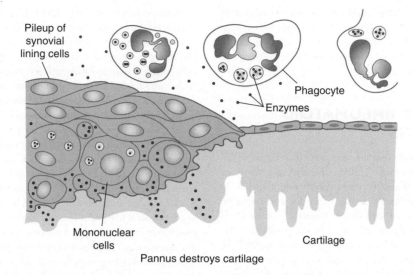

Pileup of
synovial
lining cells

Phagocyte

Enzymes

Mononuclear
cells

Cartilage

Pannus destroys cartilage

Figure 15.3 Synovial lining cells multiply, creating a mass called **pannus.** Substances in this mass further damage the underlying cartilage, which softens, weakens, and ultimately is destroyed. The waste products of cartilage cell destruction further stimulate the inflammatory process. New phagocytes rush to the area to clean up the debris. Some lymphocytes and other mononuclear cells are mistakenly rendered capable of attacking cartilage. Lysosomal enzymes and collagenase are released, thus perpetuating the abnormal process. (Reprinted with permission from the Arthritis Foundation. [1988]. *The AHPA Arthritis Teaching Slide Collection.* [2nd ed.].)

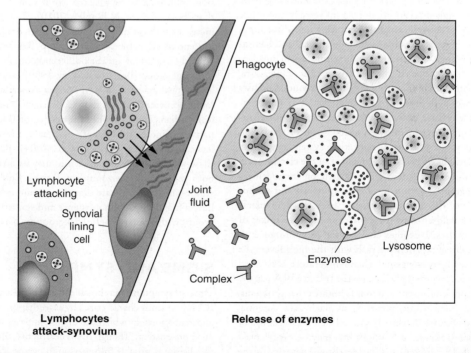

Phagocyte

Lymphocyte
attacking

Synovial
lining
cell

Joint
fluid

Lysosome

Enzymes

Complex

**Lymphocytes
attack-synovium**

Release of enzymes

Figure 15.4 In the development of inflammatory rheumatic diseases, the normal protective process of inflammation goes awry. Lymphocytes can no longer distinguish between antigens and healthy tissue, and they secrete substances that cause the synovial lining to become inflamed. Phagocytes become overloaded with immune complexes and release lysosomal enzymes into the joint fluid. The enzymes then attach to the cells of the joint lining, eventually destroying them. (Reprinted with permission from the Arthritis Foundation. [1988]. *The AHPA Arthritis Teaching Slide Collection.* [2nd ed.].)

more severe RA that could involve internal organs as well as joints. Continued research on genetic factors may facilitate genetic counseling to identify people at higher risk of developing severe forms of RA or of needing more intensive treatment.

JUVENILE RHEUMATOID ARTHRITIS

JRA is the most common rheumatic disease in childhood. The diagnostic criteria for JRA are onset at age younger than 16 years, persistent arthritis in one or more joints for at least 6 weeks, and exclusion of other types of childhood arthritis (Table 15-1) (Gewanter, Rognmann, & Baum, 2005). The three classifications for JRA are summarized in Table 15-2. Estimates of prevalence vary from 30 to 150 per 100,000 per year in Europe and the United States (Gewanter et al., 2005). There has been ongoing dialogue among pediatric rheumatologists from different parts of the world about the classification of the juvenile arthritides for several decades (Hofer & Southwood, 2002). Childhood arthritis overlaps with many other conditions, and the clinical features lack definitive laboratory test findings. The known genetic and serologic markers are not yet universally applicable or biologically meaningful. Despite these difficulties, an effort has been made to include clinical and laboratory findings, autoantibodies, systemic organ involvement, and genetic risk factors (Adib et al., 2008). The international community of pediatric rheumatologists continues to be divided by the classification criteria controversy (Hofer & Southwood). Readers of the rheumatology literature need to be cognizant of the origin of the study and the classification system employed. There will likely be more refinement of the classification system. A final system is contingent on homogeneity of subgroups defined by immunogenetics and pathogenesis of the diseases. Systemic JRA (S-JRA) affects 10% of children with JRA. Intermittent fever spikes of more than 101 degrees characterize it. Children with SJRA often experience a rash with the high fever; the rash may be present only when temperature is elevated and is most commonly seen on the trunk. SJRA usually affects multiple joints and may facilitate other problems, such as pericarditis, pleuritis, stomach pain, **anemia**, and an increase in white blood cells. General feelings of fatigue, weakness, and weight loss may be experienced as well. The prognosis is decided by the severity of the arthritis that usually develops with the fever and rash. Onset of JRA may begin at any age; however, the peak of onset is 1 to 6 years old. Boys and girls are equally affected (Colbert, 2010). Polyarticular JRA affects

approximately 40% of children with JRA and is initiated in several joints at once (five or more). The course usually involves the small joints of the hands and fingers but can also affect the weight-bearing joints. The joints are typically affected symmetrically and fevers may be present. JRA is subdivided into two groups and identified most readily by the absence or presence of **rheumatoid factor** (RF). The prognosis for those with an RF-positive factor is that they are at higher risk for erosions, nodules, growth retardation, lack of adequate bone mineralization, anemia, and poor functional status. Pauciarticular arthritis, or oligoarthritis, accounts for 50% of those with JRA. This type of JRA characteristically affects the large joints such as the knees, ankles, or elbows and engages only a few joints (four or fewer) at a time. Pauciarticular JRA is divided into two groups: late onset and early onset. Those with late-onset JRA are usually girls (outnumbering boys 4 to 1) who are very young (1 to 5 years old), have a 30% to 50% chance of developing chronic eye inflammation with complications, and have the best articular outcome. Late-onset JRA affects boys who are HLA-B27 positive and have tendonitis, with the large joints (hip and low back) of the body being the most affected (Colbert). The prevalence of JRA is approximately 1:1,000 of the childhood population, with girls being affected seven times more often than boys (Foster & Rapley, 2010). The prevalence increases with age until about the seventh decade. Eighty percent of all patients who develop RA are between 35 and 50 years of age. Sex differences diminish in the older age group (Beers & Berkow, 1999). Racial factors also appear relevant in RA. African Americans have a lower occurrence of RA than Caucasians. North American Indians have a higher prevalence of RA, whereas native Japanese and Chinese may have a lower prevalence than whites (Kasper et al., 2004). Reasons for these variations are unknown and may be attributed to both genetic and environmental factors. Epidemiologic studies in Africa indicate that climate and urbanization have a major impact on incidence and severity of RA in groups with similar genetic backgrounds (Kasper et al.).

SIGNS AND SYMPTOMS

Onset of symptoms may be sudden and may vary in degree. RA is frequently characterized by exacerbations (flare-ups) and remissions, in which the disease appears to be quiet and non-existent. Though RA is destructive, the course of the disease is variable from person to person. Some individuals experience only a mild, brief monoarticular involvement and minimal joint damage, whereas others will have an ongoing progressive arthritis with significant joint deformity. Most often, RA affects more than one joint at

TABLE 15.1 Criteria for the Diagnosis of Juvenile Rheumatoid Arthritis

I. General

The JRA Criteria subcommittee in 1982 reviewed the1977 Criteria (86) and recommended that JRA be the name for the principal form of chronic arthritic disease in children and that this general class should be classified into three onset subtypes: systemic, polyarticular, and pauciarticular. The onset subtypes may be further subclassified into subsets as indicated below. The following classification enumerates the requirements for the diagnosis of JRA and the three clinical onset subtypes and lists subsets of each subtype that may be useful in further classification.

II. General criteria for the diagnosis of juvenile rheumatoid arthritis:
    A. Persistent arthritis of at least 6 weeks duration in one or more joints
    B. Exclusion of other causes of arthritis (see list of exclusions)

III. JRA onset subtypes: The onset subtype is determined by manifestations during the first 6 months of disease and remains the principal classification, although manifestations more closely resembling another subtype may appear later.
    A. Systemic onset JRA: This subtype is defined as JRA with persistent intermittent fever (daily intermittent temperatures to 103°F or higher) with or without rheumatoid rash or other organ involvement. Typical fever and rash will be considered probable systemic onset JRA if not associated with arthritis. Before a definite diagnosis can be made, arthritis, as defined, must be present.
    B. Pauciarticular onset JRA: This subtype is defined as JRA with arthritis in four or fewer joints during the first 6 months of disease. Patients with systemic onset JRA are excluded from this onset subtype.
    C. Polyarticular JRA: This subtype is defined as JRA with arthritis in five or more joints during the first 6 months of disease. Patients with systemic JRA onset are excluded from this subtype arthritis or Still's disease. Hence reports of studies of JCA or JA cannot be directly compared with one another nor to reports of JRA or Still's disease.
    D. The onset subtypes may include the following subsets:
        1. Systemic onset
            a. Polyarthritis
            b. Oligoarthritis
        2. Oligoarthritis (pauciarticular onset)
            a. Antinuclear antibody (ANA) positive-chronic uveitis
            b. RF positive
            c. Seronegative, B27 positive
            d. Not otherwise classified
        3. Polyarthritis
            a. RF positive
            b. Not otherwise classified

(Continued)

TABLE 15.1 Criteria for the Diagnosis of Juvenile Rheumatoid Arthritis *(Continued)*

IV. Exclusions

    A. Other rheumatic diseases

        1. Rheumatic fever

        2. Systemic lupus erythematosus

        3. Ankylosing spondylitis

        4. Polymyositis or dermatomyositis

        5. Vasculitic syndromes

        6. Scleroderma

        7. Psoriatic arthritis

        8. Reiter's syndrome

        9. Sjögren's syndrome

        10. Mixed connective tissue disease

        11. Behçet's syndrome

    B. Infectious arthritis

    C. Inflammatory bowel disease

    D. Neoplastic disease including leukemia

    E. Nonrheumatic conditions of bones and joints

    F. Hematologic diseases

    G. Psychogenic arthralgia

    H. Miscellaneous

        1. Sarcoidosis

        2. Hypertrophic osteoarthropathy

        3. Villonodular synovitis

        4. Chronic active hepatitis

        5. Familial Mediterranean fever

V. Other proposed terminology for juvenile chronic arthritis, JCA and JA are new diagnostic terms currently in use in some places for the arthritides of childhood.

once. In two-thirds of patients, an exacerbation is initiated by feelings of fatigue, generalized weakness, weight loss, malaise, and vague musculoskeletal symptoms until synovitis becomes more obvious. Although joint involvement is generally symmetrical, some patients may experience an asymmetrical pattern (Kasper et al., 2004). An exploration of joint involvement can be divided into two sections: stages of inflammatory joint disease as experienced overall and specific manifestations to particular joints.

Articular and Periarticular Involvement

Table 15-3 presents the stages of the inflammatory process: (a) acute, (b) subacute, (c) chronic-active, and (d) chronic-inactive. As previously mentioned, onset may be sudden, with inflammation occurring in many joints at once. In the acute and subacute phases, fatigue may be extensive enough to cause disability from disuse of joint motion and loss of strength before joint changes actually occur. Various degrees of general soreness and aching are experienced. These are usually followed by progressive, localized symptoms of pain, inflammation, warmth, and tenderness in a joint or multiple joints. Symmetrical involvement of small hand joints, feet, wrists, elbows, and ankles is typical, though initial manifestations may occur in any joint. Pain originates primarily from the joint capsule, which is heavily supplied with pain fibers and is highly sensitive to stretching and distension. Joint swelling results from accumulation of synovial fluid, hypertrophy of the synovium, and thickening of the joint capsule. Synovial thickening, the most specific physical finding, eventually occurs in most active joints. Various degrees of generalized stiffness occur, including the gel phenomenon, which is the inability to move joints after prolonged rest. Morning

TABLE 15.2 Juvenile Rheumatoid Arthritis Subtype Characteristics

	Systemic	Polyarticular	Pauciarticular
Frequency of cases	10%	40%	50%
Number of joints with arthritis at onset	Variable	>5	<4
Gender ratio (F:M)	1:1	3:1	5:1
Frequency of uveitis	1%	5%	20%
Frequency of RF positivity	<20%	5–10%	<2%
Frequency of greater than five joints involved any time during the course of JRA	50–60%	100%	40%
Frequency of active disease >10 years follow-up	42%	45%	41%
Frequency of erosions or joint space narrowing on radiographs	45%	54%	28%
Median time to develop erosions or joint space narrowing on radiographs (years after disease onset)	2.2	2.4	5.4
Frequency of adult height <5th percentile	50%	16%	11%

stiffness that lasts longer than 1 hour is an almost universal feature of inflammatory arthritis, one that distinguishes it from noninflammatory disorders. The length and intensity of the stiffness can be used as a gross assessment of disease activity (Kasper et al., 2004). In JRA, morning stiffness or gelling after inactivity and night pain are encountered as frequently as in adult disease. Frequently, children may not discuss these symptoms with anyone, so their presence is detected only by caregiver observation. Initial presentation of disease may be detected by the child's increased irritability, joint guarding, or his or her outright refusal to walk (Gewanter, Roghmann, & Baum, 2005). Also, adults and children with RA have decreased joint motion, decreased muscle strength and endurance, and a loss of appetite and body weight. Patients frequently experience chills in their hands and feet as well as numbness and tingling. With pain limiting motion, the inflamed joint is usually held in flexion to maximize joint volume and minimize distension of the capsule. Once the acute and subacute stages have subsided, limited joint ROM causes contractures to form. Contractures are the result of adhesions that form when the patient avoids movement during the acute, painful phase.

Limitations in ROM result from **ankylosis**, subluxation, or dislocation. Muscle atrophy in chronic stages results from disuse in the earlier, more acute stages (Matschke, Murphy, Lemmy, Maddison, & Thom, 2009).

Specific Joint Manifestations: Hand

When considering the extremities, the hands are by far the most severely affected by RA (Fouque-Aubert, Chapurlat, Miossec, & Delmas, 2009). Joints with the highest synovium-to-cartilage ratio are those most frequently affected by the disease (Matschke et al., 2009). Fusiform or spindle-shaped fingers, a typical sign of RA, result from swelling in the proximal interphalangeal (PIP) joints (Fig. 15.5). This is usually related to bilateral and symmetrical swelling of the metacarpophalangeal (MCP) joints. Pressure on these joints causes tenderness. Distal interphalangeal (DIP) joints are rarely involved, which discriminates RA from osteoarthritis and psoriatic arthritis (Fowler & Nicol, 2001). Boutonniere and **swan-neck deformities** are two other common hand deformities that result from RA. A **boutonniere deformity** is a

TABLE 15.3 Stages of Inflammatory Joint Disease

Stages	Objective Signs	Subjective Symptoms
Acute	Limited ROM Fever Decreased muscle strength Possible cold, sweaty hands Overall stiffness Gel phenomenon most prominent Weight loss Decreased appetite	Pain at rest and movement most severe Inflammation most severe Hot, red joints Decreased function Tingling and numbness in hands and feet
Subacute	Decreased ROM Poor endurance Mild fever Decreased muscle strength Morning stiffness Gel phenomenon Weight loss Decreased appetite	Pain and tenderness at rest and movement decreases Joints warm and pink Inflammation subsiding Decreased function Tingling and numbness in hands and feet
Chronic-active	Decreased ROM Fever has subsided Muscle strength decreased Endurance low	Pain and tenderness at rest minimal Pain on motion decreases Inflammation low-grade Increased activity noted, owing to adjustment to pain
Chronic-inactive	Limited ROM Muscle atrophy Decreased endurance from limited activity in previous stages Residuals seen from above stages Potential contracture	Pain at motion caused by stiffness from disuse during previous stages and instability of joint No inflammation Residuals seen from above stages Functioning may be decreased due to pain

combination of PIP joint flexion and DIP joint hyperextension (Fig. 15.6). More specifically, it is flexion of the PIP joint through the detached central slip of the extensor tendon, which serves as a "button-hole" through which the joint can pop. The DIP joint is then forced into hyperextension. Swan-neck deformities result from contractures of the interosseus and flexor muscles and tendons, which in turn produce a flexure contracture of the MCP joint, compensatory hyperextension of the PIP joint, and flexion of the DIP joint (Fig. 15.7). Thumb deformities associated with RA have been classified into three categories. In type I, MCP inflammation leads to stretching of the joint capsule and boutonniere-like deformity. In type II, edema of the CMC joint leads to volar subluxation during ankylosis of the adductor pollicis. In type III, after sustained disease of both MCP joints, exaggerated adduction of the first metacarpus, flexion of the MCP joint, and hyperextension of the DIP joint result from the patient's need to establish a compensatory method to pinch (Neumann & Bielefeld, 2003). Stiffness and crepitary inflammation along the tendon sheath with limitations of flexion and extension may be exhibited (Fig. 15.8). Finger "triggering" occurs when thickening or nodule formation of the tendon interplays with tenosynovial inflammation, trapping the tendon in a flexed position. Tendon rupture most frequently occurs in the abductors

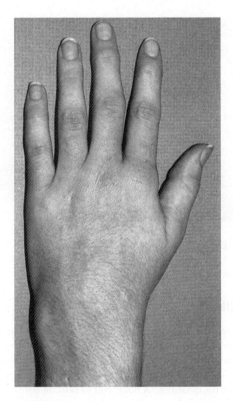

Figure 15.5 Fusiform swelling and erythema about the PIP joints, most significant in the long finger. Swelling at the MCP joints has caused loss of definition of joint margins. The extensor carpi ulnaris tendon sheath (sixth dorsal compartment of the wrist) has synovial thickening and swelling.

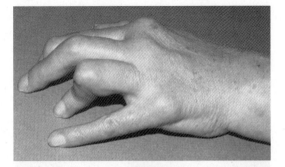

Figure 15.6 A boutonniere deformity of the ring finger, flexion deformity of the long finger PIP joint, and mild swan-neck deformity of the index finger. Extensive synovitis at the MCP joints obscures the usual definition of joint margins.

Wrist

Ulnar deviations and volar subluxation at the MCP joints or radiocarpal deviation are characteristic signs of RA at the wrist as seen in Figure 15.11. These problems develop and result from severe **tenosynovitis** and inflammation where the ligaments surround the joint and eventually lead to edema, joint laxity, erosion of the tendons and ligaments, and muscle imbalance. When ulnar deviation of the MCP is present with radial deviation at the radiocarpal joint, a "zigzag" presentation of the hand is seen (Figs. 15.12 and 15.13). Dorsiflexion of the wrist often is one of the first movements to be limited. **Carpal tunnel syndrome** is commonly diagnosed, resulting from synovial proliferations on the volar aspect of the wrist, which

of the thumb and extensor carpi ulnaris of the fourth and fifth fingers. Rupture of the latter is usually caused by a combination of synovitis in the tendon sheaths and mechanical irritation from an eroded and subluxed distal ulna (Ashe, McCauley, & Khan, 2004). **De Quervain's tenosynovitis** (Fig. 15.9), which involves extensors at the thumb, causes severe pain and discomfort, resulting in a decrease in hand function and the ability to grip. Mutilans deformity (opera glass hand) causes transverse folds of the skin of the thumb and fingers, resembling a folded telescope. Pulling on the fingers during examination may lengthen the digit much like opening opera glasses, or the joint may bend in unusual directions just by the pull of gravity. Radiographs of the fingers and thumb identify severe bone resorption, erosions, and shortening of the MCP, PIP, radiocarpal, and radioulnar joints (Fig. 15.10) (Ashe et al., 2004). The gross instability of the thumbs and severely deformed phalanges negatively affect hand function as well as participation in a wide variety of daily living activities.

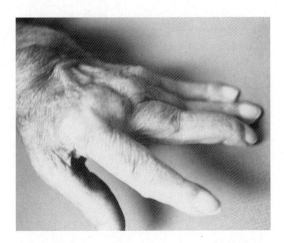

Figure 15.7 Swan-neck deformities of long, ring, and little fingers, with concomitant subluxation of the MCP joints.

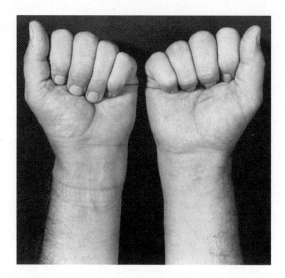

Figure 15.8 Flexor tendinitis at the wrist and in the palm leading to decreased flexion of the fingers of the left hand.

then impinge upon the median nerve (Barr, Barbe, & Clark, 2004). This causes paresthesia of the palmar aspect of the thumb, the second and third digits, and the radial aspect of the fourth digit (Fig. 15.14).

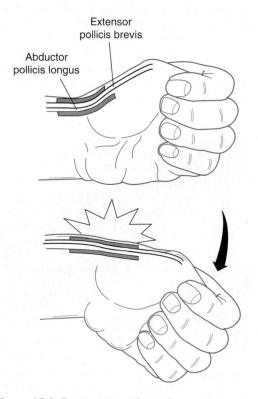

Extensor pollicis brevis

Abductor pollicis longus

Figure 15.9 Finkelstein's test for de Quervain's disease.

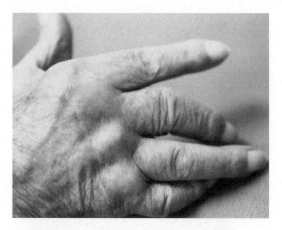

Figure 15.10 Arthritis mutilans. The long PIP joint has been destroyed by RA. Deflection of the distal portion of the phalanx is caused by the pull of gravity.

Elbow

Loss of motion because of flexion contractures in addition to inflammation is the most prevalent problem with elbow involvement. Synovial swelling and thickening may be observed in the lateral area between the radial head and the olecranon. A bulge will be seen. Synovitis in the radiohumeral joint can result in decreased motion during pronation and supination of the forearm. Lateral epicondylitis, more often referred to as tennis elbow, is reported as sharply painful when firm pressure is placed on this specific area. Other symptoms include paresthesia over

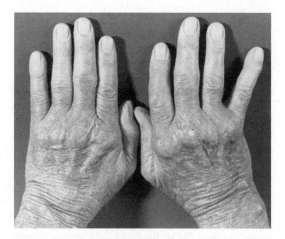

Figure 15.11 Subcutaneous tissue atrophy, MCP joint proliferation synovitis with loss of joint definition, and mild PIP joint enlargement. There is slight volar subluxation of the MCP joints and mild ulnar deviation at the MCP joints of the right hand. Involvement of the dominant (right) hand is more pronounced.

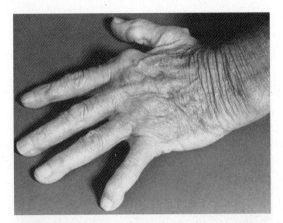

Figure 15.12 "Zigzag" deformity with ulnar deviation of the fingers at the MCP joints and clockwise rotation of carpus on the distal radius.

the fourth and fifth fingers and weakness in the flexor muscle of the fifth digit.

Shoulder

Shoulder involvement is common and can complicate significantly as RA progresses. The glenohumeral, acromiocla-

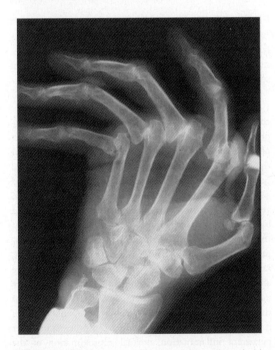

Figure 15.13 Severe MCP joint subluxations in the volar and ulnar directions. There is a concomitant clockwise rotation of the carpus on the distal radius (zigzag deformity). Erosions of the ulnar styloid and metacarpal heads are evident.

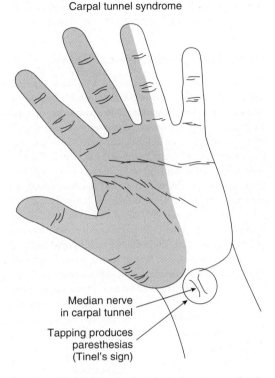

Carpal tunnel syndrome

Median nerve in carpal tunnel

Tapping produces paresthesias (Tinel's sign)

Figure 15.14 Distribution of pain or paresthesias (*shaded area*) when the median nerve is compressed by swelling in the wrist (carpal tunnel).

vicular, and thoracoscapular joints are the most susceptible. Because the shoulder capsule lies beneath the muscular rotator cuff, inflammation is difficult to detect during physical assessment. Difficulty with shoulder movement and with participation in daily living activities is usually the chief complaint, followed by pain and tenderness (Adams, Burridge, Mullee, Hammond, & Cooper, 2004). Because the shoulder relies on extensive coordinated movement, when any one of these joints becomes affected, dysfunction in activities of daily living (ADL) is seen. Impairment in ability to manage and carry out self-care tasks may be significant. Localized pain and tenderness, resulting from tendonitis in the glenohumeral area where the supraspinatus muscle or the long head of the biceps tendon inserts, are frequently seen. Rotator cuff tears are likely where the rotator cuff tendon inserts into the greater tuberosity. Erosion is triggered by the proliferative synovitis that develops there (Maloney & Ryder, 2003). Tendinitis, capsulitis, and **bursitis** (grouped under local conditions of arthritis categories) are causes of shoulder pain diagnosed more frequently than synovitis. Synovitis of the glenohumeral area is seen occasionally in those with RA and is observed as a bulge in the anterior or lateral superior area of the shoulder. Loss of motion is a complication of shoulder synovitis, which is seen in progressed cases, and is known as frozen shoulder.

Head, Neck, and Cervical Spine

The cervical spine is often involved in RA (Mink, Gordon, & Deutsch, 2003). Involvement of C1 and C2 may produce life-threatening conditions. Neck pain on motion and occipital headaches are common symptoms of cervical spine involvement and occur in those individuals who have had RA longer than 10 years (Niere & Jerak, 2004). Patients with severe deformities in their hands, as in mutilans deformity, are very likely to have had significant amounts of corticosteroids for RA management (Crowther, 2001). During radiologic examination of this area in advanced cases of RA, the lower cervical and odontoid processes often appear eroded, as do the cervical **apophyseal** and intervertebral joints. The first to fourth cervical joints are those most commonly affected by inflammation and pain (Figs. 15.15 and 15.16). Involvement of the upper cervical spine in advanced cases leads to subluxation, whereas lower cervical spine involvement produces symptoms of

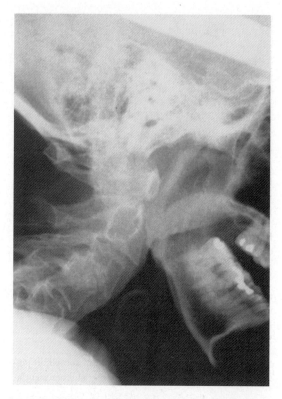

Figure 15.16 A lateral radiograph of a patient with RA who is experiencing severe upper extremity neurologic decline caused by C2–C3 and C3 and C4 anterior subluxations. The odontoid is not visible because of severe erosion.

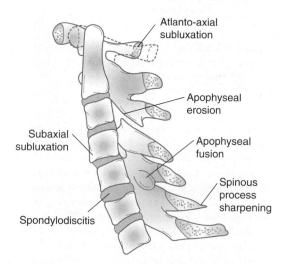

Figure 15.15 Neck abnormalities in RA. The neck is usually involved in adult and juvenile RA. The most common disorder is subluxation of the atlantoaxial joint, which occurs particularly on flexion of the neck. C1 moves forward on C2, and the odontoid process can actually cause pressure on the spinal cord posteriorly. Other findings include erosions at the apophyseal joints, fusion of the apophyseal joint, which occurs particularly in JRA, and subluxation at other levels. Disk involvement also may occur, and erosive changes and resorption can cause sharpening of the spinous process. (Reprinted with permission from the Arthritis Foundation. [1988]. *The AHPA Arthritis Teaching Slide Collection.* [2nd ed.].)

cord-root compression. For example, with a C5 root compression, problems are (a) sensation on the radial aspect of the forearm, (b) muscle weakness and abduction of the shoulder and flexion of the elbow, and (c) decreased biceps jerk reflex. Subluxation also can cause twisting and compression of the vertebral arteries, which can lead to vertebrobasilar artery insufficiency. This may be facilitated by syncope on downward gaze. Flexion and extension of the cervical spine are usually less affected. The temporomandibular joints (TMJs) have varied involvement in RA, ranging from 1% to 60% by some estimates. Women are affected three times more often than men. Both TMJs are usually involved (Melchiorre et al., 2010). Involvement of this synovial joint results in the inability to open the mouth fully because of side-to-side gliding and protrusion. After persistent inflammation, normal approximation of the upper and lower teeth may be affected. Hoarseness occurs in up to 30% of patients presenting with RA. This stems from inflamed cricoarytenoid joints, which rotate with the vocal cords as they abduct and adduct to vary pitch and tone of the voice (Berjawi et al., 2010).

Hip

Approximately half of the patients diagnosed with RA have radiographic evidence of hip disease as seen in Figure 15.17. Although hip involvement is common, early manifestations of the hip disease are typically not apparent because the location of the joint is deep within the pelvis. With progressive hip involvement, an abnormal gait pattern, possibly in the form of a limp, may be observed. This can result from a variety of factors, including pain, flexion contractures, muscle weakness, or hip instability (Williams, Brand, Hill, Hunt, & Moran, 2010). Fibrous contractures in flexion or external rotation are standard if restriction of motion is prolonged. Because the hip joint capsule is limited in its ability to stretch, severe RA involvement followed by swelling and massive effusion of synovium into the joint capsule may be extremely painful. It is also to be noted that hip involvement will result in discomfort and pain in the groin and the medial aspect of the knee. As involvement increases (e.g., increased flexion contractures), more functional problems will be experienced in all mobility activities, including donning lower extremity garments, sitting in a chair comfortably, ascending stairs, and positioning during sexual activity (Josefsson & Gard, 2010).

Knee

Hypertrophy and effusion of large amounts of synovium into the joint capsule are common in the knee joint and are more readily demonstrated in the knee than in the hip (Fig. 15.18). Greater than 5 mL of synovial fluid in the knee may be observed as a "bulge" sign; bulges occur behind the patella when fluid is pushed into the suprapatellar pouch and then back into the joint. Swelling, quadriceps muscle atrophy, ligamentous laxity, and joint instability may be more obvious when the patient stands or walks. Pain and swelling on the posterior knee may be caused by significant increases in intra-articular pressure during flexion, which produces an out-pouching, or Baker's cyst. Popliteal cysts such as these may impede superior venous flow in the thigh, producing a dilation of veins

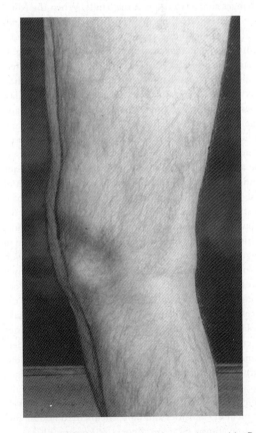

Figure 15.18 Lateral view of a patient with RA affecting the knees. There are quadriceps atrophy, significant synovial proliferation with joint effusion in the suprapatellar pouch, and fullness in the popliteal space because of a small synovial (Baker's) cyst.

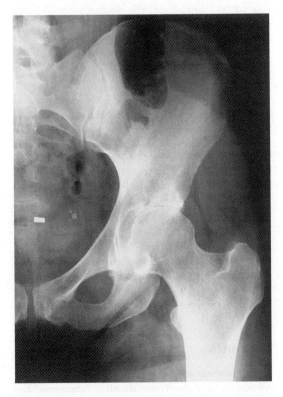

Figure 15.17 Hip radiograph of a patient with RA. There are diffuse joint space narrowing, small cysts in the femoral head and acetabulum, and little reparative bony change.

and edema (Siegel & Gall, 1999). When the joint capsule is stretched, a reflex spasm triggers in the hamstring muscles. To relieve joint pain and tension, patients will hold their hips and knees in a flexion position that facilitates contractures. These contractures will cause difficulty in all weight-bearing activities.

Ankle and Foot

True rheumatic disease is less common in the ankle than in other areas of the body and usually is not seen without concurrent midfoot or metatarsophalangeal (MTP) involvement. Tibiotalar swelling and loss of subtalar motion can develop. Ankle synovitis can be palpated in front of, behind, and below the malleoli. The ankle is often very tender and sensitive. Symptomatic involvement of the feet is reported by 30% to 90% of those who have RA (Otter et al., 2010). RA of the toes involving the MTP joints results in changes similar to those in the hands. When the MTP joints are affected, normal gait is disrupted. Problems will be exhibited during the push-off phase of ambulation, causing compensatory action with other weight-bearing joints. Characteristic manifestations of the feet include claw toes, hammer toes, cock-up toes, and hallux valgus (Costa, Rizak, & Zimmerman, 2004). Claw toes result from the hyperextension of the MTP and the flexion of the PIP and DIP joints. Hammer toes differ from claw toes in that the DIP joint is hyperextended as seen in Figure 15.19. Cocking up the toes may be associated with subluxation of the metatarsal heads and, finally, a claw-like appearance with an elevation of the tip of the toe above the surface on which the foot is resting. Hallux valgus is a common event in which the fibular deviation of the first through fourth toes occurs. This is similar to ulnar deviation of the hands as seen in Figures 15.20 and 15.21. Rheumatoid nodules develop over bony prominences that bear more than normal pressure. For individuals affected by painful forefoot weight bearing, rheumatoid nodules can occur on the heels because of increased weight bearing there (Jaakkola & Mann, 2005). Tarsal joint involvement does not occur as often as in the forefoot; however, it can be detrimental to a person's ability to ambulate. As the longitudinal arch in the foot flattens and hind foot valgus occurs, weight-bearing pressure tends to shift medially (Fig. 15.22). This, in turn, facilitates the possible development of callosities and more rheumatoid nodule formation (Burns, Scanlon, Zgonis, & Lowery, 2005).

Muscle Involvement

Most individuals with RA have muscle involvement, including muscle weakness. Researchers have suggested

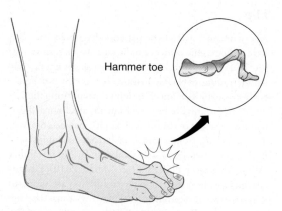

Figure 15.19 In this diagram, the second tow has a cock-up deformity, which is similar to the boutonniere abnormality of the hand. Often this deformity is associated with subluxation of the corresponding MTP joints. This deformity may be hastened in a patient who wears shoes that are too small. Rubbing of the PIP joints on other joints causes pain, callus formation, and possibly ulceration. This abnormality is not restricted to patients with RA. (Reprinted with permission from the Arthritis Foundation. [1988]. *The AHPA Arthritis Teaching Slide Collection.* [2nd ed.].)

five stages of muscle disease in the RA process, which are listed below:

1. Reduction of muscle bulk associated with muscle atrophy that accompanies the inflammatory process as a result of disuse, bed rest, vascular events, and drug effects. A muscle can lose up to 30% of its bulk in 1 week, with loss of muscle bulk being associated with decline in function.
2. Peripheral neuromyopathy, usually related to mononeuritis multiplex, which is frequently associated with rheumatoid vasculitis involving localized sensory loss.
3. Steroid myopathy.
4. Active myositis and muscle necrosis (or muscle fiber inflammation resulting in destruction of the muscle fibers).
5. Chronic myopathy resembling a dystrophic process.

Tendon

Tendon damage may result from inflammation of the synovial lining of the tendon sheath (tenosynovitis) and interferes with smooth gliding of the tendon. A lag phenomenon may be seen in patients with tendon damage or muscle weakening, displaying a significant difference between passive and active ROM.

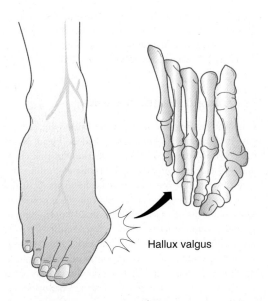

Hallux valgus

Figure 15.20 An anatomical and clinical diagram of hallux vagus. Pes planus and ligamentous laxity lead to lateral deviation of the great toe with a resultant hallux vagus. This deformity can be hastened by the wearing of narrow-toed shoes. Rubbing of the bunion on the shoe surface produced pain, and the lateral deviation of the great toe may impinge on other digits of the foot. This abnormality is not restricted to patients with RA. (Reprinted with permission from the Arthritis Foundation. [1988]. *The AHPA Arthritis Teaching Slide Collection.* [2nd ed.].)

Extra-Articular Systemic Manifestations

As has been mentioned previously in this chapter, RA affects the joint and is systemic. The number and severity of extra-articular features vary with the duration and extent of the disease and tend to occur in individuals with higher levels of RF in their blood (Hochberg, Johnston, & John, 2008). The following are additional manifestations that may exist in those with RF.

Rheumatoid or Subcutaneous Nodules

Rheumatoid nodule formation is one of the most common extra-articular manifestations of RA and occurs in up to 50% of individuals at some point during the course of the disease (Hochberg et al., 2008). Periarticular structures; extensor surfaces; and areas subject to pressure such as the olecranon (Fig. 15.23), the proximal ulna, the Achilles tendon, the occiput, and the sacrum are primary sites for those growths. Most can develop insidiously and regress at any time.

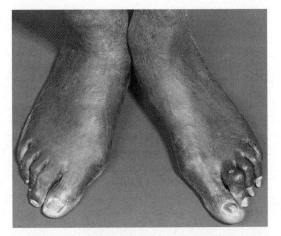

Figure 15.21 Mild hallux valgus, with dorsal subluxation of the MTP joints and resultant "hammer toe" deformities of second through fifth toes. Midfoot instability has led to eversion, with concomitant flattening of the feet.

Pulmonary Manifestations

Pleuritis, interstitial fibrosis, pulmonary nodules, pneumonitis, and other forms of pulmonary obstructive disease occur more frequently in those with RA than in the population at large (Kim, Collard, & King, 2009). Evidence of pleuritis is usually found at autopsy, because the disease is generally asymptomatic during life. In a few cases, upper-airway obstruction from cricoarytenoid arthritis or laryngeal nodules may develop. Some researchers believe that small-airway dysfunction is related to factors other than RA.

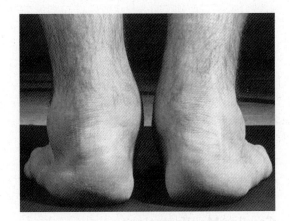

Figure 15.22 Significant ankle and midfoot synovitis. Loss of definition of the arch and eversion at the subtalar joint also are evident.

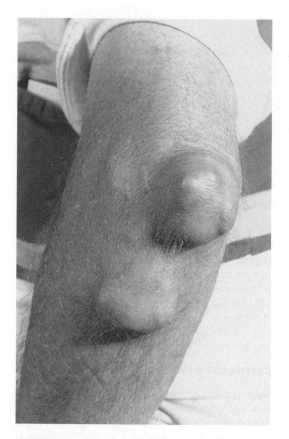

Figure 15.23 Large rheumatoid nodules in the olecranon bursa and along the extensor surface of the proximal ulna. Each mass is a collection of multiple smaller nodules. A small effusion is present in the olecranon bursa.

Felty's Syndrome

The condition of leukopenia associated with collagen-vascular disorders, called Felty's syndrome, occurs in <1% of patients with RA (Chandra, 2008). This syndrome is usually found in those who have progressed and have chronic RA as well as those who have high levels of RF (13). Splenomegaly, leukopenia, anemia, neutropenia, thrombocytopenia, and granulocytopenia also are features of this syndrome. Felty's syndrome is a disorder where patients with RA develop splenomegaly, neutropenia, and, on rare occasions, portal hypertension without underlying cirrhosis. Splenectomy is the treatment of choice for complications of portal hypertension in patients with Felty's syndrome (Stock, Kadry, & Smith, 2009).

Cardiac Manifestations

Most pericardial disease develops with synovitis several years into the course of RA. Manifestations may vary from mild to being the actual cause of death. Other forms of cardiac disease in RA include rheumatoid carditis, endocardial (valve) inflammation, conduction defects, coronary arteritis, and granulomatous aortitis (Turesson, McClelland, Christianson, & Matteson, 2007).

Neurologic Manifestations

Neurologic manifestations may be caused by cervical spine subluxation. As briefly described in "Head, Neck, and Cervical Spine" and "Wrist" sections in this chapter, nerve entrapment that is the result of proliferative synovitis or joint deformities may facilitate neuropathies of the median, ulnar, radial, or anterior tibial nerves. In aggressive forms of vasculitis (Fig. 15.24), polyneuropathy and mononeuritis multiplex may result (Harrop, Hanna, Silva, & Sharan, 2007). Direct central nervous system involvement does not appear to occur, but vasculitis and rheumatoid nodule-like granulomas can occur irregularly in the meninges (Zolcinski, Bazan-Socha, Zwolinski, & Musial, 2008).

Ophthalmologic Manifestations

The rheumatoid process involves the eye in <1% of patients. Sjögren's syndrome (Fig. 15.25) is a chronic disease of unknown etiology causing corneal and conjunctival lesions and is characterized by dry eyes and mouth (Baiza-Duran, Medrano-Palafox, Hernandez-Quintela,

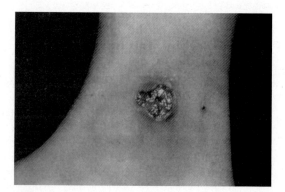

Figure 15.24 Vasculitis, defined as inflammation of the small vessels, is common in RA. The most common vascular abnormality in patients with RA is leg ulceration, which may be indolent and difficult to heal. Ulcers are not usually associated with either arterial or venous insufficiency. Other vasculitis problems among patients with RA include benign digital (fingertip) ulceration and severe systemic vasculitis similar to polyarteritis nodosa. (Reprinted with permission from the Arthritis Foundation. [1988]. *The AHPA Arthritis Teaching Slide Collection.* [2nd ed.].)

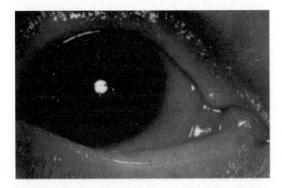

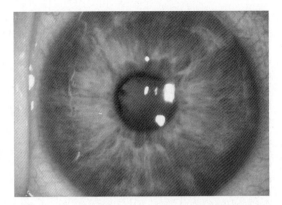

Figure 15.25 Patients with RA may also have Sjögren's syndrome. Sjögren's syndrome is a chronic inflammatory disorder characterized by diminished lacrimal and salivary gland secretions (sicca complex), resulting in keratoconjunctivitis sicca and xerostomia. Patients may complain that the eyes feel "as if they have sand in them." The syndrome also may include decreased vaginal lubrication. Keratoconjunctivitis sicca is demonstrated here by flecks of reddish-purple discoloration in the lower portion of the cornea and conjunctiva, which were stained with rose bengal dye. One-half of all patients with Sjögren's syndrome have RA or some other connective tissue disease, particularly systemic lupus erythematosus or systemic sclerosis. More than 90% of these patients are women, with a mean age of 50 years at the time of diagnosis. Keratoconjunctivitis sicca develops in 10% to #% of all patients with RA. (Reprinted with permission from the Arthritis Foundation. [1988]. *The AHPA Arthritis Teaching Slide Collection.* [2nd ed.].)

Figure 15.26 Chronic changes in the eye with JRA iritis: posterior synechiae (iris-lens adhesions at pupil margin); iris bombe (shallowing of the anterior chamber caused by blockage of aqueous flow from posterior chamber through pupil); and secondary cataract. (Reprinted with permission from Hiles D. A. (1987). Slide atlas of pediatric physical diagnosis. In: B.J. Zitelli & H. W. Davis (Eds.) *Pediatric Ophthalmology.* New York: Gower Medical Publishing.)

Lozano-Alcazar, & Alaniz-de la O, 2010). Eye discomfort includes the inability to cry and a sandy feeling when blinking. Scleritis, which involves the deeper layers of the eye, may cause pain and visual impairment. Episcleritis is a less serious inflammatory condition and is usually temporary (Nizam, Johnstone, Green, & Gough, 2009). Eye involvement occurs in 30% to 50% of early-onset JRA (Fig. 15.26). In 80% of those children who experience eye involvement, the inflammation process primarily involves the anterior chamber of the eye with minimal to no symptoms. Cases have been reported including severe, irreversible eye changes as a result of corneal clouding, cataracts, glaucoma, and partial or total loss of vision. Children with JRA should be screened at regular intervals and treated by eye specialists (Reiff, 2009).

Depression

Depression has been identified as a significant problem for those with arthritis. Researchers have determined that the greater the negative impact on an individual's ability to accomplish daily living activities, the greater the likelihood that he or she will develop symptoms of depression. Additionally, the extent of pain and fatigue experienced by an individual will have a direct correlation to their tendency to experience depression (Wolfe & Michaud, 2009).

Body Composition

Researchers at the United States Department of Agriculture (USDA) Human Nutrition Center on Aging at Tufts University and New England Medical Center found that among persons with RA, changes in their immune system and the substances it produces resulted in higher metabolism, loss of lean body mass, and loss of appetite. This, in turn, suggests that the use of measures for lean mass in those with RA might identify high-risk individuals who could then be identified for interventions, such as nutritional counseling, to improve body composition (Book, Karlsson, Akesson, & Jacobsson, 2009).

COURSE AND PROGNOSIS

The course of RA tends to vary from person to person because its effects can differ so dramatically from case to case. Physical and functional outcomes are often difficult for the clinician to predict with accuracy. Onset of the disease is usually gradual or insidious, though too it may be abrupt. As a result of the cyclical nature of the RA process, an individual's ability to function can fluctuate according to the stage and severity of the disease

(Adams et al., 2004). Approximately 20% of patients will improve spontaneously and may even achieve remission, especially in the first year of the disease. However, chronic disease progression and functional deterioration occur in the majority of all cases (Goronzy et al., 2004). Long-term studies have determined that patients with RA have greater probability of restrictions in daily activities, restrictions in activity days, and 10 times the work disability rate as the general population (Allaire et al., 2009). In children with JRA, 70% to 90% make a satisfactory recovery from their disease without serious disability. A small percentage will develop recurrence as adults (Gewanter et al., 2005). Researchers have found that some patients do experience spontaneous remission. Features that appear to have prognostic importance are (a) number and length of remissions, (b) levels of RF, (c) presence of subcutaneous nodules, (d) extent of bone erosion seen radiographically at the initial evaluation, and (e) sustained disease activity for more than 1 year. Additionally, it has been learned that in patients younger than age 50, women tend to have a worse prognosis with regard to persistence and severity (Table 15-4) (Iikuni et al., 2009). Classification and prognosis of RA also can be assessed by functional analysis as outlined in Table 15-5. The functional capacity of an individual declines as the disease becomes more prevalent. Research has established both an immediate and a long-term relationship between arthritis and limitations in function (Verschueren, Esselens, & Westhovens, 2009). Self-reported functional status and the physical demands of work are the best predictors of disability. Lack of autonomy over the work schedule, the pace of the work, and the nature of the job all increase the likelihood of becoming disabled (Kessler et al., 2008). Early mortality has been linked by researchers to functional disability (Sokka, Abelson, & Pincus, 2008). Although there is no cure for RA, treatment methods continue to improve. Data suggest that individuals currently admitted to the hospital for RA are likely to have a decreased number of contractures and less fusion of peripheral joints at admission than did a similar cohort of patients 20 years ago (Strauss, Alfonso, Baidwan, & Cesare, 2008). Upon completion of a thorough evaluation by a physician, early diagnosis can assist in the development of a treatment approach to reduce joint pain, impede the disease process, and decrease joint deformity. Early classification of the disease facilitates earlier intervention and ideally a slowing of the disease process and progress. Emotional and financial supports for treatment contribute to the prognostic outcome and performance of children and adults. Research has demonstrated a high incidence of depression, decreased self-esteem, and social withdrawal. In those individuals with a progressed case of RA, the type of treatment prescribed plays a key part in life expectancy as well as ultimate quality of life.

DIAGNOSIS

Individuals with joint disease delay seeking medical care on average for 2 to 4 years (Kumar et al., 2007). It is much more difficult to establish a diagnosis of RA in the early development of the disease than in the more progressed, later stages. Several visits to a physician for evaluation and testing may be required before a definitive diagnosis can be confirmed. The American College of Rheumatology (ACR), formerly the American Rheumatism Association (ARA), first developed diagnostic criteria for the classification of RA in 1958, with revisions in 1987 (Tables 15-6 and 15-7). Originally, these criteria were

---

TABLE 15.4 Criteria for Remission in Rheumatoid Arthritis

Five or more of the following requirements must be fulfilled for at least 2 consecutive months:

1. Duration of morning stiffness not exceeding # minutes

2. No fatigue

3. No joint pain (by history)

4. No joint tenderness or pain on motion

5. No soft tissue swelling in joints of tendon sheaths

6. Erythrocyte sedimentation rate (Westergren method) < 30 mm/hour for a female or 20 mm/hour for a male

These criteria are intended to describe either spontaneous remission or drug-induced disease suppression, which stimulates spontaneous remission. To be considered for this designation, a patient must have met the ARA criteria for definite or classic rheumatoid arthritis at some time in the past. No alternative explanation may be involved to account for the failure to meet a particular requirement. For instance, in the presence of knee pain that might be related to degenerative arthritis, a point for "no joint pain" may not be awarded.

TABLE 15.5 Classification of Functional Capacity in Rheumatoid Arthritis

Class I	Complete functional capacity with the ability to carry on all usual duties without handicaps
Class II	Functional capacity adequate to conduct normal activities despite handicap of discomfort or limited mobility of one or more joints
Class III	Functional capacity adequate to perform only a few or none of the duties of usual occupation or self-care
Class IV	Largely or wholly incapacitated, with patient bedridden or confined to wheelchair, permitting little or no self-care

guidelines for the classification of disease syndromes to allow correct diagnosis in individuals taking part in clinical research investigations. The criteria have also been used as guidelines for the specific diagnosis of individuals in general (Symmons, 2007). The ACR continues to monitor the criteria for accuracy and validity. When diagnosis is still in doubt, further biopsies should be completed, if feasible, on subcutaneous nodules to differentiate them from gouty

tophi, amyloid, and other types of nodules. Even though RA shares many characteristics of other collagen diseases, particularly systemic lupus erythematosus, the latter can usually be identified by the characteristic skin lesions on the light-exposed areas, temporal frontal hair loss, oral and nasal mucosal lesions, and joint fluid with a white blood count seen as "overlap syndrome" (Amezcua-Guerra, 2009). Diagnosis of JRA may be a long, emotionally

TABLE 15.6 Classification of Progression of Rheumatoid Arthritis

Stage I—early

1. No destructive changes on roentgenographic examination

2. Roentgenologic evidence of osteoporosis may be present

Stage II—moderate

1. Roentgenologic evidence of osteoporosis with or without slight subchondral bone destruction; slight cartilage destruction may be present

2. No joint deformities, although limitation of joint mobility may be present

3. Extensive muscle atrophy

4. Extra-articular soft tissue lesions, such as nodules and tenosynovitis, may be present

Stage III—severe

1. Roentgenologic evidence of cartilage and bone destruction in addition to osteoporosis

2. Joint deformity such as subluxation, ulnar deviation, or hyperextension, without fibrous or bony ankylosis

3. Extensive muscle atrophy

4. Extra-articular soft tissue lesions, such as nodules and tenosynovitis, may be present

Stage IV—terminal

1. Fibrous or bone ankylosis

2. Same criteria of stage III

TABLE 15.7 1987 ARA Revised Criteria for the Classification of Rheumatoid Arthritis

1. Morning stiffness	Morning stiffness in and around the joints lasting at least 1 hour before maximal improvement.
2. Arthritis of three or more joint areas	At least three joint areas at the same time have had soft tissue swelling or fluid observed by a physician. The 14 possible areas are right or left PIP, MCP, wrist, elbow, knee, ankle, and MTP joints.
3. Arthritis of hand joints	At least one area swollen in a wrist, MCP, or PIP joint.
4. Symmetric arthritis	Simultaneous involvement of the same joint areas on both sides of the body (bilateral involvement of PIPs MCPs, or MTPs is acceptable without absolute symmetry).
5. Rheumatoid nodules	Subcutaneous nodules over bony prominences or extensor surfaces or in juxta-articular regions, observed by a physician.
6. Serum RF	Demonstration of abnormal amounts of serum RF by any method for which the result has been positive in 5% of normal subjects.
7. Radiographic changes	Radiographic changes typical of RA on posteroanterior hand and wrist radiographs, which must include erosions or unequivocal bony decalcification localized in the involved joints.

charged process for a family. The diagnosis depends on symptoms experienced in the first 6 months of the illness. The primary steps include many of those taken to diagnose RA in an adult. These include the following:

- A comprehensive health history to help determine the length of time symptoms have been present.
- A physical examination to look for joint inflammation, rashes, nodules, and eye problems.
- Laboratory tests to rule out other diseases.
- Radiograph examinations of joints to identify other possible conditions.
- Tests of fluids from joints and tissues to evaluate for infections and/or inflammation.

MEDICAL/SURGICAL MANAGEMENT

The goals of medical management of RA and JRA are (a) relief of pain and stiffness, (b) reduction of inflammation, (c) preservation of muscle strength and joint function, (d) minimizing medication side effects, (e) maintenance of as much

of a normal lifestyle as possible, and, for children, (f) promotion of normal growth and development. Another objective is to attempt to resolve or modify disease progress through early, aggressive drug therapies advocated because of the diagnosis, prognosis, and reversible damage in the articular cartilage within the first 2 years of the disease (Finckh et al., 2009). Because the etiology of RA is unknown and the mechanisms of therapeutic interventions are uncertain, therapy remains essentially experimental. None of the interventions are curative; therefore, all must be viewed as palliative, aimed at relieving the signs and symptoms of the disease. A comprehensive therapeutic management program for those with JRA and RA includes (a) physical management (including occupational and physical therapies), (b) psychosocial care (including self-image, pain management work, school participation, leisure, family functioning, family education, and financial considerations), (c) nutritional aspects, (d) pharmacologic management, and (e) other medical aspects including management of comorbidities. An interdisciplinary approach that focuses on physical, functional, and psychosocial issues is common with RA patients. Physical and occupational therapy interventions, including exercise and rest strategies, and physical agent modalities, including ultrasound, heat, gentle ROM, and splinting to allow proper alignment of deformed joints, have all assisted with managing symptoms. Patient and family education centering on self-help and self-management of RA have demonstrated positive outcomes. Review of medical and patient education outcomes research shows that medications offer 20% to 50% improvement in arthritis symptoms for most patients and that patient education interventions, such as the various self-help courses available through the Arthritis Foundation, can reduce symptoms an additional #% to 30% (Lorig, Ritter, Laurent, & Plant, 2008).

Drug Therapy

A variety of different drugs are used in the medical management of RA. Five different types of drugs are important: analgesic drugs; nonsteroidal anti-inflammatory drugs (NSAIDs), including salicylates; corticosteroids; disease-modifying antirheumatic drugs (DMARDs), which are considered second-line drugs; and cytotoxics, which are considered third-line drugs. Treatment is focused on anti-inflammatory and immunosuppressive effects to both prevent destruction of the joint and give pain control. However, as mentioned earlier in this chapter, a wide variety of treatment intervention options are available to the clinician and should not necessarily be limited to drug therapy alone. During the 1980s, a "pyramid approach" to medical management began with the most conservative methods and then assumed a more aggressive approach as the disease progressed (van Vollenhoven, 2009). This thought process began to slowly change when methotrexate, a cytotoxic drug, demonstrated that it could control RA with minimal toxicity compared with other second-line DMARDs. In the 1990s, the pyramid approach was used less frequently. Instead, more aggressive therapy consisting of immunosuppressives (including cytotoxic drugs) were implemented as the first part of treatment and combined with DMARDs to obtain disease control before severe joint destruction occurred. Salicylates (e.g., aspirin) or the newer NSAIDs are the primary, and less toxic, drugs available for RA treatment. These provide relief from pain, reduce inflammation, and, though most require a physician's order, are relatively inexpensive (van Vollenhoven, 2009).

Surgery

Surgery plays a role in the management of RA in patients with severely damaged joints. Hip and knee arthroplasty and total joint replacements have offered the most positive outcomes in terms of pain relief, improved function, and maximization of mobility. The goals of surgery are (a) pain reduction, (b) correction of deformity, and (c) functional improvement. As with any major surgery, there are inherent risks that must be thoughtfully weighed. The patient must be prepared for surgery and demonstrate a willingness to be an active participant in the rehabilitation process (Grotte et al., 2010).

IMPACT ON OCCUPATIONAL PERFORMANCE

Effects on occupational performance for individuals with RA are usually disruptive, but not life threatening. A person with RA will experience varying degrees of improvement, depending on the progression of the disease, anatomical structures involved, systemic problems experienced, comorbidities, financial support available, and overall psychological outlook. Trombley calls identifying occupational performance problems as the first step in assessment a more "top-down" approach (as opposed to the "bottom-up" approach of evaluating performance components like ROM and muscle strength). Taking the top-down approach also gives the clinician a better understanding of the context within which the person functions and the priorities he or she believes are paramount (Trombley, 1995). It is important to focus on the context in which the individual must perform daily activities, as this will assist in determining the feasibility and appropriateness of intervention. Christiansen states that hand strength and dexterity limitations have an impact on all ADL and instrumental activities of daily living (IADL), carried out within a variety of contexts (Christiansen & Matuska, 2004). Considering that every object in our environment must be grasped, gripped, manipulated, moved, smoothed, or pressed, one can understand how RA or JRA can cast a wide shadow over a variety of leisure, work, and self-care activities. A variety of tools are available to assess performance deficits and assets as well as performance components. For the occupational therapy professional one area of concentrated focus may be on hand and upper extremity function. A selection of tests of hand and upper limb function for individuals with rheumatic diseases follows:

- Arthritis Hand Function Test (AHFT) (Adams, Mullee, Burridge, Hammond, & Cooper, 2010)
- Cochin Rheumatoid Hand Disability Scale (Rannou et al., 2007).
- Disabilities of the Arm, Shoulder, and Hand (DASH) Questionnaire (Raven et al., 2008)
- Michigan Hand Outcomes Questionnaire (MHQ) (Walgee, Burns, & Chung, 2010)
- Sequential Occupational Dexterity Assessment (SODA) (Rallon & Chen, 2008)

As with all assessments, formal and informal, it is important to focus on the context in which the individual must perform daily activities, as this will determine the feasibility and appropriateness of the occupational therapy intervention.

IMPACT ON CLIENT FACTORS

Sensory Functions and Pain

The processing of sensory information may be affected in the patient with RA. Tactile, proprioceptive, visual, and auditory abilities specifically seem to be those most vulnerable. Nerve impingement from the loss of soft tissue integrity can affect both tactile and proprioceptive processing throughout both proximal and peripheral joints. People with RA have an increased risk for eye problems caused by associated conditions or medication side effects. Consequent visual impairment may increase the risk of falls or difficulties self-administering medications (Piper et al., 2007). Auditory changes can occur in the individual with RA because of the inflammation of the inner ear bony joints (Murdin, Patel, Walmsley, & Yeoh, 2008).

Neuromusculoskeletal and Movement-Related Functions

By far the most significant deficit in the neuromuscular component is the decrease in both passive and active ROM in the major joints. Subsequent to the loss of ROM, an individual can likely experience loss of muscle mass and strength. Joint deformities are common, especially in the position of flexion. The inflammation of RA causes joint swelling. Joint stiffness, especially in the morning, is a commonly reported complaint (Fendler & Braun, 2009). The cumulative effects of immobility, stiffness, and pain result in generalized fatigue that exacerbates the mobility impairment. Patients may present with decreased power during formal functional strength testing. The clinician should be aware that a patient might demonstrate strength in a "good" range in the pain-free portion of joint range and a significantly lower score in painful areas of joint range. Strength and function may likewise vary during those times of the day when joint stiffness is decreased. The most significant motor impairment will be demonstrated as depressed activity tolerance because of decreased neuromuscular status in the individual presenting with RA. Fatigue should be assessed over a 24-hour period or longer in order to gain a full understanding of the client's patterns of behavior and activity participation. Energy conservation principles involve prioritizing activities; planning and pacing activities over the day, week, or month; and regular physical activity as a mainstay for sustaining endurance for all daily life activities (Cordery & Rocchi, 1998).

It is beneficial for the clinician to measure heart rate, respiratory rate, and blood pressure during functional activities. Although formal evaluation of passive and active ROM and strength is useful as baseline data, if joint pain and poor tolerance to activity are apparent, the clinician must consider incorporating a functional ROM assessment in order to determine availability of motion for performing functional activities that are relevant and necessary for the client. Documenting the time of day during which the assessment takes place can assist in determining if there are cycles or periods when stiffness and diminished functionality are more pronounced. Joint instability can be a significant deterrent to initiation and completion of many daily self-care activities. Researchers have suggested that practice, along with application of joint-protection principles, improves functional ability (Oldfield & Felson, 2008). Orthotic devices and splints can help stabilize joints, address underlying biomechanics of motion, reduce pain during activity, and improve hand strength and function (Gomes-Carreira, Jones, & Natour, 2010).

Mental Functions

RA does not have a direct effect on cognitive functioning. It has been shown in the literature that difficulty with attention span, short-term memory, sequencing, and problem solving as well as other process skills may be caused and/or exacerbated by depression. It is not unusual for an individual with RA to have disease exacerbation as a result of major psychological stressors (Hanly, Omisade, Su, Farewell, & Fisk, 2010). Breakdown in coping mechanisms may lead to feelings of hopelessness and a sense of helplessness. For some individuals a diminishment of self-concept and the ability to self-manage one's life may occur. Depression and anxiety are other potential conditions that the individual with either RA or JRA may encounter at some time during their life with their condition. It has been shown that nearly 50% of patients with RA report dysfunction in the areas of social interaction, communication with others, and other emotional behaviors (Bai et al., 2009). The individual with RA or JRA frequently has to implement changes in various aspects of his or her life. Changes in medications, exercise routines, and self-care activities can create anxiety and a sense of loss of control for the individual. Some individuals while seeking to maintain autonomy will disregard the advice and guidance of their caregivers. The caregiver must allow the individual the prerogative to make decisions regarding his or her own care and to encourage autonomy and mastery of one's self as well as one's environment. Through mutual respect, the caregiver and the individual dealing with RA or JRA can maximize function while facilitating mastery and self-directedness.

CONCLUSION

During the past several decades, the health care environment has been stressed in regard to reimbursement and funding issues related to assessment and treatment of those with RA, JRA, and all of the other forms of arthritis (Lundkvist, Kastang, & Kobelt, 2008). Joint problems are limiting the functional capacity of 43 million Americans, and according to some estimates they are more costly than cancer or diabetes. The numbers are going up steadily with each passing year. By 2025, the total is expected to top 60 million people affected. As obesity in the United States continues to grow and reach epidemic proportions, more and more individuals will suffer the effects of unrelenting wear and tear on their weight-bearing joints due to arthritis. The active generation of baby boomers now entering their retirement years will likewise be experiencing joint maladies directly attributable to the continuation of active and sometimes competitive athletics into their fifth and sixth decades. All indicators point health care providers and caregivers in the direction of needing to acknowledge the total life impact that these rheumatoid arthritic conditions can and do have on people and their ability to carry on routine daily activities. Key professionals in the care of this growing population of individuals needing care will continue to be the primary care physician, the family practice physician, physician assistants, and nurse practitioners. Physical and occupational therapists will continue to be essential team members, as will athletic trainers, rehabilitation counselors, and educators. Many people will seek and receive assessment, diagnosis, and treatment from medical specialists in the field of rheumatology. Research has shown clearly that positive outcomes have been achieved with the initiation of early, aggressive intervention. Patient-centered treatment including self-help, self-management, and education will continue to be advocated by the array of health care providers. The clinician's role in partnering with each client is to assist in the development of realistic goals, to provide encouragement, and to offer a positive environment for the exploration of the various options available now. It will be the continuing responsibility of all health care professionals involved in the assessment and treatment of all types of arthritis to remain informed and aware of advances in the field.

Case Illustrations

Case 1

Pete is a 44-year-old landscaper and lawn irrigation system installer living in New Jersey. He is married, has two children in high school, and continues to remain active in his company's softball league on weekends. His wife works part-time as a registered nurse. For the past few months Pete has experienced pain and stiffness in the small joints of his hands and stiffness in both elbows and knees. His wife also has noticed that his fingers look swollen and are warm to the touch. Pete tends to discount what he considers "minor aches and pains" and attributes his discomfort to "growing pains" and the fact that his hands are in cold water frequently when he is working. Typically, by his first coffee break at 10:# in the morning, Pete has forgotten his early morning pain and stiffness and is his usual self. After several more months of repeated complaints, Pete's wife arranged for an evaluation with their family practice physician. After a series of tests and some time, he was diagnosed with RA.

Case 2

Mora Pelladona is a 34-year-old single mother of two children; she lives in a rent-subsidized one-bedroom apartment in Staten Island, New York. Her 10-year-old son is in the fourth grade, and an 8-year-old daughter born with spina bifida attends special education class in a school across town from their home. Mora was diagnosed with RA approximately 4 years ago and has been managing her home and her self-care as well as the responsibilities inherent in caring for her young children. Recently, Mora has been experiencing exacerbation of her symptoms, flare-ups including increased joint swelling and pain. Mora prides herself on being independent and able to multitask in order to accomplish many activities in her life. In her rare free time she enjoys scrap booking and playing poker with her friends in the apartment complex. Since the onset of her most recent exacerbation, Mora has seen a significant change in her lifestyle and ability to maintain some of the routine activities necessary for balanced family life. Moderate involvement of motor and neuromuscular components affects all occupational performance areas. ROM and muscle strength is affected in all movement in her elbows, wrists, and hands. There is a slight, but noticeable ulnar drift at the MP joints bilaterally. Prehension skills are functional for routine activities of daily living, but Mora has noticed that she is having increased difficulty opening containers such as the bottle of shampoo and the dead bolt on the front door. Gross grasp is weakening, and Mora has begun purchasing milk for the children in half-gallon containers rather than the cost-saving larger gallon size. Mora is experiencing stiffness and pain in the small joints of her fingers. This limits her when she attempts to prepare some dishes for the family dinner. She is also less interested in playing cards when she is feeling this way; she says that it is harder to keep her "poker face" when she is in such discomfort. Recently Mora's sister has been helping out with grocery shopping and clothing shopping for the two children. Her sister is also willing and able to assist by taking Mora's daughter to various clinic visits when necessary. Mora can operate her own car, but her endurance can be drastically affected when the RA is in a flare-up. Mora is hesitant to apply for a handicap-parking permit, but parking and walking distances into and out of stores is getting nearly impossible to do, particularly in the damp and cold winters experienced in the New York metropolitan area. Maintaining her self-esteem and morale is becoming more and more difficult as her disease persists. Previously Mora was able to rally herself and work through her pain and the limitations this wrought on her life. Lately she has been staying in bed in the morning after the children leave for school, getting up only to answer the telephone or to make a cup of coffee for breakfast. There are some days when she does not change out of her pajamas, leaving the bedroom only to use the toilet. She can actually feel herself pulling away socially and emotionally from her sphere of friends and at times from her loving family. She feels angry and guilty about no longer being the "super person" she once thought she was. Mora never was one to look to support groups for answers to her life situation. She vowed to manage the needs of her children, especially her daughter's many physical and medical needs, without leaning on others. Now she is worried that she is losing ground, and many days she feels like she is "sinking into wet concrete." Her sister is planning to attend a local support group for family members of those with RA. The group meets monthly in the basement of a church in the city, and it is a first step toward helping Mora and her kids.

RECOMMENDED LEARNING RESOURCES

Organizations
Consumer and Professional Resources
Health Organizations
American Juvenile Arthritis Organization (AJAO)
Tel: 404-872-7100, 1-800-568-4045
www.arthritis.org
Arthritis Foundation (AF**)**
Tel: 404-872-7100, 800-568-4045
www.arthritis.org
The Arthritis Society (Canada)
393 University Avenue, Suite 1700
Toronto, Ontario M5G 1E6
Canada
Tel: 416-979-7228;
Fax: 416-979-8366
www.info@arthritis.ca
The European League Against Rheumatism (EULAR)
EULAR Executive Secretariat
Seestrasse 240
8802-Kilchberg
Switzerland
Tel: +41-44-716-30-30
www.secretariat@eular.org

Higher Education and Training for People with Handicaps (HEATH)
George Washington University
HEATH Resource Center
2121 K Street NW, Suite 220
Washington, D.C. 20037
Tel: 800-544-3284
www.heath.gwu.edu
National Chronic Pain Outreach Association (NCPOA)
P.O. Box 274
Millboro, VA 24460
Tel: 540-862-9437; Fax: 540-862-9485
www.chronic pain.org
Support Groups
Contact the Arthritis Foundation for local groups across the United States of America
Professional Organizations
American College of Rheumatology (ACR)/Arthritis Health Professionals Association (AHPA)
1800 Century Place
Suite 250
Atlanta, GA 30345
Tel: 404-633-3777; Fax: 404-633-1870

www.acr@rheumatology.org
American Occupational Therapy Association (AOTA)
4720 Montgomery Lane
P.O. Box 31220
Bethesda, MD 20824–1220
Tel: 301-652-7711, 800-377-8555 (TDD), 1-800-SAY-
AOTA
www.aota.org
The American Orthopedic Society for Sports Medicine
6300 N. River Road Suite 500
Rosemont, IL 60018
Tel: 847-292-4900
www.sportsmed.org
American Podiatric Medical Association, Inc.
9312 Old Georgetown Road
Bethesda, MD 20814–1621
Tel: 1-800-FOOTCARE
www.apma.org
American Physical Therapy Association (APTA)
111 N. Fairfax Street
Alexandria, VA 22314–1488
Tel: 1-800-999-2782, 703-683-6748 (TDD)
www.apta.org
Juvenile Arthritis Information
www.rheumatology.org/patient/jra.htm

Research Centers and Institutes

Arthritis Center
Boston University
Conte Building
71 E. Newton Street
Boston, MA 02118
Tel: 617-534-5#4
Arthritis Center
University of Missouri-Columbia
MA427 Health Sciences Center
1 Hospital Drive
Columbia, MO 65212
Tel: 314-882-8738
Missouri Arthritis Rehabilitation Research and Training
Center
Walter Williams Hall
Room 13
Columbia, MO 65211

Tel: 1-877-882-6826
marrtc@missouri.edu
National Arthritis and Musculoskeletal and Skin Dis-
eases
Information Clearinghouse (NAMSIC)
9000 Rockville Pike
PO Box AMS
Bethesda, MD 20892
Tel: 301-495-4484
www.niams.nih.gov/
University of Connecticut Health Center
School of Medicine
Division of Rheumatic Diseases
263 Farmington Avenue
Farmington, CT 06030–1310
Tel: 860-679-3605
www.penguin.uchc.edu/rheum
Adaptive Aids
These companies have catalogs that contain resources
for those with arthritis.
AliMed Rehabilitation Products, Inc.
297 High Street
Dedham, MA 02026–9135
Tel: 1-800—255-2160
www.alimed.com
Amigo Mobility International, Inc.
6692 Dixie Highway
Bridgeport, MI 48722–9725
Tel: 1-800-248-9131
info @myamigo.com
DeRoyal/LMB, Inc.
P.O. Box 1181
San Luis Obispo, CA 93406
Tel: 1–800-541-3992
Independent Living Aids, Inc.
27 East Mall
Plainview, NY 11803
Tel: 1-800-537—2118
Invacare Corporation
899 Cleveland Street
Elyria, OH

REFERENCES

Adams, J., Burridge, J., Mullee, M., Hammond, A., & Cooper, C. (2004). Correlation between upper limb functional ability and structural hand impairment in an early rheumatoid population. *Clinical Rehabilitation, 18*(4), 405–413.

Adams, J., Mullee, M., Burridge, J., Hammond, A., & Cooper, C. (2010). Responsiveness of self-report and therapist-rated upper extremity structural impairment and functional outcome measures in early rheumatoid arthritis. *Arthritis Care & Research, 62*(2), 274–278.

Adib, N., Hyrich, K., Thornton, J., Lunt, M., Davidson, J., et al. (2008). Association between duration of symptoms and severity of disease at first presentation to paediatric rheumatology: Results from the Childhood Arthritis Prospective Study. *Rheumatology, 47*(7), 991–995.

Allaire, S., Wolfe, F., Niu, J., LaValley, M. P., Zhana, B., & Reisine, S. (2009). Current risk factors for work disability associated with rheumatoid arthritis: Recent data from a US national cohort. *Arthritis Care & Research, 61*(3), 321–328.

Amezcua-Guerra, L. M. (2009). Overlap between systemic lupus erythematosus and rheumatoid arthritis: Is it real or just and illusion. *The Journal of Rheumatology, 36*(1), 4–6.

Arnett, F. (1996). Rheumatoid arthritis. In J. C. Bennett & F. Plum (Eds.), *Cecil's textbook of medicine* (Vol. 2) (20th ed.). Philadelphia, PA: WB Saunders Co.

Ashe, M. C., McCauley, T., & Khan, K. M. (2004). Tendenopathies in the upper extremity: A paradigm shift. *Journal of Hand Therapy, 17*(3), 329–334.

Baecklund, E., Askling, J., Rosenquist, R., Ekbom, A., & Klareskog, L. (2004). Rheumatoid arthritis and malignant lymphomas. *Current Opinion in Rheumatology, 16*(3), 254–261.

Bai, M., Tomenson, B., Creed, F., Mantis, D., Tsifetaki, N., Voulgan, P. V., et al. (2009). The role of psychological distress and personality variables in the disablement process in rheumatoid arthritis. *Scandivanian Journal of Rheumatology, 38*(6), 419–430.

Baiza-Duran, L., Medrano-Palafox, J., Hernandez-Quintela, E., Lozano-Alcazar, J., & Alaniz-de la O, J. F. (2010). A comparative clinical trial of the efficacy of two different aqueous solutions of cyclosporine for the treatment of moderate-to-severe dry eye syndrome. *British Journal of Opthalmology, 94*(10), 1312–1315.

Barr, A. E., Barbe, M. F., & Clark, B. D. (2004). Work-related musculoskeletal disorders of the hand and wrist: Epidemiology, pathophysiology, and sensorimotor changes. *Journal of Orthopedic Sports Physical Therapy, 34*(10), 610–627.

Beers, M. H., & Berkow, R. (Eds.) (1999). Rheumatoid arthritis. In *The Merck Manual of Diagnosis and Therapy* (17th ed.). New York, NY: John Wiley & Sons.

Berjawi, G., Uthman, I., Mahfoud, L., Husseini, S. T., Nassar, J., Kotobi, A., et al. (2010). Cricothyroid joint abnormalities in patients with rheumatoid arthritis. *Journal of Voice, 24*(6), 732–737.

Birnbaum, H., Pike, C., Kaufman, R., Maynchenko, Y., Kidolezi, Y., & Cifaldi, M. (2010). Societal cost of rheumatoid arthritis patients in the U.S. *Current Medical Research and Opinion, 26*(1), 77–90.

Bolen, J., Schieb, L., Hootman, J. M., Helmick, C. G., Theis, K., Murphy, L. B, et al. (2010). Differences in the prevalence and impact of arthritis among racial/ethnic groups in the United States, National Health Interview Survey, 2002, 2003, and 2006. *Preventing Chronic Disease, 7*(3), A64.

Book, C., Karlsson, M. K., Akesson, K., & Jacobsson, L. T. H. (2009). Early rheumatoid arthritis and body composition. *British Society of Rheumatology, 48*(9), 1128–1132.

Burns, P. R., Scanlon, R. L., Zgonis, T., & Lowery, C. (2005). Pathologic conditions of the heel: Tumors and arthritides. *Clinical Podiatric Medicine and Surgery, 22*(1), 115–136.

Centers for Disease Control and Prevention. (2003). Direct and indirect costs of arthritis and other rheumatic conditions in the United States. (1997). *Morbidity and Mortality Weekly Report, 52*, 1124–1127.

Chandra, P. A. (2008). Rituximab is useful in the treatment of Felty's Syndrome. *American Journal of Therapeutics, 15*(4), 321–322.

Christiansen, C. Matuska, K. (2004). *Ways of living: Adaptive strategies for special needs.* Bethesda: AOTA Press

Colbert, R. A. (2010). Classification of juvenile spondyloarthritis: Enthesitis-related arthritis and beyond. *Nature Reviews Rheumatology, 6*, 477–485.

Cordery, J. & Rocchi (1998). Joint protection and fatigue management. In J. Melvin & G. Jensen (Eds.), Rheumatologic Rehabilitation Series, Vol. 1: Assessment and Management. Bethesda, MD; American Occupational Therapy Association.

Costa, M., Rizak, T., & Zimmerman, B. (2004). Rheumatologic conditions of the foot. *Journal of the American Podiatric Medical Association, 94*(2), 177–186.

Crowther, C. L. (2001). The effects of corticosteroids on the musculoskeletal system. *Orthopedic Nursing, 20*(6), 33–39.

Escalante, A., & dle Ricon, I. (2001). Epidemiology and the impact of rheumatic disorders in the United States. *Current Opinions in Rheumatology, 13*, 104–110.

Fendler, C., & Braun, J. (2009). Clinical measures in rheumatoid arthritis and ankylosing spondylitis. *Clinical & Experimental Rheumatology, 27*(55), S80–S82.

Finckh, A., Bansback, N., Marra, C., Anis, A. H., Michaud, K., Lubin, S., et al. (2009). Treatment of very early rheumatoid arthritis with symptomatic therapy, disease-modifying antirheumatic drugs, or biologic agents. *Annals of Internal Medicine, 151*(9), 612–621.

Foster, H., & Rapley, T. (2010). Access to pediatirc rheumatology care-a major challenge to improving outcome in juvenile idiopathic arthritis. *The Journal of Rheumatology, 37*(11), 2199–2202.

Fouque-Aubert, A., Chapurlat, R., Miossec, P., & Delmas, P. D. (2009). A comparative review of the different techniques to assess hand bone damage in rheumatoid arthritis. *Joint Bone Spine, 77*(3), 212–217.

Fowler, N. K., & Nicol, A. C. (2001). Functional and biomechanical assessment of the normal and rheumatoid hand. *Biomechanics, 16*(8), 660–666.

Gewanter, H. L., Rohnmann, K. J., & Baum, J. (2005). The prevalence of juvenile arthritis. *Arthritis & Rheumatism, 26*(5), 599–603.

Gomes-Carreira, A. C., Jones, A., & Natour, J. (2010). Assessment of the effectiveness of a functional splint for osteoarthritis of the trapeziometacarpal joint of the dominant hand: A randomized controlled study. *Journal of Rehabilitation, 42*, 469–474.

Goronzy, J. J., Matteson, E. L., Fulbright, J. W., Warrington, K. J., Chang-Miller, A., & Hunder, G. G., et al. (2004). Prognostic markers of radiographic progression in early rheumatoid arthritis. *Arthritis & Rheumatism, 50*(1), 43–54.

Goronzy, J. J., & Weyand, C. M. (1997). Rheumatoid arthritis: Epidemiology, pathology, and pathogenesis. In H. J. Klippel, C. M. Weyand, & R. L. Wortman (Eds.), *Primer on the rheumatic diseases* (11th ed.) Atlanta: Arthritis Foundation.

Grotte, M., Garratt, A. M., Klokkerud, M., Lochting, I., Uhlig, T., & Hagen, K. B. (2010). What's in team rehabilitation care after arthroplasty for osteoarthritis? Results from a multi-center, longitudinal study assessing structure, process, and outcome. *Journal of the American Physical Therapy Association, 90*(1), 121–131.

Hanly, J. G., Omisade, A., Su, L., Farewell, V., & Fisk, D. (2010). Assessment of cognitive function in systemic lupus erythematosus, rheumatoid arthritis, and multiple sclerosis by computerized neuropsychological tests. *Arthritis & Rheumatism, 62*(5), 1478–1486.

Harrop, J. S., Hanna, A., Silva, M., & Sharan, A. (2007). Neurological manifestations of cervical spondylosis: An overview of signs, symptoms, and pathophysiology. *Neurosurgery, 60*(1), 14–20.

Helmick, C. G., Felson, D. T., Lawrence, R. C., Gabriel, S., Hirsch, R., et al. (2007). Estimates of the prevalence of arthritis and other rheumatic conditions in the United States: Part I. *Arthritis & Rheumatism, 58*(1), 15–25.

Hochberg, M. C., Johnston, S. S., & John, A. K., (2008). The incidence and prevalence of extra-articular and systemic manifestations in a cohort of newly-diagnosed patients with rheumatoid arthritis between 1999 and 2006. *Current Medical Research and Opinion, 24*(2), 469–480.

Hofer, M., & Southwood, T. R. (2002). Classification of childhood arthritis. *Clinical Rheumatology, 16*(3), 379–396.

Jaakkola, J. I., & Mann, R. A. (2005). Managing foot and ankle problems in RA. *Journal of Musculoskeletal Medicine, 22*(1), 30–32.

Josefsson, K. A., & Gard, G. (2010). Women's experiences of sexual health when living with rheumatoid arthritis-an explorative qualitative study. *Musculoskeletal Disorders, 11*, 240–248.

Joyce, A. T., Smith, P., Khandker, R., Melin, J. M., & Singh, A. (2009). Hidden cost of rheumatoid arthritis (RA): Estimating cost of co-morbid cardiovascular disease and depression among patients with RA. *Journal of Rheumatology 36*(4), 743–752.

Kasper, D. L., Braunwald, E., Fauci, A., Longo, D., Jameson, J. L., & Fauci, A. S. (Eds.) (2004). *Harrison's principles of internal medicine* (16th ed.). New York: McGraw-Hill.

Kessler, R., Maclean, J. R., Petukhova, M., Sarawate, C., Short, L., Li, T. T., & Stang, P. E. (2008). The effects of rheumatoid arthritis on labor force participation, work performance, and healthcare costs in two workplace samples. *Journal of occupational & Environmental Medicine, 50*(1), 88–98.

Kim, E. J., Collard, H. R., & King, T. E. (2009). Rheumatoid arthritis-associated interstitial lung disease: The relevance of histopathologic and radiographic pattern. *Chest, 136*(5), 1397–1405.

Kumar, K., Daley, E., Carruthers, D. M., Situnayake, D., Gordon, C., Grindulis, K., et al. (2007). Delay in presentation to primary care physicians is the main reason why patients with rheumatoid arthritis are seen late by rheumatologists. *British Journal of Rheumatology, 49*(9), 1438–1440.

Iikuni, N., Sato, E., Hoshi, M., Inoue, E., Taniguchi, A., Hara, M., et al. (2009). The influence of sex on patients with rheumatoid arthritis in a large observational cohort. *The Journal of Rheumatology, 36*(3), 508–511.

Lorig, K. R., Ritter, P. L., Laurent, D. D., & Plant, K. (2008). The internet-based arthritis self-management program: A one-year randomized trial for patients with arthritis or fibromyalgia. *Arthritis Care & Research, 59*(7), 1009–1017.

Lundkvist, J., Kastang, F., & Kobelt, G. (2008). The burden of rheumatoid arthritis and access to treatment: Health burden and costs. *The European Journal of Health Economics, 8*(2), 49–60.

Maloney, M. D., & Ryder, S. (2003). Multiple overlapping causes and symptoms can complicate the differential diagnosis and management of shoulder disorders. *Journal of Musculoskeletal Medicine, 20*(9), 412–418.

Matschke, V., Murphy, P., Lemmy, A. B., Maddison, P. J., & Thom, J. M. (2009). Muscle quality, architecture, and activation in cachetic patients with rheumatoid arthritis. *The Journal of Rheumatology, 37*(2), 282–284.

Melchiorre, D., Falcini, F., Kaloudi, O., Bandinelli, F., Naccia, F., & Cerinica, M. M. (2010). Sonographic evaluation of the temporomandibular joints in juvenile idiopathic arthritis. *Journal of Ultrasound, 13*(1), 34–37.

Mink, J. H., Gordon, R. E., & Deutsch, A. L. (2003). The cervical spine: Radiologist's perspective. *Physical Medicine and Rehabilitation Clinic of North America, 14*(3), 493–548.

Murdin, L., Patel., Walmsley, J., & Yeoh, L. H. (2008). Hearing difficulties are common in patients with rheumatoid arthritis. *Clinical Rheumatology, 27*(5), 637–640.

Neumann, D. A., & Bielefeld, T. (2003). The carpometacarpal joint of the thumb: Stability, deformity, and therapeutic intervention. *Journal of Orthopedic Sports Physical Therapy, 33*(7), 386–399.

Niere, K., & Jerak, A. (2004). Measurement of headache frequency, intensity and duration: comparison of patient report by questionnaire and headache diary. *Physiotherapy Research International, 9*(4), 149–156.

Nizam, S., Johnstone, A., Green, M., & Gough, A. (2009). Necrotising scleritis and connective tissue disease—Three cases and review. *Clinical Rheumatology, 28*(3), 339–341.

Oldfield, V., & Felson, D. (2008). Exercise therapy and orthotic devices in rheumatoid arthritis: Evidence-based review. *Current Opinion in Rheumatology, 20*(3), 353–359.

Otter, S. J., Lucas, K., Springett, K., Moore, A., Davies, K., Cheek, L. et al. (2010). Foot pain in rheumatoid arthritis prevalence, risk factors and management: An epidemiological study. *Clinical Rheumatology, 29*(3), 255–271.

Piper, H., Douglas, K., Treharne, G. J., Milton, D. L., Haider, S., & Kitas, G. D. (2007). Prevalence and predictors of ocular manifestations of RA: Is there a need for routine screening? *Musculoskeletal Care, 5*(2), 102–117.

Rallon, C. R., & Chen, C. C. (2008). Relationship between performance-based and self-reported assessment of hand function. *The American Journal of Occupational Therapy, 62*(5), 574–579.

Rannou, F., Poiraudeau, S., Berezne, A., Baubet, T., Le-guern, V., Cabane, J., et al. (2007). Assessing disability and quality of life in systemic sclerosis: Construct validities of the Cochin Hand Function Scale, Health Assessment Questionnaire (HAQ), Systemic Sclerosis HAQ, and medical Outcomes Study 36-item short form survey. *Arthritis Care & Research, 57*(1), 94–102.

Raven, E., Haverkamp, D., Sierevelt, I. N., van Montfoort, D. O., Poll, R. G., Blankevoort, L., & Tak, P. P. (2008). Construct validity and reliability of the Disability of Arm, Shoulder and Hand Questionaire for upper extremity complaints in rheumatoid arthritis. *The Journal of Rheumatology, 35*(12), 2334–2338.

Reiff, A. (2009). Ocular complications of childhood rheumatic diseases: Nonuveitic inflammatory eye diseases. *Current Rheumatology Reports, 11*(3), 226–232.

Rothchild, B. M., & Woods, R. J. (1990). Symmetrical erosive disease in Archaic Indians: The origin of rheumatoid arthritis in the New World. *Seminars in Arthritis and Rheumatism, 19,* 278–284.

Sen, M., & Carson, D. A. (2003). RA: Learning from its origins and development. *Journal of Medical Microbiology, 20*(11), 497–499, 503–506.

Siegel, L. B., & Gall, E. P. (1999). A systematic approach to the physical examination in RA: Part 2: The hip, lower extremities, and extra-articular systems. *Journal of Musculoskeletal Rehabilitation, 16*(7), 392–394.

Simkin, P. A. (1997). The musculoskeletal system: Joints. In H. J. Klippel, C. M. Weyand, & R. L. Wortman (Eds.). *Primer on the rheumatic diseases* (11th ed.). Atlanta, GA: Arthritis Foundation.

Sokka, T., Abelson, B., & Pincus, T. (2008). Mortality in rheumatoid arthritis: 2008 update. *Clinical Experimental Rheumatology, 26*(51), S35–S61.

Stock, H., Kadry, Z., & Smith, J. P. (2009). Surgical management of portal hypertension in Felty's syndrome: A case report and literature review. *Journal of Hepatology, 50*(4), 831–835.

Strauss, E. J., Alfonso, D., Baidwan, G., & Cesare, P. E. (2008). Orthopedic manifestations and management of psoriatic arthritis. *American Journal of Orthopedics, 37*(3), 138–147.

Symmons, D. P. M. (2007). Classification criteria for rheumatoid arthritis—Time to abandon rheumatoid factor? *British Journal of Rheumatology, 46*(5), 725–726.

Trombley, C. C. (1995). *Theoretical foundations for practice.* In C. A. Trombley, (Ed.), *Occupational therapy for physical dysfunction* (4th ed.) (pp. 15–27).

Turesson, C., McClelland, R. L., Christianson, T. J. H., & Matteson, E. L. (2007). Severe extra-articular disease manifestations are associated with an increased risk of first ever cardiovascular events in patients with rheumatoid arthritis. *Annals of Rheumatic Diseases, 66,* 70–75.

van Vollenhoven, R. F. (2009). Treatment of rheumatoid arthritis: State of the art 2009. *Nature Reviews Rheumatology, 5,* 531–541.

Verschueren, P., Esselens, G., & Westhovens, R. (2009). Predictors of remission, normalized physical function, and changes in the working situation during follow-up of patients with early rheumatoid arthritis: An observational study. *Scandinavian Journal of Rheumatology,* 38(3), 166–172.

Walgee, J. F., Burns, P., & Chung, K. C. (2010). Validity of the Michigan Hand Outcomes Questionnaire for rheumatoid arthritis: A multi-center study. *Plastic and Reconstructive Surgery, 125*(6), 46.

Williams, S. B., Brand, C. A., Hill, K. D., Hunt, S. B., & Moran, H. (2010). Feasibility and outcomes of a home-based exercise program on improving balance vand gait stability in women with lower-limb osteoarthritis or rheumatoid arthritis: A pilot study. *Archives of Physical Medicine and Rehabilitation, 91*(1), 106–114.

Wolfe, F., & Michaud, K. (2009). Predicting depression in rheumatoid arthritis: The signal importance of pain extent and fatigue, and co-morbidity. *Arthritis Care & Research, 61*(5), 667–673.

Zolcinski, M., Bazan-Socha, S., Zwolinski, G., & Musial, J. (2008). Central nervous system involvement as a major manifestation of rheumatoid arthritis. *Rheumatology International, 28*(3), 281–283.

16

Spinal Cord Injury

■ *Laura V. Miller*

… of the many forms of disability which can beset mankind, a severe injury or disease of the spinal cord undoubtedly constitutes one of the most devastating calamities in human life. (Guttmann, 1976)

—Sir Ludwig Guttmann, pioneer in 20th-century management of spinal cord injury

The future lies in our own hands, and if a challenge should enter our life, it is important to remember we have tremendous strength, courage, and ability to overcome any obstacle.

—Douglas Heir, Esq., Attorney-at-Law (Personal communication, December 1994)

The full impact of the preceding quotes may not strike the reader unless the whole story is known. The latter author, Doug Heir, sustained a spinal cord injury (SCI) at age 18. He dove into a pool to save a boy who appeared to be drowning. The boy was only playing, but Doug's injury resulted in tetraplegia. Decades later, Doug has become known for being many things, among them an author, the U.S. ambassador to the Soviet Union, the cover athlete for Wheaties cereal, an associate legal editor of the National Trial Lawyer, and a gold medalist in the 1988 Olympics in Seoul, South Korea—an impressive list of accomplishments for someone who sustained "one of the most devastating calamities in human life!"

The goals of the health care team should include empowering clients to take charge of their futures. To accomplish this, the health professional must understand the complexities of the diagnosis. This chapter explores the ramifications of spinal cord injuries, beginning with a brief overview of the central nervous system (CNS) and surrounding structures.

DESCRIPTION AND DEFINITIONS

Overview of CNS and Related Structures

The brain and spinal cord make up the CNS. The spinal cord receives sensory (afferent) information from the peripheral nervous system and transmits this information to higher structures (i.e., the thalamus, cerebellum, cerebral cortex) in the CNS. Descending motor (efferent) information, originating from the cortex, is also transmitted by the spinal cord back to the peripheral nervous system.

The consistency of the spinal cord has been compared to a ripe banana, and it is fortunate that the spinal cord and cerebral cortex are protected by bony structures. Whereas the skull protects the brain, the vertebral column protects the spinal cord. The vertebral column is composed of 33 vertebrae, with 7 cervical vertebrae in the neck region (C1 through C7); 12 thoracic vertebrae in the chest region (T1 through T12); 5 lumbar vertebrae in the midback region (L1 through L5); 5 sacral vertebrae (S1 through S5), which are actually fused in the lower back and pelvic region; and 4 fused coccygeal vertebrae that make up the coccyx or tailbone (Fig. 16.1). There are 31 pairs of spinal nerves, which exit from the spinal cord and branch to form the peripheral nervous system. The nerves exit through the openings formed between each two vertebrae. The spinal nerves are named according to the vertebrae above or below their point of exit. Note that spinal nerves C1 through C7 exit *above* the corresponding vertebrae, whereas the remaining spinal nerves (C8 through S5) exit *below* the corresponding vertebrae. Thus, although there are seven cervical vertebrae, there are eight cervical spinal nerves. The actual spinal cord ends just below the L1 vertebra. However, some spinal nerves continue and exit beyond the point where the spinal cord ends. Because of their visual resemblance, this bundle of nerves is referred to as the **cauda equina**, which is Latin for horse's tail (Hanak & Scott, 1983). The meningeal covering of the spinal cord, which contains the cerebrospinal fluid (CSF) that bathes the structures of the CNS, also extends past the end of the spinal cord to the L4 vertebral level. The CSF-filled meningeal space between L2 and L4, referred to as the lumbar cistern, is the site where diagnostic or therapeutic lumbar punctures, that is, spinal taps, are performed, because the spinal cord is not present, yet CSF is accessible.

Sensory and Motor Tracts

The terms tract, pathway, lemniscus, and fasciculus all refer to bundles of nerve fibers that have a similar function and travel through the spinal cord in a particular area. It is important to know the names, locations, and functions

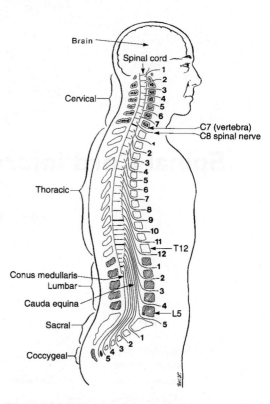

Figure 16.1 The spinal cord, spinal nerves, and vertebral column. (Reprinted with permission from the Rehabilitation Institute of Michigan.)

of these tracts to understand the possible outcomes of an SCI at a given level. Figure 16.2 shows the location of major tracts within a cross section of the spinal cord.

Two basic types of nerve tissue make up the spinal cord. Gray matter is located centrally and resembles a butterfly in cross sections of the cord. Gray matter is composed of cell bodies and synapses. White matter encompasses most of the periphery of the cord and contains the ascending and descending pathways. Table 16-1 provides a more detailed description of the functions of the various sensory and motor pathways that travel through the white matter of the spinal cord. It may be helpful to remember that many pathways are named according to their origin and the location of their final synapse (e.g., spinocerebellar, corticospinal).

Specific motor and sensory information is carried by each pair of spinal nerves. In general, the cervical nerves (C1 through C8) carry afferent and efferent impulses for the head, neck, diaphragm, arms, and hands. The thoracic spinal nerves (T1 through T12) serve the chest and upper abdominal musculature. The lumbar spinal nerves (L1 through L5) carry information to and from the legs and a portion of the foot, and the sacral spinal nerves (S1 through S5) carry impulses for the remaining foot musculature, bowel, bladder, and the muscles involved in sexual

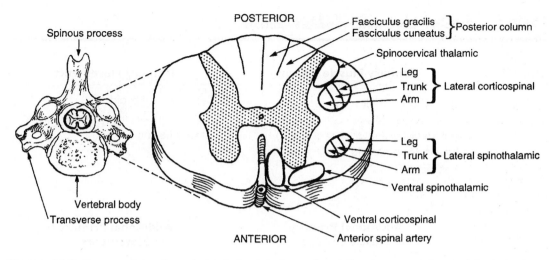

Figure 16.2 Cross section of cervical spinal cord, shown in relation to surrounding vertebral structures. Selected ascending and descending pathways are illustrated. (Adapted with permission from Rehabilitation Institute of Michigan.)

functioning. Table 16-2 and Figure 16.3 present a more detailed outline of muscles innervated by each level of the spinal cord and a dermatomal segmentation (sensory map) of the body.

Reflex Arc

Most nerve impulses move up the spinal cord to the brain and back through the cord to the peripheral nerves.

However, some impulses directly enter the cord through the dorsal nerve root, synapse, and exit by the ventral nerve root. This causes certain muscle functions or responses to occur without direction from the brain. A simple example of this "looping" can be seen in the knee-jerk reflex. If the knee is tapped with a reflex hammer, the knee will extend without any influence from the brain. The stimulation by the hammer causes afferent impulses to enter the cord, synapse, and exit, causing a contraction

TABLE 16.1 Noninclusive Listing of Ascending and Descending Pathways

Ascending Afferent (Sensory) Pathways	Function
Spinocerebellar	Nonconscious proprioception
Lateral spinothalamic	Pain, temperature
Ventral spinothalamic	Touch, pressure
Fasciculus gracilis/fasciculus cuneatus[a]	Two-point tactile discrimination, vibration, conscious proprioception stereognosis
Spinocervicothalamic	Touch, proprioception, stereognosis, vibration
Descending efferent (motor) pathways	Function
Lateral corticospinal	Movement to extremities
Ventral corticospinal	Movement of neck and trunk
Vestibulospinal	Equilibrium
Reticulospinal	Autonomic functions: motor respiratory functions

[a]Called the posterior column.

TABLE 16.2 Spinal Cord Innervations/Function

Spinal Cord Level	Primary Muscle Groups	Primary Movements
C1-3	Infrahyoid muscles Head/neck extension Rectus capitis (anterior and lateral) Sternocleidomastoid Longus colli Longus capitis Scaleni	Depression of hyoid Neck extension, flexion, rotation, and lateral flexion
	Additional Primary Muscle Groups	**Additional Primary Movements**
C4	Trapezius Upper cervical paraspinals Diaphragm	Shoulder elevation, scapular adduction, and depression Independent breathing
C5	Rhomboids Deltoids Rotator cuff muscles (partially—some nerve supply is at C6 level) Biceps Brachialis (partially) Brachioradialis (partially)	Scapular downward rotation Weak shoulder external rotation, flexion, and extension Shoulder abduction and rotation Weak approximation of humeral head to glenoid fossa Elbow flexion
C6	Rotator cuff muscles (complete innervation) Serratus anterior (partially) Pectoralis (clavicular segments) Total innervation of elbow flexors Supinators Extensor carpi radialis Flexor carpi radialis	Full shoulder rotation, adduction, flexion, extension Scapular abduction Horizontal shoulder adduction Strong elbow flexion and supination Wrist extension (weak) Tenodesis action of hand Very weak wrist flexion
C7	Latissimus dorsi Pectoralis major (sternal portion) Triceps Pronator teres Flexor carpi radialis Flexor digitorum superficialis Extensor digitorum (partially) Extensor pollicis longus and brevis	Elbow extension Forearm pronation Wrist flexion Finger flexion (trace) Finger extension (weak) Thumb extension (weak)

TABLE 16.2 Spinal Cord Innervations/Function *(Continued)*

Spinal Cord Level	Primary Muscle Groups	Primary Movements
C8	Flexor carpi ulnaris	Complete wrist extension, adduction, and abduction
	Extensor carpi ulnaris	Finger flexion (stronger)
	Flexor digitorum profundus and superficialis	Thumb flexion, abduction, adduction, and opposition
	Flexor pollicis longus and brevis	Weak flexion at MCP with IP extension
	Abductor pollicis longus	
	Abductor pollicis	
	Opponens policies	
	Lumbricals (partially)	
T1	Dorsal interossei	Finger abduction
	Palmar interossei	Finger adduction
	Abductor pollicis brevis	Thumb abduction (strong)
	Lumbricals (complete innervation)	MCP flexion with IP extension (strong)
	Erector spinae muscles (partially)	Thoracic spine extension
	Intercostal muscles (partially)	Increased respiratory function with presence of intercostals
T4-8	Erector spinae muscles (partially)	Stronger thoracic spine extension
	Intercostal muscles (partially)	Stronger respiratory function
	Abdominal muscles (beginning at T7)	Thoracic flexion
		Weak trunk flexion
T9-12	Lower erector spinae muscles	Strong thoracic spine extension
	Lower intercostal muscles Abdominal muscles	Trunk flexion, extension, rotation, and stability
	Quadratus lumborum (partially)	Pelvic control and stability
L1-3	Quadratus lumborum (full innervation)	Pelvic elevation
	Iliopsoas	Hip flexion
	Erector spinae (lumbar segment)	Lumbar extension
L4-5	Lumbar erector spinae	Lumbar extension and stability
	Hip adductors	Hip adduction
	Hip rotators	Hip rotation
	Quadriceps	Knee extension
	Hamstrings (partially)	Knee flexion (weak)
	Tibialis anterior	Ankle dorsiflexion (weak)

(Continued)

TABLE 16.2 Spinal Cord Innervations/Function *(Continued)*

Spinal Cord Level	Primary Muscle Groups	Primary Movements
S1-2	Hip extensors	Hip extension
	Hip abductors	Hip abduction and stability
	Hamstrings (complete innervation)	Knee flexion
	Plantar flexors	Ankle plantar: flexion
	Invertors of ankle	Ankle inversion and stability
	Evertors of ankle	Ankle eversion and stability
S2-5	Bladder	Genitourinary functions
	Lower bowel	Bowel functions
	Genital innervations	

MCP, metacarpophalangeal; IP, interphalangeal.

of the muscle fibers (Fig. 16.4). This activity is called a **reflex arc**. In persons with an intact spinal cord, afferent nerve impulses also travel to the brain almost instantaneously. This allows an awareness, or "feeling," of the initial stimulation (knee tap) and subsequent response (knee jerk). This concept is important to an understanding of SCIs. It explains why some individuals with SCI continue to have reflexes, but do not have voluntary control of their muscles. It also explains why others have no reflexes at all below the level of their injury. This is discussed in much greater detail in the section on classification of injuries.

ETIOLOGY

Historically, many demographic sources attempted to count the number of persons who have sustained SCIs. Since 1973, the National Spinal Cord Injury Database has been in existence, making strides in collecting comprehensive data on a national level. In 1985, the Centers for Disease Control and Prevention began promoting surveillance mechanisms at state and national levels for the collection and reporting of these data. Prior to this time, data related to etiology and incidence of SCI in the United States were inconsistently collected and lacked uniformity; advancements are continuing to be made in this area.

The leading cause of SCI in the United States is motor vehicle accidents, followed by falls and acts of violence (Fig. 16.5). Sports-related injuries account for most of the remaining SCIs, with diving being historically the most common (and preventable) cause (Table 16-3).

Analyzing the etiology of SCIs helps target prevention programs. Public awareness of the effects of using substances while operating a vehicle is certainly heightened. Tougher penalties for driving under the influence of cognitive altering substances have been enacted, and many states have adopted seat belt, child restraint, and "distracted" driving legislation. All of these efforts have the potential to reduce the leading cause of SCI. Grant monies have even been awarded to hospital-based programs that evaluate the home environments of senior citizens for safety. Their recommendations may reduce the risk of falls—a major cause of SCI in the elderly. An innovative effort sponsored by the University of Michigan Health System involves airing public service announcements on the prevention of diving injuries before the "coming attractions trailers" at popular movies for teens during the summer months.

Although much of the literature focuses on trauma, there are many nontraumatic causes of spinal cord damage (http://www.spinalcord.uab.edu). Developmental conditions such as spina bifida, **scoliosis**, and spinal cord agenesis may yield many of the same clinical signs as traumatic SCI. Acquired conditions, such as bacterial or viral infections, benign or malignant growths, embolisms, thromboses, hemorrhages, and even radiation or vaccinations, can also lead to damage of spinal cord tissue.

INCIDENCE AND PREVALENCE

Incidence rates for SCI in the United States are estimated at 40 cases/million population/year, excluding those who die at the scene of an accident (http://www.spinalcord.uab.edu). This translates to about 12,000 new cases of SCI every year. The statistics indicate that over 80% of persons who sustain spinal cord injuries are male; notably, the mean age at the time of injury has increased from 28.7 years in the 1970s to the

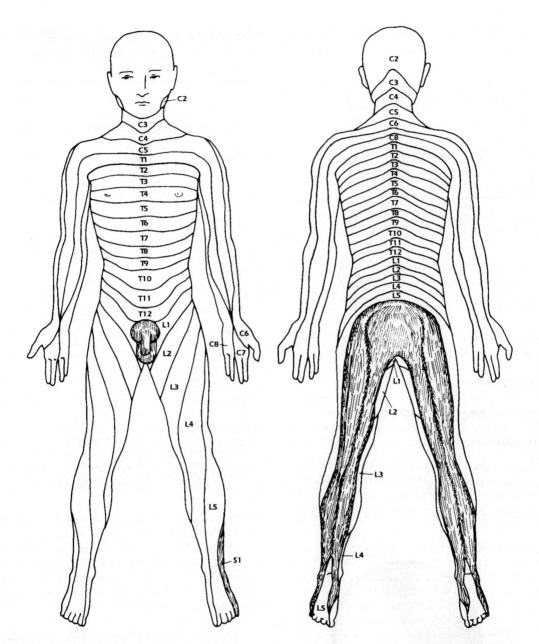

Figure 16.3 Dermatome map. (Reprinted with permission from Hammond, M., Umlauf, R. L., Matteson, B., & Perduta-Fulginiti, S. (Eds.). (1989). *Yes You Can! A Guide to Self Care for Persons with Spinal Cord Injury.* Washington, DC: Paralyzed Veterans of America.)

present mean age of 40.2 years (National Spinal Cord Injury Statistical Center, 2009a). Seasonal sports cause fluctuations in etiology and incidence statistics throughout a given year, and some urban hospitals are reporting that a disproportionate number of their SCI cases are caused by acts of violence (National Spinal Cord Injury Statistical Center b). In the United States, of the spinal cord injuries reported to the national database since 2005, 66.2% of individuals were identified as Caucasian, 27% African American, 2% Asian, and 7.9% Hispanic (http://www.spinalcord.uab.edu). One may be tempted to conclude from these statistics that Caucasians are at higher risk for sustaining spinal cord injuries, but this would be erroneous. When compared to the composition of the general population, spinal cord injuries have a higher incidence among non-Caucasians (http://www.spinalcord.uab.edu.; Fine, Kuhlemeier, Devivo, & Stover, 1979).

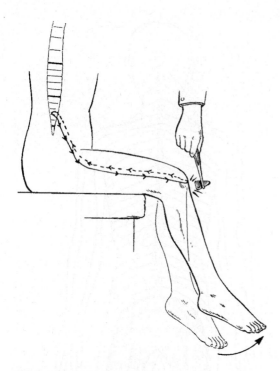

Figure 16.4 Knee-jerk reflex.

SIGNS AND SYMPTOMS

Sensory Functions

The two major classifications of SCI are complete and incomplete. A complete SCI occurs with a complete transection of the cord. In this case, all ascending and descending pathways are interrupted, and there is a

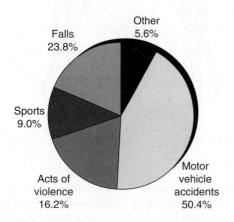

Figure 16.5 Etiologic distribution of SCI since 2005. (Adapted from Spinal Cord Injury Facts and Figures at a Glance, 2010, a publication of the National Spinal Cord Injury Statistical Center. (2010). Birmingham, AL: University of Alabama at Birmingham.)

TABLE 16.3 Comparison of Select Sports-Related Spinal Cord Injuries

Sport	No. of Reported Injuries—2009	Percentage
Diving	1,676	59.4
Bicycling	328	11.6
Football	136	5.7
Snow skiing	127	4.5
Horseback riding	121	4.3
Other winter sports	115	4.1
Surfing	98	3.5
Wrestling	83	2.9
Trampoline	60	2.1
Gymnastics	48	1.7
Waterskiing	30	1.1

Developed with data from The National Spinal Cord Injury Statistical Center. (2008). Annual Statistical Report (p. 32). University of Alabama at Birmingham.

total loss of motor and sensory function below the level of injury. The injury also may be referred to as an upper motor neuron (UMN) injury, if the reflex arcs are intact below the level of injury but are no longer mediated by the brain. UMN lesions are characterized by (a) a loss of voluntary function below the level of the injury, (b) spastic paralysis, (c) no muscle atrophy, and (d) hyperactive reflexes (Fig. 16.6).

Complete injuries below the level of the conus medullaris (see Fig. 16.1) are referred to as lower motor neuron (LMN) injuries, because the injury has affected the spinal nerves after they exit from the cord. In fact, injuries involving spinal nerves after they exit the cord at any level are referred to as LMN injuries. In these injuries, the reflex arc cannot occur, because impulses cannot enter the cord to synapse. As a result, LMN injuries are characterized by (a) a loss of voluntary function below the level of the injury, (b) flaccid paralysis, (c) muscle atrophy, and (d) absence of reflexes.

UMN and LMN injuries may be complete or incomplete. There also may be a mixture of UMN and LMN

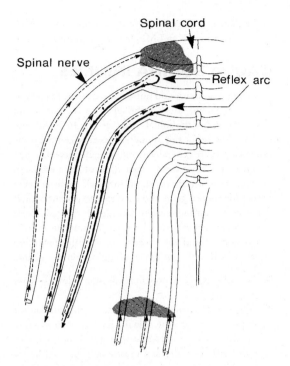

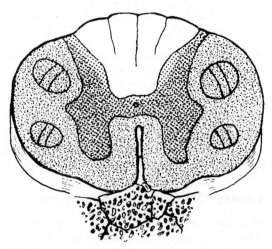

Figure 16.7 A cross section of the spinal cord illustrating the damage that causes anterior cord syndrome. The anterior artery is involved, resulting in damage to most areas, with the exception of the posterior columns. (Reprinted with permission from the Rehabilitation Institute of Michigan.)

Figure 16.6 A diagrammatic representation of the reflex arc. The shaded lesion above denotes a UMN lesion, with the exception of the spinal nerve entering at the level of the lesion. The shaded lesion below represents an LMN lesion. (Reprinted with permission from the Rehabilitation Institute of Michigan.)

signs after an incomplete lesion in the lower thoracic/upper lumbar region. The following section discusses incomplete injuries in greater detail.

Incomplete Injuries

If damage to the spinal cord does not cause a total transection, there will still be some degree of voluntary movement or sensation below the level of injury. This is known as an incomplete injury, which may be further categorized according to the area of the spinal cord that was damaged and the clinical signs that are present.

Anterior Cord Syndrome

This syndrome results from damage to the anterior spinal artery or indirect damage to anterior spinal cord tissue (Fig. 16.7). Clinical signs include the following:

■ Loss of motor function below the level of injury. Loss of thermal, pain, and tactile sensation below the level of injury.

■ Light touch and proprioceptive awareness are generally unaffected (Hayes, Hsieh, Wolfe, Potter, & Delaney, 2000).

Brown-Séquard Syndrome

This syndrome occurs when only one side of the spinal cord is damaged (Fig. 16.8). A hemisection of this nature frequently is the result of a penetrating (e.g., stab,

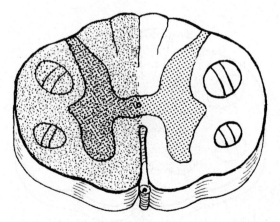

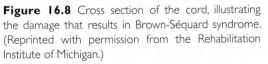

Figure 16.8 Cross section of the cord, illustrating the damage that results in Brown-Séquard syndrome. (Reprinted with permission from the Rehabilitation Institute of Michigan.)

gunshot) wound. The clinical signs of Brown-Séquard syndrome generally include

- Ipsilateral loss of motor function below the level of injury
- Ipsilateral reduction of deep touch and proprioceptive awareness (There is a reduction rather than loss as many of these nerve fibers cross.)
- Contralateral loss of pain, temperature, and touch

Clinically, a major challenge presented by Brown-Séquard syndrome is that the extremities with the greatest motor function have the poorest sensation.

Central Cervical Cord Syndrome

In this lesion, the neural fibers serving the upper extremities (UEs) are more impaired than those of the lower extremities (LEs) (Fig. 16.9). This occurs because the fibers that innervate the UEs travel more centrally in the cord, and, as the name of the syndrome implies, the central structures are the ones that are damaged (see Fig. 16.2). Injury to the central portion of the spinal cord is often seen, along with structural changes in the vertebrae. Most commonly, hyperextension of the neck, combined with a narrowing of the spinal canal, results in this type of injury. Because arthritic changes can lead to spinal canal narrowing, this syndrome is more prevalent in aging populations. The signs of central cord syndrome often include

- Motor and sensory functions in the LEs are less involved than those in the UEs. Improvements in intrinsic hand function are generally evidenced last, if at all (Merriam, Taylor, Ruff, & McPhail, 1986; Roth, Lawler, & Yarkony, 1990).
- A potential for flaccid paralysis of the UEs, as the anterior horn cells in the cervical spinal cord may

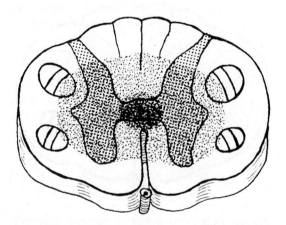

Figure 16.9 Cross section of the cord, illustrating the damage resulting in central cervical cord syndrome. (Reprinted with permission from the Rehabilitation Institute of Michigan.)

be damaged. Because these are synapse sites for the motor pathways, an LMN injury may result.

CAUDA EQUINA INJURIES

Cauda equina injuries do not involve damage to the spinal cord itself, but rather to the spinal nerves that extend below the end of the spinal cord (see Fig. 16.1). Injuries to the nerve roots and spinal nerves that comprise the cauda equina are generally incomplete. Because this type of injury actually involves structures of the peripheral nervous system (exiting spinal nerves), there is some chance for nerve regeneration and recovery of function if the roots are not too severely damaged or divided. These injuries are usually the result of direct trauma from fracture dislocations of the lower thoracic or upper lumbar vertebrae. Clinical signs of cauda equina injuries include

- Loss of motor function and sensation below the level of injury.
- Absence of a reflex arc, as the transmission of impulses through the spinal nerves to their synapse point is interrupted. Motor paralysis is of the LMN type, with flaccidity and muscle atrophy seen below the level of injury. Bowel and bladder functions are also areflexic (American Spinal Injury Association [ASIA], 2008).

COMPLETE VERSUS INCOMPLETE INJURIES

In both complete and incomplete injuries, the terms quadriplegia, tetraplegia, and paraplegia may be used to further describe the impact of the injury. Quadriplegia refers to lost or limited function of all extremities as a result of damage to cervical cord segments. The American Spinal Injury Association (ASIA) advocates the term tetraplegia over quadriplegia. Tetraplegia refers to impairment or loss of motor or sensory function in the cervical segments of the spinal cord that is the result of damage of neural elements within the spinal canal. Tetraplegia causes impairment of function in the arms as well as in the trunk, legs, and pelvic organs. It does not include brachial plexus lesions or injury to peripheral nerves outside the neural canal (American Spinal Injury Association/ International Medical Society of Paraplegia, 1992). Paraplegia, which refers to lost or limited function in the LEs and trunk depending on the level of injury, occurs after lesions to thoracic, lumbar, or sacral cord segments.

Spinal cord injuries are frequently classified further, based on the ASIA Impairment Scale (American Spinal Injury Association/International Medical Society of Paraplegia, 1992), which contains the following categories:

A = Complete; no motor or sensory function is preserved in the sacral segments S4 through S5.

B = Incomplete; sensory but not motor function is preserved below the neurologic level and extends through the sacral segments S4 through S5.

C = Incomplete; motor function is preserved below the neurologic level, and the majority of key muscles below the neurologic level have a muscle grade <3.

D = Incomplete; motor function is preserved below the neurologic level, and the majority of key muscles below the neurologic level have a muscle grade of ≥3.

E = Normal; motor and sensory function is normal.

A manual muscle test is performed to assess the strength of muscles and aid in the determination of the extent and nature of injury. Usually, strength is graded on a six-point scale (Aids to Investigation of Peripheral Nerve Injuries, 1943; Brunnstrom & Dennen, 1931; Hislop, Montgomery, & Connelly, 1995; Lovett, 1917).

0 = Total paralysis

1 = Palpable or visible contraction

2 = Active movement, full range of motion (ROM) with gravity eliminated

3 = Active movement, full ROM against gravity

4 = Active movement, full ROM against moderate resistance

5 = Normal active movement, full ROM against full resistance

NT = Not testable

COURSE AND PROGNOSIS

A prognosis implies that one can forecast or predict the outcome and chances for recovery from a particular disease or traumatic injury. That is somewhat challenging for SCIs. Although some aspects of SCI are highly predictable (e.g., specific muscle functions impaired with a complete lesion at C5), other aspects are much more vague.

Part of the ambiguity lies in the definitions of the term "recovery." One definition is to get back, or regain, which tends to be the client's focus. Another definition for recovery stresses compensation, which is often the thrust of the health care professional working with SCI. While the physiologic prognosis of SCI will be discussed here, the clinician should always be aware, and acknowledge the validity, of the client's perspective on recovery. To "regain" and to "compensate for" are dramatically different frames of reference. When discussing prognosis with a person who has survived an SCI, the clinician should always be truthful, but must also be acutely aware of the impact of what the client is hearing. Perhaps the most crucial indicators of an individual's functional outcome are personal characteristics such as motivation, use of support systems, and coping mechanisms. The clinician must be skilled at fostering these strengths while at the same time providing accurate information.

POSTTRAUMATIC COMPLICATIONS

Spinal Shock

The period of altered reflex activity immediately after a traumatic SCI is known as **spinal shock**. As a result of injury, spinal cord segments below the level of the lesion are deprived of excitatory input from higher CNS centers. What is observed clinically during this phase is a flaccid paralysis of muscles below the level of injury and an absence of reflexes (Yashon, 1986). The bladder is also flaccid, requiring **catheterization**, and there is no voluntary control of the bowel. Depending on the level of the injury, the person with an SCI may require a ventilator because of lost or temporarily interrupted innervation to the diaphragm, intercostals, and abdominal muscles.

Spinal shock generally lasts from 1 week to 3 months after injury. Once spinal shock subsides, the areas of the spinal cord above the level of the lesion operate as they did premorbidly. Below the level of the lesion, reflexes will resume if the reflex arc is intact. This is an important concept to understand. Unlike a plant, which may die entirely if its stem is cut in half, the spinal cord is still alive and functional above and below the level of injury. The problem is one of communication; the brain cannot receive sensory information beyond the lesion site and cannot volitionally control motor function below that point.

After spinal shock subsides, there is often an increase in spasticity, especially in the flexor muscle groups. The reflex arc "fires" and the brain is unable to interfere. After this phase, there may be a period of 6 to 12 months after injury when an increase in the spasticity of the extensor groups is common. Usually, after 1 year postinjury, the wide fluctuations in tone will cease.

An array of complications can greatly affect the prognosis of a person who has sustained an SCI. Some of the more common medical complications are addressed in the next section.

Respiratory Complications

Persons with spinal cord injuries at or below the level of T12 generally have a normal respiratory status. Injuries above that level, however, compromise the respiratory system to some degree. The abdominal musculature is innervated by segments T7 through T12, the intercostal muscles are served by segments T1 through T12, and the diaphragm is innervated by C4. Persons with complete injuries above C4 usually need a respirator. Some may be candidates for a phrenic nerve stimulator if the nerve shows the ability to conduct an impulse. Generally, persons with complete injuries at C4 and below do not use respirators, but respiratory complications may persist. Breathing may be shallow, and the ability to cough productively may be compromised. Various deep-breathing and assisted-coughing techniques may be taught, along with other procedures to keep the lungs clear. Prevention and early management of respiratory complications is crucial. Currently, respiratory complications are the most common cause of death following SCI.

Autonomic Dysreflexia (Hyperreflexia)

As implied by its name, **autonomic dysreflexia (hyperreflexia)** involves an exaggerated response of the autonomic nervous system (ANS). A function of the ANS is the integration of body functions in the "fight-or-flight" response—heart rate, blood vessel constriction/dilation, regulation of glands, and smooth muscle. Autonomic dysreflexia usually occurs in persons with spinal cord injuries above the T6 level. Signs to look for include a sudden, pounding headache; diaphoresis; flushing; goose bumps; and tachycardia followed by bradycardia. These signs are caused by an irritation of nerves below the level of injury. Common sources of irritation include an overfull bladder or bowel, urinary tract infections (UTIs), or **decubitus ulcers.** Even irritations such as ingrown toenails can trigger the response. These irritations would be bothersome to a person with an intact spinal cord—he or she would feel uncomfortable and act to remedy the situation. But the person with an SCI lacks this feeling, and autonomic dysreflexia is the body's way of warning that something is wrong below the level of the injury.

The most important aspect of managing autonomic dysreflexia is to find the cause and alleviate it. This may require emptying the bladder, checking for obstructions in external urinary drainage tubing, assessing for bowel impaction, or evaluating for other factors. It helps to decrease blood pressure if the person assumes an upright position. Most persons with tetraplegia will experience an episode of autonomic dysreflexia at least once, but if the signs of autonomic dysreflexia appear frequently, medication may be indicated. Autonomic dysreflexia may appear suddenly and must be managed promptly. Because the blood pressure may elevate dramatically, there is risk of stroke or death if the situation is ignored or mismanaged. Although autonomic dysreflexia may be more prevalent in the initial months following injury, it has the potential of being an ongoing complication, and persons with SCI must be educated about symptoms and management (McQuillan, VonReuden, Hartsock, Flynn, & Whalen, 2002).

Postural Hypotension

In contrast to autonomic dysreflexia, blood pressure decreases in postural hypotension. This condition, often seen in persons who have sustained cervical or thoracic SCIs, also may be referred to as orthostatic hypotension (Bloch & Basbaum, 1983). Blood tends to pool distally in the LEs as a result of reduced muscle tone in the trunk and legs. The symptoms of postural hypotension frequently occur when a person attempts to sit up after prolonged periods of bed rest. Symptoms include lightheadedness, dizziness, pallor, sudden weakness, and unresponsiveness. Preventive measures include the use of antiembolism hosiery and abdominal binders, which externally assist circulation. Also, assuming an upright position slowly can help avoid these symptoms. If symptoms do occur, a semireclined or reclined position should be maintained until the symptoms subside.

Deep Vein Thrombosis

Deep vein thrombosis (DVT) can be a serious complication in many types of medical conditions. It is a potential complication in SCI for three main reasons: reduced circulation caused by decreased tone; frequency of direct trauma to legs, causing vascular damage (e.g., repeated trauma during transfer or bed mobility activities); and prolonged bed rest. Edema is often seen in SCI for the same reasons. Clinical signs of DVT may include swelling in the LEs, localized redness, and a low-grade fever. However, a DVT may be relatively asymptomatic on bedside evaluation. Vigilant medical screenings for DVT should be performed in all cases of SCI. An undetected and unmanaged DVT may result in an embolism and death. In persons with SCI, it appears that the greatest risk of DVT is seen within the initial 2 weeks postinjury (ASIA, 2008; Consortium for Spinal Cord Medicine, 1997; Fowler, 1995; McQuillan et al., 2002; Ragnarsson, Hall, & Wilmot, 1995).

Thermal Regulation

It has already been seen that damage to the spinal cord can disrupt the ANS, possibly resulting in autonomic dysreflexia. Thermal regulation is another function of the ANS that can be disturbed after SCI. Maintaining the appropriate body temperature is often a problem for persons whose injuries are above T6. During the first year after injury, the body tends to assume the temperature of the external environment. This condition is called poikilothermia (Hanak & Scott, 1983). In time, some adjustment usually occurs. Cold weather often causes discomfort, as blood vessels below the level of injury do not constrict sufficiently to conserve the body's heat. Conversely, excessive sweating may occur above the level of injury in warmer weather but not below, which hampers the body's efforts to prevent hyperthermia. Because of this, extreme temperatures should be avoided, and attention should be given to the extent and type of clothing worn in all conditions.

Musculoskeletal Complications

Spasticity

In persons who have UMN lesions, increased tone appears in muscles below the level of injury after spinal shock subsides. Virtually all individuals with cervical cord injuries experience spasms; 75% of those with thoracic lesions, <58% of those with lumbar injuries, and <25% of those with cauda equina injuries report spasms (Burke & Murray, 1975). An increase in spasticity can be triggered by a variety of factors including infections, positioning, pressure sores, UTIs, and heightened emotional states. Spasms are not necessarily disadvantageous. The ability to trigger their spasms can help some individuals maintain muscle bulk, circulation, bowel and bladder management, transfers, and other activities of daily living (ADL). Excessive spasticity, however, may result in contractures, pain, and a reduced ability to participate in activities. At this point, pharmacologic or surgical options may be recommended.

Heterotopic Ossification (Ectopic Bone)

Heterotopic ossification (HO) refers to the abnormal formation of bone deposits on muscles, joints, and tendons. It occurs most often in the hip and knee and less frequently in the shoulder and elbow. It has been estimated that 20% of all persons with SCI have some degree of ectopic bone growth (Hernandez, Fjorner, & DeLaFuente, 1978). Clinical signs of HO may include heat, pain, swelling, and a decrease in active or passive ROM. These signs should always alert the clinician, as they may also indicate other serious complications such as a DVT. Many facilities that specialize in the care of persons with SCI routinely provide prophylactic medications that have shown promise in halting this abnormal calcification. In extreme cases in which ROM is permanently and severely limited by HO, surgery may be indicated.

Genitourinary Complications

UTIs are a common and dangerous complication of SCI. Prior to modern medical management, many persons with SCI who survived the initial trauma died within a few years after injury, with one of the most common causes being kidney failure as a result of chronic UTI. For several reasons, individuals with SCI are prone to UTI or bladder infections. The bladder is composed of smooth muscle, innervated by sacral segments of the spinal cord. As such, it is affected by a loss of sensory and motor function, as are other parts of the body, depending on the level and extent of injury. The nature of bladder function will depend on whether the injury caused LMN or UMN deficits (Fig. 16.10). Injury at point A yields a UMN bladder, also referred to as a reflex or spastic bladder. In this case, the bladder can contract and void reflexively.

Although this action is involuntary, some persons with SCI can trigger the reflex through various stimuli, much as the knee-jerk reflex being triggered by tapping with a reflex hammer. This is because impulses can still enter the cord below the level of injury, synapse, and exit.

Persons with a UMN bladder may use various types of catheters and additional techniques to ensure that the bladder does not become distended or retain urine. They generally cannot rely on sensation to alert them that the bladder has exceeded its normal capacity; rather, they must rely on an established voiding schedule.

An LMN bladder may also be referred to as a nonreflex or flaccid bladder. This type of bladder function is usually seen during the spinal shock phase and may remain if the injury has affected the cauda equina area. An injury at point B or C (see Fig. 16.10) can result in an LMN bladder. With this type of injury, a reflexive emptying of the bladder cannot occur, as the reflex arc is destroyed. Because the bladder is flaccid and does not spontaneously empty, urine will accumulate continuously. Persons with an LMN bladder must catheterize according to a schedule or must apply external pressure to force urine from the bladder. The application of external pressure on the abdomen with their fists, starting at the umbilicus and pressing downward, is called **Credé's maneuver**. Another technique for generating force is called the Valsalva maneuver, which involves closing the glottis and contracting the abdominal muscles, as if resisting a forceful exhilation (Somers, 2010). Chronic use of Credé's maneuver may

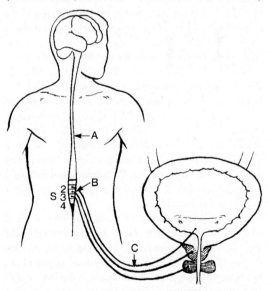

Figure 16.10 Bladder and corresponding spinal segment innervations. Injuries at point A would result in a UMN or spastic bladder. Injuries at point B or C would result in LMN, or flaccid, bladder function. (Reprinted with permission from the Rehabilitation Institute of Michigan.)

lead to multiple complications, including inguinal hernias, hemorrhoids, and vesicouretral reflux (Chang, Hou, Dong, & Zhang, 2000; Consortium for Spinal Cord Medicine, 2006; Somers, 2010).

With either type of bladder (UMN or LMN), voiding must occur routinely and completely. Chronic overstretching of the bladder will reduce its ability to empty adequately. Residual urine is a breeding ground for infections that can spread to all structures in the urinary system, including the ureters and kidneys. Chronic infections can lead to renal calculi (kidney stones), kidney failure, and, potentially, death. Warning signs of a UTI include urine that appears cloudy or has excessive particles, dark or foul-smelling urine, an elevated fever, chills, or an increase in spasticity. The best treatment of UTI is prevention—adhering to an effective voiding schedule, using clean or sterile techniques, maintaining a proper diet and adequate fluid intake, and prompt attention to warning signs.

Complications Associated with the Bowel

Normally, elimination occurs when stool is present in the rectum. Nerves in the rectal musculature are stimulated, triggering a reflexive **peristalsis** and a relaxation of the rectal sphincters. A bowel movement may be prevented at this step of the process if the brain overrides this reflex, sending down an impulse to tighten the sphincter muscles until an appropriate time. We have all experienced the sensation of urgency caused by a full rectum, but perhaps we have not fully appreciated our brain's ability to allow us to forestall the process until a socially acceptable time.

Unfortunately, an SCI can interfere with bowel function in much the same way as it impedes the bladder. The bowel can become spastic or flaccid. A reflex bowel can be caused by a lesion at point A (Fig. 16.11). In this case, stool can be eliminated reflexively if nerves located in the rectum are stimulated. This stimulation may be done manually through digital stimulation or in conjunction with the use of suppositories. Establishing and following a regular schedule for bowel management can reduce occurrences of incontinence.

The bowel is usually flaccid during the phase of spinal shock and may remain in that state if the injury involves the areas illustrated at points B and C (see Fig. 16.10). As with the flaccid bladder, the flaccid bowel cannot be stimulated to empty reflexively. Stool often remains in the rectum after attempts at evacuation, and it may be necessary to remove it manually to prevent impaction.

Constipation or impaction may result if elimination does not occur regularly. In addition to the general discomfort associated with this, autonomic dysreflexia may be triggered in persons with lesions above the T6 level.

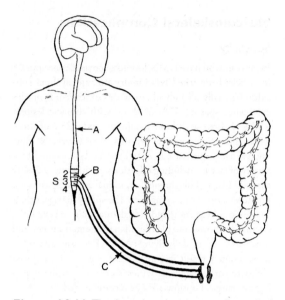

Figure 16.11 The bowel and corresponding spinal segment innervations. Injuries at point A would result in a UMN or spastic bowel. Injuries at point B or C would result in LMN, or flaccid, bowel function. (Reprinted with permission from the Rehabilitation Institute of Michigan.)

Diarrhea is another complication that can be particularly frustrating for the person with an SCI who is trying to establish a set schedule for bowel management. This condition is always frustrating, but the majority of the general population have the benefit of intact sensation to provide a warning. The best strategies to prevent diarrhea for persons with an SCI include making sure to use (not overuse) laxatives if they are prescribed, eating a proper diet, maintaining adequate hydration, and following a scheduled bowel program that reduces the chance of impaction, which can result in diarrhea.

Dermal Complications

The skin is the largest organ of the body, and it performs essential functions in maintaining health. Skin assists in thermal regulation, providing insulation in cold weather and sweating to prevent hyperthermia during hot conditions. Aside from literally keeping the body together, skin acts as a barrier to the external environment. At the cellular level, skin provides the site for O_2/CO_2 exchange through the capillary system. Keeping skin intact is essential and requires conscious effort by a person with an SCI, as sensations that would normally provide warning of potential skin damage, such as pain and extremes in temperature, are not perceived below the level of injury.

Damage to the skin as a result of pressure sores, or decubitus ulcers, is a major reason for hospital admissions in SCI populations. The mechanism of injury is continued pressure due to lack of movement. Circulation is impaired because of the pressure, and capillary exchange is impeded. This can result rapidly in tissue necrosis. The severity of pressure sores can be classified into four stages:

Stage I. Clinical signs are reddened or darkened skin. Damage is limited to more superficial (epidermal and dermal) layers. At this stage, tissue breakdown can be halted merely by removing pressure until the skin returns to its normal color.

Stage II. The skin now appears reddened and open. A blister or scab is present. The scab is not a sign of healing; rather, the tissue beneath it is necrotic. This involves the epidermal and dermal layers as well as deeper adipose tissue. Wound dressings may be involved at this stage, and it is imperative that pressure be kept off the site.

Stage III. The skin breakdown is deeper, and the wound is now draining. Muscle may be visible through the open wound. An ulcer is developing in the necrotic tissue. In addition to wound dressings, surgical intervention may be indicated if more conservative treatment is unsuccessful.

Stage IV. All structures, from the superficial levels to the bone, are destroyed. Infection and bone decay occur. Surgical intervention is likely, and the person with a decubitus ulcer at this stage often must spend weeks after a skin graft, with pressure totally removed from the involved site (Cassell, 1986).

Pressure sores are preventable with diligent attention and preventative strategies. A person with SCI can use, or instruct another person to assist with, a variety of pressure relief methods. Also, visual skin inspections should be performed at least twice daily, taking particular note of areas most prone to breakdown. These would include areas where bony prominences (e.g., the sacrum, ischium, calcaneus, and scapula) can add to pressure. Proper nutrition also should be needed, as healthy skin is less apt to break down and is more responsive to healing in early stages of pressure sore development.

Other dermal complications, such as burns or frostbite, are prevented by attentiveness and common sense. Even commonly encountered things, such as space heaters or exposed plumbing under a sink, can cause severe burns to persons with an SCI without their immediate knowledge. It is important to be aware of the environment and to rely on other, intact senses to avoid injury.

MEDICAL/SURGICAL MANAGEMENT

Medical management of an SCI should begin immediately at the onset of injury. As typically injuries occur outside a hospital setting (roadways, lakes, sporting events), often first responders are not medical personnel. Any person with a suspected SCI should be immobilized with a backboard and neck brace before transport (Cooper, 2006). Diagnostic evaluation of the vertebral column and spinal cord must be completed to determine the next steps of intervention. Injuries may require surgical or nonsurgical intervention to decompress, realign, and stabilize the spine (McQuillan et al., 2002). Surgical procedures such as laminectomies may be performed to remove the cause of pressure on the cord (such as a bony fragment or bullet) (Hanak & Scott, 1993). Spinal fusion may also be required to achieve stability. External alignment devices may be used following spinal surgery or may be sufficient substitutes for surgery (Hanak &Scott, 1993). In thoracic injuries, a thoraco-lumbar-sacral-orthosis or clamshell brace is often used. This device is a "total-contact" molded two-piece brace, applied to the anterior and posterior of an individual to limit trunk movement (Beets, Faisant, Houghton, & Schlich, 1987). Multiple devices also exist for external stabilization of cervical injuries. These orthoses typically restrict the chin and the posterior aspect of the skull, restricting cervical motion (Somers, 2010). Among the most restrictive cervical devices is the "halo" orthosis. This is comprised of a metal ring affixed directly to the skull with screws (called "pins") at occipital and temporal points and steel bars mounted to a body vest (Somers, 2010; Hanak & Scott, 1993). The determination of the need and/or type of orthosis required demands careful assessment of vertebral stability and the nature of movement the device is able to restrict.

Concurrent with spinal decompression, realignment, and stabilization, prompt pharmacologic management is vital (McQuillan et al., 2002). In the most acute stages following injury, recent research headlines have reported that the use of steroids—specifically, methylprednisolone—may improve neurologic outcomes of patients with SCI if administered within the first 8 hours after injury (Bracken, Holeord, & Shepard, 1990). Additionally, select experimental drugs administered soon after injury, such as GM-1 ganglioside (Sygen) and 4-AP, were hoped to aid in the preservation of damaged nerves and insulating them from the toxic level of chemicals the body releases during trauma and possibly reduce cell death (http://www.spinalcord.org/news). Study outcomes to date relating to the benefit of these drugs are mixed, and some concerns have been raised about potential adverse effects versus limited functional gains with some of these protocols. Another very recent acute experimental intervention that has been tried to mitigate spinal cord damage and hopefully improve outcomes is "therapeutic hypothermia." This process involves lowering the core body temperature to discourage spinal cord edema and reduce metabolic demands soon after injury occurs (Cappuccino, 2008). While this technique has been used historically for other diagnoses, its consideration in the management of SCI is relatively new. Perhaps the first introduction to this technique for many was during the 2007 National Football League season opening game, when millions watched live as Buffalo Bills' tight end Kevin Everett was involved in helmet-to-helmet contact that resulted in a cervical SCI. The team orthopedic surgeon administered almost-immediate hypothermic intervention. The technique, which Everett has credited with his positive outcomes, was described for days in the media (Higgins, 2007). Certainly, significant additional research needs to be conducted in all aspects of the very acute management of SCI, but improved initial treatments hold promise for better long-term outcomes.

On other fronts, while fetal stem cell research relating to spinal cord regeneration is prevalent in the news, meaningful functional outcomes have been limited. However, newer research related to stem cells found in a living donor's brain, spinal cord, or other structures may hold greater promise and potentially avoid problems of cell rejection found with fetal stem cells (http://www.spinalcord.uab.edu). Headlines were made in the recent past regarding the treatment of spinal cord injuries with the use of stem cells from umbilical blood. This process reportedly resulted in a South Korean woman who had been paralyzed for 20 years being able to perform some level of ambulation with assistance (http://chinadaily.com.cn/english/doc/ 2004–11/29/ content_395570.htm). Autologous (self-donated) bone marrow stem cell transplants have also been shown in select reported case studies to result in functional gains and quality-of-life improvements in spinal cord injured recipients (Geffner, Santacruz, & Izurieta, 2008). Additional research is being aimed at a variety of strategies, including pharmacologic and enzyme therapy, cloning of nerve cells, and the highly sophisticated altering of the cellular environment to encourage actual regeneration. As stated earlier, the spinal cord is alive above and below the level of injury; one goal of current research is to encourage functional reconnection of the disrupted pathways.

Aside from research on actual spinal cord regeneration, significant work is also being done with highly technical devices to compensate for paralysis. Functional electrical stimulation (FES) is one example. Persons with UMN injuries have experienced increases in their functional abilities (improved ability to productively cough, UE function, standing ability, ambulation) with the external application of electrodes that stimulate muscle contraction. Although some may feel that the FES apparatus is cumbersome, unsightly, time consuming, and difficult to apply, refinements are ongoing. Many persons with SCI feel that, although not ideal, the technology provides an appealing alternative to outcomes from traditional methods of rehabilitation. Another technologic development is the use of neuroprosthetic devices, which are surgically implanted FES systems. One device, the Freehand System, combines internal electrodes, stimulators, sensors, and transmission coils within an external control box. It allows a person with tetraplegia to achieve a degree of functional prehension, enhancing such ADL as eating, writing, and phone and computer use. Select studies have shown gains in the functional performance of individuals with C5-6 tetraplegia utilizing this system (Taylor, Esnouf, & Hobby, 2002).

A different picture is presented with cauda equina injuries or injuries involving the nerve root. These types of injuries carry the potential for regeneration if the nerve roots are not severely damaged or divided. The degree of regeneration that can be expected is very difficult to predict, which must be done on an individual basis after extensive medical testing.

Overall, although actual regeneration of the cord may not be on the immediate scientific horizon, the advances in all phases of SCI management are promising. Everyone has the right to hope for what is not yet reality, without being said to have unrealistic expectations. Assisting someone to be hopeful, while simultaneously working to maximize today's function, is to truly master the art of the therapeutic relationship.

IMPACT OF CONDITION ON OCCUPATIONAL PERFORMANCE

Performance in areas of occupation relates to a person's ability to engage in activities that are essential and meaningful. Performance in areas of occupation include ADL, instrumental activities of daily living (IADL), education, work, play, leisure, and social participation. Clearly, an SCI can have a catastrophic effect on a person's ability to function in these areas, because it can affect body function categories that support the ability to participate in these activities. Body function categories that may be impacted by an SCI include sensory functions and pain, voice and speech functions, functions of cardiovascular and respiratory systems, genitourinary and reproductive functions, neuromusculoskeletal and movement-related functions, functions of the skin and related structures, and select mental functions. The importance of understanding the theory of occupational performance cannot be overstated. We cannot begin to holistically treat a person with SCI until we can visualize the impact that this diagnosis has on the various aspects of that person's life. The following sections explore occupational performance areas and components to present a comprehensive view of the impact of SCI. Table 16-4 shows generally expected functional outcomes at various levels of complete injuries.

TABLE 16.4 Expected Functional Outcomes of Various Levels of Complete Injury (Noninclusive)

Last Spinal Cord Level Intact (Spared)	Expected Functional Outcome
C1-3	Requires 24-h availability of caregiver.
	Generally ventilator-dependent; some individuals at C3 may be successfully weaned from a ventilator.
	Requires maximal assistance of another for pressure relief or requires an adapted switch and reclining chair.
	May propel power chair independently with adapted switches (pneumatic, chin, head, mouthstick); requires maximal setup.
	Maximal assistance needed for transfers, positioning, bed mobility, dressing, feeding, hygiene, grooming, and bowel/bladder care.
	Dependent with driving.
C4	Requires 24-h availability of caregiver.
	Generally able to be weaned from a ventilator; continued difficulty with productive coughing and deep breathing.
	Pressure relief, wheelchair propulsion, transfers, bed mobility, dressing, hygiene, bowel/bladder care, and driving status comparable to C1-3 level.
	Adaptive feeding and grooming devices are available; they require setup and are very time-consuming and exhaustive for a person at this level and generally do not result in task independence.
C5	May require 24-h availability of caregiver.
	Decreased respiratory endurance, but not using ventilator.
	A strong person with a C5 injury may be independent in pressure relief by leaning side to side; a weaker person may require maximal assistance.
	Independent on level surfaces with a power chair and occasionally wrist/forearm supports; a manual wheelchair with rim adaptations may be used by a strong person for short distances, but is typically not a reasonable mobility strategy.
	Moderate to maximal assistance is required for all transfers, and generally a sliding board or mechanical lift is used.
	Moderate assistance is required for bed mobility.
	A strong person with a C5 injury may assist with some dressing, hygiene, and grooming activities with the aid of adapted equipment. Feeding is generally possible with the use of adapted utensils and setup.
	Driving is feasible at this level (in the absence of additional complications such as extensive UE tone/contractures); a person may be able to drive with specially adapted steering, braking, and acceleration hand controls, and due to transfer limitations would drive directly from the wheelchair.

(Continued)

TABLE 16.4 Expected Functional Outcomes of Various Levels of Complete Injury (Noninclusive) *(Continued)*

Last Spinal Cord Level Intact (Spared)	Expected Functional Outcome
C6	Amount of assistance needed from another person varies from moderate to minimal with just a few specific activities. Some decreases in respiratory capacity and productive cough. Has potential for independence in pressure relief. Independently uses a manual wheelchair on level surfaces and gradual inclines; rim adaptations improve propulsion abilities. Generally requires a power wheelchair for long distances or rough terrain. Ability to transfer varies. Some strong persons with C6 injuries are able to transfer independently with the use of a sliding board to a car, chair, bed, commode, or tub seat. Has the potential for independent bed mobility and positioning with rails, power controls, and trapeze. With some adapted devices, usually independent with hygiene, shaving, and grooming. Potential for independence in bathing and bowel/bladder care with equipment. Generally independent with UE dressing, and potential for independence in LE dressing with adaptive devices, although often the latter is quite time consuming. Independent with feeding, although a wrist-hand orthosis and setup may be required. Generally able to drive independently using hand controls and adaptive devices; if transfers are challenging/inconsistent, driving directly from the wheelchair is indicated.
C7-8	May be able to live independently without attendant care, although assistance required for high/low/heavy tasks. Some decreased respiratory endurance. Independent in pressure relief. Independently uses manual wheelchair. Generally able to transfer without a sliding board, depending on the surface characteristics. Generally independent with positioning, bed mobility, hygiene, feeding, shaving, hair care, dressing, bathing, cooking, and light housekeeping. Generally independent with bowel/bladder care using adaptive equipment/techniques. Drives independently with hand controls/steering adaptations. Generally able to stand in parallel bars once assisted to upright position, with the use of a knee-ankle-foot orthosis (KAFO).
T1-3	Can live independently, although assistance required for high/low/heavy tasks. Respiratory capacity and coughing abilities significantly improved compared to previous levels. All transfers generally independent unless other complicating factors (e.g., excessive tone challenges, contractures, shoulder dysfunction).

TABLE 16.4 Expected Functional Outcomes of Various Levels of Complete Injury (Noninclusive) *(Continued)*

Last Spinal Cord Level Intact (Spared)	Expected Functional Outcome
	Independent with all self-care.
	Finger dexterity, strength, and coordination are functional.
	Drives independently with hand controls. Typically able to stow certain types of manual wheelchairs in a car, but may be excessively time consuming, energy depleting, and adversely impacting shoulders, and as such a van may be indicated.
	Able to stand with minimal assistance, KAFO, and use of walker or parallel bars. Ambulation is generally not practical because of reduced trunk control/balance and high energy expenditure.
T4-8	Can live independently, although assistance required for high/low/heavy tasks.
	Respiratory status stronger than T1-3 level; only slightly decreased pressure relief, wheelchair use, positioning, bad mobility, and self-care all independent.
	Driving: comparable to T1-3 level.
	May have potential to ambulate short distances with the use of a walker or Lofstrand crutches and KAFO on level surfaces only; however even if able, high energy output is required, and wheelchair use remains predominant form of mobility.
T9-12	Respiration is functional.
	Pressure relief, wheelchair use, transfers, positioning, bad mobility, self-care, homemaking (except heavy tasks) all independent.
	Able to drive with hand controls.
	Generally able to ambulate with KAFO and Lofstrand crutches as noted above, with somewhat less energy demands; wheelchair use remains predominant form of mobility.
L1-3	Same as T9-12 level with the addition of improved ambulation distances; a wheelchair is often required for long distances.
L4-5	Same as above, with exceptions: Driving may be independent without adaptive devices; strength of ankle dorsiflexion and tone must be assessed. Generally able to ambulate with ankle foot orthosis and canes. Wheelchairs generally not needed for household ambulation, but may be indicated for longer distances.
S1-2	A person with an S2-spared injury has the potential to ambulate without devices or orthoses.
	A wheelchair is generally not required. Hip extensors/abductors, knee flexors, and ankle plantar flexors are weak at the S1 level of injury. As with all other preceding levels, bowel and bladder function is impaired but managed independently at the level through adapted devices/techniques.

Developed with material from the Rehabilitation Institute of Michigan, 1996.

Instrumental Activities of Daily Living

Grooming, Oral Hygiene, Eating, Bathing, Dressing

For a person with tetraplegia, grooming, oral hygiene, and eating may be extremely laborious. The use of extensive adaptive devices or reliance on a caregiver may be necessary because of deficits in sensory and neuromuscular performance components. Persons with paraplegia are generally independent in these tasks, but they must often think ahead, making sure that items are available and sufficient time is allocated. Bathing and dressing present major challenges for persons with quadriplegia. With higher-level injuries (C1 through C4), total assistance is required. At lower levels of injury, with varying amounts of adaptive equipment and assistance from others in some task components, the person with quadriplegia can be a more active participant. It is extremely important for the person's own goals to be acknowledged. A small but revealing study documented that individuals with a complete C6 injury typically required from 20 to 60 minutes to dress with the use of adaptations, yet none of the 10 patients in the study reported dressing themselves routinely after discharge from the hospital (Weingarden & Martin, 1989). They sought assistance from others because of feelings that the task was too time consuming and exhausting. The question becomes, "Is this functional?" If a person is attempting reentry into the work force or return to school, is it "functional" to spend an entire hour, as well as all the physical energy, in just getting dressed? Or is it a sign of greater autonomy to delegate some tasks to a caregiver to allow participation in activities that are more meaningful?

Secondary conditions aside, individuals with paraplegia are usually independent in bathing and dressing. Some even have the strength to transfer to the bottom of a tub without assistive devices.

Toileting

Managing altered bowel and bladder function is a challenge for virtually everyone with SCI. The two aspects to this challenge are the actual physiologic management and the various techniques and equipment used in the toileting process.

Medications may be required for physiologic management. Stool softeners are used, as well as suppositories to assist in evacuation. A goal of effective bowel management is to eliminate or reduce reliance on medications. For persons with injuries at C7 or below, independence in toileting can usually be achieved with an array of equipment that may include suppository inserters, digital stimulators (devices that trigger reflexes to relax the rectal sphincter in UMN injuries), catheterization devices, leg separators, mirrors, and adapted commode chairs that allow access to the perianal area for bowel-training procedures.

Aside from medications and equipment, additional strategies include maintaining a specific schedule for elimination, eating a healthy diet that promotes regularity, assuming positions that facilitate elimination, and using Credé's method. If toileting appears to be tiring, then it has been portrayed correctly! But many persons with SCI become adept at its management. It may be a very different picture, though, when a person attempts these procedures in a community environment (i.e., rest rooms at work or school), due to accessibility, availability of equipment, and time limitations. In order to promote greater freedom and independence, some individuals opt to explore alternatives—such as undergoing surgical urinary diversion. Surgeries such as the Mitrofanoff procedure create a permanent stoma in the abdomen, which can allow an individual to catheterize through their navel. This presents benefits of easier anatomical access and significantly less adjustment of clothing versus traditional catheterizing. While not every individual is a candidate, and the procedure is certainly not without risk and potential long-term complication, studies have revealed that many who undertake it have been highly satisfied with the degree of freedom and independence it has allowed them (Merenda, Duffy, & Betz, 2007).

The person with a higher-level cervical injury faces greater challenges. Although the bowel- and bladder-management concepts are the same, neuromuscular deficits limit performance of the tasks, even with adaptive equipment. Generally, persons with injuries above the C6 level require a caregiver to assist with or perform functions such as transfers to adaptive commode chairs, suppository insertion, digital stimulation, catheterization, and general perianal care. The person with an SCI must indicate who the caregiver will be, particularly for tasks that are socially sensitive. Even though family members may be willing to assist, it is perfectly justifiable for the person to request someone else as a caregiver. Some persons may have no reservations about who assists them, whereas others may feel strongly that it would negatively affect established roles. Whatever the case, whenever feasible, the preferences of the person with an SCI should be the deciding factor in selecting caregivers for various tasks.

Personal Device Care

The extent of personal and adaptive devices required by an individual with an SCI can generally be predicted by the level of injury (see Table 16-4). Additional complications, such as reduced ROM resulting from contractures, may require the use of more extensive devices than are typically seen at a particular level. Usually, personal device care is performed by others for those with injuries at C4 and above. Those with injuries at the C5 level and below have progressively more ability to assist in personal device care and use, but this fluctuates greatly depending on the individual's endurance, motivation, resources, and priorities.

Health Maintenance

Fostering a healthy lifestyle is critical, but often challenging, after an SCI. Most persons with an SCI are advised to follow lifelong exercise programs to preserve and enhance ROM and strength as well as to promote good cardiovascular fitness and weight management. Many individuals report weight gains in the months after injury, as their energy demands are greatly altered in great part by use of a wheelchair for mobility. Attention also must be given to proper nutrition for weight management, impact on skin integrity, and bowel and bladder management. As mentioned earlier, routine attention to skin condition is crucial to avoiding dermal complications. A health maintenance routine may require the assistance of others, depending on the level of injury, for such activities as setting up weights and equipment, performing passive ROM, pressure relief, and aiding in skin inspection.

Socialization, Functional Communication, and Emergency Response

With a singular diagnosis of SCI, no cognitive deficits are inherent that would preclude a person from socializing in an appropriate contextual manner. What is challenging, though, are the variety of barriers that may inhibit socialization. Architectural, environmental, and transportation barriers; reduced endurance; and increased reliance on others may discourage or actually prevent someone from traveling to the places where they socialized before their injury. Psychological barriers also may prevent reintegration into a premorbid social support system, and these "barriers" are as real as physical ones.

In all but the highest of injuries, verbal communication is functional. Persons with injuries at C7 or below are generally independent with a variety of forms of communication (e.g., writing, keyboard use, phone use) without the use of adaptive equipment. Above this level, however, adaptive devices are progressively required.

The need to request assistance in emergencies is possible at virtually all levels of injury, depending on the environment and adaptive equipment available. For persons with higher-level injuries, adaptive phone devices, emergency call systems, and environmental control units make contact with emergency agencies feasible. At the level of C4 and above, however, the availability of a caregiver 24 hours a day remains the most appropriate safety option. Individuals with injuries below this level may use a phone independently with possible adaptations but may be limited in other emergency responses, such as exiting a dwelling or attending to the physical needs of another injured person.

Functional Mobility

Persons with complete injuries at the thoracic levels of injury and above usually rely on wheelchairs for household and community mobility. Those with injuries at C6 or above may require additional assistance in manual wheelchair management; they may utilize a manual wheelchair with power-assist wheels or a power wheelchair. Individuals with higher-level quadriplegia may use adapted orthotic devices to aid in controlling a power wheelchair or alternative interfaces such as "puff and sip" or chin controls to maneuver the wheelchair in the absence of sufficient UE function. Even at lower levels of injury, while an individual may be able to navigate a manual wheelchair under certain conditions, power wheelchairs may be considered due to community access needs (e.g., the need to navigate a large college campus routinely). Persons with lower-level thoracic injuries may be able to ambulate short distances with ambulation devices such as walkers or Lofstrand (forearm) crutches and LE orthotic devices; however, the practicality of this in household and community settings must be evaluated. It is important to consider the need to avoid repetitive motion disorders in the UEs, which can become problematic if overused during ambulation activities. Persons with sacral injuries often can ambulate community distances without orthoses or devices.

Sometimes it is not so much the ability or inability of the person with an SCI but the inaccessibility of the environment that limits functional mobility. Whereas the home environment can be modified through creative thoughts, planning, and finances, the community environment is much harder to change. Although the Americans with Disabilities Act celebrated its 20th anniversary of enactment on July 26, 2010, most would agree that compliance with and enforcement of barrier-free environments are less than ideal. Many physically challenged persons continue to fight discriminatory situations (e.g., inaccessible public transportation, restaurants, offices, classrooms). A lighter side of the inaccessibility issue was recalled by Ed Roberts, founder of the first Center for Independent Living. He reminisced that early protestors in the disability rights movement were released from police custody because jail cells were inaccessible (Price, 1990)! In the vast majority of situations, however, an inaccessible environment is frustrating, demeaning, and personally violating. The health care team can do its part by helping physically, emotionally, or cognitively challenged persons to be aware of their rights, as well as by providing them with information on advocacy groups.

Functional mobility includes driving as a consideration for many. A strong C5-injured person may be able to drive with specially adapted low-effort steering, braking, and acceleration hand controls. Usually, those with injuries above the C5 level cannot drive because of physical and respiratory limitations. Persons with C6 injuries and below may be able to drive independently using hand controls and adaptive steering devices. A van with a power lift or ramp may be recommended for someone who has difficulty transferring from their wheelchair or independently stowing their wheelchair in a vehicle. Often, finances more than need may dictate the type of transportation used, and clinicians can be invaluable in helping clients identify what financial and community resources may be available to help them meet their mobility needs.

Sexual Expression

As with bowel and bladder function, most persons with SCI experience alterations in their ability to perform sexually as compared with their premorbid status. The nerves that innervate the genital area (both motor and sensory components) originate at the sacral spinal cord levels, so in the great majority of SCI cases, sexual function is affected.

For the most part, a person can participate in a variety of sexual activities despite SCI, although the level of sensation and motor response will vary, depending on the extent and level of injury. Medications, surgical implants, and sexual enhancement devices may be recommended by specialists, but this is highly individualized.

Advances in the field of fertility have improved the chances for a spinal cord–injured male to father a child. Although fertility rates for men with SCI are estimated at <10%, techniques such as electrostimulation to induce ejaculation in paraplegics have proven successful in many cases (Perkash, Martin, & Warner, 1990). Men may be well advised to delay a decision about surgical penile implants until at least 1 year after injury. This allows time to evaluate the full impact of the SCI on sexual function and to determine the extent, if any, of sensory or motor return in an incomplete injury. The reproductive capabilities of women are generally unaltered by an SCI, and women and their partners should be made aware that the potential for pregnancy exists (Sipski, 1991).

Addressing sexual function should be an integral part of each person's treatment plan, but a distinction should be made between purely physiologic sexual performance—arousal, orgasm, and ejaculation—and sexuality, which is the totality of a person's attractiveness, personality, and self-perception as a sexual being. Sexuality does not have to rely on physiology. Whereas performance may be hampered as a result of an SCI, one's sexuality can be quite healthy and intact. The health care provider must make accurate information available and identify sources of more detailed information or expertise. It is entirely at the discretion of the person with an SCI to explore, or not explore, options available to them.

Home Maintenance

Tasks such as household maintenance, meal preparation, shopping, cleaning, clothing care, and safety procedures are included within the general category of home maintenance. Usually, persons with a C6-level injury or above require assistance with all of these activities and need some personal attendant care. Persons with injuries at C7 or lower can often live independently (without attendant care) as they are able to perform their basic ADL tasks in accessible environments. However, they typically require assistance with heavier home-maintenance tasks or activities requiring access to high or low areas.

Care of Others

An SCI can certainly make caring for others difficult, particularly if the injured person had been the primary caregiver for a child, spouse, or parent. Although a major goal of those with SCI is mastering personal self-care, a concurrent goal may be the introduction of activities (e.g., diapering, bathing a child) that can allow them to assume some premorbid roles. Often, many of these previous responsibilities must be delegated to others. In these cases, it is ideal if the person with SCI retains the responsibility for the verbal direction of care.

Education

Persons with SCI can generally resume educational activities, even while still inpatients in rehabilitation facilities. Many specialty hospitals retain the services of teachers from local school districts—or encourage the involvement of a student's premorbid teachers—and educational instruction is often scheduled along with other therapies for elementary, secondary, and high school students, encouraging smoother reintegration after discharge. The length of hospital admission following an SCI has decreased dramatically in the nearly three decades since more reliable statistics have been available; currently, the average length of combined acute/inpatient rehabilitation hospitalization following an SCI is 49 days (http://fscip.org//facts.htm). Certainly, a variety of factors can impact the length of hospitalization (e.g., level of injury, secondary diagnoses, complications, availability of specialty hospital resources), but the overall trend toward reduced inpatient hospitalization allows for individuals to reintegrate back into their premorbid roles and support systems much more rapidly than in the past. There are certainly advantages, but some inherent concerns, for children and adolescents returning more quickly to their previous school environments after the significant life changes brought on by an SCI. The ongoing support of the health care team can be critical in promoting successful reintegration.

College students would most likely be able to resume their studies following an SCI. Depending on their level of injury; however, persons may reevaluate their course of study to prepare for a more feasible career.

Adaptive writing devices, page turners, recording devices, and computers have made returning to the classroom less intimidating. Laws have also improved the accessibility of public buildings. It is challenging, though, for a student with an SCI to manage bowel and bladder schedules, adjustment of clothing, eating devices, and so forth, but with planning and the assistance of others if needed, many individuals have successfully returned to the classroom.

Vocational

It is appropriate for a person with any level of SCI to begin to formulate vocational options, even as an inpatient, with the members of the health care team. Individual situations are so variable—premorbid occupation, level of injury, educational level, other vocational interests, family support, cognitive abilities, motivation, financial resources—making it impossible to say whether a person with a certain level of SCI can or cannot be gainfully employed. However, legislation mandates that work sites be accessible within reason. Also, many employers recognize the importance of a trained employee and will make additional accommodations to return a valued person to the workplace.

As we move from an industrial to an information society, the job market will continue to change, with positions requiring less physical labor than in the past. Job requirements will increasingly demand analytical thought, problem solving, and creativity, all of which are certainly intact after an SCI!

Leisure Activities

For most people, leisure pursuits are an integral part of a meaningful life. Although an SCI can alter the way in which one participates in leisure activities, it does not have to change the intensity of participation.

Sports, both individual and team, are excellent leisure pursuits that are growing in popularity for persons with SCI. Virtually any sport can be undertaken, from basketball to tennis to archery. Adaptive equipment and modified regulations help make some sports more feasible for persons with an SCI, and these modifications should not be viewed as detracting from the competitiveness of the sport. Consider that athletes in the general population use adaptive equipment all the time. How long would a catcher last in a baseball game without a mitt or a mask? Adaptive equipment need not detract from the legitimacy of the contest. It is heartening to see that, even internationally, the wheelchair athlete is recognized for excellence, with designated events in the Olympic games. Persons with an SCI who want to participate have numerous avenues open to them.

Aside from sports, opportunities for social activities from square dancing to traveling abound. Travel agencies and tour groups have recognized the market created by the wheelchair traveler and have responded. Most hospitals with specialized SCI rehabilitation units have well-established programs that help persons get involved with special interest groups. Often, during the acute phase of SCI, persons cannot envision themselves participating again in the things they enjoy. The health care professional must be available for these individuals to encourage renewed interest in favorite leisure activities.

Several resources related to leisure activities, as well as other issues, have been discussed in this chapter. The reader is encouraged to consult the references and suggested readings at the end of this chapter for more information. Additionally, Table 16-4 gives an overview of specific expected outcomes for each level of SCI.

Case Illustrations

Case 1

M.L. is a 24-year-old woman who sustained an SCI during a motor vehicle accident while on her honeymoon. Her husband was thrown from the vehicle but received only minor injuries. M.L. was transported by emergency medical services to the local emergency department. She was diagnosed with a C5 through C6 vertebral subluxation and a C6 crush injury, resulting in a complete (ASIA-A) C6 SCI. She also sustained a left clavicular fracture. She received nasal O$_2$ for respiratory support. Once stabilized, she was transferred to the specialized trauma center near her home. A halo vest was applied, which stabilized her cervical spine. No operative procedures were indicated at that time. After 22 days, her endurance improved so that she could tolerate sitting upright in a chair for up to 1 hour. She was transferred to the nearby rehabilitation facility's SCI unit. During her 12 weeks there, the only complications she experienced were two episodes of autonomic hyperreflexia (apparently secondary to hard stool in the lower rectum) and a mild UTI. Spasticity developed in her wrists, elbows, and LEs.

Before her injury, M.L. was a recently graduated college student with a liberal arts degree. She and her new husband had recently signed a 1-year lease on an upstairs apartment close to the university, as she was anticipating pursuing graduate studies. She had been totally independent in all of her ADL and home-management activities. Her leisure pursuits included recreational team sports (particularly softball) and more sedentary activities like reading and gourmet cooking. She was also involved with her family, particularly two sisters and her parents, who live close by.

Many body functions are significantly affected by M.L.'s injury. Her sensorimotor deficits are consistent with those anticipated for a C6 complete quadriplegia.

M.L. is challenged by the psychosocial/psychological issues facing her as a result of her SCI. She feels that her role has changed significantly, especially in her relationship with her husband. He has been willing to assist her in those activities in which she is physically limited; however, his assistance in some activities—particularly bowel management—has been difficult for her to accept. This has been a source of frustration for her, and she has discussed with him the possibility of hiring an attendant on a limited basis to assist with specific activities. He resists this idea, stating that it is his desire and duty to care for her. He took a temporary leave of absence from the family-owned landscaping company where he is employed when she was discharged 2 weeks ago. There is no definite timetable for his return. M.L. also is concerned about her ability to express herself sexually, as well as her potential to have children in the future. She attended classroom sessions on these topics in the rehabilitation facility, but she did not seek any individual counseling. M.L. states that she probably was not ready to hear anything specific then, but she now wishes she had someone to whom she could ask questions.

M.L. has not begun to consider her work activities or return to school. Even before her accident, she had been undecided about a career path. She has expressed interest, however, in exploring possible alternatives.

M.L. has stated that eventually she might like to get involved in team sports again. In the 2 weeks since her discharge, though, her main leisure pursuits have been reading and watching television.

Case 2

H. B. is a 6-year-old boy who sustained an incomplete (Brown-Séquard) SCI, as the result of being struck by a stray bullet during a drive-by shooting in early August. He did not lose consciousness during transport to the emergency department. It was determined radiologically that the bullet, which entered from the right near the base of his neck/upper back, was lodged in the C7/C8 cervical spinal canal, and surgery was performed to remove the bullet soon after admission. H.B. is now 2 weeks postinjury and exhibits a loss of voluntary movement, reduced touch, and proprioceptive sensation on the right below the level of C7. He exhibits reduced pain, reduced thermal, and some reduction in touch awareness on the left below the level of C7. The levels of C7 and above appear intact for both motor and sensory function. H.B. has had an uncomplicated hospital admission at this time. It is anticipated that he will remain in the acute children's specialty hospital for at least another 2 weeks and then transfer to the inpatient pediatric rehabilitation unit.

At the time of his injury, H.B. was living with his maternal grandmother, who is also his legal guardian. H.B. had been cocaine-positive at birth, and his biologic mother had relinquished her parental rights shortly after he was born. H.B.'s biologic father is unknown. H.B.'s grandmother is also caring for another of H.B.'s siblings, an 8-year-old sister. H.B.'s grandmother reports that prior to his injury, he did not appear to have any overt behavioral/cognitive challenges and had successfully completed kindergarten. She related that he was a "normal, active boy," and enjoyed playing any type of outdoor games as well as watching television. She states he did not have much exposure to computers or video games, as the family did not own these items. She states he had been looking forward to starting first grade, which is scheduled to begin in his district next week.

H.B. has been very cooperative with all of the health care providers working with him; he appears to enjoy the attention he is receiving from the staff as well as the visitors from the neighborhood, his grandmother's church, and police department. His grandmother has expressed many concerns to the health care professionals working with H.B. Her overriding concern is fear that she will be unable to provide sufficient care—both from a physical and financial perspective—for H.B. following his inpatient rehabilitation stay. She related that the family residence is an older, rented duplex, with seven steps leading up to the front porch. She stated the interior of the residence is not conducive to any type of mobility devices, as the hallways and doorways are narrow, and all the bedrooms are on the second story of the unit. She also states concern about how he will be treated when he eventually starts school; although his older sister is in the same elementary school, H.B.'s grandmother states she has had very limited contact with teachers/administrators at the school and has no idea what resources are available to help him. She expressed frustration that H.B.'s shooter has not been apprehended and shared feelings of hopelessness and helplessness in her ability to protect H.B. and his sister from harm in the future.

RECOMMENDED LEARNING RESOURCES

Americans with Disabilities Act, http://www.ada.gov. Accessed June 17, 2010.

General Texts/Resources Relating to SCI

American Spinal Injury Association/International Medical Society of Paraplegia. (1992). *International standards for neurological and functional classification of spinal cord injury.* Chicago: American Spinal Injury Association.

Berczeller, P. H., & Bezkor, M. F. (1986). *Medical complications of quadriplegia.* Chicago: Yearbook Medical Publishers.

Buchanan, L. E. & Nawoczenski, D. A. (1987). *Spinal cord injury: Concepts and management.* Baltimore, MA: Williams & Wilkins.

Field-Fote, E. C. (2009). *Spinal cord injury rehabilitation.* Philadelphia: F.A. Davis Co.

National Institute of Neurological Disorders and Stroke. Retrieved from http://www.ninds.gov. Accessed July 22, 2005.

National Spinal Cord Injury Statistical Center (NSCISC). 619 19th Street South, SRC 515, Birmingham, Alabama, 35249–7330. Retrieved from http://www.spinalcord.uab.edu. Accessed August 12, 2010.

Ozer, M. N. (1988). *The management of persons with spinal cord injury.* New York: Demos Publications.

Somers, M. F. (2010). *Spinal cord injury: Functional rehabilitation (3rd ed.).* Upper Saddle River, NJ: Pearson.

Treischmann, R. (1988). *Spinal cord injuries: Psychological, social and vocational rehabilitation (2nd ed.).* New York: Demos Publications.

Whiteneck, G., Lammertse, D., …Manley, S. (1989). *The Management of High Quadriplegia.* New York: Demos Publications.

Yashon, D. (1986). *Spinal injury (2nd ed.).* East Norwalk, CT: Appleton-Century-Crofts.

Patient/Family Resources

Alpert, M., & Wisnia, S. (2008). *Spinal cord injury and the family: A new guide.* Boston, MA: Harvard University Press.

Christopher Reeve Foundation P.O. Box 277, FDR Station, New York, NY 10150–0277. Retrieved from www.apacure.com

Corbet, B. (1980). *Options: Spinal cord injury and the future.* Denver: A.B. Hirschfield.

Hammond, M., Umlauf, R. L., Matteson, B., & Perduta-Fulginiti, S. (Eds.). (1989). *Yes you can! A guide to self care for persons with spinal cord injury.* Washington, DC: Paralyzed Veterans of America.

Phillips, L., Ozer, A., … Axelson, P. (1987). *Spinal cord injury: A guide for patient and family.* New York: Raven Press.

Spinal Cord Injury Information Network. Retrieved from www.spinalcord.uab.edu. Accessed July 29, 2010.

The Miami Project to Cure Paralysis. University of Miami School of Medicine. P.O. Box 0#960, Mail Locator R-48, Miami, FL 33101. Retrieved from www.miamiproject.miami.edu. Accessed August 14, 2010.

General Neuroanatomy

Barr, M. L. (1979). *The human nervous system: An anatomic viewpoint.* (3rd ed.). New York, NY: Harper & Row.

Liebman, M. (1986). *Neuroanatomy made easy and understandable.* (3rd ed.). Rockville, MD: Aspen Publishers.

REFERENCES

Aids to Investigation of Peripheral Nerve Injuries. (1943). *Medical research council war memorandum* (2nd ed.). Revised. London: HMSO.

American Spinal Injury Association (ASIA). (2000, reprinted 2008). *American spinal injury association international standards for neurological classification of spinal cord injury.* Atlanta, GA: American Spinal Injury Association.

American Spinal Injury Association/International Medical Society of Paraplegia. (1992). *International standards for neurological and functional classification of spinal cord injury.* Chicago, IL: American Spinal Injury Association.

Beets, C. L., Faisant, T., Houghton, V., & Schlich, C. M. (1987). The anterior shell orthosis: An alternative TLSO. *Clinical Prosthetics and Orthotics, 11*(2), 95–100.

Bloch, R. F., & Basbaum, M. (1983). *Management of spinal cord injuries* (pp. 53–154). Baltimore, MD: Williams & Wilkins.

Bracken, M., Holeord, T., & Shepard, M. J. (1990). A randomized, controlled trial of methylprednisolone or naloxone in the treatment of acute spinal cord injury. *New England Journal of Medicine, 322*(20), 1405–1411.

Brunnstrom, F., & Dennen, M. (1931). *Round table on muscle testing.* Annual Conference of American Physical Therapy Association, Federation of Crippled and Disabled, Inc., New York, 1–12.

Burke, D. C., & Murray, D. D. (1975). *Handbook of spinal cord medicine* (67). New York, NY: Raven Press.

Cappuccino, A. (2008). Moderate hypothermia as treatment for spinal cord injury. *Orthopedics,* March, 2008. Retrieved from http://www.orthosupersite.com/view.aspx?rid=26905. Accessed May 18, 2010.

Cassell, B. L. (1986). Treating pressure sores stage by stage. *RN, 49*(36).

Chang, S. M., Hou, C. L., Dong, D. Q., & Zhang, H. (2000). Urologic status of 74 spinal cord injury patients from the 1976 Tangshan Earthquake, and

Managed for over 20 years using the Credé Maneuver. *Spinal Cord, 38*(9), 552–554.

Consortium for spinal cord medicine: Bladder management for adults with spinal cord injury: A clinical practice guideline for health-care providers. (2006). Washington, DC: Paralyzed Veterans of America.

Consortium for spinal cord medicine: Prevention of thromboembolism in spinal cord injury. (1997). Washington, DC: Paralyzed Veterans of America.

Cooper, G. (2006). Essential physical medicine and rehabilitation. Totowa, NJ: Humana Press.

Fine, P. R., Kuhlemeier, K. V., Devivo, M. J., & Stover, L. (1979). Spinal cord injury: An epidemiological perspective. *Paraplegia, 17,* 237–250.

Fowler, S. B. (1995). Deep vein thrombosis and pulmonary embolism in neuroscience patients. *Journal of Neuroscience in Nursing 27,* 224–228.

Geffner, L. F., Santacruz, P., & Izurieta, M. (2008). Administration of autologous bone marrow stem cells into spinal cord injury patients via multiple routes is safe and improves their quality of life: Comprehensive case studies. *Cell Transplantation, 17,* 1277–1293.

Guttmann, L. (1976). *Spinal cord injuries.* Oxford, England: Blackwell Scientific.

Hanak, M., & Scott, A. (1983). *Spinal cord injury: An illustrated guide for health care professionals.* New York: Springer Publishing.

Hayes, K. C., Hsieh, J. T., Wolfe, D. L., Potter, P. J., & Delaney, G. A. (2000). Classifying incomplete spinal cord injury syndromes: algorithms based on the international standards for neurological and functional classification of spinal cord injury patients. *Archives of Physical Medicine and Rehabilitation, 81,* 644–652.

Hernandez, A. M., Fjorner, J. V., & DeLaFuente, T. (1978). The para-articular ossifications in our paraplegics and tetraplegics: A survey of 704 patients. *Paraplegia,* 272–275.

Higgins, M. (2007, September 12). Doctor's say Bills' Everett will walk again. *The New York Times.* Retrieved from http://www.nytimes.com/2007/09/12/sports/football/12everett.html?_r=1. Accessed April 30, 2010.

Hislop, H., Montgomery, J., & Connelly, D. (Eds.). (1995). *Muscle testing: Techniques of manual examination* (6th ed.). Philadelphia: WB Saunders Co.

Lovett, R. (1917). *The treatment of infantile paralysis* (2nd ed.) (136). Philadelphia: P. Blakiston's Son.

McQuillan, K., VonRueden, K., Hartsock, R., Flynn, & Whalen, E. (2002). *Trauma nursing from resuscitation through rehabilitation* (3rd ed.). Philadelphia: WB Saunders Co.

Merenda, L., Duffy, T., & Betz, R. (2007).Outcomes of urinary diversion in children with SCI. *Journal of Spinal Cord Medicine, 30*(Suppl 1), 41–47.

Merriam, W. F., Taylor, T. K., Ruff, S. J., & McPhail, M. J. (1986). A reappraisal of acute traumatic central cord syndrome. *Journal of Bone and Joint Surgery, 68,* 708–713.

National Spinal Cord Injury Statistical Center. (2009a). *2009 Annual Statistical Report.* Birmingham, AL: University of Alabama at Birmingham.

National Spinal Cord Injury Statistical Center. (2009b). *2009 Facts and Figures at a Glance.* Birmingham, AL: University of Alabama at Birmingham. Retrieved from http://fscip.org/facts.htm. Accessed August 14, 2010.

Perkash, I., Martin, D., & Warner, H. (1990). Electroejaculation in spinal cord injury patients: Simplified new equipment and techniques. *Journal of Urolology, 143,* 305–307.

Price, D. (1990, March 18). *Building lives with no barriers* (pp. 17–23A). Detroit News Washington Bureau.

Ragnarsson, K., Hall, K., & Wilmot, C. (1995). Management of pulmonary, cardiovascular and metabolic conditions after spinal cord injury. In S. L. Stover, J. A. DeLisa, & G. G. Whiteneck (Eds.). *Spinal cord injury: Clinical outcomes from the model systems.* (pp. 79–99). Gaithersburg, MD: Aspen.

Roth, E., Lawler, M., & Yarkony, G. (1990). Traumatic central cord syndrome: Clinical features and functional outcomes. *Archives of Physical Medicine and Rehabilitation, 71,* 18–23.

Sipski, M. L. (1991). The impact of spinal cord injury on female sexuality, menstruation and pregnancy: A review of the literature. *Journal of the American Paraplegic Society, 14,* 122–126.

Somers, M. F. (2010). *Spinal cord injury functional rehabilitation* (3rd ed.). Upper Saddle River, NJ: Pearson.

Spinal cord injury facts and figures at a glance—February 2010. (2010). *Spinal cord injury information network.* Retrieved from http://www.spinalcord.uab.edu. Accessed August 13, 2010.

Spinal cord injury treatment and cure research fact sheet. (2007). *The National Spinal Cord Injury Association, July 2007.* Retrieved from http://www.spinalcord.org/news. Accessed June 19, 2010.

Stem Cell Therapy Brings Paralyzed to Feet. (2004). Retrieved from http://chinadaily.com.cn/english/doc/ 2004–11/29/ content_395570.htm. Accessed December 21, 2004.

Taylor, P., Esnouf, J., & Hobby, J. (2002).The functional impact of the freehand system on tetraplegic hand function: Clinical results. *Spinal Cord, 40,* 560–566.

University of Alabama. Research in Spinal Cord Injury. (1998). SCI info sheet#18. Spinal Cord Injury Information Network. RRTC in Secondary Complications of SCI at the University of Alabama at Birmingham, Department of PM&R, December, 1998. Retrieved from http://www.spinalcord.uab.edu. Accessed November 5, 2004.

Weingarden, S., & Martin, C. (1989). Independent dressing after spinal cord injury: A functional time evaluation. *Archives of Physical Medicine and Rehabilitation, 70,* 518–519.

Yashon, D. (1986). *Spinal injury* (2nd ed.) (pp. 35–36). East Norwalk, CT: Appleton-Century-Crofts.

17

Orthopedics

■ *Heather Javaherian-Dysinger*
■ *Sharon Pavlovich*

KEY TERMS

Arthroplasty
Closed fracture
Colles' fracture
Comminuted fracture
Complex regional pain syndrome (CRPS)
Compound fracture
Delayed union
Distal radius fracture
Ecchymosis
Greenstick fracture
Heterotopic ossification
Humeral fracture
Malunion
Nonunion
Open fracture
Open reduction internal fixation (ORIF)
Osteoarthritis
Osteopenia
Osteoporosis
Pathologic fracture
Remodeling
Smith's fracture
Volkmann's deformity

Mary is a 68-year-old widow who lives alone in a small two-story home. Though obese and managing diabetes, she is very active. She volunteers at her church and the community hospital. She loves to garden, walk, play cards with her friends, and do crossword puzzles. At home she cooks simple meals and does light housework as the pain in her hip and hands makes it too difficult to carry out the activities that she did in the past. Mary was an avid square dancer, but with the hip pain and loss of her husband, she gave up dancing, a valued occupation.

After much encouragement from her friends and children, Mary finally went to the doctor and told him about the severity of her pain. After a few tests he diagnosed her with arthritis. She started anti-inflammatory medication to manage her pain and discomfort. Over the past year, however, her right hip became more and more painful. She had difficulty getting out of bed in the morning and had to ask her children to help with the housework and gardening. She cried on the phone as she told her daughter, "I can't do anything anymore." She missed being out in her garden and tending to the plants as it gave her peace and helped her feel connected to the memories of her husband. She also missed socializing, walking, and playing cards with her friends. When they came over to check on her, they encouraged her to talk to her doctor again.

After seeing her doctor, who confirmed that she had severe arthritis in her hip and degeneration, Mary chose to have an elective total hip replacement (THR). Plain radiographs obtained from the right hip revealed severe arthritic changes. Her physician thoroughly discussed the benefits and risks of the surgery with her. She was seen for preassessment training, which involved meeting with several members of the orthopedic total joint team. During this time she met with both an occupational and a physical therapist. The occupational therapist asked her several questions about her postoperative goals, the design of her home, her family support, and the activities in which she liked to engage. The occupational therapist explained that she would receive occupational therapy after the surgery to help her regain independence in daily activities while safely following her hip precautions. The occupational therapist told her that it would take about 6 weeks to recover and that she should be walking with her friends, meeting them for card night, working in the garden with possible modifications, and, most importantly, enjoying life again.

DESCRIPTION AND DEFINITION

Orthopedic conditions involve injury and disease of bones, joints, and their related structures, which include ligaments, tendons, and muscles. The severity of the injury determines the extent of involvement of those supporting structures. Orthopedic conditions may be caused through a variety of circumstances and diseases including traumatic injury, motor vehicular accident (MVA), or arthritis. Injuries during sports such as snowboarding, leisure activities including hiking, and unexpected falls that happen while going about one's day contribute to many of the conditions we see in occupational therapy. Orthopedic conditions may also be caused by rheumatic diseases such as **osteoarthritis** and **osteoporosis**. As a result of these diseases, people may need a joint replacement or **arthroplasty** to promote participation in daily activities and to help improve their quality of life with severe arthritis.

One of the most common orthopedic conditions is a fracture, which is a break in the continuity of the bone. When one considers the forces involved in an injury such as the impact to the wrist as an older woman tries to protect herself from falling or from the force of a door crushing against a finger, it is easy to understand that the ligaments and tendons surrounding the involved joint or bone are often injured as well. Though this is common in orthopedic conditions, the focus of this chapter is on conditions related directly to bones and joints.

ETIOLOGY

Fractures

Fractures are caused by a trauma or disease of the bone or joint. There are two critical factors involved in the determination of a fracture: (1) the amount of force applied to the bone and (2) the strength of the bone (Kunkler, 2002). Forces can be high energy such as those experienced in a motor vehicle accident (MVA) or low energy such as those experienced in a fall or through chronic stress as seen in long distance running. Consequently, these are called stress fractures. The second determining factor is bone strength, which may be normal or weakened from pathologic conditions such as tumors or osteoarthritis and osteoporosis. In addition, the age of a person and the size of the bone further influence the bones' ability to withstand a force. These factors negatively affect bone density, elasticity, and supportive structures, thus making the bone more vulnerable to fracture. For example, an older adult who has decreased bone density from osteoporosis has a weak bone that may be unable to sustain normal forces experienced during daily activities. Thus, the bone may fracture while the person simply bends over or gets out of bed. This type of fracture is called a **pathologic fracture**. Osteoarthritis and osteoporosis are common conditions that contribute to a pathologic fracture.

Osteoarthritis

Osteoarthritis, also referred to as degenerative joint disease, is a noninflammatory joint disease that results in deterioration of articular cartilage and the formation of new bone or osteophytes on the joint surface. These changes often result in pain, joint edema, and impaired participation in life activities. Osteoarthritis is the most common joint disease in the upper extremity. Osteoarthritis of the knee tends to cause the most disability as it impacts one's ability to walk, go up and downstairs, and engage in leisure and work activities. As a result of osteoarthritis, many individuals seek elective surgery for hip and knee replacements to return to a more active and pain-free lifestyle. In the United States, approximately 773,000 total hip and knee replacements are performed annually, with this number expected to increase with the aging of the population (National Institute of Arthritis and Musculoskeletal and Skin Diseases, 2009). The technology of joint replacements continues to evolve, making them essential in promoting participation in daily activities and improving quality of life in people with severe arthritis.

Other Orthopedic Conditions

Osteoporosis is a disease characterized by low bone density and deterioration of bone. It is common in postmenopausal women due to the cessation of estrogen production. The National Osteoporosis Foundation (2010) estimates that over 10 million people in the United States have osteoporosis. A person with osteoporosis may fracture a bone through normal movement such as turning to reach an item of clothing when getting dressed in the morning. The most common sites for these fractures according to data gathered in 2005 are the vertebrae, the wrist, the hip, and pelvis, with approximately 547,000 vertebral fractures, 397,000 wrist fractures, and 297,000 hip fractures (National Osteoporosis Foundation, 2010).

Osteopenia is a reversible weakening of the bone that may be diagnosed through a bone density scan just as osteoporosis. It is estimated that nearly 34 million people have low bone mass (National Osteoporosis Foundation, 2010). As osteopenia is a reversible condition, it is important to take advantage of bone density screenings offered at health fairs and follow up with your physician. Measures to help decrease the risk of osteopenia and halt further progression into osteoporosis include a balanced diet, supplements, weight-bearing exercise, and bone density screenings.

Heterotopic ossification (HO) is an orthopedic condition resulting in abnormal bone formation in extraskeletal soft tissues (Moore & Cho). This condition is often associated with traumatic injuries including severe burns, spinal cord injuries, and head injuries as well as other bone-forming diseases such as ankylosing spondylitis (Moore & Cho, 2010). The exact cause and pathophysiology of HO is still unclear. The massive trauma sustained by the body creates a whole body response, and in some instances, fibroblasts inappropriately start forming bone (Matityahu, et al, 2006). This results in excessive bone growth near joints causing stiffening and loss of movement. This painful and debilitating condition is still not clearly understood, but it can have a significant impact on a person's functional abilities.

INCIDENCE AND PREVALENCE

Fractures

In 2007, the National Center for Injury Prevention (NCIP) reported unintentional falls as the leading cause of nonfatal injuries in the United States across all age groups. The most common fractures that result from falls are those of the humerus, wrist, pelvis, and hip. Falls are the leading cause of fractures among older adults (Bell, Talbot-Stern, & Hennessy, 2000). In 2001, more than 1.6 million older adults were treated for fall-related injuries, which included fractures and other conditions. The 2000 census reported that there are 360,000 to 480,000 fall-related fractures in older adults per year involving the hip, wrist, humerus, vertebrae, and pelvis, with the most serious being a hip fracture (National Center for Injury Prevention and Control, 2004). Older adult women sustain approximately 80% of all hip fractures (Stevens & Olson, 2000). Population studies projected significant increases in rates of hip fractures, with the rising number of older

adults. Fortunately, the hip fracture rate decreased by 25% from 1996 to 2004 (CDC, 2009a). Hip fractures, however, continue to be a significant condition contributing to high costs in health care and changes in quality of life (Cummings, Rubin, & Black, 1990; CDC, 2009a).

Hip fractures are one of the primary causes of disability and mortality in the older adults. Statistics suggest that one in five people dies within the first year of sustaining a hip fracture (Gillespie, 2002). Some people will not return to their premorbid functional level and may rely on adaptive equipment or modifications to their daily activities (Crotty et al., 2010; Hall, Williams, Senior, Goldswain, & Criddle, 2000; Koval, Skovron, Aharonof, & Zuckerman, 1998; Magaziner et al., 2000; Marottoli, Berkman, & Cooney, 1993). A randomized trial by Hagsten, Svensson, and Gardulf (2004), however, found that occupational therapy intervention increased a patient's ability to perform activities of daily living (ADL) sooner than those who did not receive occupational therapy. Thus, patients receiving occupational therapy were more likely to return to an independent living situation and require less postoperative care. This charges occupational therapy practitioners with the role of promoting life participation and well-being among individuals who are recovering from fractures as well as other orthopedic conditions.

Osteoarthritis

Arthritis is one of the leading causes of disability impeding people's capacity to engage in meaningful and necessary daily occupations due to pain, weakness, and loss of range of motion (ROM) (Healthy People 2010, 2010). According to the CDC (2009b), 51.2 million people have arthritis. In the United States alone, it is estimated that 27 million people have osteoarthritis (National Institute of Arthritis and Musculoskeletal and Skin Diseases, 2002). Osteoarthritis typically affects the knee, distal interphalangeal joints, proximal interphalangeal joints, and the first carpal metacarpal joint.

Other Orthopedic Conditions

According to the National Osteoporosis Foundation, 10 million people have osteoporosis, of which 80% are women (National Osteoporosis Foundation, 2010). Early signs of osteoporosis are seen in younger women in the form of osteopenia. This trend emphasizes the importance of prevention and lifestyle management as once the disease progresses beyond osteopenia to osteoporosis, bone regeneration is no longer reversible. The significantly weakened bone contributes to an increased risk of fractures seen in older adults (Greenspan et al., 1994) and impacts participation in meaningful activities and quality of life (Kotz, Deleger, Cohen, Kamigaki, & Kurata, 2004).

HO is a common complication after traumas such as fractures, arthroplasties, traumatic amputations, spinal cord injuries, head injuries, and burns, with the incidence varying depending on the injury. Though it is a common complication, only 10% to 20% of people who develop HO will have significant functional limitations (Bruno-Petrina, 2008; Wheeless, 2010). Most people will be asymptomatic and most likely diagnosed when it is seen on a film. HO usually occurs 1 to 4 months after the traumatic injury (Wheeless). HO may occur after a fracture especially in those who have an **open reduction internal fixation (ORIF)** (Bruno-Petrina). In injuries and fractures to the elbow, the incidence may be as high as 90% (Bruno-Petrina). The incidence of HO in hip arthroplasties is generally 50%, although only one-third of the people experience clinically significant symptoms such as limited ROM and pain (Kocic, Lazovic, Mitkovic, & Djokic, 2010; Wheeless). Revisions to hip and knee replacements increase the risk of developing HO (Barrack, Brumfield, Rorabeck, Cleland, & Myers, 2002; Moore & Cho, 2010). With the increase in combat-related injuries over the last several years, we have seen more soldiers with traumatic amputations. The incidence of HO in these amputations was found to be 63%, which is much higher than that previously expected (Potter, Burns, Lacap, Granville, & Gajewski, 2007). Fortunately, the majority of the cases are successfully managed or the soldiers are asymptomatic. HO occurs in 40% to 50% of people who have a spinal cord injury, with it primarily affecting the knee, pelvis, and hip (Moore & Cho; Wheeless). Research suggests that it also occurs in 20% of people who have a traumatic brain injury (Bruno-Petrina). The incidence of HO appears to be much higher in fractures and neurologic injuries involving spasticity than it does in burns. A previous study found a 1.2% incident rate in 1,478 people admitted to a burn center (Peterson, Mani, Crawford, Neff, & Hiebert, 1989).

SIGNS AND SYMPTOMS

Fractures

The general symptoms of a break are localized pain at the fracture site, deformity, edema, and **ecchymosis**, which is often seen after 24 to 48 hours of onset (Altizer, 2002). A physician performs a clinical evaluation obtaining information on the signs and symptoms and the circumstances surrounding the fracture. The physician usually refers the person to radiology to confirm and determine the degree and classification of the fracture. The radiologist also evaluates for other associated findings such as a pathologic fracture (bone weakened by a tumor), stress fracture, or other preexisting conditions that may have affected the integrity of the bone. The diagnosis is commonly confirmed through plain films or x-ray, though other studies

may be ordered depending on the physician, suspected injury, and location of the suspected injury.

There are several types of fractures. A **closed fracture** refers to a fracture that has not broken through the skin, whereas in an **open fracture** the bone breaks through the skin surface. Open fractures, also known as **compound fractures**, have an increased chance for infection. The term comminuted is applied to fractures that have two or more fragments. A displaced fracture involves segments that have become separated or shifted from the bone (Altizer, 2002). **Greenstick fractures** are often seen in children whose bones are still soft and growing. Rather than snapping into two, the bone breaks on one side and bends on the other. It is similar to how a young twig or tree limb breaks, thus the name greenstick fracture.

Fractures are further described by the type of fracture line. A complete fracture involves a break in the full continuity of the bone. An incomplete fracture involves a partial disruption in the continuity of the bone. Such breaks are often called cracks or hairline fractures (Altizer). A transverse fracture occurs when the fracture line is at a right angle to the longitudinal axis of the bone. An oblique fracture involves a fracture line that is diagonal or slanted. Torsional stress applied to bone causes a twisting fracture line, which is called a spiral fracture.

Distal Radial Fractures

Distal radial fractures may cause loss of sensation, strength, movement, and limited functional use of the hand and possibly the arm. As most of these injuries are caused by a fall on an outstretched arm, the entire upper extremity should be examined for injury. A **Colles' fracture** will reveal "dorsal displacement, dorsal comminuting, and radius shortening" (Laseter, 2002). This is often referred to as a dinner fork deformity given its resemblance to an upside down fork (Fig. 17.1). A **Smith's fracture** is the reverse of a Colles' fracture; therefore, the deformity displaces toward the volar or palmar aspect of the wrist (Laseter, 2002) (Fig. 17.2).

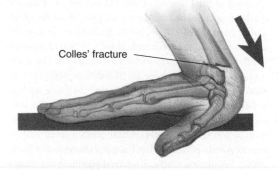

Figure 17.1 Colles' fracture.

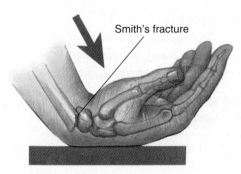
Smith's fracture

Figure 17.2 Smith's fracture.

Hip Fractures

A hip fracture generally refers to a fracture of the proximal femur. It may be intracapsular or extracapsular. Intracapsular fractures involve the femoral neck such as a subcapital or transcervical fracture (Fig. 17.3). Extracapsular fractures involve the trochanters such as a subtrochanteric or intertrochanteric fracture. An individual with a hip fracture may experience referred pain to the knee, may be unable to bear weight on the involved lower extremity, and will often have a leg-length discrepancy.

Humeral Fractures

The incidence of **humeral fractures** in the United States has increased as a result of the aging of its population, increased participation in sports, and the rise of osteoporosis (Gill, 2002). A humeral fracture may present with humeral displacement and malposition of the distal limb. Radial nerve injury is found in approximately 18% of humeral shaft fractures (Wheeless, 2004). A spiral fracture may lacerate the radial nerve, or it may be damaged by displaced bony segments. Clinical signs of radial nerve involvement include loss of wrist extension and impaired sensation on the dorsal aspect of the wrist. Seventy-five to ninety percent of individuals who have closed humeral fractures have recovery of the radial nerve in 3 to 4 months (Wheeless).

Fractures that occur at the distal end of the humerus just above the medial and lateral condyles are referred to as supracondylar fractures. These fractures are commonly known as elbow fractures. The medial and lateral condyles serve as an origin site for many muscles of the forearm and have bony connections to the radius and ulna of the forearm. Nerves and arteries pass along this area; therefore, a supracondylar fracture can also result in injury to muscles, nerves, and tissue that further affect the function of the entire arm. Understandably, it is associated with a high risk for complications such as **malunion** and **Volkmann's deformity**. Volkmann's deformity is a condition that results from severe damage to tissues and muscles

caused by increased pressure in the forearm compartments (Kare, 2008). Increased compartmental pressures may be caused by several factors such as ischemia, compartmental bleeding, and excessively tight bandages (Kare, 2008). Signs of ischemia include pale or bluish skin, absence of radial pulse, decreased sensation, and severe pain. Suspected cases of increased compartmental pressure should be immediately reported to the physician as it can result in nerve damage and necrosis.

Scaphoid Fractures

The position of the scaphoid in the proximal row of the carpal bones makes it particularly vulnerable to injury. It is the most commonly fractured bone in the wrist, with an incidence of 35,000 to 50,000 fractures annually (Dell & Dell, 2002). Scaphoid fractures are commonly seen in young males with a sports injury, resulting in wrist hyperextension with radial deviation. Fractures of the middle and proximal poles of the scaphoid are susceptible to avascular necrosis because of its poor blood supply (Dell & Dell, 2002). Plain radiographs are commonly used to classify the scaphoid fracture; however, other radiographic procedures may be necessary to evaluate its healing.

Arthritis

There are other conditions in addition to fractures that affect the integrity of the bone, such as rheumatic diseases. Rheumatic diseases include an array of progressive conditions leading to impairments in joints and soft tissue. Examples include osteoarthritis and osteoporosis. Rheumatic diseases are closely associated with the term arthritis, which means joint inflammation. Arthritis is a general term used to describe a host of conditions characterized by joint pain, redness, swelling, and stiffness (Deshaies, 2006).

Osteoarthritis symptoms build up gradually and often begin with notable aches with movement especially after inactivity. Osteoarthritis is often characterized by joint pain, inflammation, stiffness, tenderness, limited ROM, and crepitus, which is an audible or palpable crunching or popping in the joint caused by the irregularity of opposing cartilage surfaces (Hochberg as cited in Deshaies, 2006).

Other Orthopedic Conditions

Osteoporosis is gradual and somewhat silent as it emerges. In the early stages of osteoporosis, symptoms are not usually present. Over time, however, advanced symptoms present themselves through pain, height loss, and kyphosis. The primary clinical signs of osteoporosis include skeletal fractures and recurring pathologic fractures (Dal Bello-Haas, 2009). Osteopenia is a predecessor to osteoporosis. Even more silent, there are no clinical signs or presentation for osteopenia. Osteopenia is often evident

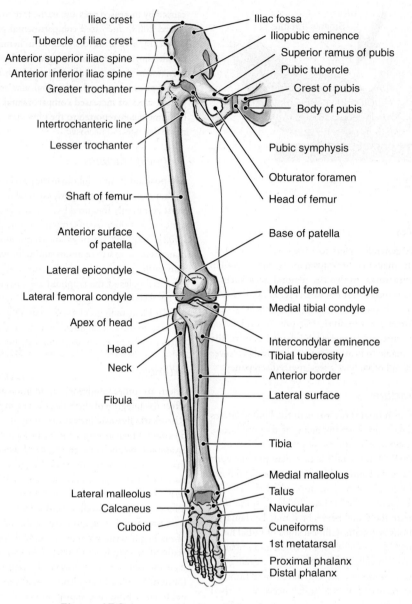

Figure 17.3 Lower extremity, anterior view.

in bone scans, which may be used to confirm the diagnosis (Li, Smith, Tuohy, Smith, & Koman, 2010). It may be initially diagnosed in health screenings or when an adult has several risk factors such as being female, smoking, consuming excessive alcohol, having a low body weight (U.S. Department of Health & Human Services, 2005), and a parent who has had a hip fracture due to osteoporosis (Ahlborg et al., 2010; Khosla & Melton, 2007; National Osteoporosis Foundation, 2010).

HO usually begins with pain, joint warmth, swelling, and decreased ROM approximately 1 to 4 months after

an injury (Adler, 2006). There may be a palpable mass, which becomes harder as the bone forms. HO can be diagnosed by a radiologist through bone scan, ultrasonography, or CT scan (Moore & Cho, 2010).

COURSE AND PROGNOSIS

The prognosis and functional outcomes for orthopedic conditions varies depending on the condition itself and the health of the person. The general course and prognosis of fractures are dependent upon several factors: age, type of fracture, fracture location, severity of the fracture, and the patient's intrinsic motivation and premorbid health status. It is important to note, however, that considering all of the orthopedic conditions, hip fractures are the leading cause of morbidity and mortality in older adults (Hall et al., 2000; Stevens & Olson, 2004; Wolinsky, Fitzgerald, & Stemp, 1997). Therefore, occupational therapy practitioners should work closely with the referring physician for the appropriate protocol and precautions. This statistic also emphasizes the importance of addressing fall prevention and community wellness programs for older adults.

The way in which the bone heals influences the patient's course and prognosis. There are two types of tissues that form bone: cancellous and cortical. Cancellous bone or spongy bone is the inner layer, which houses the bone's vascular supply. It is essential for nutrients to help form strong healthy bones. Cortical bone is the hard outer layer of the bone that provides support and protection. The periosteum is a dense fibrous membrane consisting of connective tissues, elastic fibers, and nerve fibers, which line the outer surface of most bones (Gray, 2004). A fractured bone normally takes 6 to 12 weeks to heal (Kunkler, 2002).

To achieve optimal healing, it is important that the fracture site receive immediate vascular circulation and appropriate immobilization. The healing process involves five stages (Kunkler, 2002). First, a hematoma forms and seals the damaged blood vessels; then osteoclasts reabsorb the damaged bone and tissue. The second stage is the formation of a granular or fibrocartilage tissue, which increases the stability of the bone fragments. The third stage involves the formation of a callus. This takes place between 2 and 6 weeks. The formation of the callus has a significant influence on the outcome of the fracture. The fourth stage is ossification and the formation of a bony union. The fifth or final stage is often referred to as consolidation and **remodeling** occurring between 6 weeks and 1 year. To reiterate, the amount of healing time depends on the severity of the fracture and any premorbid health conditions. During remodeling, the bone is ideally reshaped to its original form to enable it to resume its intended function as best as possible.

In some instances, the bone heals abnormally. Abnormal healing can be caused by several factors including an open fracture, severe soft tissue damage, infection, poor vascularization, nerve damage, phlebitis, or compartment syndrome. Such complications can result in **delayed union**, malunion, and **nonunion**. A delayed union is when the bone takes more time to heal than is expected; it heals slowly. It may be suspected when pain and tenderness persist at the fracture site 3 months to 1 year after the injury (Kunkler, 2002). Delayed unions may be caused by several factors including infection, poor vascularization, or inadequate immobilization. Once the causing factor is identified and corrected, the bone will typically heal. In a malunion fracture, the fracture heals in an abnormal or deformed position. Contributing factors include muscle imbalance and inadequate protection and positioning of the fracture (Altizer, 2002). A malunion fracture has significant functional implications as the person will often experience limited ROM, strength, and coordination. Nonunion fractures refer to a fracture in which the bone is not healing. A nonunion fracture may be caused by several factors such as vascular and tissue damage, poor alignment, stress to the fracture site, and infection (Altizer, 2002). The scaphoid bone has a high risk for nonunion due to its limited blood supply.

Arthritis

The course and prognosis of arthritis varies. Idiopathic osteoarthritis, which is the most common, may show itself by osteophytes or "bone spurs" on the proximal interphalangeal joints (Bouchard's nodes) and distal interphalangeal joints (Herberden's nodes). These may become painful and inflamed, limiting functional use. In cases where there is significant pain and joint degeneration, an arthroplasty may be warranted. This is most common in the carpal metacarpal joint of the thumb (Cooper, 2008).

Other Orthopedic Conditions

Osteopenia may progress to osteoporosis if untreated through lifestyle changes including calcium supplements, a calcium-enriched diet, and added weight-bearing exercise. As mentioned before this condition is silent and will transform into osteoporosis without any signs. Osteoporosis is irreversible. In regards to prognosis, a person can live a productive and active life but will need to take extra caution in joint protection and fall prevention to avoid a resulting fracture due to the weakened bone.

In the case of HO, 10% to 20% of patients will have permanent functional loss (Bruno-Petrina, 2008; Wheeless, 2010). The severity of the functional limitations will depend on the joints involved. For instance, there may be more functional implications for a person who has had a burn and develops HO in the dominant upper extremity versus if it develops in the hip joint of someone who has paraplegia. The course of the condition, however, can be complicated if there is additional nerve compression due to the ossification and lymphedema. Medical management, which will be covered in the next section, is important in maintaining ROM and decreasing functional limitations and pain.

MEDICAL AND SURGICAL MANAGEMENT

The medical management of orthopedic conditions varies depending on the specific condition. Some require conservative treatment consisting of over-the-counter medications, splinting, and home exercise programs, while others may require surgery. Below, we have provided a brief summary of the medical management of the more common conditions that we have discussed this chapter.

Fractures

Hip Fractures

Most hip fractures require surgical intervention. The type of procedure depends on several factors such as the severity of the fracture, prefracture functional level of the patient, age of the patient, the presence or absence of comorbid conditions, and the preference of the surgeon (Beloosesky et al., 2002; Lowe, Crist, Bhandari, & Ferguson, 2010). Patients who are more active prior to their fracture often have fewer complications and more positive results after surgery, thus emphasizing the importance of a healthy lifestyle (Beloosesky et al., 2002). There is still mixed-evidence on the morbidity and mortality rates and surgical approach for the very elderly (Bhandari et al., 2005; Lowe et al., 2010). Therefore, physicians will carefully consider these factors and make necessary preoperative referrals to medically stabilize the patient while keeping in mind complications and further discomfort that might arise with a delay in surgery (Holt, Smith, Duncan, & McKeown, 2010).

The goal of surgical intervention for a hip fracture is to align and immobilize the fracture site to allow for normal healing. Hip fractures are treated with closed reduction and immobilization or ORIF. Closed reduction involves realigning the fracture fragments through manual manipulation or traction, which may be done under general or local anesthesia (Kunkler, 2002). Immobilization can be accomplished through casts, traction, splints, or braces. Open reduction, on the other hand, involves surgically opening and reducing the fracture site. Internal fixation is commonly done after an open reduction to secure the fracture. Internal fixation involves securing the fracture site with pins, rods, plates, and screws. This promotes healing and allows for early mobilization, which can reduce complications often associated with immobility. Some hip fractures such as an intracapsular femoral neck fracture may be treated with hemiarthroplasty or

a THR (Brunner & Eshilian-Oates, 2003; Wheeless, 2010). A hemiarthroplasty is a partial joint replacement in which the femoral head and neck are replaced by a metal prosthesis. A total arthroplasty or THR may be indicated depending on the patient's age and whether the femur and acetabulum were damaged from the injury or a preexisting disease.

Distal Radial Fractures and Humeral Fractures

Distal radial and humeral fractures may be reduced or realigned manually or with surgery. Closed fractures may be reduced manually and immobilized with a cast. Fractures that are unstable or cannot be manually reduced require surgery. This procedure is called an ORIF, which secures the fracture site with screws, pins, plates, and rods. Open and **comminuted fractures** often require ORIF. Figure 17.4 is a radiograph of an ORIF in which two plates and screws were used to surgically stabilize displaced fractures of the radius and ulna of a woman who had been in an MVA. Some **distal radius fractures** may occasionally require a long arm cast to prevent forearm rotation that involves movement of the humerus, ulna, and radius. This movement can result in displacement and impact the healing process (Laseter, 2002). For open and closed fractures a splint may be worn for the first few days after surgery to allow for natural swelling. A cast is then worn approximately 4 to 6 weeks depending upon the physician, type of fracture, and healing process. Following bone healing, external fixators are often removed after 6 to 8 weeks depending upon fracture consolidation. Some fractures that are relatively stable may require splinting for as little as 3 weeks (Laseter).

Scaphoid Fractures

A nondisplaced scaphoid fracture is typically immobilized with a thumb spica cast for approximately 8 to 10 weeks (Dell & Dell, 2002) (Fig. 17.5). Proximal scaphoid fractures may require a long arm-thumb spica cast followed by the use of a short-arm-thumb spica cast to promote healing for as long as 6 weeks to 6 months. Displaced or unstable scaphoid fractures require an ORIF with a compression screw (Dell & Dell).

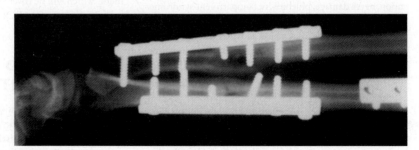

Figure 17.4 Open reduction internal fixation.

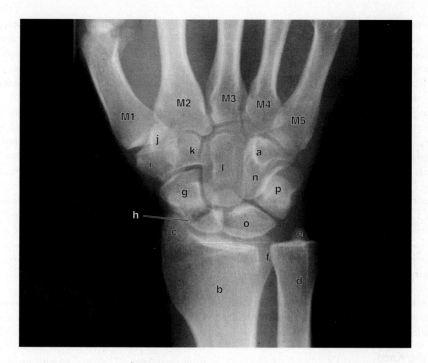

Figure 17.5 Scaphoid fracture.

Following the ORIF, a wrist splint should be used for 2 to 6 weeks or until the bony union is formed. A percutaneous fixation technique using a Herbert screw is a common and effective approach used in the treatment of acute scaphoid fractures. This technique has been found to be associated with a more rapid return of hand function, higher client satisfaction, and minimal complications (Jeon et al., 2003). The physician and therapist should closely monitor the fracture to ensure proper vascularization.

Arthritis

Arthritis may be controlled with various medications, and patients should be followed closely by a rheumatologist. Arthroplasty may be indicated in joints that have severe pain and joint deterioration that significantly limits participation in daily activities. Arthroplasties or joint replacements may be done in the hands, shoulder, and other joints though it is most common in the hip and knee as they are our weight-bearing joints.

Arthritis of the Hip

THRs are typically indicated for those who have severe arthritis causing pain and stiffness that significantly limits the person's participation in daily activities, or as mentioned above, when there is damage to the acetabulum or femur during a fall. This is a common condition seen by occupational therapy practitioners working in acute

care and in-patient rehabilitation. THRs are often seen in individuals 55 years and older. The procedure involves replacement of the acetabulum and ball of the femur with artificial implants. These may be secured by bone cement or a cementless prosthesis, which allows for bone growth. Hip replacements or arthroplasties generally last for 10 to 25 years (Roberts, 2002); though researchers continue to evaluate implant wear.

Following a THR, there are several precautions that a patient must follow for 6 to 8 weeks after the surgery (Maher & Bear-Lehman, 2008; Rasul & Wright, 2010). These precautions include no hip adduction and rotation of the operated leg and no hip flexion beyond 90 degrees of the operated leg (Table 17.1). If the surgeon uses an anterior approach, the patient must also avoid hip extension. Oftentimes, therapists will encourage their clients to avoid hip rotation in general to ensure that the surgical hip is protected. These precautions are

TABLE 17.1 Total Hip Precautions

1. Avoid hip flexion beyond 90 degrees

2. Avoid hip rotation of operated leg

3. Avoid hip adduction of operated leg (avoid crossing legs)

currently the standard of care; however, recent research suggests that an anterolateral surgical approach rather than strict adherence to traditional hip precautions was more likely to be associated with a low rate of dislocation (Peak et al., 2005). Depending on the severity of the condition, the surgical approach and procedure, and the orthopedic surgeon, there may be weight-bearing precautions for patients who undergo a THRs and ORIFs. Common weight-bearing statuses include non–weight bearing, touchdown or toe-touch weight bearing, partial weight bearing, weight bearing as tolerated, and full weight bearing (Table 17.2).

Hip precautions have functional implications for the person in a variety of daily activities. Occupational therapy practitioners must educate clients on the hip precautions and teach them adaptations for sitting, dressing, bathing, reaching for items, and driving among others. In regards to driving, patients are to avoid driving for 4 to 6 weeks following surgery (Ganz, Levin, Peterson, & Ranawat, 2003). At this time, most patients have reached their preoperative driving reaction time and continue to show improvements in reaction time for up to 1 year.

Arthritis of the Knee

The first line of management of arthritis of the knee is conservative treatment, which often begins with over-the-counter anti-inflammatory medications and heat and ice. If pain and functional limitations progress, the patient's primary physician or rheumatologist may prescribe medications to effectively control the arthritis. When conservative treatment does not work, the patient may be a candidate for a partial or total knee replacement (TKR).

This is also referred to as a knee arthroplasty. A TKR involves resurfacing the entire knee joint with metal and plastic prosthetic components. The procedure typically involves a femoral component, a tibial plate, and a patellar button (Roberts, 2002) and may be done unilaterally or bilaterally.

After surgery, it is important to begin the rehabilitation process (Bade, Kohrt, & Stevens-Lapsley, 2010; Rasul & Wright, 2010). Treatment involves pain medication and early mobilization to strengthen the quadriceps and prevent loss of ROM. A continuous passive motion machine may be prescribed while in the hospital or at home to help improve circulation and movement at the knee joint depending on the patient's postoperative health and functional abilities. Initial rehabilitation goals include independence in bed mobility, knee flexion to approximately 90 degrees, knee extension, and to walk with crutches or a walker (American Academy of Orthopaedic Surgeons, 1995–2009).

To maximize the results of the surgery and functional outcomes, the patient needs education on several precautions such as avoiding putting a pillow under the knee while in bed, resting both feet on the floor when sitting to increase knee ROM, and wearing an immobilizer as instructed by the physician to protect the knee joint until the muscle is strong enough to support it (Erickson & Perkins, 1994; Rasul & Wright, 2010). The immobilizer may be required when walking, while in bed, or at all times. Kneeling should be avoided. Other considerations include not driving, running, and jumping until cleared by the physician. Generally, patients are able to return to most of their normal daily activities after 3 to 6 weeks

TABLE 17.2 Weight-Bearing Status

Weight-Bearing Status	Percentage and Description
Non–weight bearing	0%. No weight bearing on the operated leg; it should not touch the floor.
Touchdown or toe-touch weight bearing	10%–15%. Foot of operated leg may rest on floor.
Partial weight bearing	30%–50%. Patient may put 30%–50% of weight through the operated leg.
Weight bearing as tolerated	Patient may put as much weight through operated leg as tolerated without unnecessary pain or discomfort.
Full weight bearing	75%–100%. Patient bears full weight on the operated leg.

Modified from Goldstein, T. S. (1999). *Geriatric orthopedics: Rehabilitative management of common problems* (2nd ed.). Gaithersburg, MD: Aspen.

though high-impact activities may need to be modified. Driving may be resumed around 4 to 6 weeks as long as the patient is able to bend his or her knee enough to get in and out of the car and have appropriate muscle strength and control to operate the pedals. Patients need to follow up with their physician to monitor for complications and ensure continued progress.

IMPACT ON OCCUPATIONAL PERFORMANCE

Occupational therapy practitioners use a holistic approach to examine specific client factors residing within the person to understand their impact on occupational performance (American Occupational Therapy Association [AOTA], 2008). Systems of values, beliefs and spirituality; body functions, and body structures are client factors that are often affected by illness or disability (AOTA, 2008). Client factors are an important consideration when working with a person who has an orthopedic condition to help them engage in daily occupations such as dressing, working, managing the home, and leisure pursuits. We will discuss client factors that are commonly affected by an orthopedic condition.

During the initial evaluation it is important to carefully assess the nature and circumstances surrounding the onset of the orthopedic condition. For example, children and adults are likely to sustain fractures during play and sports activities, whereas older adults may experience a fracture as a result of a fall or osteoporosis. In some circumstances, however, a fracture may also be a result of child abuse or domestic violence. The nature of the circumstance surrounding the injury or condition may impact secondary injuries and psychosocial involvement. It is important therefore to conduct a thorough history of the fall and a radiologic analysis of the fracture (American Academy of Pediatrics, 2000) and, for children, to ascertain their developmental level.

Orthopedic conditions may compromise participation in several areas of occupation including ADLs, instrumental activities of daily living, sleep, education, work, play, leisure, and social participation (AOTA, 2008). The degree of impairment depends upon the severity of the injury, location of the injury, and the client's premorbid health status. Several client factors may be compromised by orthopedic conditions (Table 17.3). The main client factors that will affect one's participation in occupation are neuromusculoskeletal and movement-related functions and structures and sensory and pain functions and

---

TABLE 17.3 Client Factors Commonly Involved in Orthopedic Conditions

1. Values, beliefs, and spirituality

2. Body functions
   (a) Mental functions
   (b) Sensory functions and pain
      (i) Vestibular function (balance)
      (ii) Pain
      (iii) Protective functions of the skin
   (c) Neuromusculoskeletal and movement-related functions
      (i) Joint mobility
      (ii) Joint stability
      (iii) Muscle power
      (iv) Muscle tone
      (v) Muscle endurance
   (d) Skin and related structure functions
      (i) Repair function of the skin

3. Body structures
   (a) Structures related to movement
   (b) Skin and related structures

From American Occupational Therapy Association (AOTA). (2008). Occupational therapy practice framework: Domain and process (2nd ed.). *American Journal of Occupational Therapy, 62*, 625–683.

structures. Joint mobility, stability, and alignment are directly affected by a fracture or a condition such as osteoarthritis. Therefore, in the case of fractures, it is necessary to reduce or realign them in a timely manner. Limited joint mobility may affect an individual's ability to participate in daily activities such as dressing, cooking, and cleaning. This in turn can affect one's role performance. For example, a woman with a distal radius fracture may initially have difficulty fulfilling her mothering role with an infant. Until the pain and swelling are reduced and the fracture is stabilized, she may be unable to lift her baby and have difficulty doing things such as changing diapers.

Muscle strength and endurance are often affected by orthopedic conditions as a result of immobilization of a joint during recovery. These limitations may also be caused and worsened by disuse of the involved extremity. A person will often hold his or her involved extremity in a dependent or guarded position and refrain from using it. This further compounds the patient's symptoms and often leads to loss of ROM, strength, and pain in other joints and musculature that were initially uninvolved. Limitations in muscle strength and endurance directly impact one's performance and participation in daily activities. A person recovering from a humeral fracture may find it difficult to golf or may find that his or her arm tires easily when painting or doing household chores.

Orthopedic conditions may affect sensation function and pain in the areas of balance, sensation, and pain. When recovering from a THR or hip fracture, an individual may struggle with balance as he or she tries to walk, move around in the bathroom, and get dressed while following weight-bearing precautions. As a result, the individual may need to modify how he or she does certain activities in order to prevent a fall. Sensation may be affected if there is nerve involvement at the fracture site. Depending on the degree of sensory involvement, an individual may have difficulty picking things up. Pain, as noted earlier in the discussion, is a common sign of an injury. Pain will vary depending on the person, severity of the injury, and complications. Sharp or continuous pain may affect an individual's ability to complete daily tasks. The pain experienced by people who develop **complex regional pain syndrome (CRPS)** can be so overwhelming that it affects their ability to work and carry out their life roles.

Joint pain, inflammation, and limited ROM from osteoarthritis often affect participation in daily life activities as the integrity of the bone is compromised Yasuda, (2008). As such, an individual may require the use of adaptive equipment to help with tasks such as dressing and grooming. Fluctuations in movement-related functions can vary from day to day secondary to medications, pain, and efforts put forth in energy conservation and work simplification techniques.

In addition, functions of the skin and related structures and mental functions may be impacted by orthopedic conditions. Compound fractures that break through the skin will result in a wound at risk for infection. This type of fracture will involve more medical management and may consequently limit an individual's ability to participate in a variety of daily occupations due to pain, wound care procedures, and type of fixator.

Mental functions such as one's self-concept, motivation, and interests may be impacted by an orthopedic condition. A distal radius fracture, for example, may present with skin changes, edema, and severely limited movement in the fingers. As a result, the individual may have difficulty doing many tasks such as dressing, grooming, and writing. The inability to perform these daily tasks that we often take for granted may impair one's self-concept and thus affect a person's motivation such as when one withdraws from activities that he or she is normally interested in. This emphasizes the importance for the occupational therapy practitioner to continually assess and address the person's values, beliefs, and spirituality as these factors will impact the person's coping strategies and mental well-being throughout the healing process.

Case Illustrations

Case 1

Distal Radial Fracture

Josh is a 16-year-old man who enjoys participating in several sports during the winter months. On a recent snowboarding venture Josh was taken to a local emergency room (ER) after he fell on his right arm while performing an air stunt. The on-call physician evaluated Josh and ordered x-rays to confirm a distal radial fracture. After confirmation of a closed fracture, the physician manually reduced the fracture and immobilized Josh with a cast. After 5 weeks the cast was removed and occupational therapy was ordered to address ADL.

The occupational therapy evaluation found Josh to have impaired strength and limited ROM in his forearm. Josh reported having difficulty turning his forearm to dress and shares that his arm does not feel strong enough to hold all of his school books.

Case 2

Supracondylar Fracture of the Humerus

Ana is a 57-year-old woman who fractured her humerus in an MVA. She was taken to the ER where the physician conducted a clinical assessment and ordered x-rays to confirm the suspected fracture. The radiologist report confirmed that there was a closed transverse fracture of the middle third of the right humeral shaft. The physician was able to reduce the fracture without surgery. He immobilized the arm in a sling. Four weeks later, Ana still had significant pain and tenderness in her upper arm. Radiologic tests revealed that the bone was forming a malunion. The physician determined that it was necessary to surgi-

cally reduce the fracture and stabilize it with internal fixation. Radiologic studies showed signs of healing 6 weeks after the second reduction as well as signs of osteopenia. The physician wrote a prescription for occupational therapy.

The occupational therapist evaluated Ana. He noted that she held her arm in a dependent position and was very hesitant to move it or let him examine it. She reported significant pain and had atrophy of her upper arm and forearm muscles. Her skin appeared shiny in comparison to her left arm. Ana had limited movement and reported that her husband had to help her with everything. She had been unable to return to work as an office manager because the pain was just too great.

RECOMMENDED LEARNING RESOURCES

Books

Bonder, B. R., & Dal Bello-Haas, V. (2009). *Functional performance in older adults.* Philadelphia, PA: F.A. Davis.

Mackin, E. J., Callahan, A. D., Osterman, L., Skirven, T. M., & Schneider, L. (2002). *Rehabilitation of the hand and upper extremity* (5th ed.). St. Louis, MO: Mosby.

Radomski, M. V., & Trombly-Latham, C. A. (2007). *Occupational therapy for physical dysfunction* (6th ed.). Philadelphia, PA: Lippincott Williams & Wilkins.

Journals

American Journal of Occupational Therapy
www.aota.org
American Journal of Orthopedics
http://www.amjorthopedics.com/
Journal of American Geriatrics Society
http://www.wiley.com/bw/journal.asp?ref=0002-8614&site=1

Orthopaedic Nursing
http://journals.lww.com/orthopaedicnursing/pages/default.aspx

Web sites

American Occupational Therapy Association. Evidence-Based Practice & Research
http://www.aota.org/Educate/Research.aspx
Centers for Disease Control and Prevention
http://www.cdc.gov
Healthy People 2020
http://www.healthypeople.gov/hp2020/
Lewis, W. H. (Ed.). *Gray's anatomy (12th ed.).* New York, NY: Bartleby.com. Retrieved from http://www.bartleby.com/107
United States Department of Health & Human Services
http://www.hhs.gov/
Wheeless, C. R. (2010). *Wheeless' textbook of orthopaedics.* http://www.wheelessonline.com

REFERENCES

Adler, C. (2006). Spinal cord injury. In M. B. Early (Ed.), *Physical dysfunction practice skills for the occupational therapy assistant* (2nd ed., pp. 528–550). St. Louis, MO: Mosby.

Ahlborg, H., Rosengren, B., Jarvinen, T., Rogmark, C., Nilsson, J., Sernbo, I., & Karlsson, M. (2010). Prevalence of osteoporosis and incidence of hip fracture in women—Secular trends over 30 years. *BMC Musculoskeletal Disorders, 11*(1).

Altizer, L. (2002). Fractures. *Orthopaedic Nursing, 21,* 51–59.

American Academy of Pediatrics. (2000). Diagnostic imaging of child abuse. *Pediatrics, 105,* 1345–1348.

American Occupational Therapy Association (AOTA). (2008). Occupational therapy practice framework: Domain and process (2nd ed.). *American Journal of Occupational Therapy, 62,* 625–683.

Bade, M. J., Kohrt, W. M., & Stevens-Lapsley, J. E. (2010). Outcomes before and after total knee arthroplasty in health adults. *Journal of Orthopaedic Sports Physical Therapy, 40*(9), 559–567. http://www.jospt.org/

Bhandari, M., Devereaux, P., Tornetta, P., Swiontkowski, M., Berry D., Haidukewych, G.,... Guyatt, G. (2005). Operative management of displaced femoral neck fractures in elderly patients. An international survey. *Journal of Bone and Joint Surgery (America), 87*(9), 2122–2130.

Barrack, R., Brumfield, C., Rorabeck, C., Cleland, D., & Myers, L. (2002). Heterotopic ossification after revision total knee arthroplasty. *Clinical Orthopaedics & Related Research, 404,* 208–213. DOI: 10.1097/01.blo.0000030497.43495.3f.

Beloosesky, Y., Grinblat, J., Epelboym, B., Weiss, A., Grosman, B., & Hendel, D. (2002). Functional gain of hip fracture patients in different cognitive and functional groups. *Clinical Rehabilitation, 16,* 321–328.

Bell, A. J., Talbot-Stern, J. K., & Hennessy, A. (2000). Characteristics and outcomes of older patients presenting to the emergency department after a fall: A retrospective analysis. *eMedical Journal of Australia, 173,* 179–182. Retrieved from www.mja.com.au. *The Journal of Bone and Joint Surgery (American)* 2007;89:476–486. doi:10.2106/JBJS.F.00412

Brunner, L. C., & Eshilian-Oates, L. (2003). Hip fractures in adults. *American Family Physician, 67,* 537–542.

Bruno-Petrina, A. (2008). Posttraumatic heterotopic ossification. *Emedicine.* Retrieved from http://emedicine.medscape.com/article/326242-overview

Centers for Disease Control and Prevention (CDC). (2009a). Arthritis: Morbidity. *Summary Health statistics for US Adults: National Health Interview Survey, 2008.* Retrieved from www.cdc.gov/nchs/fstats/arthrits.htm on March 31, 2010.

Centers for Disease Control and Prevention (CDC). (2009b). *Injury prevention and control: Home and recreational safety: Hip fractures among older adults.* Retrieved August 26, 2010, from http://www.cdc.gov/HomeandRecreationalSafety/Falls/adulthipfx.html

Cooper, C. (2008). Hand impairments. In M. V. Radomski & C. A. Trombly Latham (Eds.), *Occupational therapy for physical dysfunction* (6th ed.). Philadelphia, PA: Lippincott Williams & Wilkins.

Crotty, M., Unroe, K., Cameron, I. D., Miller, M., Ramirez, G., & Couzner, L. (2010). Rehabilitation interventions for improving physical and psychosocial functioning after hip fracture in older people. *Cochrane Database Systematic Review, 1,* CD007624.

Cummings, S. R., Rubin, S. M., & Black, D. (1990). The future of hip fractures in the United States: Numbers, costs, and potential effects of postmenopausal estrogen. *Clinical Orthopaedics & Related Research, 252,* 163–166.

Dal Bello-Haas, V. (2009). Neuromusculoskeletal and movement function. In B. R. Bonder & V. Dal Bello-Haas (Eds.), *Functional performance in older adults* (pp. 130–176). Philadelphia, PA: F.A. Davis.

Dell, P. C., & Dell, R. B. (2002). Management of carpal fractures and dislocations. In Mackin, E. J., Callahan, A. D., Osterman, L., Skirven, T. M., & Schneider, L. (Eds.). *Rehabilitation of the hand and upper extremity* (5th ed.). St. Louis, MO: Mosby.

Deshaies, L. (2006). Arthritis. In H. M. Pendleton & W. S. Krohn (Eds.), *Occupational therapy practice skills for physical dysfunction* (pp. 950–982). St. Louis, MO: Mosby.

Erickson, B., & Perkins, M. (1994). Interdisciplinary team approach in the rehabilitation of hip and knee arthroplasties. *American Journal of Occupational Therapy, 48*(5), 439–445.

Ganz, S. B., Levin, A., Peterson, M. G., & Ranawat, C. S. (2003). Improvement in driving reaction time after total hip arthroplasty. *Clinical Orthopaedics, 413,* 192–200.

Gill, M. (2002). Managing distal and humeral shaft fractures. *Journal of the National Association of Orthopedic Technologists, 4,* 1–4.

Gillespie, W. (2002). Hip fractures. *Clinical Evidence, 8,* 1126–1148.

Gray, H. (2004). Bone. In W. H. Lewis (Ed.), *Gray's anatomy* (12th ed.). New York, NY: Bartleby.com. Retrieved from http://www.bartleby.com/107

Greenspan, W., Myers, E., Maitland, L., Kido, T., Krasnow, M., & Hayes, W. (1994). Trochanteric bone mineral density is associated with type of hip fracture in the elderly. *Bone and Mineral, 9,* 1889–1894.

Hagsten, B., Svensson, O., & Gardulf, A. (2004). Early individualized postoperative occupational therapy training in 100 patients improves ADL after hip fracture. *Acta Orthopaedica, 75,* 177–183.

Hall, S. E., Williams, J. A., & Senior, J.A., Goldswain, P. R., & Criddle, R. A. (2000). Hip fracture outcomes: Quality of life and functional status in older adults living in the community. *Australian New Zealand Journal of Medicine, 30,* 327–332.

Healthy People 2010. (2010). Arthritis, osteoporosis, and chronic back conditions. Retrieved July 26, 2010, from www.healthypeople.gov/document/html/volume1/02arthritis.htm

Holt, G., Smith, R., Duncan, K., & McKeown, D. (2010). Does delay to theatre for medical reasons affect the peri-operative mortality in patients with a fracture of the hip? *Journal of Bone and Joint Surgery (British), 92*(8), 835–841.

Kare, J. A. (2008). Volkmann contracture. *Emedicine.* http://www.emedicine.com/orthoped/topic 578.htm

Jeon, I.,Oh, C., Park, B., Ihn, J. Kim P.(2003). Minimal invasive percutaneous Herbert screw fixation in acute unstable scaphoid fracture. *Hand Surgery, 8,*213–218.

Khosla, S., & Melton, J. (2007). Osteopenia. *The New England Journal of Medicine*, 356(22), 2293–2300. www.nejm.org

Kocic, M., Lazovic, M., Mitkovic, M., & Djokic, B. (2010). Clinical significance of the heterotopic ossification after total hip arthroplasty. *Orthopedics*, doi: 10.3928/01477447-20091124-13.

Kotz, K., Deleger, S., Cohen, R., Kamigaki, A., & Kurata, J. (2004). Osteoporsis and health-related quality-of-life outcomes in the Alameda County study population. *Preventing Chronic Disease: Public health Research, Practice, and Policy*, 1(1), 1–9. http://www.cdc.gov/pcd/issues/2004/jan/03_0005.htm

Koval, K. J., Skovron, M. L., Aharonof, G., & Zuckerman, J. D. (1998). Predictors of functional recovery after hip fractures in the elderly. *Current Orthopaedic Practice*, 348. http://journals.lww.com/c-orthopaedicpractice/pages/default.aspx

Kunkler, C. E. (2002). Fractures. In A. B. Maher, S. W. Salmond & T. A. Pellino (Eds.). *Orthopedic nursing*. Philadelphia: Saunders.

Jagmin, M. G. (2002). Assessment and management of immobility. In A. B. Maher, S. W. Salmond, & T. A. Pellino (Eds.). *Orthopedic nursing*. Philadelphia, PA: Saunders.

Laseter, G. F. (2002). Therapist's management of distal radius fractures. In E. J. Mackin, A. D. Callahan, L. Osterman, T. M. Skirven & L. Schneider (Eds.). *Rehabilitation of the hand and upper extremity* (5th ed.). St. Louis, MO: Mosby.

Li, Z., Smith, B. P., Tuohy, C., Smith, T. L., & Koman, L. A. (2010). Complex regional pain syndrome after hand surgery. *Hand Clinics*, 26(2), 281–289. doi:10.1016/j.hcl.2009.11.001.

Lowe, J., Crist, B., Bhandari, M. & Ferguson, T. (2010). Optimal treatment of femoral neck fractures according to patient's physiologic age: an evidence-based review. *Orthopedic Clinics of North America*, 41, 2, 157-66.

Magaziner, J., Hawkes, W., Hebel, J. R., Zimmerman, S. I., Fox, K. M., Dolan, M., et al. (2000). Recovery from hip fracture in eight areas of function. *Journal of Gerontology: Medical Sciences*, 55(9), M498–M507. doi: 10.1093/gerona/55.9.M498.

Maher, C., & Bear-Lehman, J. (2008). Orthopaedic conditions. In M. V. Radomski & C. A. Trombly Latham (Eds.). *Occupational therapy for physical dysfunction* (6th ed.). Philadelphia, PA: Lippincott Williams & Wilkins.

Marottoli, R. A., Berkman, L. F., & Cooney, L. M. (1993). Decline in physical function following hip fracture. *Journal of American Geriatrics Society*, 40(9), 861–866.

Matityahu, A., Bruck, N., & Miclau, T. (2006). Heterotopic ossification and acetabular fractures. *Current Opinions in Orthopaedics*, 17(1), 34–37. doi: 10.1097/01.bco.0000192520.48411.fa.

Moore, D. S., & Cho, G. (2010). Heterotopic ossification. *eMedicine*. Retrieved from http://emedicine.medscape.com/article/390416-overview

National Center for Injury Prevention and Control. Office of Statistics and Programming, NCIP, CDC. (2007). *Ten leading causes of nonfatal injury, United States*. Retrieved from http://www.cdc.gov/ncipc/wisqars/nonfatal/quickpicks/quickpicks_2007/allinj.htm

National Institute of Arthritis and Musculoskeletal and Skin Diseases. (2002, Revised 2006). Osteoarthritis. NIH Publication No. 06-4617. Retrieved from http://www.niams.nih.gov/Health_Info/Osteoarthritis/default.asp

National Institutes of Arthritis and Musculoskeletal and Skin Diseases. (April 2009). *Arthritis*. NIH Publication No. 09-5149.

National Osteoporosis Foundation. (2010). *Fast facts on osteoporosis*. Retrieved August 16, 2010, from http://www.nof.org/osteoporosis/diseasefacts.htm

Peak, E., Parvizi, J., Ciminiello, M., Purtill, J. J., Sharkey, P. F., Hozack, W. J., et al. (2005). The role of patient restrictions in reducing the prevalence of early dislocation following total hip arthroplasty. A randomized, prospective study. *Journal of Bone and Joint Surgery American Volume*, 87(2), 247–253. http://www.ejbjs.org/

Peterson, S., Mani, M., Crawford, C., Neff, J., & Hiebert, J. (1989). Postburn heterotopic ossification: Insights for management decision making. *Journal of Trauma-Injury Infection & Critical Care*, 29(3), 365–369. http://journals.lww.com/jtrauma/pages/default.aspx

Potter, B., Burns, T., Lacap, A., Granville, R., & Gajewski, D. (2007). Heterotopic ossification following traumatic and combat-related amputations prevalence, risk factors, and preliminary results of excision. *Journal of Bone and Joint Surgery (American)*, 89, 476–486. doi:10.2106/JBJS.F.00412.

Rasul, A. T., & Wright, J. (2010). Total joint replacement rehabilitation, *eMedicine*. Retrieved September 17, 2010, from http://emedicine.medscape.com/article/320061-overview

Roberts, D. (2002). Degenerative disorders. In A. B. Maher, S. W. Salmond & T. A. Pellino (Eds), *Orthopedic nursing*. Philadelphia, PA: Saunders.

Stevens, J. A., & Olson, S. (2000). *Reducing falls and resulting hip fractures among older women*. National Center for Injury Prevention and Control. Retrieved from http://www.cdc.gov/mmwr/preview/mmwrhtml/rr4902a2.htm

U.S. Department of Health & Human Services. (2005). *Osteonecrosis, osteoporosis, and osteopenia*. Retrieved September 16, 2010, from http://www.aidsinfo.

nih.gov/ContentFiles/OsteonecrosisOsteoporosis-Osteopenia_FS_en.pdf

Wheeless, C. R. (2010). Fractures of the humerus. *Wheeless' textbook of orthopaedics*. Retrieved from http://www.wheelessonline.com

Wolinsky, F. D., Fitzgerald, J. F., &Stump, T. E. (1997). The effects of hip fractures on mortality, hospital-ization, and functional status: A prospective study. *American Journal of Public Health, 87,* 398–403.

Yasuda, Y. L. (2008). Chapter 44: Rheumatoid arthritis, osteoarthritis, and fibromyalgia. In M. V. Radomski & C. A. Trombly-Latham (Eds.), *Occupational therapy for physical dysfunction* (6th ed.). Philadelphia, PA: Wolters Kluwer, Lippincott Williams & Wilkins.

Low Vision Disorders

■ *Diane K. Dirette*

George was leading a leisurely retirement and enjoying the time he had to kick back and do all the things he couldn't do while he was working. He was finally able to spend time fishing at his cottage and taking care of his grandkids when his daughter needed his help. George knew his vision wasn't what it used to be, but he started using reading glasses and felt like he was getting by. One day while driving home from the store, he stopped at a four-way intersection and then drove straight into the side of a car that had stopped before him. Luckily no one was hurt, but after that his daughter insisted that he should see an ophthalmologist who diagnosed him with a low vision disorder called age-related macular degeneration (AMD). George was devastated. He feared he would become blind and lose his ability to live alone.

Low vision disorders are progressive diseases that lead to chronic loss of sight and limit everyday function. Low vision disorders are one of the most common causes of disability in the United States with an estimated 3 million people 40 years and older affected (Rosenberg & Sperazza, 2008). It is estimated that 80% of the population of people with low vision is over 65 years old (Massof, 2002). Because of the aging of the population, the number of people with low vision disorders is expected to continue to increase with projected estimations of 5.5 million people in the United States by the year 2020 (Rosenberg & Sperazza). In the United States, the three most common causes of low vision for people who are over 40 years old are macular degeneration, glaucoma, and cataracts (Rosenberg & Sperazza). Because of the prevalence of these diagnoses, most occupational therapists will work with people who have one of these disorders as either a primary or a secondary diagnosis.

Low vision is the third most common cause of impaired function in people who are older than 70 years (Rossenberg & Sperazza, 2008). Low vision disorders not only limit a person's ability to function independently but also increase the risk of depression, social isolation, fall injuries, and a general decline in overall health (Massoff, 2008;

301

Rosenberg & Sperazza). There is also a fear of blindness among people with low vision. Blindness is one of the most feared diseases in the United States (Burack-Weiss, 1992).

MACULAR DEGENERATION

Description and Definitions

AMD is a low vision disorder that results from loss of function of the macula, which is the center of the retina (Bressler & Gills, 2000). There are two types of AMD including dry AMD (atrophic) and wet AMD (neovascular/exudative). Dry AMD is atrophy of the macula and wet AMD is an ingrowth of new blood vessels that bleed into the subretinal space (Chong et al., 2008; Hirami et al., 2009).

AMD is also classified as either early or late. Early AMD is considered the beginning sign that the disease is developing, and late AMD is when the disease has progressed to the macula (Chong et al., 2008). Early AMD is when the retina is unhealthy and predisposed to visually threatening complications or late AMD (Fig. 18.1).

Etiology

Research indicates that the cause of AMD is probably a combination of genetic and environmental factors (Chong et al., 2009; Wang et al., 2008). The complement factor H gene and gene variants BF and C2 have been associated with higher rates of AMD (Wang et al.). Many environmental factors including smoking, diet, and ultraviolet (UV) light exposure have also been linked to the development of AMD. Cigarette smoking has been found to trigger or promote the development of AMD or contribute significantly to higher risks for AMD (Wang et al.). Diets high in red meat consumption are associated with early AMD (Chong et al., 2009) and diets high in fish consumption are associated with decreased risk for late AMD (Montgomery et al., 2010; Wang et al., 2008).

Incidence and Prevalence

AMD is the leading cause of severe vision loss for people older than 50 years in the United States and other developed countries (Friedman et al., 2004). Because the population is continuing to age, the prevalence of AMD is increasing with an expected rise of 3 million cases of late AMD in the United States by the year 2020. Dry AMD accounts for 80% of AMD cases in Western countries, whereas other parts of the world have higher incidence of wet AMD (e.g., Japan) (Hirami et al., 2009). In general, AMD is more common in women and Caucasians.

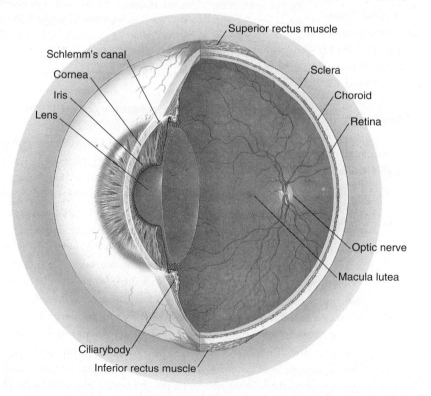

Figure 18.1 Anatomy of the eye.

Signs and Symptoms

The primary symptom of wet AMD is acute loss of central vision that becomes permanent as the retina atrophies and is replaced by fibrous tissue. Dry AMD can also result in the loss of central vision, but the progression is much slower taking years to develop. Initially, a person with AMD may by asymptomatic. Over time, loss of visual acuity for discrimination of details, metamorphopsia (distortion of objects), central scotomas, increased glare sensitivity, decreased contrast sensitivity, and decreased color vision can develop (Rosenberg & Sperazza, 2008).

Although the loss of vision can be profound and greatly impair function, people with AMD frequently do not notice the symptoms in the early stages. The visual loss does not result in black or white spots, but in spotty loss that is filled in by the surrounding vision that is still intact (Table 18-1).

Course and Prognosis

The course of AMD varies from person to person. Dry AMD does not always advance into wet AMD, but wet AMD always is preceded by dry AMD. The timeline for this process, however, is variable. Some people have dry AMD for years before it develops into wet AMD, and others develop wet AMD right away (Mogk & Mogk, 2003).

The prognosis for loss of central vision due to AMD also varies. For some people loss of central vision will proceed rapidly and others will have AMD for years and still maintain a functional level of central vision (Mogk & Mogk, 2003). Regardless of the speed of progression, AMD does not cause total blindness. AMD results in loss of central vision, but it does not affect peripheral vision. Therefore, the person will retain peripheral vision even if he or she has late AMD.

Diagnosis

The signs of AMD are detected through examination by an ophthalmoscope. In early AMD, the formation of drusen, small yellow deposits in the center of the retina, can be seen when the pupil is dilated (Bressler & Gills, 2000). In wet AMD, abnormal new blood vessels in the choroidal layer of the eye that nourish the outer retina grow and proliferate with fibrous tissue within the drusen material. The bleeding accumulates within and beneath the retina and the retina atrophies or becomes replaced with fibrous tissue. In dry AMD, the pigmented layer of the retina slowly atrophies.

Medical/Surgical Management

Although there are no treatments to cure or reverse the vision loss due to AMD, there are some treatments aimed at preserving the central vision for as long as possible. Current treatments of AMD include medications and laser treatment. Photodynamic therapy and intravitreal injections of antivascular endothelial growth factor and corticosteroids have shown promise for some people with AMD. In addition, high-dose regimens of zinc and antioxidants (vitamin C, vitamin E, and

TABLE 18.1 Signs and Symptoms of Low Vision Disorders

Macular Degeneration	Glaucoma	Cataracts
Acute loss of central vision	Slow loss of peripheral vision	Decreased visual acuity
Loss of visual acuity	Decreased ability to see in dim light	Cloudy, blurry, or foggy vision
Metamorphopsia (distortion of objects)	Decreased contrast sensitivity	Decreased contrast sensitivity
Central scotomas	Poor adaptation to changes in lighting	Increased glare sensitivity
Increased glare sensitivity	Increased glare sensitivity	Near-sightedness (myopia)
Decreased contrast sensitivity	Blurred vision	Decreased color perception
Decreased color vision	Decreased depth perception Ocular pain Eventual loss of central vision	Especially to blue hues

beta-carotene) are recommended (Rosenberg & Sperazza, 2008). Lipid-lowering drugs such as statins have been tested as a treatment for AMD, but have not been found to be effective in the treatment or prevention of AMD (Chuo, Wiens, Etminan, & Maberley, 2007).

Laser treatments are used for wet AMD including laser treatments which aim to burn the area of the retina with neovascularization, and photodynamic therapy which uses the drug verteporfin with the laser treatment to selectively destroy lesions (Bressler & Gills, 2000). This treatment is usually repeated every three or four months to prevent growth of blood vessels.

In addition to medical treatments, people with AMD are assessed for impairments in mobility and activities of daily living with a referral to physical therapy (PT) or occupational therapy (OT) if necessary. They may also benefit from psychological evaluation for anxiety or depression as persons with AMD have been found to have significant emotional distress and profoundly reduced quality of life (Rosenberg & Sperazza, 2008; Williams, Brody, Thomas, Kaplan, & Brown, 1998).

GLAUCOMA

Description and Definitions

Glaucoma is a low vision disorder characterized by progressive loss of the ganglion cell layer of the retina usually caused by increased intraocular pressure (IOP) (Rosenberg & Sperazza, 2008; Wittstrom et al., 2010). Three types of glaucoma include open-angle glaucoma, angle-closure glaucoma, and neovascular glaucoma. Angle-closure glaucoma is the obstruction by the iris to the outflow pathway of aqueous humor at the angle between the peripheral cornea and the iris (Subak-Sharpe, Low, Nolan, & Foster, 2009). In open-angle glaucoma there is not an obstruction of the aqueous humor, but the damage to the retina is caused by increased IOP. Neovascular glaucoma is a secondary disorder that results from other diseases, such as diabetes mellitus or tumors, which cause new blood vessels to grow and obstruct the outflow of aqueous humor (Shazly & Latina, 2009). See Figure 18.2.

Etiology

As with AMD, glaucoma is thought to be caused by a combination of genetic and environmental factors. A family history of glaucoma increases a person's chances of developing the disease. Although several genes have been identified in relation to glaucoma, they account for only a small portion of cases (Leske, 2007). Other factors that may contribute to glaucoma include abnormal blood pressure, diabetes, cataracts, and hypothyroidism (McDaniel & Besada, 1996; Subak-Sharpe et al., 2009).

Several pharmacological interventions have also been linked to angle-closure glaucoma (Subak-Sharpe et al., 2009).

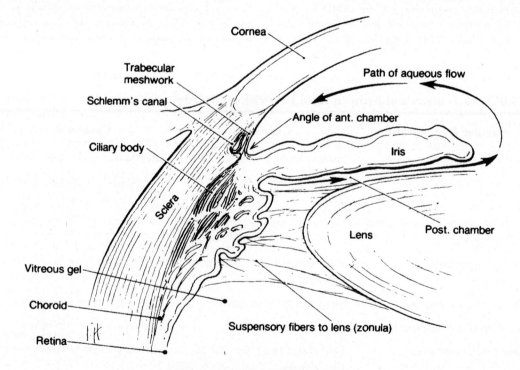

Figure 18.2 Path of aqueous flow.

Bronchodilators, antidepressants, anticholinergics (used for overactive bladder), antihistamines, botulinum toxin, and sildenafil (Viagra) are all pharmaceuticals that have been linked to angle-closure glaucoma. Also, recreational drug use of cocaine and ecstasy has been shown to cause angle-closure glaucoma.

Incidence and Prevalence

Glaucoma is the second most common cause of blindness worldwide accounting for 4.5 million people or 12% of cases, but it is the leading cause of blindness among people of African descent accounting for 32% of cases (Leske, 2007; Lin & Yang, 2009). Open-angle glaucoma is the most common form of glaucoma in Western cultures, but angle-closure glaucoma accounts for 50% of blindness worldwide and is more common in Asian populations (Leske, 2007; Subak-Sharpe et al., 2009). Although variation is noted, most studies report higher incidence and prevalence of glaucoma in men than in women (Leske, 2007) and higher incidence and prevalence in people of African descent (Rosenberg & Sperazza, 2008).

There is a marked increase in the prevalence of glaucoma among people older than 40 years. Variations in the prevalence of open-angle glaucoma among people older than 40 years can be seen throughout the world with estimates of 1% to 5% in the United States, 1% to 3% in Europe, 1% to 4% in Asia, 1% to 8% in Africa and 2% to 3% in Australia (Leske). The highest prevalence is in the Caribbean with 7 % to 9%. Most people in the Caribbean have ancestry linked to West Africa where open-angle glaucoma is very common.

Signs and Symptoms

Open-angle glaucoma begins with a slow loss of peripheral vision that can eventually lead to loss of central vision (Rosenberg & Sperazza, 2008). Other symptoms include decreased ability to see in dim light, decreased contrast sensitivity, poor adaptation to changes in lighting, sensitivity to glare, blurred vision, and decreased depth perception (Lin & Yang, 2009). In the early stages, however, many of these symptoms may not occur or may develop so gradually that people are not aware of their condition (Beleforte et al., 2010). By the time visual loss appears, there is usually already significant and permanent damage. The symptoms of closed-angle and neovascular glaucoma, however, usually have a more rapid onset. The symptoms include significant ocular pain and loss of vision.

Course and Prognosis

Angle-closure glaucoma has three stages. The first stage is marked by contact between the peripheral iris and the trabecular meshwork. This progresses to the formation of adhesions, which cause increased IOP. If not treated, this may progress to cause glaucomatous optic neuropathy which causes significant functional impairment of the vision (Subak-Sharpe et al., 2009). Open-angle glaucoma tends to progress at a slower rate and the patient may not notice that he or she has lost vision until the disease has progressed significantly. Neovascular glaucoma begins when a fibrovascular membrane initially obstructs aqueous outflow in an open-angle fashion and later contracts to produce secondary angle-closure glaucoma (Shazly & Latina, 2009).

If left untreated, glaucoma will lead to blindness. If treated, however, people with glaucoma usually retain some level of functional vision for their whole life (Ang & Eke, 2007).

Diagnosis

Early diagnosis and treatment are important to prevent vision loss. Diagnosis of open-angle glaucoma is based on visual field defects, disc defects, and abnormally increased IOP (Sonnsjo & Krakau, 1993). There is some debate about the use of IOP in the diagnosis of glaucoma because this increase is not always seen (Leske, 2007). When increase IOP is detected, however, it is used to aid in the diagnosis. Angle-closure glaucoma is diagnosed using gonioscopy or other screening techniques to examine the anterior chamber angle for contacts or adhesions (Subak-Sharpe et al., 2009). Neovascular glaucoma is diagnosed through the detection of new blood vessels in the iris, a closed anterior chamber angle, and high IOP (Shazly & Latina, 2009).

Medical/Surgical Management

Glaucoma is treated with topical ocular medications, oral medications, laser therapy, and surgery. A trabeculectomy, the removal of part of the trabecular meshwork, is the most common surgical procedure used to reduce IOP. Glaucoma filtration surgery may also be used to decrease IOP pressure in open-angle glaucoma (Winnstrom et al., 2010). Laser surgery, such as a goniopuncture, may be used to perforate the trabecular meshwork to increase aqueous flow.

For angle-closure glaucoma, surgical procedures may include an iridotomy or an iridoplasty (Subak-Sharpe et al., 2009). An iridotomy is a procedure in which a laser is used to create a hole in the iris to allow for drainage of the aqueous humor and an iridoplasty is a procedure in which a laser is applied to the peripheral iris to remove adhesions to the trabecular meshwork and open the angle. Topical ocular medications may be given to constrict the pupil and thus pull the peripheral iris away from the trabecular meshwork. Oral medications may also be given to reduce IOP for all types of glaucoma.

CATARACTS

Description and Definitions

Cataracts are opacifications of the crystalline lens of the eye, which result in a decreased amount of light reaching the retina. The incoming light is scattered and visual acuity is decreased. While there are some variant cataract conditions such as congenital cataracts due to rubella, the focus of this chapter will be on the most common type, age-related cataracts.

Etiology

As with other low vision disorders, the cause of cataracts is a combination of factors. Risk factors for the development of cataracts include aging, cigarette smoking, ocular UVB and radiation exposure, drug use, systemic diseases (e.g., diabetes), and dietary nutritional intake with increasing age being the strongest risk factor by far (Rosenberg & Sperazza, 2008). Some of the drugs associated with increased cataract risk are corticosteroids, antipsychotics, chemotherapy agents, cholesterol-lowering medications, and tranquilizers. Lutein (found in dark green leafy vegetables and eggs), vitamin C, and vitamin E intake have shown some associations with reduced risks for the development of cataracts (Lyle, Mares-Perlman, Klein, Klein, & Greger, 1999). Iodine deficiency and injuries to the lens are also risk factors for cataracts.

Incidence and Prevalence

Cataracts are the third leading cause of blindness in the United States, accounting for about 9% of all cases (Sperduto, 1994). They are more prevalent among females than males and are more prevalent among people of African decent (Rosenberg & Sperazza, 2008; Sperduto, 1994). Cataracts also vary in prevalence among different age groups with approximately 4% of people ages 52 to 64 years, 28% of people ages 65 to 74 years, and 46% of people ages 75 to 85 years.

As the population ages, the number of people worldwide who will be blind due to cataracts is expected to increase dramatically over the next few decades (Sperduto, 1994). The number of people who are blind due to cataracts could reach close to 40 million by the year 2025. As the ozone layer is depleted, there is an increase in UV radiation and this is expected to also increase the incidence of c ataracts worldwide.

Signs and Symptoms

Decreased visual acuity, decreased contrast sensitivity, glare disability, near-sightedness (myopia), and decreased color perception, especially to blue hues, are all common symptoms of cataracts (Rosenberg & Sperazza, 2008). Complaints of cloudy, blurry, or foggy vision are often noted. Some people may experience temporary improvement in near acuity as the shape of the lens is changed by the cataract.

Course and Prognosis

When a person is young, the lens is transparent and incoming light has no difficulty reaching the retina. Over time, however, the lens becomes less transparent as a cloudy, opaque cataract develops in the lens. One eye is usually affected earlier than the other, but eventually, both eyes are usually involved. If left untreated, cataracts may lead to blindness or develop into other eye diseases such as AMD or glaucoma (Rosenberg & Sperazza, 2008).

Diagnosis

A diagnosis of cataracts is done using pupil dilation, acuity charts, and tonometry. Tonometry is done to examine ocular fluid pressure inside the eye. Some cataracts can be detected with a visual examination that reveals a cloudy lens, but pupil dilation is done to further examine the back of the eye.

Medical/Surgical Management

Initially, the cataracts may be managed by prescription lenses, tobacco cessation, and UV protection, but the only medical treatment for cataracts is the surgical removal of the lens. When the cataract has advanced to a stage that interferes with a person's ability to function, surgery is usually recommended (Sperduto, 1994).

IMPACT OF CONDITIONS ON CLIENT FACTORS AND OCCUPATIONAL PERFORMANCE

Visual function is the client factor that is impaired in low vision disorders. The extent of the impact on occupational performance depends on the type of low vision disorder, the stage of progression of that disorder, and the treatment that has been received. Loss of central vision is the main concern for people with AMD and cataracts, and loss of peripheral vision is the main concern for people with glaucoma. For most people, cataracts will be surgically removed when they interfere with the person's ability to function. There are standardized assessments, such as the Impact of Vision Impairment Scale and the Visual Functioning Questionnaire, which may be useful to help therapists ascertain the impact of a person's visual loss on occupational performance (Lamoureux et al., 2008; Magacho et al., 2004).

Activities of Daily Living

Because of the loss of central vision, the self-care skills that require visual acuity are most affected by AMD and cataracts. These include skills such as makeup application, dental care, nail care, and shaving. Management of medications may be difficult due to difficulty reading labels and identifying various medications. Eating may also be visually challenging in advanced stages of the disorders.

Safety during functional mobility is a concern for all low vision disorders. The loss of central vision in AMD and cataracts and the loss of peripheral vision in glaucoma can impact a person's ability to safely navigate both within and outside the home. Within the home, entryways and stairs are especially difficult particularly at night. Adaptations, such as increased lighting, railings, and visual contrasts may need to be made to increase safety. Outside the home, unfamiliar places may pose challenges for both locating points of interest and negotiating varying surfaces.

Instrumental Activities of Daily Living

Driving is impacted by all low vision disorders. Because driving represents independence for most people, it can also be the most difficult occupation to address. In addition, driving is necessary for most other IADLs such as shopping, going to the post office, and making appointments.

Home management, including cleaning, doing laundry, making home repairs, and maintaining a yard, can all be impacted by low vision disorders. Being able to perform meal preparation accurately and safely are also concerns as loss of visual acuity will interfere with seeing food items, utensils (i.e., knives, measuring spoons, measuring cups), appliance settings, and recipes.

Money management for reading bills, paying bills, keeping records, and identifying and handling money can all be impacted by a loss of central vision. Large-print electronic systems may be useful for assisting with money management.

Education

Because all of these low vision disorders are likely to be age related, most people with these disorders will have completed their formal education. If participation in education is still essential, functional mobility and reading may interfere with successful completion of education-related occupations.

Work

The age of retirement has progressively increased and therefore the person may still be involved in work occupations when low vision disorders progress to the point that they interfere with function. Depending on the area of work in which the person participates, visual deficits in central and peripheral vision can impact the person's ability to successfully complete work tasks. Work-related activities such as reading, working on the computer, using the telephone, working on an assembly line, and driving can all be impaired by visual deficits.

Play and Leisure

Many leisure activities can be affected by low vision disorders. Many people with low vision disorders are retired and fill their time with leisure activities. In addition, these leisure activities may be part of the person's identity providing life purpose and satisfaction. Painting, knitting, sewing, gardening, playing games, completing puzzles, watching television, reading, and participating in sports are just some of the many leisure activities that may be difficult for a person with a low vision disorder.

Social Participation

Low vision disorders can impact social function in many ways. People with AMD frequently complain about difficulty recognizing faces, which may lead to feelings of humiliation and embarrassment is social situations. People with low vision disorders may also have difficulty negotiating crowded places such as concerts, restaurants, and ceremonies. In restaurants, they may have difficulty reading the menu in addition to navigating the physical layout. They may become distressed if they collide with people or objects. All of these factors may lead the person into a life with more isolation. The combination of the loss of independence and anxiety about the ability to function in social situations can often lead to depression. When the person becomes depressed, he or she is less likely to pursue social contact, and a cycle of isolation and depression can be worsened.

Case Illustrations

Case 1: Macular Degeneration

Mary is a 72-year-old female who has been referred to OT due to vision loss. Mary was diagnosed with wet AMD two years ago and is having difficulty functioning in her home. The recent death of her husband, who was able to help her in the home, has left her trying to find ways to manage on her own. She has two children. Her daughter lives about one hour away with her three children and her son lives about two hours away in a large urban area. Her children are reportedly concerned that she is no longer safe to live independently.

Mary worked for many years as a legal assistant until she retired at age 62. Since then, she has been enjoying traveling with her husband, spending time with her grandchildren, and participating in various leisure activities, such as knitting, reading, and gardening. She was once an avid tennis player, but had to stop playing due to her vision loss.

Mary now lives alone in a four-bedroom, split-level home and would like to remain there for as long as possible. She is having difficulty accepting the fact that driving is dangerous for her and she tries to get by using a GPS. She also becomes embarrassed when she doesn't recognize people, so she has started to avoid social situations where she is expected to interact with people who don't know about her vision loss.

She has undergone three laser treatments since she was diagnosed, but because they don't improve her vision, she has difficulty understanding why she needs more treatments. She is also taking high doses of zinc, vitamin C, vitamin E, and beta-carotene, but she states that sometimes she is not sure if she has taken the right pills.

Mary has been referred to OT for evaluation and treatment. Her primary goal is to maintain her current lifestyle as long as possible.

Case 2: Glaucoma

Bob is known amongst his friends as Bob the Builder. He retired from his job as a site manager 10 years ago, but has been busier than ever helping his friends with home improvement projects. Bob's wife states "he is so busy helping their friends, that he never has time to get to their own home improvement needs." Bob and his wife, Sharon, live in a four-bedroom century-old farmhouse that they have been fixing up since they moved in 10 years ago. Their home is on a 40-acre lot, but they rent out the land to a local farmer.

Bob and Sharon have been married for 15 years. They don't have children of their own, but both have children from previous marriages. All of their four children live within an hour of them and they have seven grandchildren among them.

Last year, Bob went to his eye doctor for a routine check up. It had been about five years since his last checkup. His kids were teasing him about his outdated glasses and he decided to get a new style. Bob hadn't noticed any significant changes in his vision. He knew he was having some difficulty seeing when it was dim lighting, but he thought this was just due to his eyes getting older. He was very surprised when the eye doctor told him that he suspected that he had glaucoma.

The eye doctor referred him to a specialist who confirmed the diagnosis. The ophthalmologist explained that he had what is called open-angle glaucoma and showed him diagrams of how much peripheral vision he had already lost. Bob and his family were surprised. Bob felt healthy and never really noticed the significant loss of vision. His mother had glaucoma, but he didn't connect that to the possibility that he would one day develop it, as well.

Bob uses eye drops and recently underwent surgery to reduce the pressure in his eye. He has been referred to OT to see if adaptation can be made to his environment and lifestyle to help him maintain as much function as possible in the coming years.

Case 3: Cataracts

Elizabeth, who is known as Beth to her family and friends, has been dealing with increasingly limited vision due to cataracts. Beth is 68 years old and has lived with her partner, Sue, for the last 26 years in a high-rise condo in an urban area. Beth has a daughter from a previous relationship and she lives within walking distance to her mother's home. Beth is retired from her career as an architect, but Sue still works as a teacher and has an hour commute to and from work.

Since her retirement, Beth spends most of her time participating in leisure activities. She loves to paint, swim, and work out in the building's gym facilities. She is also an avid reader, but has been frustrated with her visual deficits when trying to read. Her daughter owns and operates a local coffee shop, so she frequently stops by there to hang out or help out her daughter as needed.

Beth has been very aware of her increasingly limited vision over the past several years. She describes her vision as cloudy, blurry, and sensitive to "bad lighting." She started wearing glasses a few years ago, but now her vision loss is starting to interfere with her ability to function around the home and within her community.

Beth's eye doctor discussed routine eye surgery to remove the cataracts from both eyes. Once the eye doctor discovered that Beth had scarring on her retina in the right eye due to an old injury, however, she decided that the surgery would only benefit the left eye. Beth, therefore, will continue to have a significant loss of vision in her right eye even after the surgery is done.

Beth was referred to OT for an evaluation and intervention to assist her in making any adaptation necessary to increase her ability to function independently in her home and her community.

RECOMMENDED LEARNING RESOURCES

American Academy of Ophthalmology
http://www.aao.org
American Council of the Blind
http://www.acb.org
American Foundation for the Blind
http://www.afb.org
Macular Degeneration
MedlinePlus
www.nlm.nih.gov/medlineplus/maculardegeneration.html
MayoClinic.com
www.mayoclinic.com/health/macular-degeneration/DS00284
Macular Degeneration Foundation
www.eyesight.org/
Glaucoma

Glaucoma Research Foundation
www.glaucoma.org/
MayoClinic
www.mayoclinic.com/health/glaucoma/DS00283
National Eye Institute
www.nei.nih.gov
Cataracts
MedlinePlus
www.nlm.nih.gov/medlineplus/cataract.html
National Eye Institute
www.nei.nih.gov
MayoClinic
www.mayoclinic.com/health/cataracts/DS00050

REFERENCES

Ang, G. S., & Eke, T. (2007). Lifetime visual prognosis for patients with open-angle glaucoma. *Eye, 21,* 604–608.

Beleforte, N. A., Moreno, M. C., de Zavalia, N., Sande, P. H., Chianelli, M. S., Keller Sarmiento, M. I., et al. (2010). Melatonin: A novel neuroprotectant for the treatment of glaucoma. *Journal of Pineal Research, 48,* 353–364.

Bressler, N. M., & Gills, J. P. (2000). Age related macular degeneration: New hope for a common problem comes from photodynamic therapy. *British Medical Journal, 321,* 1425–1427.

Burack-Weiss, A. (1992). Psychological aspects of aging and vision loss. In E. Faye & S. Stuen (Eds.), *The aging eye and low vision: A study guide for physicians* (pp. 29–34). New York, NY: Lighthouse.

Chong, E. W. -T., Simpson, J. A., Robman, L. D., Hodge, A. M., Aung, K. Z., English, D., R., et al. (2008). Red meat and chicken consumption and its association with age-related macular degeneration. *American Journal of Epidemiology, 169*(7), 867–876.

Chuo, J. Y., Wiens, M., Etminan, M., & Maberley, D. A. L. (2007). Use of lipid-lowering agents for the prevention of age-related macular degeneration: A meta-analysis of observational studies. *Ophthalmic Epidemiology, 14*(6), 367–374.

Friedman, D. S., O'Colmain, B. J., Munoz, B., Tomany, S. C., McCarty, C., de Jong, P. T., et al. (2004). Prevalence of age-related macular degeneration in the United States. *Archives of Ophthalmology, 122*(4), 564–572.

Hirami, Y., Mandai, M., Takahashi, M., Teramukai, S., Tada, H., & Yoshimura, N. (2009). Association of clinical characteristics with disease subtypes, initial visual acuity, and visual prognosis in neovascular age-related macular degeneration. *Japanese Journal of Ophthalamology, 53,* 396–407.

Lamoureux, E. L., Pallant, J. F., Pesudova, K., Tennant, A., Rees, G., O'Connor, P. M., et al. (2008). Assessing participation in daily living and the effectiveness of rehabilitation in age related macular degeneration patients using the impact of vision impairment scale. *Ophthalmic Epidemiology, 15,* 105–113.

Leske, M. C. (2007). Open-angle glaucoma- an epidemiological overview. *Ophthalmic Epidemiology, 14,* 166–172.

Lin, J., & Yang, M. (2009). Correlation of visual function with health-related quality of life in glaucoma patients. *Journal of Evaluation of Clinical Practice, 16,* 134–140.

Lyle, B. J., Mares-Perlman, J. A., Klein, B. E. K., Klein, R., & Greger, J. L. (1999). Antioxidant intake and rick of incident age-related nuclear cataracts in the Beaver Dam eye study. *American Journal of Epidemiology, 149*(9), 801–809.

Magacho, L., Lima, F. E., Nery, A. C. S., Sagawa, A., Magacho, B., & Avila, M. P. (2004). Quality of life in glaucoma patients: Regression analysis and correlation with possible modifiers. *Ophthalmic Epidemiology, 11*(4), 263–270.

Massof, R. W. (2002). A model of the prevalence and incidence of low vision and blindness among adults in the U.S. *Optometry and Vision Science, 79,* 31–38.

McDaniel, D., & Besada, E. (1996). Hypothyroidism—A possible etiology of open-angle glaucoma. *Journal of the American Optometric Association, 67*(2), 109–114.

Mogk, L. G., & Mogk, M. (2003). *Macular degeneration: The complete guide to saving and maximizing your sight.* New York, NY: Random House.

Montgomery, M. P., Kamel, F., Pericak-Vance, M. A., Haines, J. L., Postel, E. A., Agarwal, A., et al. (2010). Overall diet quality and age-related macular degeneration. *Ophthalmic Epidemiology, 17*(1), 58–65.

Rosenberg, E. A., & Sperazza, L. C. (2008). The visually impaired patient. *American Family Physician, 77*(10), 1431–1438.

Shazly, T. A., & Latina, M. A. (2009). Neovascular glaucoma: Etiology, diagnosis and prognosis. *Seminars in Ophthalmology, 24,* 113–121.

Sonnsjo, B., & Krakau, C. E. T. (1993). Arguments for vascular glaucoma etiology. *Acta Ophthalmologica, 71,* 433–444.

Sperduto, R. D. (1994). Age-related cataracts: Scope of problem and prospects for prevention. *Preventive Medicine, 23,* 735–739.

Subak-Sharpe, I., Low, S., Nolan, W., & Foster, P. J. (2009). Pharmacological and environmental factors in primary angle-closure glaucoma. *British Medical Bulletin, 93,* 125–143.

Wang, J. J., Rochtchina, E., Smith, W., Klein, R., Klein, B. E. K., Joshi, T., et al. (2008). Combined effects of complement factor H genotypes, fish consumption, and inflammatory markers on long-term risk for age-related macular degeneration in a cohort. *American Journal of Epidemiology, 169*(5), 633–641.

Williams, R. A., Brody, B. L., Thomas, R. G., Kaplan, R. M., & Brown, S. I. (1998). The psychosocial impact of macular degeneration. *Archives of Ophthalmologie, 116,* 514–520.

Wittstrom, E., Schatz, P., Lovestram-Adrian, M., Ponjavic, V., Bergstrom, A., & Andreasson, S. (2010). Improved retinal function after trabeculectomy in glaucoma patients. *Graefes Archive for Clinical and Experimental Ophthalmology, 248,* 485–495.

19

Infectious Diseases

■ *Karin J. Opacich*

An occupational therapist is working for a migrant health center clinic. Most of the clients work on farms either planting and harvesting or caring for livestock. Among the largest employers is a thoroughbred breeding farm that employs 15 men and women to clean stalls, feed, and attend to the mares and foals. Over the last week, three workers from this farm have been treated for severe gastrointestinal distress. The pathogen was determined to be *Salmonella,* and it was discovered that one of the mares and her newborn foal have also been diagnosed with *Salmonella.*[1] These three workers have been sharing a dormitory room and two had been directly responsible for cleaning the infected mare's stall or handling the mare and her foal. The workers have no health insurance and no other means of financial support. They are all receiving treatment through the migrant health clinic, but they have to return to work since they have no health benefits and they do not get paid unless they work.

Cumulative discoveries and advancements in science have revealed the underlying mechanisms of infectious diseases that threaten the life and well-being of individuals and global populations. Infectious diseases may cause minor acute discomfort to chronic conditions to life-ending systemic damage. Vivid descriptions of infectious diseases have appeared in literature from ancient Greece to modern times. Hippocrates (400 BC), in a collection of ancient accounts entitled, *Of the Epidemics,* described the courses of individual sickness in painstaking detail trying to identify commonalities, patterns, and sources of illness affecting the whole community. Although much has been learned about causality since the days of Hippocrates, c. 400 BC, even recent history is replete with accounts of superstitions and misunderstanding about infectious diseases, none more poignant than the maltreatment of people with Hansen's disease (leprosy) in Hawaii in the 20th century (Gugelyk & Bloombaum,

---

[1] Three to six percent of the mare population have been found to be silent salmonella carriers who can transmit the infection to their foals in utero (Ward, Alinovi, Couetil, & Wu, 2005).

1979). While hundreds of infectious diseases have been identified and demystified, new pathogens that compromise human, animal, and environmental health are always evolving. The Center for Disease Control (CDC) now publishes a journal titled *Emerging Effective Diseases* (listed in Recommended Learning Resources section at the end of this chapter), which is entirely devoted to disseminating information about evolving or resurgent diseases such as **HIV**/AIDS, avian flu, West Nile virus, and tuberculosis (TB).

Each wave of illness has led to new knowledge and technology giving rise to the field of **epidemiology**, a scientific discipline devoted to studying the patterns of communicable diseases in order to predict, contain, and ultimately prevent the spread of disease. The famous account of Dr. John Snow, the scientist regarded as the father of modern epidemiology, chronicles the investigation that pinpointed the contaminated water pumps that spread cholera killing hundreds of people in London in 1854 (Snow, 1965). Recognizing the value of efficient disease tracking and information sharing, the U.S. Centers for Disease Control was authorized in 1946 to accumulate statistics on **incidence**, **prevalence**, **morbidity**, and **mortality** associated with major communicable diseases. Nearly 70 distinct diseases have been listed for surveillance and mandatory reporting in 2011 and these can be found at the CDC website listed in the recommended learning resources at the end of this chapter. The data collected serve to identify populations most vulnerable to infection and informs the development of individual and population interventions to curtail the spread of disease. National agencies, state departments of health, and city public health agencies may all collect and house health and communicable disease statistics. Geographic information systems (GIS) have improved the ability of these agencies to track, collect, and analyze data from broad geographic regions to areas as small as neighborhoods. Multilevel data are especially important for scientists to decipher disease trends, associations, and disparities on global, national, municipal, and in some cases even neighborhood levels.

This chapter will provide explanations by way of examples of infectious disease, TB, and HIV that affect occupational performance. Recognizing the inextricable connection between individual well-being and community health, occupational therapy practitioners are apt to acknowledge the importance of addressing transient disruptions and lasting effects of infectious diseases that impact occupational performance. Using TB and HIV as metaphors, infectious disease is explored from both population and individual perspectives from which the reader will develop a basic understanding of causative organisms, routes of infection, manifestations of illness, and medical interventions. Occupational therapy practitioners will find it necessary to take into account the context in which individuals experience their illnesses to fully address the occupational lives of their clients. The following exemplars can serve as templates for broadening our understanding of other infectious diseases encountered in occupational therapy practice.

DESCRIPTION AND DEFINITIONS OF INFECTIOUS DISEASES

Infectious diseases are characterized by a set of symptoms attributable to the introduction of a specific **pathogen**, a microorganism that compromises the health of an individual. Most pathogens fall into three general categories: bacteria, viruses, and fungi. Pathogens may be transmitted by direct contact (*in utero*, sexual activity, or nonsexual physical contact), aspiration (airborne), or ingestion (water or food). See Table 19.1 for examples of some of the infectious diseases of most interest to the Centers for Diseases Control (CDC), the associated pathogens, and routes of transmission. Tracking these diseases over time yields the evidence necessary to develop interventions and policies that protect individuals and populations from contracting and spreading infectious diseases. For instance, the preponderance of data pertaining to foodborne infections resulted in a new federal legislation, The Food and Drug Administration Food Safety Modernization Act (2010), imposing higher standards and penalties for the protection of consumers. Since food preparation and eating are fundamental human occupations, practitioners might consider how food safety is integrated into patient, family, and community habits and routines.

The scientific literature reveals that severity of illness in any individual is contingent upon multiple factors including the virility of the pathogen, the inherent **disease trajectory**, the premorbid health status of the

TABLE 19.1 Pathogens, Vectors, and Cases in 2008 for 10 Infectious Diseases

Disease	Pathogen	Vector	New US Cases (in 2008)[a]
HIV Stage III (formerly AIDS)	Human immunodeficiency virus	Sexually transmitted, injecting drug use, contaminated blood products	39,202
Chlamydia	*Chlamydia trachomatis*	Sexually transmitted	1,210,523
Gonorrhea	*Neisseria gonorrhoeae*	Sexually transmitted	336,742
Hepatitis B	Hepatitis B virus	Blood-borne	4,033
Lyme disease	*Borrelia burgdorferi*	Blood-borne, commonly transmitted by infected deer tick	35,198 (28,921 confirmed)
Pertussis	*Bordetella pertussis*	Inspiration of infectious mucus, close contact	13,278
Salmonellosis	*Salmonella*	Food-borne, contact with infected feces	51,040
Syphillis	*Treponema pallidum*	Sexually transmitted	46,277
Shigellosis	*Shigella*	Food-borne, waterborne, contact with infected feces	22,625
Tuberculosis	*Mycobacterium tuberculosis*	Airborne, sputum	12,904

[a]Infectious disease data from: CDC. (2008). MMWR summary of notifiable diseases, Retrieved from http://www.cdc.gov/mmwr/preview/mmwrhtml/mm5754a1.htm

infected person, health-related resources, and access to quality care. Furthermore, not only personal attributes and behaviors but also the social capital of the community can mitigate **risk factors** influencing both vulnerability to infectious diseases and health outcomes. Some populations bear a disproportionate **burden of disease**, which means that a group experiences an illness to a greater degree than other subgroups. When a given population or group sharing a constellation of characteristics manifests lower health status and poorer health outcomes proportionate to the population as a whole, that finding is said to represent **health disparity**. Disparities have been identified in association with several infectious diseases such as **tuberculosis (TB)**, a serious and highly contagious, airborne infection usually affecting the lungs caused by *Mycobacterium tuberculosis*. Studies of TB have shown that impoverished people who live in densely populated housing, for example, agricultural migrant

worker camps, low-income housing developments, and correctional institutions, are more likely to be exposed to TB (Shrestha-Kuwahara et al., 2004).

Highlighting another disparity, poor women of color are infected with HIV disproportionate to their numbers in the census. According to the CDC, over 1 million people were living with HIV in the United States in 2008 with 56,300 new infections projected to occur every year. In 1985, women represented 8% of all HIV infections, but they now manifest 25% of total cases (more than 300,000) with the trend continuing upward (Kaiser Foundation, 2008). For 80% of new cases among women, the route of transmission was heterosexual sex. According to 2006 CDC surveillance data, new infections for black females were 14.7 times higher than that of white females and for Hispanic females 3.8 times higher than that of white females (Dean, Steele, Satcher, & Nakashima, 2005;

TABLE 19.2 CDC Disease Definition for Tuberculosis

Tuberculosis *(Mycobacterium tuberculosis)*, **2009 Case Definition**

CSTE Position Statement Number: 09-ID-65

Clinical description

A chronic bacterial infection caused by *M. tuberculosis*, usually characterized pathologically by the formation of granulomas. The most common site of infection is the lung, but other organs may be involved.

Clinical case definition

A case that meets ***all*** the following criteria:

- A positive tuberculin skin test or positive interferon gamma release assay for *M. tuberculosis*

- Other signs and symptoms compatible with tuberculosis (TB) (e.g., abnormal chest radiograph, abnormal chest computerized tomography scan or other chest imaging study, or clinical evidence of current disease)

- Treatment with two or more anti-TB medications

- A complete diagnostic evaluation

Laboratory criteria for diagnosis

- Isolation of *M. tuberculosis* from a clinical specimen

- Demonstration of *M. tuberculosis* complex from a clinical specimen by nucleic acid amplification test,[b]

- Demonstration of acid-fast *Bacilli* in a clinical specimen when a culture has not been or cannot be obtained or is falsely negative or contaminated

Comment

- A case should not be counted twice within any consecutive 12-month period. However, a case occurring in a patient who had previously verified TB disease should be reported and counted again if more than 12 months have elapsed since the patient completed therapy. A case should also be reported and counted again if the patient was lost to supervision for greater than 12 months and TB disease can be verified again.

Mycobacterial diseases

- Each case other than those caused by *M. tuberculosis* complex should not be counted in TB morbidity statistics unless there is concurrent TB.

CDC 2008). The determinants of these disparities continue to be explored and explained in the literature, and there is a National Center for Minority Health and Health Disparities within the National Institutes of Health (http://www.nimhd.nih.gov/about_ncmhd/mission.asp) devoted to supporting research and interventions to eliminate health disparities.

When developing occupational therapy interventions, practitioners will find it necessary to familiarize themselves with the causes, disease trajectories, and precautions for the communicable diseases at hand in order to implement relevant therapeutic strategies that pertain to the individual in his or her living context. A well-regarded reference book for infectious diseases is *Principles and*

Practice of Infectious Diseases, 7th edition (Mandell, Douglas, & Bennett, 2010). Therapists may also find *Emerging Infectious Diseases: A Guide to Diseases, Causative Agents, and Surveillance* (Beltz, 2011) to be useful for reference.

In 1997 the CDC established uniform criteria for reporting cases of infectious disease. Each communicable disease has its own specific criteria (definition) that is periodically revisited and redefined as knowledge accumulates.

COURSE AND PROGNOSIS OF INFECTIOUS DISEASE

Each disease is characterized by an intricate biologic mechanism designed to perpetuate itself, and any individual's **immune response** or immunity, which reflects one's defense or resistance against infection and plays a role in the expression of illness. Some pathogens are very hardy and can live on inanimate surfaces for long periods, for example, *Staphylococcus*, while others, for example, human immunodeficiency virus (HIV), are quite fragile and generally require blood-to-blood contact to survive. The amount of pathogen necessary to produce infection is called the **inoculum dose**, and this dosage varies depending on the virility of the pathogen itself and on the efficiency of one's immune system to recognize, isolate, and destroy the foreign intruder. Some infectious pathogens are fragile and require ideal conditions to flourish. In contrast, the pathogen associated with hantavirus, a disease contracted from dried droppings or secretions from infected rodents, can survive for days under normal conditions, and a tiny inoculum dose can create biologic havoc in humans through hanta pulmonary syndrome (CDC, 2005a). HIV is an example of a pathogen that requires a small inoculum dose, but the virus itself is rather fragile. It is most efficiently transmitted by blood-to-blood contact through small lesions during sexual intercourse or by injection drug use or accidental needle sticks (Blanchard & Arai, 2010). Some infectious agents are quite hardy and can linger on inanimate surfaces until they come into contact with a hospitable host. *Staphylococcus* bacteria are fairly common and can cause illness from skin rashes to respiratory ailments. When staph (short for *Staphylococcus*) comes into contact with more vulnerable hosts, like the wounds of postsurgical patients, it can be far more dangerous especially when the strain of staph is resistant to customary antibiotics, for example, methicillin-resistant *Staphylococcus aureus* or **MRSA** (Enright et al., 2002).

When a pathogen enters the body, the immune system attempts to interfere with its reproduction and exacerbation. This typically entails a chain of microbiologic events: recognition of the pathogen as foreign, isolation of the pathogen, and destruction of the pathogen. Microorganisms called **antigens**, uniquely configured proteins attached to the pathogen, stimulate the body's production of **antibodies**, again typically proteins, that recognize and attach to the disease-producing entity marking it for destruction by phagocytes. The immune system is challenged to conduct this molecular activity efficiently enough to limit the replication of the cells that threaten the integrity of the body and produce the symptoms we recognize as illness. Some pathogens, for example, retroviruses like HIV, are especially equipped to insinuate themselves into the cellular reproductive mechanism commandeering the RNA to reproduce viral cells and ultimately turning the immune system into a factory for reproducing itself.

Pharmacologic science has rendered antibiotic, antiviral, antiretroviral, and antifungal drugs to assist the immune system in combating disease-producing pathogens, thus minimizing effects of infections that may have been historically fatal. George Washington is widely believed to have died at age 67 from a sore throat, specifically epiglottitis, attributable to *Haemophilus influenzae* type B, a bacterial infection now curable with antibiotics and for which children are routinely inoculated (Anderson, 2005). Practitioners are advised to consult medical reference books that address both the microbiologic mechanisms and the symptoms specific to any individual's infectious illness. Despite progress, not all infectious diseases are curable even with drug intervention, but by and large, their exacerbation can be managed to yield a much better quality of life for the infected individual.

Some infectious diseases are not only curable but also preventable by vaccination. Using minute amounts of live or killed pathogen, vaccinations trigger immune responses that either prevent the illness or minimize its effect in the vaccinated individual. Children are now routinely immunized for measles, mumps, pertussis, diphtheria, polio, and other potentially dangerous diseases. When critical masses of people (or other animal species) are rendered immune to a communicable disease, the rampant spread of infection is curtailed, a phenomenon known as **herd immunity**. All vaccinations are accompanied with risks, and some cultural groups are leery about immunization altogether; however, historical data regarding vaccination campaigns, for example, poliomyelitis, have shown to be highly successful in minimizing what were once devastating levels of mortality and morbidity (Graham, Ledgerwood, & Nabel, 2009).

TUBERCULOSIS (TB)

Definition and Description of TB

Mycobacterium tuberculosis is the pathogen that is present in the sputum of actively infected people, other animals, and birds. Among humans, the droplets that are emitted when coughing during the infectious stage can transmit the disease to others. TB is a **zoonotic infection**, which means that it can cross species. For instance, research has demonstrated that bovine TB may be contracted through the milk of infected cows which is thought to account for much of the TB in Southeast Asia (DeKantor, LoBue, & Thoen, 2010). TB most often affects the lungs by causing tubular inflammation and eventual scar tissue that impedes respiration. Untreated, TB can cause protracted illness and painful deterioration involving all organ and skeletal systems until eventual death.

Incidence and Prevalence of TB

TB is on the list of notifiable diseases that must be reported to the CDC. Although the prevalence of TB has declined steadily in the United States from a rate of 52.6 per 100,000 in 1952 to 3.8 per 100,000 in 2009 or 11,545 active cases, it is still among the most prevalent diseases globally (World Health Organization, 2010). The greatest proportion of active TB infections worldwide occur in Southeast Asia and Africa. TB is an **opportunistic infection** affecting society's most vulnerable people, those who are already ill, weak, impoverished, or marginalized from mainstream society (Shrestha-Kuwahara et al., 2004). In the United States, 29% of reported TB in 2009 occurred among people of Hispanic or Latino ethnicity, 26% among Black or African Americans, and 26% among Asians. Cities with the highest number of reported cases of active TB in 2009 were New York City, Los Angeles, Houston, and Chicago (CDC, 2009).

Signs and Symptoms of TB

People who contract TB may experience an array of symptoms including fever, weight loss, and night sweats. Because TB usually affects the respiratory system, symptoms commonly include coughing, chest pain, and bloody expectorant. Like other infections, TB triggers an immune response, and initial symptoms may abate. Without appropriate treatment, TB can exist in a dormant state known as **latent tuberculosis** until an individual's immune system is compromised for another reason, for example, HIV or hepatitis. Although TB in its latent form is not transmitted to others, if left untreated it poses a lifetime risk to the infected individual.

Medical/Surgical Management of TB

A simple skin test is commonly used to screen for TB. It entails administration of a droplet of Mantoux tuberculin intradermally by syringe, and it reveals exposure to *M. tuberculosis* through the appearance of a localized inflammatory response. The next level of detection entails chest radiograph to reveal the presence of tubules in the lungs. The standard for determining the presence and specific configuration of the latent tuberculosis infection is the QuantiFERON-TB Gold blood test (CDC, 2005b). Once diagnosed, an infected person is engaged in a strict daily pharmaceutical regimen, and the medications commonly administered are isoniazid, rifampin, ethambutol, and pyrazinamide. Treatment entails taking at least two medications religiously for a period of 6 to 12 months (Lobue, Enarson, & Thoen, 2010). These drugs are sometimes associated with unpleasant side effects contributing to noncompliance. Because strict adherence to the drug protocol is critical for eradicating the infection, people may be directly observed taking the daily medication. Poor adherence can result in multidrug-resistant disease and persistent infection (Horsburgh et al., 2010). In the United States, TB screening leads to early medical intervention and helps to prevent the long-term and devastating multisystem destruction that can result if not treated appropriately. It is understood that adherence to the prescribed medication regimen is of utmost importance, because nonadherence can lead to persistent infection in turn resulting in wasting and painful damage to all organ systems and the skeletal system. Therapists working in third-world countries or with immigrants from these countries may see more advanced disease symptoms. Access to treatment and adherence may be more complicated for social, political, and economic reasons. For those who are interested in learning about the global picture of infectious diseases, Dworkin's book, *Outbreak Investigations Around the World: Case Studies in Infectious Disease Field Epidemiology* (2010) may be enlightening.

Social and Behavioral Considerations of TB

It is important to understand the underlying social and economic conditions that render certain populations more vulnerable to TB and some other infectious diseases. Risk factors including poor nutrition, crowded housing, and poor sanitation have also been recognized as contributing to the spread of TB. These conditions have been and continue to be associated with poverty in both industrialized countries and developing nations. Population density in settings such as dilapidated housing structures, migrant worker camps, and prisons where people live in close proximity increases the likelihood of transmission in the presence of infection. Unwillingness to admit illness for economic reasons or lack of access to medical care may delay health-seeking behavior. To reiterate, TB, like many other infectious diseases, is opportunistic, and people who may be poorly nourished or who are experiencing other health challenges may not have robust immune systems to ward off infection.

Lifestyles, cultural interpretations, and mistrust of health care providers can impose barriers to detection and treatment as well (Shrestha-Kuwahara et al., 2004). Fear, stigmatization, and poor health literacy among disparity populations must be overcome to improve individual and population health. Readers who are interested in learning more about TB may benefit from CDC's online course, *Interactive Core Curriculum on Tuberculosis: What the Clinician Should Know*, accessible free of charge at http://www.cdc.gov/tb/webcourses/CoreCurr/index.htm.

The TB case at the end of the chapter relays some specific facts in terms of prevalence, disease trajectory, and medical management, but the process of information gathering can be applied to any infectious disease. Occupational therapy practitioners can access timely information from the CDC and other credible Web sites and references to understand how the infection can affect individual and community occupations.

HUMAN IMMUNODEFICIENCY VIRUS (HIV)

Definition and Description of HIV

The origin of what has become known as HIV appears to have been the slaughter of chimpanzees infected with a virus that crossed species, mutated, and spread through human behavior. Retrospective studies indicate that HIV entered the United States sometime in the 1970s, and that the male homosexual population initially experienced the greatest burden of disease (Curran, 2003; Armstrong, Calabrese, & Taege, 2005). Most common routes of transmission include unprotected sex, receiving contaminated blood products, injection of illicit drugs, and perinatal transmission from mother to child.

Incidence and Prevalence of HIV

As of 2010, the CDC estimates that over 1 million people in the United States are HIV infected, further hypothesizing that one in five of these people remain unaware of their status. In terms of risk behaviors, approximately 12% of these cases are attributed to injection drug use. Although men who have sex with men still represent the largest cohort of people infected with HIV in the United States, the proportion of heterosexual infection has risen to 31% with women representing 27% of new cases (CDC, 2008b, 2010). The aforementioned distribution of disease is unique to the United States and varies globally where HIV is largely transmitted through unprotected heterosexual sex (UNAIDS, 2010). The number of infants diagnosed with HIV in the United States, has declined due to perinatal screening and intervention (Panel on Treatment of HIV-Infected Pregnant Women and Prevention of Perinatal Transmission, 2010).

Signs and Symptoms of HIV

Flu-like symptoms are reported and frequently overlooked by people initially infected with HIV. Definitive diagnosis of HIV infection entails a blood test. One of two commonly used blood tests, ELISA, is a sensitive screening test that detects and confirms exposure to HIV through the presence of antibodies. A more specific test, the Western Blot, determines the presence of actual virus. As in the above scenario, HIV may be diagnosed secondary to another presenting problem, like another STD or pneumonia (Divisions of HIV/AIDS Prevention, 2010). HIV is a retrovirus, meaning that it reverses the usual pattern of replication by using the host cell's DNA to manufacture viral RNA that can then be incorporated into DNA and insinuated into healthy cells. Once the virus enters the bloodstream, it assaults the immune system proliferating until the CD4 and T helper cells can no longer defend the person from illness. Unless this process is halted, HIV infection can progress to autoimmune syndrome now called HIV Stage 3 (AIDS) and usually occurs over a period of several years. The official criteria for a diagnosis of HIV Stage 3 (AIDS) include a T cell count below 200 and the presence of at least one opportunistic illness (CDC, 2008a). Commonly reported symptoms of AIDS include weight loss, fevers and sweats, weakness, persistent rashes or infections, opportunistic infections (e.g., candidiasis, TB), memory impairment, depression, irritability, cognitive deterioration, and others.

Course and Prognosis of HIV

Improved interventions have resulted in longer life for many people with HIV. For those with access to resources, years of quality life may be extended for 15 or more years beyond diagnosis. Consequently, HIV is now considered a chronic rather than a fatal disease. Among the treatment options, highly active antiretroviral therapy (HAART) protocols include multiple drugs with different actions to stop the proliferation of HIV at different points in the reproductive cycle of the virus (May et al., 2007). However, not all people with HIV are responsive to these protocols, and the drugs may be associated with unpleasant side effects such as nausea, diarrhea, mood disorders, or fevers that can affect quality of life. In the case scenario, the experience of drug-related symptoms may be an issue for Joseph. Should his HIV infection continue to progress rapidly to Stage 3, Joseph may experience musculoskeletal wasting, cognitive impairment, neuropathies, and neurologic symptoms of greater magnitude. He may also suffer from rare cancers and opportunistic infections due to the impairment of the immune system to recognize and destroy pathogens and aberrant organisms.

Social and Behavioral Considerations of HIV

People with HIV are at risk for stigmatization and isolation. Beyond providing information and education to the HIV+ person, health practitioners may be involved in educating partners, families, and communities about the disease. In Case 2, Joseph's fiancée is 3 months pregnant. Ethically and legally, she must be informed of her HIV risk and the potential risk to her unborn fetus. Screening for HIV is important because perinatal treatment can prevent the baby from seroconversion and undo suffering (Birkhead et al., 2010).

Joseph will have little chance of living well with HIV unless he ceases to use illicit drugs. Sharing needles is also the likely source of his HIV infection, and even if he continues to use drugs, Joseph must alter these practices to avoid putting others at risk of infection. If Joseph remains committed to sobriety, there are clearly additional issues that must be addressed for him to be restored to a state of occupational coherence. He may need psychological counseling and peer support to deal with both his military experiences and his HIV diagnosis. All health practitioners need to be prepared to counsel and assist people with HIV who may be suffering from isolation or stigmatization (Duffy, 2005).

IMPACT ON CLIENT FACTORS AND OCCUPATIONAL PERFORMANCE

"Participation in activities and occupations that are meaningful to the client involves emotional, psychosocial, cognitive, and physical aspects of performance. This participation provides a means to enhance health, well-being and life satisfaction" (American Occupational Therapy Association, 2004, p. 673).

The cases challenge the occupational practitioner to think broadly about the impact of an infectious disease on individuals in a community context. Focusing first on the two children who have been identified with active TB, school and home occupations and issues for others

in the community will also be considered. This approach is consistent with an ecologic approach to both infectious disease and human occupation.

Disease investigation will clarify the source of infection for the two school-age children. Whatever the source, the children must be treated to prevent spreading TB. It is likely that the children will be confined at home until acute symptoms have abetted, but all school personnel including the occupational therapy practitioner will be expected to comply with screening and observing for further indications of the spread of disease (Lazar, Sosa, & Lobato, 2010). Because of preconceived notions about TB or fear of stigmatization, some people may be reluctant to be tested or to seek appropriate care. Astute occupational therapy practitioners will be sensitive to the needs of the community and will interact with cultural humility.

Both for individuals and for the community, adherence to prevention measures will be necessary. The occupational therapy practitioner should reinforce hygienic behaviors for all school children and especially children participating in therapy, for example, covering the mouth when coughing or sneezing, disposing tissues, and washing hands routinely. Students should be discouraged from sharing food and utensils with simple explanations of how germs are passed from one person to another. All toys and surfaces where sputum might transmit bacteria should be cleaned with an appropriate disinfectant between clients. Children in group treatments should be closely monitored for attention to hygiene and for signs of illness.

It is of utmost importance for the entire health and education team to collaborate to provide relevant information about TB and to prevent stigmatizing the infected children and their families. The school nurse is likely to be the person who will observe the children taking their daily medication, at least during the school week, to assure adherence. Discretion will be important to keep the children from suffering negative social consequences, so their daily school routines should be planned with this in mind. Age-appropriate explanations and health education should be anticipated, and all staff should be attentive to issues of self-esteem and potential bullying. Communication with the families of schoolchildren and particularly the families of the children with TB is of critical importance, and the family liaison, whoever that might be, must be prepared to ascertain cultural beliefs and interpretations of TB.

The occupational therapy practitioner can be helpful in addressing daily routines and habits both at school and at home. Infected individuals are likely to be fatigued and to experience malaise, but those symptoms should abet with treatment. Because the children may experience unpleasant side effects of the medications, they may need encouragement and rewards for persevering. Every effort should be made to empower affected children to participate willingly in their own care. Once the acute illness is addressed and the children are determined to be noninfectious, there is no reason to exclude them. If during their usual school activities they appear to have lost strength and endurance or manifest other enduring symptoms of illness, the occupational therapist may be involved in resolving these.

In her book, *An Occupational Perspective of Health*, Ann Wilcock (2006) builds connections among epigenetic inheritance, biologic drives for survival, social determinants of health, and human occupational needs. Theoretical perspectives that acknowledge health as a state produced by the interaction of multiple systems are generally categorized as ecologic models (Smedley & Syme, 2000). Rather than a narrow, causative view of disease more commonly associated with bench sciences and medicine, Wilcock embraces an ecology of health with meaningful occupation at its core. Wherever the intervention occurs along the illness trajectory, occupational therapy aimed at meaningful doing entails analysis with information gleaned from several disciplines, for example, biology, medicine, sociology, anthropology, geography, public health.

Unlike the early years of the epidemic, people who expected to die have found themselves reprieved and facing the challenge of reconstructing their lives after HIV infection. Along with accommodating the demands of the disease, this may entail developing new occupational roles and behaviors (Kielhofner et al., 2004). Since his discharge from the armed services, it is likely that Joseph's role exploration and development of life skills during emerging adulthood were derailed. Once sober, he may need to reassess his interests and capacities to establish a progenerative life plan. Given his recent dysfunctional

behavior, he is likely to need assistance building a trusting intimate relationship as well as preparing to be a parent. Joseph is likely to need support to restore or establish healthy friendships and will need to contemplate with whom, when, and how he will share his HIV status.

For the remainder of his life, Joseph will need to minimize the potential of exposing others to infection as well as protecting himself from dangerous illness. First and foremost, Joseph will need to commit to practicing safe sex. Especially in his present state of health, Joseph is vulnerable to opportunistic infections including pneumonia and TB. Joseph will need to establish additional routines and habits like adhering to his drug treatment program, his medication regime, and ongoing medical monitoring. Many people with HIV find that psychosocial therapy, nutritional counseling, vocational counseling, and alternative therapies are helpful.

If Joseph is to thrive, he will need to resume role exploration and a means of supporting himself and potentially a family. Given his aspiration to work in construction, Joseph may need assistance in assessing the demands and tasks entailed in the work. Joseph will need to rebuild strength and endurance since he is currently debilitated. Periods of fatigue and weakness may be associated with both the disease and the treatment which may require a flexible work schedule, and realistically, Joseph may need to explore less physically demanding and safer roles within or outside the construction industry.

The following two cases illustrate a process of information gathering focusing on how infectious diseases express themselves in individuals and impact communities. Using the cases as prototypes for building insight into the biology and epidemiology for other communicable diseases, occupational therapy practitioners can further explore the impact of these and other infections on client factors in order to address occupational performance.

Case Illustrations

Case 1

An itinerant occupational therapist sees children at three different elementary schools. One of these, Central Elementary, serves a high number of immigrant families. Most of these families originate from rural areas where they are engaged in agricultural work. The population in the school district as well as school enrollment has increased rapidly over the past 5 years. Housing in the surrounding community is older construction largely designed for single-family occupancy, but it is now common for extended families to live together to share expenses and responsibilities.

Upon arriving at Central Elementary on this particular day, the occupational therapist is informed that two children seen by the school nurse for respiratory infections last week were diagnosed with active TB. TB is on the list of mandatory reportable diseases, so the state Department of Health (DPH) has been notified, and treatment has been initiated for the two children. Nurses and technicians from the state DPH are at the school on this day conducting TB screening tests for students and families and providing educational materials. All school personnel are undergoing screening as well. Results are to be interpreted 3 days from now, and public health nurses will be back on site to examine the skin tests and to draw blood from those whose tests are positive. The occupational therapist was treating both children for significant developmental delays affecting school performance.

Case 2

Joseph enlisted in the army immediately upon graduation from high school. After returning from a 2-year tour of duty in the army, Joseph had difficulty readjusting to civilian life. He had hoped to get a job in the construction industry, but the housing downturn resulted in many fewer jobs. Joseph found himself with few marketable job skills and fewer opportunities. He self-managed his temper and his anxiety with opioids and used drugs intravenously for a period of nearly a year. Joseph had lost considerable weight, lost his job stocking auto parts, and lost many of his friends by the time his family and fiancée convinced him to enter a drug treatment program.

Joseph was hospitalized for detoxification before entering the Live Free Center that includes occupational therapy among its services. During that initial hospitalization, it was discovered that he was also HIV+ and that his T cell count was 300. Joseph was referred to an HIV program where it was decided that he be placed on a protocol for HAART. During his second week in the drug treatment center, Joseph's fiancée informed him that she is 3 months pregnant. Joseph is consumed by guilt, depressed, and worried that he may have infected his girlfriend and child.

SUMMARY

Given the wide variability in cause, presentation, and sequelae of infectious diseases, occupational therapy practitioners can expect to encounter these illnesses in a range of settings whatever the context of their clients' lives. In order to develop responsible occupational interventions, practitioners will need to approach each situation asking a set of questions. These questions should yield information about critical epidemiology, physical manifestations of infectious disease, and medical interventions. Consistent with the tenets of occupational therapy, practitioners must also consider the social and behavioral parameters associated with the specific infectious diseases including the impact on the individual, the family, and the community in which the person receiving therapy conducts his or her daily life. Adding to this information the unique client factors, the practitioner can most successfully collaborate with the individual to develop a plan for achieving meaningful goals for occupational performance.

RECOMMENDED LEARNING RESOURCES

Center for Disease Control Centers for Disease Control and Prevention (CDC)
Department of Health and Human Services
600 Clifton Rd.
Atlanta, GA 30333
Tel: 800-233-4636
cdcinfo@cdc.gov
Emerging Effective Diseases
Center for Disease Control Centers for Disease Control and Prevention (CDC)
Department of Health and Human Services
600 Clifton Rd.
Atlanta, GA 30333

Tel: 800-233-4636
http://www.cdc.gov/ncidod/EID/index.htm
Institute of Medicine (IOM)
2100 C. Street, NW
Washington, DC
Tel: 202-334-2000
www.iom.edu
World Health Organization (WHO)
Avenue Appia 20
1211 Geneva 27
Switzerland
Tel: + 41 22 791 21 11
www.who.int/en

REFERENCES

American Occupational Therapy Association. (2004). Occupational therapy scope of practice. *American Journal of Occupational Therapy, 58*, 673–677.

Anderson, Virginia (2005, February 22). Healthy living: Bye, George. *The Atlanta Journal—Constitution.*

Armstrong, W., Calabrese, L., & Taege, A. J. (2005). HIV update 2005: Origins, issues, prospects, and complications. *Cleveland Clinic Journal of Medicine, 72*(1), 73–78.

Beltz, L. A. (2011). *Emerging infectious diseases: A guide to diseases, causative agents, and surveillance.* Jossey-Bass and APHA Press.

Birkhead, G. S., Pulver, W. P., Warren, B. L., Klein, S. J., Parker, M. M., Caggana, M., & Smith, L. (APA rules indicate that you all names up to 7 authors). (2010, January 1). Progress in prevention of mother-to-child transmission of HIV in New York State: 1988–2008. *Journal of Public Health Management and Practice, 16*(6), 481–491.

Blanchard, J. F., & Arai, S. O. (2010). Emergent properties and structural patterns in sexually transmitted infection and HIV research. *Sexually Transmitted Infections, 86*, iii4–iii9.

Broome, C. (2009). Effective global responses Broome C. (1998), Effective global response to emerging infectious diseases. *Emerging Infectious Diseases, 4*(3):358–9.

CDC. (2005a). *All about hantaviruses: Technical information.* Retrieved January 31, 2011, from http://www.cdc.gov/ncidod/diseases/hanta/hps/noframes/phys/printtechsection.htm

CDC. (2005b). Guidelines for the investigation of contacts of persons with infectious tuberculosis and guidelines for using the QuantiFERON-TB Gold test for detecting *Mycobacterium tuberculosis* infection, United States. *MMWR, 54*(RR-15), 49–55.

CDC. (2008a). *Case definitions for infectious conditions under public health surveillance. Human immunodeficiency virus infection.* Retrieved February 4, 2011, from http://www.cdc.gov/osels/ph_surveillance/nndss/casedef/aids2008.htm

CDC. (2008b). Subpopulation estimates from the HIV incidence surveillance system—United States, 2006. *MMWR, 57*(36), 985–989.

CDC. (2009). *Reported Tuberculosis in the United States 2009, Division of Tuberculosis Elimination.* Retrieved January 25, 2011, from http://www.cdc.gov/tb/statistics/reports/2009/pdf/report2009.pdf

CDC. (2010b). *HIV in the United States, July 2010, Fact Sheet, National Center for HIV/AIDS, Hepatitis, STD, and TB Prevention, Division of HIV/AIDS Prevention.* Retrieved February 25, 2011, from http://www.cdc.gov/hiv/resources/factsheets/us.htm

Curran, J. W. (2003). Reflections on AIDS, 1981–2031. *American Journal of Preventive Medicine, 24*(3), 281–284.

Dean, H., Steele, C., Satcher, A., & Nakashima, A. (2005). HIV/AIDS among minority races and ethnicities in the United States, 1999–2003. *Journal of the National Medical Association, 97*(Suppl. 7), 5S–12S.

DeKantor, I. N., LoBue, P.A., & Thoen, C. O. (2010). Human tuberculosis caused by Mycobacterium bovis in the United States, Latin America, and the Carribean. *International Journal of Tuberculosis and Lung Disease, 14*(11), 1369–1373.

Divisions of HIV/AIDS Prevention, National Center for HIV/AIDS, Viral Hepatitis, STD, and TB Prevention. (2010). Basic information about HIV and AIDS. Retrieved March 4, 2011, from http://www.cdc.gov/hiv/topics/basic/index.htm

Duffy, L. (2005). Suffering, shame, and silence: The stigma of HIV/AIDS. *Journal of the Association of Nurses in AIDS Care, 16*(1), 13–20.

Dworkin, Mark. (2010). *Outbreak investigations around the world: Case studies in infectious disease field epidemiology.* Sudbury, MA: Jones & Bartlett Publishers, LLC.

Enright, M. C., Robinson, D. A., Randle, G., Feil, E. J., Grundmann, H., & Spratt, B. G. (2002). The evolutionary history of methicillin-resistant *Staphylococcus aureus* (MRSA). *PNAS, 99*(11), 7687–7692.

Food and Drug Administration. (2011, January 4). FDA Food Safety Modernization Act, Public Law 111–353. Retrieved February 25, 2011, from http://www.gpo.gov/fdsys/pkg/PLAW-111publ353/pdf/PLAW-111publ353.pdf

Graham, B. S., Ledgerwood, J. E., & Nabel, G. J. (2009). Vaccine development in the twenty-first century: Changing paradigms for elusive viruses. *Clinical Pharmacology and Therapeutics, 86*(3), 234–236.

Gugelyk, T., & Bloombaum, M. (1979). *Ma ʻi Ho ʻoka ʻ awake: The separating sickness.* Bangkok: Anoi Press.

Hippocrates. (400 B.C.). *Of the Epidemics.* Retrieved on February 25, 2011, from http://www.greektexts.com/library/Hippocrates/Of_The_Epidemics/eng/index.html

Horsburgh, C. R., Goldberg, S., Bethel, J., Chen, S., Colson, P. W., Hirsch-Moverman, Y., et al. (2010). Latent tuberculosis infection treatment acceptance and completion in the United States and Canada. *Chest, 137*(2), 401–409.

Kaiser Family Foundation. (2008, May). *Women and HIV/AIDS in the United States, HIV/AIDS Policy Fact Sheet.* Retrieved on February 25, 2011, from http://www.kff.org/hivaids/upload/6092-04.pdf

Kielhofner, G., Braveman, Finlayson, M., Paul-Ware, A., Goldbaum, L., & Goldstein, K. (2004). Outcomes of a vocational program for persons with AIDS. *American Journal of Occupational Therapy, 58*(1), 64–72.

Lazar, C. M., Sosa, L., & Lobato, M. N. (2010). Practices and policies of providers testing school-aged children for tuberculosis, Connecticut, 2008. *Journal of Community Health, 35*, 495–499.

LoBue, P. A., Enarson, D. A., & Thoen, T. C. (2010). Tuberculosis in humans and its epidemiology, diagnosis and treatment in the United States [Serialized article. Tuberculosis: a re-emerging disease in animals and humans. Number 2 in the series]. *International Journal of Tuberculosis and Lung Disease, 14*(10), 1226–1232.

Mandell, G. L., Douglas, & Bennett, J. E. (2010). *Principles and practice of infectious diseases* (7th ed.) [Expert Consult Premium Edition—Enhanced Online Features and Print By Gerald L. Mandell, John E. Bennett, & Raphael Dolin]. Philadelphia, PA: Churchill Livingstone/Elsevier.

May, M., Sterne, J. A., Sabin, C., Costagliola, D., Justice, A. C., Thiébaut, R., et al. (2007). Prognosis of HIV-1-infected patients up to 5 years after initiation of HAART: collaborative analysis of prospective studies. *AIDS, 21*(9), 1185–1197.

Panel on Treatment of HIV-Infected Pregnant Women and Prevention of Perinatal Transmission. (2010, May 24). *Recommendations for use of antiretroviral drugs in pregnant HIV-1-infected women for maternal health and interventions to reduce perinatal HIV transmission in the United States.* pp. 1–117. Available at http://aidsinfo.nih.gov/ContentFiles/PerinatalGL.pdf. Retrieved March 4, 2011.

Shrestha-Kuwahara, R., Wilce, M., Joseph, H. A., Carey, J. W., Plank, R., & Sumartojo, E. (2004). Tuberculosis research and control. In Carol R. Ember & Melvin Ember (Eds). *Encyclopedia of medical anthropology: Health and illness in the world's cultures* (pp. 28–542). New York: Kluwer Academic.

Smedley B. D., & Syme, S. L. (Eds.), (2000). Institute of Medicine. *Promoting health: Strategies from social and behavioral research.* Washington, DC: National Academies Press.

Snow, J. (1965). *On the mode of communication of cholera* (2nd ed.). New York: Hafner Publishing Co. (Reprinted from *Snow on Cholera*, 1854)

UNAIDS. (2010). *UNAIDS Report on the global AIDS epidemic 2010.* Retrieved March 7, 2011, from http://www.unaids.org/globalreport/Global_report.htm

Ward, M. P., Alinovi, A. A., Couetil, L. L., & Wu, C. C. (2005). Evaluation of a PCR to detect *Salmonella* in fecal samples of horses admitted to a veterinary teaching hospital. *Journal of Veterinary Diagnostic Investigation, 17*, 18–123.

Wilcock, A. (2006). *An occupational perspective of health* (2nd ed.). Thorofare, NJ: Slack, Inc.

World Health Orgnaization. (2010). *Global Tuberculosis Control 2010.* Retrieved on February 25, 2011, from http://whqlibdoc.who.int/publications/2010/9789241564069_eng.pdf

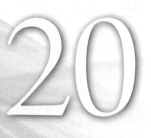

Developmental Trauma Disorder

- *Ben Atchison*
- *Brandon Morkut*

According to his foster mother, 6-year-old Travis was removed from his birth home 1 year and 3 months before the date of this report, based on evidence that his biological father isolated Travis for hours in a small closet in his home. In one of many incidents of maltreatment, Travis describes his father "swinging me around the room and hitting me against the wall." His foster mother also reports that Travis' biological mother attempted to "sell him for drugs" but it is not certain that this in fact occurred. Travis' father is reportedly intellectually disabled, with an IQ of 70 and is living with his parents. His parental rights have been terminated and he has had no contact with Travis. His mother died a year ago from cardiac complications due to extensive use of crack cocaine. Travis is described by his foster mother as having significant learning difficulties—he is in kindergarten with a 1:1 aid to support him. He has had episodes of "destructive often," going on "rampages" in the classroom. She also notes that he is "hypervigilant," seeming to wait for the "next bad thing to happen" and will stay very close to her at all times when they are together. This is Travis' third permanent foster home since he was removed 1 year ago. A permanent, adoptive home is being sought by the Department of Human Resources.

DESCRIPTION AND DEFINITION

It was not until the 19th century that children were granted the same legal status as domesticated animals with regard to protection against cruelty and/or neglect. Until that time child abuse was not only acceptable but also was, essentially, legally sanctioned. It wasn't until 1962 that the term *battered child syndrome* became part of the medical vocabulary and not until 1976 that all of the states in the United States had adopted laws mandating the reporting of suspected child abuse.

Traumatic stress occurs when children and adolescents are exposed to traumatic events or traumatic situations that overwhelm their ability to cope (National Children's Traumatic Stress Network [NCTSN], 2011). **Trauma,** from the Greek word meaning *wound,* was originally used in medicine for a serious physical injury but it is more widely used to refer to emotional shock following a stressful event or to an experience that is deeply distressing. The *American Heritage Dictionary* defines trauma as a serious injury or shock to the body, as from violence or an accident which is what comes to mind when thinking of "trauma care" or a "trauma unit." This chapter is focused on the second component of this definition, which is "an emotional wound or shock that creates substantial, lasting damage to the psychological development of a person, often leading to neurosis, and an event or situation that causes great distress and disruption" (*American Heritage,* 2011).

The construct of child trauma has historically been thought of in the context of isolated, single episodes of exposure to violence, abuse, and neglect rather than a series of chronic, pervasive incidents that occur in relational situations. **Developmental trauma disorder** (DTD) describes clinically significant patterns of behavior or syndromes that occur in an individual as a result of persistent and chronic exposure to violent episodes including physical, sexual, and emotional abuse resulting in functional impairment in one or more important areas. These patterns of behavior and or syndromes are observed in maladaptive psychobiological responses and capacities that are not culturally exclusive. (van der Kolk, 2005).

As of the date of the publication of this chapter, the diagnosis of DTD has been submitted and is being considered for official inclusion in two major diagnostic reference sources. These are the *Diagnostic and Statistical Manual of Mental Disorders* (DSM-IV) (American Psychiatric Association, 2000) which is most significant in the United States, and the *International Statistical Classification of Diseases and Related Health Problems* (World Health Organization, 2007). Clinicians, including occupational therapists, who treat children with a history of chronic trauma, have increasingly called for a diagnosis that more adequately addresses the multiple domains of concern that results from developmentally adverse interpersonal trauma. The criteria that have been proposed for DTD have been gathered by extensive clinical data provided by clinicians within major national organizations including the National Child Traumatic Stress Network, American Psychiatric Association, American Psychological Association, other mental health profession's lead organizations, and from advocacy organizations such as the National Alliance for Mental Illness.

The diagnosis of DTD considers the impact of chronic, persistent exposure to trauma rather than acute, episodic events such as the destruction of the Financial Trade Center in New York City on September 11, 2001 or the impact of exposure to the many natural disasters that have occurred in this decade. Currently, posttraumatic stress disorder (PTSD) is the only trauma-related diagnosis in the DSM-IV and it is used for both children and adults. It was created and published in the DSM-III in 1980 in response to the large number of Vietnam veterans returning home with psychiatric problems. The three main symptom clusters developed to describe PTSD including reexperience, avoidance, and hyperarousal, are virtually unchanged in the current DSM-IV (van der Kolk, 2005). For the most part, traumatized children diagnosed as having PTSD are essentially measured against criteria developed around the experience of male combat veterans over 30 year ago.

In summary, the definition of DTD as stated in the proposal for the DSM-V inclusion is as follows:

The child or adolescent has experienced or witnessed multiple or prolonged adverse events over a period of at least one year beginning in childhood or early adolescence including: (1) Direct experience or witnessing of repeated and severe episodes of interpersonal violence, and (2) Significant disruptions of protective caregiving as the result of repeated changes in the primary caregiver; repeated separation from the primary caregiver; or exposure to severe and persistent emotional abuse. (van der Kolk et al., 2009, p. 6)

ETIOLOGY

DTD is related to events occurring within the context of the external environment and the type of child-caregiver relationship including repetitive, unpredictable, uncontrollable, and violent environments in conjunction with inconsistent protective caregiving. The abuse, whether it is physical, sexual, or emotional, and neglect a child experiences from a caregiver are often **transgenerational,** that is, the caregiver's actions are based on his or her own previous parenting experiences (Perry, 2001). The most deadly form of child trauma is caused by neglect, as death can occur by accidents due to absence of supervision or abandonment and from failure to seek medical attention provided in cases of injury, illness, or a medical condition. Fatal injuries from trauma are caused by varied actions including severe head trauma such as violent shaking of an infant or small child; forceful punching of the fist to the abdomen, chest, or head; scalding; intentional drowning; suffocation; poisoning; and starvation.

Several risk factors related to DTD have been identified (Sedlak, et al, 2010):

- Over 75% of inflicted abuse is a result of parental action. Parental risk factors include young or single parents, those who did not graduate from high school, and those who either were abused themselves as children or endured a severely dysfunctional home life.

■ Adults with psychiatric disorders such as depression and bipolar disorder (BPD) are more likely to abuse children.

■ A common theme when interviewing abusive individuals is their unrealistic expectations of infant or child development. Often they expect maturation of developmental milestones significantly beyond the age of the child. This is especially true for toilet training expectations.

■ Commonly, the child is incapable of providing what many parents anticipate to be unconditional love. The normally self-centered nature of childhood behavior clashes with the abusive adult's expectations and does so with disastrous results.

■ The perpetrator's childhood: Approximately 80% of offenders were themselves abused as children.

■ Substance abuse: Children in alcohol-abusing families are nearly four times more likely to be mistreated, almost five times more likely to be physically neglected, and 10 times more likely to be emotionally neglected than children in non–alcohol-abusing families. In fact, 85% of cases in which parents' rights are terminated are a result of an inability of the parents to resolve substance addiction.

■ Family support systems: The disintegration of the nuclear family and its inherent support systems is believed to be associated with child abuse.

■ Social forces: Experts debate whether a presumed reduction in religious/moral values coupled with an increase in the depiction of violence by the entertainment and informational media may increase child abuse.

■ Children at higher risk for abuse include infants who are felt to be "overly fussy," as well as children with congenital anomalies, chronic/recurrent conditions, and children with chronic diseases as well as children with learning disabilities, speech/language disorders, and intellectual disability.

■ Specific "trigger" events that occur just before many fatal parental assaults on infants and young children include an infant's inconsolable crying and feeding difficulties, a toddler's failed toilet training, and exaggerated parental perceptions of acts of "disobedience" by the child.

■ Family income strongly correlates with incidence rates. Children from families with annual incomes below $15,000 per year are more than 25 times more likely than children from families with annual income above $30,000 to be harmed or endangered by abuse or neglect. Poverty clearly predisposes to child abuse. However, it must be recognized that all data available can only be based on reported cases. It is very likely that trauma exposure exists among other classes as well but those families are often protected by position and wealth and thus their cases do not necessarily become part of a community's child protective services (CPS) system.

■ According to the statistics, the majority of perpetrators of child mistreatment (77%) are parents and another 11% are other relatives of the victim. People who are in other caretaking relationships to the victim (for example, child-care providers, foster parents, and facility staff) account for only 2% of the offenders.

■ About 10% of all perpetrators are classified as noncaretakers or unknown. In many states, child abusers by definition must be in a caretaking role.

■ An estimated 81% of all offenders are under age 40. Overall, approximately 61% of perpetrators are female, although the gender of the abuser differs by the type of mistreatment. Neglect and medical neglect are most often attributed to female caretakers, while sexual abuse is most often associated with male offenders.

■ Younger children are at risk: 67% of abused children are less than 1 year old; 80% are less than 3 years.

■ Repeated abuse has been shown to occur more than 50% of the time; repeatedly abused children have a 10% chance of sustaining a lethal event.

■ Adopted and foster children are at higher risk.

INCIDENCE AND PREVALENCE

Child abuse is a worldwide problem affecting children from birth to 18 years of age. The U.S. Department of Health and Human Services Fourth National Incidence Study (NIS-4) of Child Abuse and Neglect (NIS-4) was published in 2010 (Sedlak et al., 2010). The Endangerment Standard Database includes both those cases where harm has been demonstrated and cases in which harm is not clearly observed but there is reason to believe that the possibility of maltreatment endangered the children; the data indicate that nearly 3 million children (an estimated 2,905,800) experienced maltreatment during the 2005–2006 study year which translates to one child in every 25 in the United States. While approximately one-third, or 835,000 children, were abused, an estimated 2,251,600 children, or 77%, were neglected. The majority of abused children (57%, or 476,600 children) were physically abused, more than one-third (36%, or 302,600 children) were emotionally abused, and less than one-fourth (22%, or 180,500 children) were sexually abused. More than one-half of the neglected children were physically neglected (53%, or 1,192,200 children) and a similar percentage were emotionally neglected (52%, or 1,173,800), whereas 16% (an estimated 360,500) were educationally neglected. Further, 1,460 children (four children per day) died in 2005 as a result of inflicted trauma with more than 77% of these deaths in children less than 4 years of age. A parent or primary caretaker was identified as the perpetrator in 83% of the cases reported, and almost half of those were reported as abused or neglected again within a 5-year period. This study also found that children younger than 3 years of age were most likely to be victims of recurring maltreatment and that when the perpetrator of abuse or neglect was exclusively the mother, there was a much higher risk of repeated abuse. Studies have shown a consistent pattern regarding the abuse and neglect inflicted on children of different genders. Approximately 75% of sexual abuse is inflicted upon girls. Girls also are more likely to suffer from sexual abuse, emotional abuse, and neglect. Boys, on the other hand, are more likely to experience physical trauma (other than sexual abuse). When focusing solely on cause of death, studies indicate fathers are more likely to kill their child via physical abuse, while mothers cause fatalities by reason of willful neglect (for example, starvation).

In a survey of clinicians within the National Children's Trauma Stress Network NCTSN (2003) interpersonal victimization uniformly emerged as the most prevalent form of trauma exposure, typically occurring in the home. Each of the following types of trauma exposure was reported for approximately one-half of the children the clinicians treated, indicating multitraumatic experiences:

- Psychological maltreatment, that is, verbal abuse, emotional abuse, or emotional neglect
- Dependence on an impaired caregiver, that is, parental mental illness or substance abuse
- Domestic violence
- Sexual maltreatment/assault
- Neglect (i.e., physical, medical, or educational neglect)
- Physical maltreatment/assault

Forms of trauma exposure not involving interpersonal victimization were significantly less common, as fewer than 1 in 10 children included in the NCTSN survey had been exposed to serious accidents, medical illness, or disaster. The survey further revealed that a large percentage of trauma-exposed children exhibit several forms of posttraumatic symptoms and signs not captured by standard PTSD, depression, or anxiety disorder diagnoses.

Interestingly, 50% or more of the cases in the survey were reported to exhibit significant disturbances in the following domains: affect regulation, attention and concentration, negative self-image, impulse control, and aggression or risk taking. In addition, approximately one-third of the sample exhibited significant problems with **somatization**, which occurs when mental and emotional stresses become physical complaints in the absence of an explained diagnosis as well as attachment dysfunction. The one-third of this sample also included conduct disorder, increased sexual interest, activity or avoidance, and **dissociation**, which in its most severe form is essentially an "out-of-body experience" in which the person detaches from an event that is overwhelmingly stressful.

Complicating the collection of data to provide incidence and prevalence data is the general underreporting of child abuse. Very young children are incapable of verbally communicating the harm inflicted on them. Other factors such as fear, guilt, or confusion about the abuser's erratic behaviors may also hinder younger children from informing on their abuser. While reports of alleged child abuse are not always substantiated during the investigation process, most authorities nevertheless believe that a large underreporting bias is inherent in the data. The NIS-4 also reported that three times as many children are maltreated as are reported to CPS agencies (Sedlak et al., 2010).

SIGNS AND SYMPTOMS

There are three major categories in which the signs and symptoms of DTD cluster. Those include **affective and physiologic dysregulation**, **attentional and behavioral dysregulation**, and **self- and relational dysregulation** (van der Kolk et al., 2009). Based on extensive evidence to date and the continuing efforts of trauma researchers to legitimize the need for a more comprehensive diagnosis for trauma, the proposed criteria for the inclusion of DTD in the DSM-V are described in this section, which illuminates the chronic and pervasive nature of trauma and the complexity of its impact on one's life (van der Kolk, et al., 2009).

Affective and Physiologic Dysregulation

Behaviors include difficulty with arousal regulation and modulation and toleration and recovery from extreme affective states such as fear, anger, and shame that emerge from chronic trauma exposure, manifested by prolonged and extreme emotional tantrums on one side of the spectrum to catatonic-like immobilization. Disorders of bodily functions may occur including disturbances in sleeping, eating, and elimination (Egger, Costello, Erkanli, & Angold, 1999; Glod, Teicher, Hartman, & Harakal, 1997; Noll, Trickett, Susman, & Putnam, 2006). Sensory processing disorders such as overreactivity or underreactivity to touch and sounds has been reported along with diminished awareness of and or dissociation of sensations (Atchison, 2007; Richardson, Henry, Black-Pond, & Sloane, 2008). Signs of disorganized behaviors during routine transitions are often mistakenly identified among children with DTD as attention deficit disorder (ADD) or attention deficit hyperactivity disorder (ADHD), when in fact the behaviors are manifestations of neural dysfunction directly related to chronic trauma exposure (Alessandri, 1991; Perry, 2001). **Alexithymia**, or the impaired capacity to describe emotions or bodily states, is a persistent sign of affective dysregulation. This includes difficulty describing internal states and communicating basic needs such as hunger or elimination, as well as expressing emotions, wishes, and desires. (Sayar, Kose, Grabe, & Topbas, 2005; Way, Yelsma, Van Meter, & Black-Pond, 2007).

Attentional and Behavioral Dysregulation

Signs and symptoms include impairment in those competencies related to sustained attention, learning, or coping with stress. An inability to sustain goal-directed behavior may include a lack of curiosity, difficulties with planning or completing tasks, or avolition. The capacity to focus on and complete tasks as well as capacity to plan and anticipate affects nearly half of those exposed to chronic trauma. In addition, children and adolescents with a chronic history are twice as likely as other trauma-exposed children to have impairments in their ability to organize behavior to achieve rewards in the environment (Nolin & Ethier, 2007).

A persistent sense of threat or impaired capacity to perceive threat may be observed as the child may misread cues related to safety and danger. The child demonstrates an impaired capacity or misperception of risk, combined with poor impulse control and difficulty understanding consequences. When experiencing a sense of threat, maladaptive attempts at self-soothing may manifest by substance abuse and rhythmical maladaptive actions such as head banging, body rocking, and compulsive masturbation (Ford et al., 2000). Self-harm among chronically traumatized children and adolescents has been described in the literature. These include dangerous actions such as setting fires; sexual promiscuity; and actions of self-harm such as cutting, picking, and burning one's skin; and other self-mutilation actions (Brown, Houck, Hadley, & Lescano, 2005).

Self- and Relational Dysfunction

One of the most significant signs of the developmental impact of trauma is maladaptive behaviors related to disruption of attachment. The type of relationship between a child and a caregiver influences how a child responds to present and future emotional and physical experiences.

A normal child-caregiver relationship develops into a secure attachment in about 55% to 65% of the general population (NCTSN, 2003). In a secure attachment, the caregiver responds to stressful situations by providing the child a safe environment and a sense of protection, which in turn influences the child's ability to appropriately regulate affect and behavior. Over 80% of children who experience chronic trauma demonstrate insecure attachment patterns (NCTSN, 2003). Repeated exposure to unpredictable and uncontrollable stressful environments in conjunction with erratic, hostile, rejecting, or abusive caregiving, are precursors to an insecure child-caregiver attachment (Cook et al., 2007). Insecure attachment and associated signs can be subcategorized into three typologies: avoidant, ambivalent, and disorganized.

Avoidant attachment develops as a result of persistent caregiver rejection and failure to provide basic emotional and physical support to their child. These children often become skilled at distrusting their emotions in conjunction with avoiding establishment of meaningful relationships with peers and adults. Children with ambivalent attachment experience parents who demonstrate predictable patterns of detachment and neglect to excessive intrusiveness. The first sense that an important adult is rejecting or overly engaging facilitates the child's maladaptive coping response which is an act of separating from others (Cook, Blaustein, Spinazzola, & van der Kolk, 2003). Disorganized attachment develops when children are traumatized by repeated exposure to uncontrollable and unpredictable stress, for example, physical or sexual abuse, in conjunction with consistent absence of a caregiver who is nurturing, reliable, and protective. These children who demonstrate difficulty organizing an adaptive response to daily experiences due to childhood trauma display significant challenges regulating their emotions, problem-solving through the use of language, managing stress, and developing empathy (Cook et al., 2007). It has been hypothesized that disorganized attachment interferes with efficient neurodevelopmental connections between the right and left hemispheres of the orbital prefrontal cortex, which is responsible for regulating emotions, conscious decision making, and social behavior (Cook et al., 2003). Other brain structures associated with the development of attachment that can be affected by complex trauma include the amygdala, that is, threat detection, hippocampus, that is, new memory and learning, hypothalamic-pituitary-adrenal (HPA) axis, that is, response to perceived threat, and neurotransmitters, that is, oxytocin, dopamine, norepinephrine, and others (Henry, Sloane, & Black-Pond, 2007). Attachment dysfunction leads to intense preoccupation with safety of the caregiver or other loved ones or difficulty tolerating reunion with them after separation.

Other signs that emerge in self- and relational dysfunction include the following:

- Persistent negative sense of self, including self-loathing, helplessness, worthlessness, ineffectiveness, or defectiveness
- Extreme and persistent distrust, defiance, or lack of reciprocal behavior in close relationships with adults or peers
- Reactive physical or verbal aggression toward peers, caregivers, or other adults
- Inappropriate (excessive or promiscuous) attempts to get intimate contact(including but not limited to sexual or physical intimacy) or excessive reliance on peers or adults for safety and reassurance
- Impaired capacity to regulate empathic arousal as evidenced by lack of empathy for, or intolerance of, expressions of distress of others, or excessive responsiveness to the distress of others

COURSE AND PROGNOSIS

The course of DTD is marked by observable changes in behavior across multiple domains with prognosis directly related to the extent of exposure, the application of appropriate interventions, and **resiliency** factors. Signs and symptoms and associated impairments have been shown to be characterized by progressive deterioration with episodic signs of symptom severity in childhood and adolescence, as well as persistent challenges across the lifespan in many cases. The multiple consequences that emerge as a result of chronic trauma and impact on the course are detailed in a seminal white paper by the NCTSN Complex Trauma Task Force titled *Complex Trauma in Children and Adolescents* (Cook et al., 2003). Two major considerations for course and prognosis are directly related to the extent of neurobiologic damage and resiliency factors.

Neurobiologic

The impact of chronic trauma on brain development has been reported in the literature with the primary benefit of these studies being a better understanding of the scope of the problems associated with trauma exposure as well as informing clinicians about the intervention approaches necessary to improve the prognosis for healing and recovery. Ito, Teicher, Glod, and Harper (1993) reported that children exposed to chronic trauma had left hemisphere EEG abnormalities in anterior, temporal, and parietal areas. Taylor, S., Eisenberger, N., Saxbe, D., Lehmna, B, & Lieberman, M., (2006) found decreased amygdala activation among children who experienced detached emotional

engagement from parents. The amygdala is necessary to perceive such emotions as fear and to respond to those feelings in a protective manner. In a task requiring identification of emotions, Taylor also found a significant positive correlation between the activation of the amygdala and right ventrolateral prefrontal, a finding which indicates reduced inhibition of the amygdala.

Curtis and Cicchetti (2007) found that maltreated children categorized as nonresilient had decreased left hemisphere activation when compared to resilient maltreated children, and decreased left parietal activity compared to nonmaltreated children. Neuroendocrine changes have been documented in the aftermath of childhood interpersonal trauma.

Bevans, Cerbone, and Overstreet (2008) found that exposure to childhood trauma was related to alterations in diurnal cortisol variation. Cortisol, a steroid hormone, is released in response to stress and acts to restore homeostasis. However, prolonged cortisol secretion results in significant physiologic changes including immunologic and neurologic changes.

Cicchetti and Rogosch (2001) found that maltreated children with internalizing problems and coexisting internalizing and externalizing problems had elevated cortisol compared to nonmaltreated children. Neuroimaging studies have indicated reduced growth of the hippocampus and limbic abnormalities as well as diminished growth in the left hemisphere and compromised function of the corpus callosum, the structure which allows for efficient interhemispheric connectivity (Teicher, 2000). Henry et al. (2007) summarized brain structures affected as a result of chronic trauma, which are illustrated in Table 20-1.

Recognition of the brain-behavior connection by becoming aware of the increasing evidence linking trauma and neurodevelopmental function is critical to occupational therapists working with this population so that appropriate intervention is provided to improve the prognosis for healing and engagement and participation in occupations.

Resiliency Factors

The concept of resilience is central to understanding the course and prognosis of DTD. *Human resiliency* refers to the ability of an individual to recover from adverse or traumatic events in a manner that is adaptive and nonpathologic. While the risk of pathologic responses are indeed great among children who have experienced trauma, there is the potential to gain competence across a variety of domains if provided with the necessary intervention, including those that address both internal and external factors (Masten & Coatsworth, 1998). Resilience is most threatened by the loss of organic and relational protective

TABLE 20.1 Impact of DTD on Specific Brain Areas

Area	Function
Attachment	
Neurotransmitters	Enables communication of different areas of brain structures
HPA axis	Allows response to perceived threats "fight/flight/freeze" response
Amygdala	Primary role is threat detection—initiates the "fight/flight/fright/freeze" response; connected to many other brain structures
Hippocampus	New memory and learning
Corpus callosum	Connects cerebral hemispheres to smoothly integrate functions; emotional regulation
Fusiform face area	Facial recognition; especially important for infant recognition of caregiver
Affect Regulation	
Locus ceruleus	Located in brainstem—arousal and alertness
Thalamus	"Relay station" screening and distribution of sensory input to other brain areas
Striatum	Reward center of brain
Orbitofrontal cortex (OFC)	Regulation of emotion, decision making, social behavior
Information Processing	
Amygdala and hippocampus	New memory formation
Anterior cingulated	Associated with conflict mentoring, resolution, and executive function
OFC	Conscious decision making

systems which occur in response to traumatic events. The extent of brain damage and associated cognitive, perceptual, and self-regulatory dysfunction, along with severely compromised caregiver relationships are key factors that compromise resilience (Teicher, Anderson, & Polcari, 2002). In addition, loss of motivation to seek out interpersonal relationships, to interact with one's environment, and to learn and to develop new skills greatly inhibits recovery while supportive relationships, family connections, and cognitive resources help protect one and serve as "inoculations against adversity" (Kagan, 2004). Several factors have been found to be the most critical for promoting resilience, including (a) positive attachment and connections to emotionally supportive and competent adults within a child's family or community, (b) development of cognitive and

self-regulation abilities, (c) positive beliefs about oneself, and (d) motivation to act effectively in one's environment (Luthar, Cichetti, & Becker, 2000; Werner & Smith, 1992; Wyman, Sandler, Wolchik, & Nelson, 2000).

MEDICAL MANAGEMENT

Due to the impact of chronic trauma on multiple developmental domains, the child may demonstrate signs of comorbid psychiatric disorders. These common mental health disorders include PTSD, depression, ADHD, oppositional-defiant disorder, anxiety disorders, BPD, dissociative disorders, and personality disorders,

Traditional medical management of trauma will include psychopharmacological intervention which, in best practice, is prescribed as an adjunct to psychosocial treatment modalities and not as a free-standing approach. Medication should only be used in conjunction with trauma-specific treatment and not in the absence of it.

In a survey sample representing 1,699 children, (Pynoos et al., 2008) ages infancy through 18, who were exposed to chronic trauma, it was determined that most trauma intervention occurs in an outpatient setting with the frequency of intervention modalities identified as follows:

- Weekly psychotherapy (78%)
- Self-management/coaching (62%)
- Family therapy (56%)
- Play therapy (55%)
- Expressive therapies (41%)
- Pharmacotherapy (27%)
- Community outreach (25%)

The majority of those responding to this survey included psychiatrists, social workers, and psychologists and are representative of traditional models. Traditional models of intervention are typically provided by either a social worker or psychologist, however there are existing models of assessment and intervention that are grounded in interdisciplinary and transdisciplinary approaches that include several professional disciplines on a team including occupational therapy (Hyter, Atchison, Henry, Sloane, & Black-Pond, 2001; Koomar, 2009).

IMPACT ON CLIENT FACTORS AND OCCUPATIONAL PERFORMANCE

As a result of DTD, there are significant disturbances across many of the client factors and performance skills described in the occupational therapy practice framework (AOTA, 2002). As described in the section on signs and symptoms, client factors include dysfunction in global and specific mental functions, sensory functions and pain, some functions of the cardiovascular and respiratory systems, immunologic and digestive systems, and speech functions, particularly that related to fluency. Evidence of compromised performance skills has been determined including those related to motor and praxis skills, sensory-perceptual skills, emotional regulation skills, cognitive skills, and communication and social skills that impact all areas of occupation (Richardson et al., 2008; Atchison, 2007; Pynoos et al., 2008).

Personal Activities of Daily Living

Bathing

As a result of physiologic manifestations of stress, regulation of bodily functions is compromised leading to difficulties in personal activities of daily living (PADLs). Stress responses are especially impacted by children with a history of sexual abuse while being bathed as well as being physically abused by immersion in hot or cold water.

Toileting

Encopresis, or the act of passing feces in inappropriate places such as in clothing or other places, is known to occur more frequently among children who have experienced sexual abuse, although it is not a specific indicator of child abuse. Enuresis, or the repeated voiding of urine in the clothing and in inappropriate places, often accompanies encopresis among traumatized children. Whether intentional or not, it is essentially an expression of the child's only mechanism of control in the midst of complete submission to the perpetrators of abuse.

Feeding and Eating

There are many relational factors between a primary caregiver and a child with regard to nutritional intake, beginning in the initial attachment process in infancy. A negative nurturing relationship with an infant including lack of attunement, irritability, depression, and other maternal problems will result in significant maladaptive, disorganized responses by the infant including difficulty with oral mechanisms such as suckling, sucking, swallowing and breathing rhythm, food refusal, and overactive response to certain smells and tastes. Toddlers will often present with severe dental decay, or "bottle rot," a condition resulting from being bottle-fed with high concentrates of sugar while dental development is taking place and at times is a major source of nutrition. Children exposed to chronic trauma are at a higher risk for developing an eating disorder as they grow older. In a home where physical or sexual abuse is taking place, the child may turn to an eating disorder to gain a sense of control. Similar to the psychodynamics associated with encopresis and enuresis—the lack of control in terms of what is happening to their bodies—they are unable to control their food intake or their weight. Children who are compulsive eaters or those who hoard and hide food are usually using food to help them deal with feelings of anger, sadness, hurt, loneliness, abandonment, fear, and pain.

Personal Hygiene and Grooming

DTD often results in children who lack the attention needed to provide proper hygiene and grooming, which often comes to the attention of school personnel and may facilitate a referral to CPS. This may be the result of incompetent parenting who lack the intellectual requirements to facilitate a child's awareness of healthy grooming or willful neglect of one, but not all, children among a set of siblings.

Sexual Activity

Reactions to chronic sexual abuse naturally include significant dysfunction in sexual activity including age-inappropriate sexual activity, the most frequent being sexualized behavior including a preoccupation with sexual organs of self, parents, and others expressed in drawings and in language. Children with a history of molestation are seven times more likely to become drug/alcohol dependent (Pynoos et al., 2008). In a sexual abuse effects study of 938 adolescents admitted to residential, therapeutic communities for the treatment of substance abuse and related disorders, 64% of the girls and 24% of the boys reported histories of sexual abuse (Hawke, Jainchill, & DeLeon, 2000).

Instrumental Activities of Daily Living

DTD has a significant impact on instrumental activities of daily living (IADL). A common occurrence among a group of siblings in an abusive and neglectful environment is for one child, usually the oldest, to take on the role of a parent, referred to as **parentification** as there is an absence of an adult careprovider willing or able to provide care for others. Oftentimes, neglected children are exposed to dangerous in home situations such as fire hazards, firearms, insect and animal infestation, from parents operating methamphetamine labs. Parents might become physically or mentally unable to care for a child. Other times, alcohol or drug abuse may seriously impair judgment and the ability to keep a child safe.

Rest and Sleep

Exposure to trauma often results in significant difficulty with rest and sleep patterns as the child often exhibits **hypervigilance** and overactivity. Multiple exposures to violence and trauma result in autonomic and endocrine hyperarousal which are observed overreactions to stimuli. This may include being easily startled, craving high-risk, stimulating, or dangerous activity—all of which impair the balance of play, work, and rest. The NCTSN clinician survey (Pynoos et al., 2008) found that 73% of children with DTD experienced sleep disturbances, a finding that has been supported by additional studies (Egger et al., 1999; Glod et al., 1997; Noll et al., 2006). While not a common occurrence, victims of chronic abuse may experience "sleep terrors" which are also called "night terrors." In a typical episode, an individual will sit up in bed and begin to scream or shout which may include kicking and thrashing. The child may say or shout nonsensible exclamations with an intense fearful expression with eyes wide open and heart racing. In addition, the child may sweat, breathe heavily, and be very tense.

Education

In a study that included a sample of 9,336 children receiving trauma intervention across the United States, 41% had academic problems including behavior problems in school/daycare (Pynoos et al., 2008). Academic functioning is a significant area of developmental competence beginning with preschool to higher education. In addition to intellectual abilities, success is significantly tied to a child's ability to regulate internal events or experience and to effectively interact with peers and teachers. By preschool, trauma-exposed children demonstrate problems in both of these areas as demonstrated by poor frustration tolerance, a higher incidence of anger and noncompliance, and significantly higher dependency on others for support (Egeland, Sroufe, & Erikson, 1983; Vondra, Barnett, & Chichetti, 1990). In elementary school, they are less persistent on and more likely to avoid challenging tasks and are overly reliant on teachers' guidance and feedback (Shonk & Cicchetti, 2001). By middle school and high school, they are more likely to be considered having a lack of motivation, learning below average, and there is a higher incidence of disciplinary referrals and suspensions (Eckenrode, Laird, & Doris, 1993). Developmental delays and emotional/behavioral dysregulation, learning disabilities, and intellectual impairment that cannot be accounted for by neurologic or other factors that are experienced by children exposed to trauma can profoundly affect their school performance (Atchison, 2007). A cycle often is created whereby a student's lack of success in school reduces his or her self-esteem and increases a lethargy often perceived as laziness or willful disobedience by adults. The student's poor self-concept then further exacerbates limited school functioning. If this cycle continues, the student may face significant challenges as he or she plans for the future. A variety of school intervention programs, with a focus on creating trauma-informed or trauma-sensitive classrooms, have been utilized and are described in the literature as a means of addressing these students' needs (Atchison, 2011; Katoaka, et al, 2003 Macy, Macy, Gross, & Brighton, 2003; Stein et al., 2003). The key components of a trauma sensitive classroom that emerge from descriptions of intervention programs for children exposed to chronic trauma include

- Establishing and maintaining safety
- Relational engagement
- Acquiring affective regulation skills
- Participation in and enhancement of their own learning
- Assistance in making meaning of students' experiences

Unfortunately, there exists a paucity of awareness in most school systems regarding the need for classroom-based intervention that addresses the child as the victim of chronic abuse. The child, because of the many challenges he or she has in response to trauma experiences, acts out and behaves in ways that are interpreted as willful and thus being labeled as *oppositional-defiant* or other diagnoses that lay blame solely on the child, leading to continuous conflicts with school personnel. The lack of appropriate intervention leads to academic underperformance, non-attendance, disciplinary problems, a high drop-out rate, failure to complete diplomas which ultimately leads to poor success in vocational pursuits.

Work

Persons with DTD typically show disinterest in work, with ill-defined employment interests and poor employment-seeking skills or vocational interests. The lack of antecedent behaviors which are necessary for job performance skills leads to the inability to acquire and maintain employment. Persistent conflict with coworkers or supervisors is also a significant barrier to successful work performance.

Play and Leisure

The lack of acquisition in the components of interpersonal competence, poor self-concept, difficulty with social communication, sensory processing disorders, and intellectual impairment have a significant impact on play exploration, constructive play, and symbolic play. Typical early childhood behavior among those with DTD will often reflect traumatic events which may include sexual acting out or violent play with dolls, seemingly disorganized and nonpurposeful interaction with items that may indicate a reenactment of events. Persistent themes may be noted as the child is essentially reliving the event in an attempt to

control or gain mastery over fears that continue to create fear or that overwhelm the child. The child may be easily triggered by environmental stimuli, including other children and adults, which result in rage and physical aggression during play sessions with other children or alone. At later ages, the pursuit of leisure interests, which rely on intrinsic motivation and engagement in self-selected activities are typically not healthy or productive as would be other children with a firm foundation built from successful play experiences and development of competence in play.

Social Participation

In a sample of 9,336 children with a history of trauma who were receiving intervention across the United States, 48% were reported to have had difficulty with social engagement within the home and in the community (Pynoos et al., 2008). Within peer groups, there is a significant degree of isolation, deviant affiliations, persistent physical or emotional conflict, avoidance/passivity, involvement in violence or unsafe acts, and age-inappropriate affiliations or style of interaction. Family interaction is marked by interpersonal conflict, avoidance/passivity, running away, detachment and surrogate replacements, attempts to physically or emotionally hurt family members, and nonfulfillment of responsibilities within the family. Many individuals with a history of DTD are at high risk for dysfunctional social participation within their communities including a high incidence of arrests and recidivism, detention, convictions, incarceration, violation of probation or other court orders, increasingly severe offenses, crimes against other persons, and disregard or contempt for the law or for conventional moral standards (Pynoos et al., 2008).

Case Illustrations

Case 1

Derrick is a 3-year, 4-month-old boy who has been living in his current foster care home since he was 1 year 6 months old. While Derrick was living with his biological father, he struck Derrick's legs and buttocks "to get him to sit still" during diapering. The foster mother reported that Derrick's biological mother and father placed him in his room each day at 6:00 p.m., leaving him there for the rest of the evening, into the morning. Both biological parents were reportedly intoxicated often, with consistent physical altercations with

one another in the presence of Derrick and his brother Jason. Jason is four years old and is living in a different foster home while Derrick's biological mother has been diagnosed with BPD and has a history of severe physical abuse by her own biological mother prior to being adopted as a child. Reportedly, she was drinking heavily and using crack cocaine during the first and second trimesters of her pregnancy. Derrick's biological parents were recently released from prison and are pursuing custody. During the weekly 2-hour supervised visitation with them and his brother, Derrick tends to gravitate toward his case worker rather than actively engaging with his brother or his parents and shows little reaction when the session has ended and his parents and brother leave the room.

Derrick's foster mother is concerned about his difficulty with regulation of his mood. He is described as having severe tantrums in which he will scream in response to loud noises and voices and unexpected movements by others. He is described as "being upset about 70% of the time" requiring significant time and effort to calm him.

The foster mother reports that Derrick is in Head Start and is having difficulty with typical developmental tasks expected for a child his age. A recent assessment by an occupational therapist placed him at 16- to 19-month developmental age range across all domains including gross and fine motor, perceptual, cognitive, language, and self care. Observations of his play skills, based on the Knox Play Scale, correlate with this range across all four domains. He is not yet independent in toileting, and is reported to be aggressive with his peers, hitting or kicking others if he wants a toy or a snack that another child has. His foster mother states that if he doesn't like a toy or food he is given, he will throw it and fall down crying and kicking his feet on the floor.

Case 2

Kayla is a 14-year-old who is currently living with her adoptive mother and her live-in female partner, who is concerned about her daughter's difficulty in school as well as her hypersexuality as noted by inappropriate and indiscriminate self-stimulation and persistent sexual themes expressed during conversations about boys at school such as "He's hot … I would do him" and "Look at that guy … I'd like to make out with him." She reports that Kayla was removed from her biological mother at age six and lived in five different foster homes until she was adopted at age 9. The identity of her biological father is unknown. Removal from her home was followed by termination of her mother's parental rights due to substantiated sexual abuse of Kayla by a live-in boyfriend, who was subsequently imprisoned for 16 to 20 years on charges of first-degree sexual misconduct. In addition to active substance abuse, including use of methamphetamine and alcohol while in a drug treatment program, Kayla's biological mother was charged with having failed to protect her daughter from repeated sexual abuse that occurred in the home while she was present. In addition to charges of sexual abuse, it was determined that Kayla was frequently slapped by her mother and in one incident, she pushed Kayla to the floor where she put her foot on the side of her face, leaving an imprint. Kayla is repeating the eighth grade and is struggling academically in all subjects except art, which she enjoys. A recent assessment by a trauma assessment team indicated that she has a composite IQ score of 78 (verbal = 75, nonverbal = 76) and scored low in the areas across developmental domains including fine motor, visual processing, receptive language, memory, attention, and higher level cognitive functioning. In addition to her academic concerns, her teacher reports that Kayla is resistive to completion of assignments in class, is inattentive, and often sent to the principal's office for behavioral problems such as swearing at other students, asking to copy homework, taking pencils and pens from others, and threatening to "slap you silly" to a student who told her to stop bothering her during class. A referral for special education evaluation has been made to determine if Kayla qualifies for support services. She is also reported to have significant aversion to certain smells and tastes, often threatening to "throw up" if an odor she perceives as offensive is detected.

Kayla's adoptive mother reports that Kayla is "gothic" and resists attempts to "tone down her dress attire." She fears that Kayla may be "running with a fast crowd" and is concerned that she may be sexually active.

RECOMMENDED LEARNING RESOURCES

American Professional Society on the Abuse of Children (APSAC)
350 Poplar Avenue
CHO 3B-3406
Elmhurst, IL 60126
Tel: 877- 402-7722
www.apsac.org

The Annie E. Casey Foundation
701 St. Paul Street
Baltimore, MD 21202
The Child Trauma Academy
5161 San Felipe, Suite 320
Houston, TX 77056
Tel: 866-943-9779

www.childtrauma.org
The Doris Duke Charitable Foundation
650 Fifth Avenue, 19th Floor
New York, NY 10019
Tel: 212-974-7000
www.ddcf.org
National Children's Traumatic Stress Network
Center for Mental Health Services
Substance Abuse and Mental Health Services Administration

Department of Health and Human Services
5600 Fishers Lane
Parklawn Building, Room 17C-26
Rockville, MD 20857
www.nctsn.org
The National Institute for Trauma and Loss in Children
42855 Garfield Road
Suite 111
Clinton Township, MI 48038
www.starrtraining.org/contact-tlc

REFERENCES

Alessandri, S. (1991). Play and social behavior in maltreated preschoolers. *Development and Psychopathology, 3*(2), 191–205.

American Heritage Dictionary (4th ed.). (2006). Boston, MA: Houghton Mifflin Company.

American Occupational Therapy Association. (2002). Occupational therapy practice framework: Domain and process. *American Journal of Occupational Therapy, 56,* 609–639.

American Psychiatric Association. (2000). *Diagnostic and statistical manual of mental disorders* (Rev. 4th ed). Washington, DC: American Psychiatric Association.

Atchison, B. (2007). Sensory modulation disorders among children with a history of trauma: A frame of reference for speech pathologists. *Language, Speech, and Hearing Services in Schools, 38,* 109–116.

Atchison, B. (2011). *Creating trauma-informed classroom: the school intervention project.* National Child Traumatic Stress Network Webinar Series. Retrieved February 12, 2011, from http://learn.nctsn.org/course/category.php?id=3

Bevans, K., Cerbone, A., & Overstreet, S. (2008). Relations between recurrent trauma exposure and recent life stress and salivary cortisol among children. *Development and Psychopathology, 20*(1), 257–272.

Brown, L.K., Houck, C.D., Hadley, W.S., & Lescano, C.M. (2005). Self-Cutting and sexual risk among adolescents in intensive psychiatric treatment. *Psychiatric Services, 56*(2), 216–218.

Cicchetti, D. & Rogosch, F. (2001). The impact of child maltreatment and psychopathology on neuroendocrine functioning. *Development and Psychopathology,* 13:783–804.

Cook, A., Blaustein, M., Spinazzola, J., & van der Kolk, B. (Eds.) (2003). *Complex trauma in children and adolescents.* National Child Traumatic Stress Network. http://www.NCTSNet.org

Cook, A., Spinazzola, J., Ford, J., Lanktree, C., Blaustein, M., & Sprague, C. (2007). Complex Ttrauma in Children and Aadolescents. *Focal Point, 21*(1), 4–8.

Curtis, W. J., & Cicchetti, D. (2007). Emotion and resilience: A multilevel investigation of hemispheric electroencephalogram asymmetry and emotion regulation in maltreated and nonmaltreated children. *Development and Psychopathology, 19*(3), 811–840.

Eckenrode, J., Laird, M., & Doris, J. (1993). School performance and disciplinary problems among abused and neglected children. *Developmental Psychology, 29,* 53–62.

Egeland, B., Sroufe, A., & Erickson, M. (1983). The developmental consequence of different patterns of maltreatment. *Child Abuse & Neglect, 7,* 459–469.

Egger, H. L., Costello, E. J., Erkanli, A., & Angold, A. (1999). Somatic complaints and psychopathology in children and adolescents: Stomach aches, musculoskeletal pains, and headaches. *Journal of the American Academy of Child & Adolescent Psychiatry, 38*(7), 852–860.

Ford, J. D., Racusin, R., Ellis, C., Daviss, W. B., Reiser, J., Fleischer, A., et al. (2000). Child maltreatment, other trauma exposure, and posttraumatic symptomatology among children with Oppositional Defiant and Attention Deficit Hyperactivity Disorders. *Child Maltreatment, 5,* 205–217.

Glod, C. A., Teicher, M. H., Hartman, C. R., & Harakal, T. (1997). Increased nocturnal activity and impaired sleep maintenance in abused children. *Journal of the American Academy of Child & Adolescent Psychiatry, 36*(9), 1236–1243.

Hawke, J., Jainchill, N., & DeLeon, G. (2000). School professionals' attributions of blame for child sexual abuse. *Journal of Child and Adolescent Substance Abuse, 9*(3), 35–47.

Henry, J., Sloane, M., & Black-Pond, C. (2007). Neurobiology and neurodevelopmental impact of childhood traumatic stress and prenatal alcohol exposure. *Language, Speech, and Hearing Services in Schools, 38,* 99–108.

Hyter, Y., Atchison, B. Henry, J., Sloane, M. & Black-Pond, C. (2001). A response to traumatized children: Developing a best practice model. *Occupational Therapy in Health Care, 15*(3), 113–140.

Ito, Y., Teicher, M. H., Glod, C. A., & Harper, D. (1993). Increased prevalence of electrophysiological abnormalities in children with psychological, physical, and sexual abuse. *Journal of Neuropsychiatry & Clinical Neurosciences, 5*(4), 401–408.

Kagan, R. (2004). Rebuilding attachment with traumatized children: Healing from losses, violence, abuse and neglect. Philadelphia, PA: Haworth Press.

Kataoka, S. H., Stein, B. D., Jaycox, L. H., Wong, M., Escudero, P., Tu, W., Zaragoza, C., & Fink, A. (2003) A School-Based Mental Health Program for Traumatized Latino Immigrant Children. *Journal of American Child & Adolescent Psychiatry, 42*(3), 311–318.

Koomar, J. A. (2009, December). Trauma- and attachment-informed sensory integration assessment and intervention. *Sensory Integration Special Interest Section Quarterly, 32*(4), 1–4.

Luthar, S. S., Cicchetti, D., & Becker, B. (2000). The construct of resilience: A critical evaluation and guidelines for future work. *Child Development, 71,* 543–562.

Macy, R. D., Macy, D. J., Gross, S. I., & Brighton, P. (2003). Healing in familiar settings: Support for children and youth in the classroom and community. *New Directions for Youth Development, 98,* 51–79.

Masten, A., & Coatsworth, J., (1998). The development of competence in favorable and unfavorable environments: Lessons from research of successful children. *American Psychologist, 53,* 205–220.

National Children's Traumatic Stress Network. *What is Trauma?* Retrieved January 15, 2011, from http://www.nctsn.org/content/defining-trauma-and-child-traumatic-stress

Nolin, P., & Ethier, L. (2007). Using neuropsychological profiles to classify neglected children with or without physical abuse. *Child Abuse & Neglect, 31*(6), 631–643.

Noll, J. G., Trickett, P. K., Susman, E. J., & Putnam, F. W. (2006). Sleep Disturbances and Childhood Sexual Abuse. *Journal of Pediatric Psychology, 31*(5), 469–480.

Perry, B. D. (2001). *Bonding and attachment in maltreated children: Consequences of emotional neglect in childhood.* The Child Trauma Academy. Retrieved October 11, 2010, from: http://www.childtrauma.org/images/stories/Articles/attcar4_03_v2_r.pdf

Pynoos, R., Fairbank, J. A., Briggs-King, E. C., Steinberg, A., Layne, C., Stolbach, B., et al. (2008). *Trauma exposure, adverse experiences, and diverse symptom profiles in a national sample of traumatized children.* Paper presented at the 24th Annual Meeting of the International Society for Traumatic Stress Studies, Chicago, IL, November 15, 2008.

Richardson, M., Henry, J., Black-Pond, C., & Sloane, M. (2008). Multiple types of maltreatment: Behavioral and developmental impact on children in the child welfare system. *Journal of Child & Adolescent Trauma, 1,* 1–14.

Sayar, Kose, Grabe, H., & Topbas. (2005). Alexithymia and dissociative tendencies in an adolescent sample from Eastern Turkey. *Psychiatry and clinical neurosciences, 59*(2), 127–134.

Sedlak, A. J., Mettenburg, J., Basena, M., Petta, I., McPherson, K., Greene, A., et al. (2010). *Fourth National Incidence Study of Child Abuse and Neglect (NIS–4): Report to Congress, Executive Summary.* Washington, DC: U.S. Department of Health and Human Services, Administration for Children and Families.

Shonk, S. M., & Cicchetti, D. (2001). Maltreatment, competency deficits, and risk for academic and behavioral maladjustment. *Developmental Psychology, 37,* 3–17.

Spinazzola, J., Ford, J. D., Zucker, M., van der Kolk, B. A., Silva, S., Smith, S. F., et al. (2005). Survey evaluates complex trauma exposure, outcome, and intervention among children and adolescents. *Psychiatric Annals, 35*(5), 433–439.

Stein, B. D., Jaycox, L. H., Kataoka, S. H., Wong, M., Tu, W., Elliott, M. N., et al. (2003). A mental health intervention for schoolchildren exposed to violence. *Journal of American Medical Association, 290,* 603–611.

Teicher, M. (2000). Wounds that won't heal: The neurobiology of child abuse. *Cerebrum, 2* (4) 50–62.

Taylor, S., Eisenberger, N., Saxbe, D., Lehman, B, and Lieberman, M. (2006). Neural responses to emotional stimuli are associated with childhood family stress. *Biological Psychiatry, 60:* 296-301.

Teicher, M. H., Andersen, S. L., & Polcari, A. (2002). Developmental neurobiology of childhood stress and trauma. *Psychiatric Clinics of North America, 25, Special Issue: Recent advances in the study of biological alterations in post-traumatic stress disorder,* 397–426.

van der Kolk, B. A. (2005). Developmental trauma disorder: toward a rational diagnosis for children with complex trauma histories. *Psychiatric Annals, 35*(5), 2–8.

van der Kolk, B. A., Pynoos, R., Cicchetti, M., Cloitre, M., D'Andrea, W., Ford, J. et al. (2009). *Proposal to include a developmental trauma disorder diagnosis for children and adolescents in DSM-V.* National Children's Traumatic Stress Network. Retrieved June 9, 2011, from http://www.nctsn.org/sites/default/files/assets/pdfs/ComplexTrauma_All.pdf

Vondra, J. I., Barnett, D., & Cicchetti, D. (1990). Self-concept, motivation, and competence among preschoolers from maltreating and comparison families. *Child Abuse & Neglect, 14,* 525–540.

Way, I., Yelsma, P., Van Meter, A., & Black-Pond, C. (2007). Understanding alexithymia and language skills in children: Implications for assessment and intervention. *Language, Speech and Hearing Services in Schools, 38,* 128–139.

Werner A. A., & Smith A. E. (1992). *High risk children from birth to adulthood.* Ithaca, NY: Cornell University Press.

World Health Organization. (2007). *International statisti-cal classification of diseases and related health problems (ICD-10).* World Health Organization: Geneva.

Wyman, P. A., Sandler, I., Wolchik, S., & Nelson, K. (2000). Resilience as cumulative competence promotion and stress protection: Theory and intervention. In D. Cicchetti & J. Rappaport (Eds.), *The promotion of wellness in children and adolescents* (pp. 133–184). Washington, DC: Child Welfare League of America.

21

Muscular Dystrophy

- *Jennifer L. Forgach*
- *Andrea L. Washington*

J.B. is 6 years old. He has a 3-year-old brother and 1-year-old sister. J.B.'s mother is concerned because he does not seem to be "keeping up" with his peers. He gets tired quickly, has had an increased number of falls, and has never learned how to jump. J.B. recently had to quit his soccer team due to increased fatigue. J.B.'s mother takes him to his pediatrician who notes that J.B. has enlarged calves, proximal muscle weakness, and uses Gower's maneuver to rise off the floor. The pediatrician refers J.B. and his siblings for blood work, genetic testing, and to neurology/muscular dystrophy (MD) specialty clinic for further assessment.

J.B. arrives to the MD clinic. The neurologist meets with J.B. and his family. J.B.'s blood work shows elevated **creatine kinase** (CK) levels greater than 6,500 IU/L, while his 3-year-old brother's are normal at around 150 IU/L. Genetic testing reveals that J.B. is positive for Duchenne muscular dystrophy. His younger brother tests negative and his 1-year-old sister is found to be a carrier. J.B. is referred to occupational and physical therapy and is recommended to follow up with the physician in 6 months. Although the above scenario illustrates one type of MD, MD is not strictly *one* disease.

MD is one of the most prolific **neuromuscular disorders**. It is actually a grouping of nine different disorders with more than 30 different subtypes. MD can broadly be defined as a group of hereditary diseases that weaken the muscles. They are characterized by **progressive** muscle weakness, defects in muscle protein, and/or the death of muscle cells and tissues. The progressive muscle weakness is caused by the lack, or absence, of the structural protein dystrophin. **Dystrophin** is a vital part of the intracellular protein complex that is responsible for maintaining the shape and structure of the muscle fiber. In general terms, dystrophin acts as the "glue" to hold the muscle together. Without this "glue," the muscle breaks down causing the progressive weakness that is the hallmark characteristic of MD (Emery, 1994, 2001; http//:www.mda.org, 2010). It is the distribution and the progression of the muscle weakness that is used to distinguish between the nine types (Fig. 21.1). The nine main types of MD that have been identified are (http//:www.mda.org, 2010) as follows:

- Duchenne muscular dystrophy (DMD)
- Becker muscular dystrophy (BMD)
- Emery-Dreifuss muscular dystrophy (EDMD)
- Limb-girdle muscular dystrophy (LGMD)
- Facioscapulohumeral muscular dystrophy (FSHD)
- Myotonic muscular dystrophy (MMD)
- Oculopharyngeal muscular dystrophy (OPMD)
- Distal muscular dystrophy (DD)
- Congenital muscular dystrophy (CMD)

Although there are currently nine identified forms of the disease, this chapter highlights six types of MD most commonly seen by occupational therapists.

DESCRIPTION AND DEFINITION

Duchenne Muscular Dystrophy

Although DMD is genetically present at birth, symptoms of the disease may not present themselves until the child is 3 to 4 years of age. DMD affects only males and, as discussed later, is an **x-linked** recessive inherited condition (Biggar, 2006). DMD is caused by an absence, or deficiency, of dystrophin. Initial symptoms include are delayed motor development, proximal weakness, and increased fatigue. These symptoms manifest themselves

as a waddling gait, enlarged calf muscles, increased falls, and failure to develop the ability to run or jump (Emery, 1994, 2001). Also present in 90% of males with DMD is the **"valley sign."** This is a depressed area on the posterior axillary fold that can be seen when the patient abducts shoulders to 90 degrees, elbows flexed to 90 degrees, with bilateral hands pointing upward (Fig. 21.2).

The pattern of muscle weakness is always bilateral and symmetrical. It progresses from proximal to distal, and affects the lower extremities prior to upper extremities. The rate of progression varies from person to person. The individual can alternately go through periods of both rapid progression and slowed or no progression. Most individuals with DMD will be wheelchair dependent by 12 years of age. DMD affects all voluntary skeletal muscles, as well as cardiac and pulmonary muscles (Emery, 2001). Of note, up to one-third of the individuals with DMD may have cognitive impairments. Current research indicates that this *may* also be related to the lack of dystrophin (Ashraf & Wong, 2005; Emery, 1994, 2001).

As muscle wasting progresses, active range of motion (ROM) decreases, and the individual can be left with **contractures** at the elbows, hips, and knees, as well as severe spinal deformities. The joint contractures are often at a 90-degree angle later in the disease process, indicative of prolonged wheelchair use.

Becker Muscular Dystrophy

Like DMD, BMD is characterized by progressive muscle weakness, affecting only males, as an x-linked recessive inherited condition. BMD is also genetically present at birth, but onset of symptoms can vary widely from 2 to 40 years of age. Symptoms most often appear, however, between 6 and 18 years of age. Individuals with BMD often demonstrate delayed ambulation, difficulty climbing

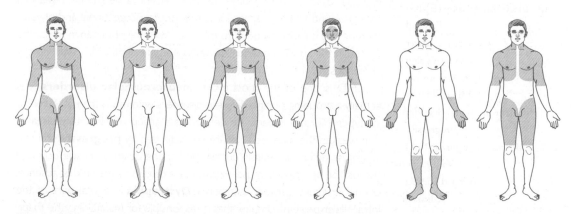

Figure 21.1 Typical distribution of muscle weakness seen in different types of MD. Left to right: Duchenne/Becker, Emery-Dreifuss, limb-girdle, facioscapulohumeral, distal, oculopharyngeal.

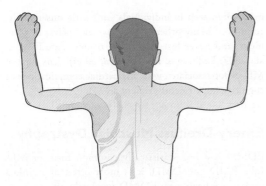

Figure 21.2 The valley sign. Note the depressed area of the left posterior axillary region seen beneath the deltoid when the individual abducts shoulders to 90 degrees, elbows flexed to 90 degrees, with bilateral hands pointing upward.

stairs, "toe walking," muscle cramps, and fatigue as their early symptoms (http//:www.mda.org, 2010; Emery, 1994, 2001; Stockley, Akber, Bulgin, & Ray, 2006).

Muscle wasting/weakness progresses from proximal to distal and generally occurs at a slower rate than DMD (Stockley et al., 2006). It is usually symmetric, starting in the muscles of the pelvic girdle and thighs. Eventually it extends to the trunk and upper extremities. The calves and forearms remain preserved until later stages of the disease. Facial muscles are not affected. Eventually, heel cord contractures (from toe walking) and **lumbar lordosis** are seen due to the individual attempting to compensate for pelvic weakness (Emery, 2001).

Affected men can become wheelchair dependent in their 30s. Some may never require the use of a wheelchair, managing daily life with the use of **compensation** and adaptations.

Limb-Girdle Muscular Dystrophy

LGMD accounts for approximately half of the identified subtypes of MD (Cardamone, Darras, & Ryan, 2008). LGMD is classified based on age of onset, rate of progression, and type of inheritance. Most forms of LGMD are of **autosomal recessive** inheritance while up to 10% of cases are **autosomal dominant**. The autosomal recessive forms exhibit more severe symptoms with a faster decline and loss of function, with an onset usually in childhood (http://www.mda.org, 2010; Emery, 2001).

Other forms of LGMD have their onset in later adolescence, or even into adulthood. Adult-onset forms of LGMD are less severe and progress more slowly. Childhood forms can clinically resemble DMD. Males and females are equally affected. Dystrophin levels are normal; however, there is a lack of structural, dystrophin-associated glycoproteins. There are no associated cognitive deficits with LGMD (Bonnemann, 2005).

Progression of muscle weakness is not always symmetrical. It first affects the muscles of the pelvis and shoulders, "the limb-girdle." Muscle wasting is usually slow, but variable. While individuals with severe cases can lose the ability to ambulate in their early adolescence, others may never have more than complaints of muscle cramping in their lower extremities. Cardiopulmonary complications may appear in later stages of the disease (Bonnemann, 2005; http://www.mda.org, 2010; Emery, 2001).

Typical presentation includes enlarged calves, severe lordosis with scoliosis, proximal muscle weakness, and a positive **Gower's sign**. **Gower's maneuver** can be described as the inability to rise off the floor without using the upper extremities to "walk up" the thighs to assist with hip extension (Fig. 21.3). When

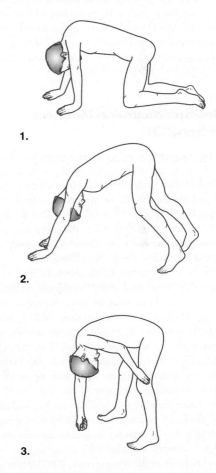

1.

2.

3.

Figure 21.3 The Gower's maneuver: the sequence of movements utilized by individuals with proximal weakness needed to rise off the floor. Named for William Richard Gower who first described this technique in 1879 (1).

a person is observed to use this technique to get up off the floor, it is documented as having a positive Gower's sign (Bonnemann, 2005).

Myotonic Muscular Dystrophy

MMD is marked by teen or adult onset. Only 50% of the individuals affected live beyond 50 years of age. MMD is an autosomal dominant inherited disorder affecting both males and females. Progression of muscle weakness is slow (http://www.mda.org, 2010; Emery, 1994).

Muscle wasting/weakness begin in the face, lower legs, forearms, hands, and neck. Delayed relaxation after muscle contraction is a common symptom. This can be seen by "locking up" of the muscles, followed by a slowed relaxation (McNally & Pytel, 2007; Emery, 1994). In addition, MMD affects the gastrointestinal system, vision, heart, and/or respiratory system. Thirty percent of individuals affected with MMD will die from cardiac complications. Cardiac symptoms often precede neurological symptoms. Cognitive impairments may also be associated with this type of MD (McNally & Pytel, 2007).

Facioscapulohumeral Muscular Dystrophy

FSHD is the third most common type of the dystrophies (Padberg & van Engelen, 2009). It is an autosomal dominant inherited disorder affecting both males and females. Onset of symptoms is quite variable, appearing anywhere from the age of 7 to the age of 20. The earlier the disease onset, the more severe the symptoms, and the faster the disease will typically progress (Van der Maarel, Frants, & Padberg, 2007).

It initially affects the facial, shoulder, and upper arm muscles with progressive weakness. Weakness begins with the facial muscles and progresses down the body (Padberg & van Engelen, 2009). Weakness, unlike the other dystrophies, is not usually symmetrical, with one side more affected than the other. Presentation of facial symptoms include the inability or difficulty with closing the eyes, asymmetry of the mouth with smiling, drooping of the corners of the mouth at rest, inability to whistle or pucker, and **atrophy** of the facial muscles (Emery, 1994; Wohlgemuth et al., 2006). As the disorder progresses into the shoulder region, **winged scapulae** with severe muscle atrophy is present (Van der Maarel et al., 2007). Shoulders appear depressed due to severe muscle weakness (especially in the biceps and triceps), and the individual is ultimately unable to raise his or her arms against gravity. With some individuals the disease can progress to pelvic muscles and eventually affect their gate. This is

most often seen in individuals with early onset of the condition. Many others never have any pelvic involvement, and never lose the ability to ambulate (Iosa et al., 2007; Padberg & van Engelen, 2009). This type of MD is not associated with any cardiac complications or cognitive impairments (Emery, 1994).

Emery-Dreifuss Muscular Dystrophy

EDMD is a less statistically common form of MD. Like BMD and DMD, it is most often of x-linked recessive inheritance. EDMD primarily affects boys. Individuals with EDMD display a unique pattern of muscle weakness characterized by the formation of muscle contractures before any significant muscle weakness is recognized by the individual. Contractures of the heel cords, elbows, and muscles of the posterior neck are most common. Tightness of the heel cords may result in toe walking and an increased number of trips and/or falls. Elbows that are contracted to a 90-degree angle are the "most important diagnostic clue" of EDMD to physicians (Brown, Piercy, Muntoni, & Sewry, 2008). Eventually, rigidity of the spine and posterior neck prevents an individual from flexing his or her body forward. Formation of contractures and the subsequent muscle weakness are generally symmetrical on the body (Brown et al., 2008; http://www.mda.org, 2010; Emery, 1994; Yazdanpanah, Javan, Nadimi, & Ghaffarain Shirazi, 2007).

Significant cardiac complications are also highly characteristic of EDMD. It is often necessary to surgically implant a pacemaker to regulate heart and pulse rate. Similar to the other forms of MD, it is often the cardiac and pulmonary complications that cause death in mid-adulthood (Gayathri, Taly, Sinha, Suresh, & Gorai, 2006). It is important to note, however, that with early intervention and proper medical management, individuals with EDMD may live an average life span (Emery, 1994).

ETIOLOGY

Most MDs are **familial**, meaning there is some family history of the disease. All of the MDs are inherited genetic disorders. MDs can be inherited in one of three ways as listed below. It is important to note, however, that some forms may be inherited in multiple ways (Cardamone et al., 2006; http://www.mda.org, 2010; Emery, 2001; Yazdanpanah et al., 2007).

X-linked recessive

■ Also referred to as *sex-linked*, occurs when a mother who carries the affected gene passes it onto her son.

Although the mother carries the affected gene on one of her X chromosomes, she may never show symptoms since it is a recessive trait.

■ MDs inherited this way: Duchenne, Becker, Emery-Dreifuss

Autosomal recessive

■ Occurs when both parents carry and pass on the affected gene
■ MD inherited this way: Emery-Dreifuss, limb-girdle, oculopharyngeal, distal, congenital

Autosomal dominant

■ Occurs when a child inherits a normal gene from one parent and an affected gene from the other parent
■ MDs inherited this way: Emery-Dreifuss, limb-girdle, facioscapulohumeral, myotonic, oculopharyngeal, distal, congenital

INCIDENCE AND PREVALENCE

It is estimated that at least 1 in every 5,000 people in the population are currently affected with some form of MD. The actual prevalence of the disease is most likely higher than this as many forms of MD are often misdiagnosed or not yet identified. Therefore, specific current statistical information is difficult to obtain (Cardamone et al., 2008; Emery, 1994, 2001; Kohler et al., 2009; McNally & Pytel, 2007). Table 21.1 is an *approximation* of available statistical figures in research literature today. It should be used only as a tool to compare the occurrence of one type of MD to another.

It is most important to recognize from Table 21.1 that DMD and BMD are by far the most common types and affect only males. Other forms, like LGMD and EDMD, have statistically unknown or unreliable data. This may be due to EDMD being less common than the other forms, and the many different subtypes of LGMD. MD

occurs worldwide affecting all races, ages, and genders. Depending on the region of the world, or country, a certain form of MD may be very common or very rare.

SIGNS AND SYMPTOMS

Refer to each of the individual descriptions of the different types of MD for specific signs and symptoms as it relates to each of the various subtypes. As mentioned, decreased strength, muscle cramping, and decreased gross motor skills are the common link between all forms, with each form having its own unique presentation. As previously defined, the Gower's maneuver and the "valley sign" are two key clinical indicators that may be evident in any form of MD with proximal muscle weakness (Emery, 1994, 2001).

There are other progressive neuromuscular disorders that mimic MD and are often mistaken for MD in their early stages. Some of these include **spinal muscular atrophy (SMA)** and its subtypes myasthenia gravis (MG), Pompe disease, **Charcot Marie Tooth (CMT)**, mitochondrial myopathy, and **amyotrophic lateral sclerosis (ALS)**. These disorders exhibit the same symptoms at onset including muscle cramping, generalized progressive weakness, and joint stiffness and are often treated in neurological clinics alongside individuals with MD (http://www.mda.org, 2010).

DIAGNOSIS

MD is often first suspected by a primary care physician when a patient presents with complaints of muscle weakness, increased falls, muscle cramps or increased fatigue. It is at that point that clinical assessment becomes a vital part of the diagnostic process.

The patient is physically assessed by the physician. Based on the distribution of the weakness in conjunction

TABLE 21.1 Incidence and Prevalence of Specific Types of muscular dystrophy

Type of MD	Incidence	Prevalence
Duchenne MD	1 in 3,500 males	1 in 4,000 males
Becker MD	1 in 30,000 males	1 in 20,000 males
Facioscapulohumeral MD	1 in 22,000 males and females	1 in 50,000 males and females
Myotonic MD	1 in 8,000 males and females	1 in 20,000 males and females
Limb-girdle MD	Statistically unknown	1 in 25,000 males and females
Emery-Dreifuss MD	Statistically unknown	1 in 100,000 males and females

with other aforementioned physical symptoms, MD may be suspected. At this point, the physician will begin to order more testing to confirm diagnosis.

The following three diagnostic tests are typically used to confirm or rule out an MD diagnosis (Emery, 1994, 2001; Stockley et al., 2006):

- Blood work to perform genetic testing and reveal creatine kinase levels. Creatine kinase levels become elevated when there is muscle damage in the body; therefore, elevated levels will indicate that there is muscle wasting occurring. Normal CK levels average around 100 to 200 IU/L. The levels in DMD, in comparison, can be elevated 50 to 100 times this amount (Biggar, 2006; Emery, 1994, 2001).
- **Electromyography (EMG)** to evaluate the current electrical activity produced by the skeletal muscles. An EMG examination can be used to confirm the diagnosis of dystrophy and distinguish this from other types of neuromuscular diseases. It cannot reveal what type of dystrophy a patient may have (Emery, 2001).
- **Muscle biopsy** used to examine the cellular makeup of the muscle tissue, and look at the differences in muscle fibers, fiber size, fiber splitting, and fiber necrosis. Muscle biopsy can be used to distinguish the type of dystrophy, based on subtle differences in the muscle tissues (Emery, 1994).

These are not stand-alone tests; therefore, it is important to complete a thorough clinical and neurological exam to identify any patterns of muscle weakness, test reflex responses and coordination, and identify contracted muscles (Wren, Blumi, Tseng-Ong, & Gilsanz, 2007). If one child is diagnosed with MD, all siblings and parents should be tested for the condition as well.

COURSE AND PROGNOSIS

Each of the MDs follows its own unique course. Each type has a variable prognosis with most ultimately resulting in a shortened lifespan. Prognosis will depend not only on the primary diagnosis but also on what specific subtype of the disorder is present. For instance, LGMD has up to 15 different subtypes. Some of these subtypes have a normal life expectancy, while others have a shortened lifespan. The course and prognosis of each of the MDs examined in this chapter are discussed individually below. While the figures represent an average of current statistical data, research and medical advances are beginning to extend life expectancies (http://www.mda.org, 2010).

DMD: Males affected with DMD have an average life expectancy of late teens to early 20s. The cause of death is usually secondary to respiratory and/or cardiac complications (Biggar, 2006; Emery, 1994, 2001; Kohler et al., 2009).

BMD: Less severe than DMD, males affected with BMD demonstrate a much slower progression. Life expectancy varies greatly, but average is between middle and late adulthood, approximately 25 to 30 years after onset of the condition (Emery, 2001; Stockley et al., 2006).

EDMD: Disease progresses slowly, often with cardiac and respiratory complications. Individuals may live an average lifespan if proper cardiac management is received (Cardamone et al., 2008; Chen, 2008).

LGMD: Progresses slowly. Although symptoms may appear in childhood, they often do not appear until adolescence or even adulthood. If muscles deteriorate rapidly, life expectancy may be only into early 30s. Otherwise, an individual may live a normal lifespan. The course of LGMD is by far the most variable of the dystrophies (Bonnemann, 2005; http://www.mda.org, 2010; Emery, 1994, 2001).

FSHD: Symptoms appear around age 20. Disease progresses slowly with some periods of rapid decline. Course of disease may spread over many decades, with life expectancy being normal (Padberg & van Engelen, 2009; Van der Maarel et al., 2007).

MMD: Disease progresses slowly with course spanning up to 50 to 60 years. Life expectancy may be typically into late adulthood (Cardamone et al., 2008).

MEDICAL/SURGICAL MANAGEMENT

Currently there is no cure or specific treatment that can reverse or stop the progression of any form of MD. Symptom management will have the greatest impact on enhancing a person's quality of life and possibly increasing his or her life expectancy. The primary goal of treatment with MD is maintenance of independence for as long as possible (Emery, 2001).

Respiratory Maintenance

As mobility and muscle functioning decrease, respiratory maintenance becomes increasingly difficult. The individual will have decreased ability to use the voluntary muscles of the thorax to fully inhale, or cough, causing inability to keep the lungs clear. The individual may require suctioning, cough assist, or antibiotics to preserve lung function. They are high risk for pneumonia and other respiratory infections. Monitoring for signs/symptoms of aspiration is an important part of pneumonia prevention (Kohler et al., 2009; Thompson, 1999).

Skin Integrity

Skin integrity becomes a risk factor with decreased mobility. When skin integrity is compromised, the individual is at increased risk for infection, further tissue damage, and loss of joint mobility. Careful skin inspection should be incorporated into one's daily routine. Severe infections can lead to death if not properly managed.

Pain

Pain should be assessed in all individuals with MD. While most types of MD are not directly associated with pain, some physical symptoms may contribute to discomfort (Emery, 1994). Initial feelings of muscle cramping or spasms may occur. The pain cycle may initially worsen when a stretching or strengthening program is initiated. It is advantageous to complete these exercises on a regular basis as the body will tolerate the stretches with less discomfort. In fact, it is common for an individual with MD to request joint stretching as a source of pain relief. As the disease progresses, pain levels should be continually monitored and assessed as increased or localized pain could be indicative of further concerns. Adequate pain management is essential to quality of life as well as promoting maximum participation in daily tasks.

Nutrition

Good nutrition and hydration are essential to maintaining overall health and can aid in the maintenance of skin integrity. Nutrition can also assist in controlling obesity which can be detrimental to function and mobility. People with MD are at high risk for obesity, secondary to lack of mobility and loss of muscle function. *Safe* maintenance of nutrition becomes a priority as oral and pharyngeal musculature may also be weakened in some forms of MD. As a result, swallowing can become unsafe. Individuals should be closely monitored for signs of dysphagia so that diet can be modified or a feeding tube inserted (Cardamone et al., 2008; Thompson, 1999).

Occupational and/or Physical Therapy

Therapy should be initiated as soon as diagnosis is confirmed to train the patient and family in an extensive home exercise program. A baseline of activities of daily living (ADL) skills and mobility performance should also be obtained. It is important to initiate therapy prior to the formation of contractures or muscle tightness (Thompson, 1999). Therapy is an essential component in preventing or slowing loss of strength, ROM, and function. Another major role of therapy is to assess current equipment needs for home and community use. This role becomes increasingly important as the disease progresses and specific individual needs change. Evaluation and provision of splints and orthotics as needed to prevent joint contracture formation should further be considered at the time of the evaluation.

Drug Intervention

Corticosteroids *may* decrease muscle damage and assist with preserving respiratory function. Although they present possible benefits, they are often associated with side effects that must be closely monitored, including the tendency to gain weight. While corticosteroids are widely used, there continues to be controversy. Significant research is being conducted regarding whether the use of steroids has any effect on life expectancy. In addition to corticosteroids, there are other medications that are often prescribed by a physician for treatment of MD. Immunosuppressant drugs can be used to delay muscle degeneration. Anticonvulsants can be used to control muscle activity. Antibiotics can be used to control respiratory infections. Over-the-counter analgesics can be used for pain management and cramping (Biggar, 2006).

Surgical Management

Surgical management often includes corrective and/or preventative surgeries. Some of these may include, but are not limited to, contracture release, scoliosis repair, cardiac stability, respiratory assist, or spinal stabilization. Spinal deformities can physically reduce a person's ability to breathe, and should be closely monitored. Pacemakers can be surgically implanted to control heart rhythms as needed. Tracheostomies may need to be performed if a person requires ventilator assistance or suctioning of secretions. Feeding tubes, either temporary or permanent, may need to be considered if dysphagia is a concern (Kohler et al., 2009; Thompson, 1999).

IMPACT OF CONDITIONS ON CLIENT FACTORS

All occupational performance areas and performance components may be affected by MD. These are most dependent on the type and the stage of the disease. As previously mentioned, each type of MD has its own unique progression and variable severity.

Activities of Daily Living

The individual with MD may initially be independent with his or her ADL skills; however, a decline in function is anticipated, especially with more severe forms. Maintaining the basic underlying skills of strength and ROM will keep the individual independent longer. As active movement becomes more difficult, the person will require assistance from a caregiver to complete basic tasks such as dressing, grooming, and bathing. Toileting may become a cumbersome task. This can be due to physical limitations making toilet transfers difficult; or due to loss of muscle control causing incontinence. Often with more severe forms of MD the individual is required to wear protective toileting garments.

Eventually, the use of adaptive equipment such as commode chairs, shower chairs, bathing aides, mechanical lifts, ADL equipment, and wheelchairs/mobility equipment may be necessary. These pieces of equipment will help increase independence and make caring for the individual easier and safer. Home modifications such as ramps, grab bars, and bedrails should be considered to promote independence and safety within an individual's home environment.

In less severe forms, the individual may maintain the ability to complete the task himself or herself, but may require increased time to do so. Energy conservation, or task adaptation, should be a consideration for these individuals (Kohler et al., 2009).

School

School is a major concern as the majority of MD cases are diagnosed in early childhood or early adolescence. Most forms of MD do not involve cognitive impairments and therefore, physical limitations ultimately become the barrier at school (Donders & Taneja, 2009; Thompson, 1999). Often the child with MD fatigues quickly, has difficulty keeping up with his or her peers and may require physical assistance to get through the school day. A one-on-one aid may be necessary to assist with maneuvering their wheelchair, toileting, assisting with meals, and completing basic educational tasks.

Increased absences due to illness may be common. This, combined with wheelchair/adaptive equipment use and the decreased physical ability to participate in the same activities as their peers, may contribute to social isolation.

Work

Older individuals may face many of the same barriers as children in school. Social isolation, environmental barriers, fatigue, an inability to keep up with work activities, and requiring physical assistance for some basic tasks may be common in the workplace.

Obtaining and maintaining employment and having the ability to change jobs are more difficult for these individuals due to physical limitations, decreased job opportunities, and employer misperceptions. Some individuals with severe MD may lose, or never have, the physical ability to work. Others may maintain employment with altered responsibilities/adaptations or with relatively little interruption at all.

Play/Leisure

A child's primary responsibility is to play. Many individuals diagnosed with MD are children and this area becomes a significant area of concern. It is important to encourage play, in any capacity, to ensure pleasure, learning, and development. A child with physical impairments may require modifications to their leisure activities to promote success and enjoyment.

For individuals of all ages, leisure activities such as computer and video game play, text messaging, and reading are commonly enjoyed as hand function is often preserved well enough to complete these tasks. It is beneficial to also incorporate and encourage gross motor movements into leisure activities (i.e., balloon volleyball, painting on an easel, etc.) as a means to preserve muscle strength and function (Thompson, 1999).

Psychosocial

MD affects everyone within the family, not solely the affected individual. The emotions, fears, and anxieties experienced by the individual are shared by the entire family. Parents often face feelings of guilt, helplessness, and fear over the anticipated loss of their child. Fear and anxiety are often a concern for the younger sibling as they watch the deterioration of their older sibling, with the anticipation that they will soon, too, face the same fate.

As the affected individual loses function, and the loss of independence becomes more evident, the individual often struggles with anger and frustration. Individuals who face severe functional loss often experience feelings of depression. Suicidal ideations may become a concern as the individual faces the loss of their perceived role (Bostram & Ahlstrom, 2005; Chen, 2008; Poysky & Kinnett, 2008).

ACKNOWLEDGMENTS

We would like to thank Lawrence C. Banko for his contributions. Lawrence was responsible for drawing all sketches/illustrations used in this chapter.

Case Illustrations

Case 1

A.F. is 32 years old. When she was 13 years old, she began to notice that her hips and lower back would fatigue quickly and that she was having minor trouble with her balance. Her primary care physician felt that it was "growing pains" and told her that he was sure it would pass. A year later, A.F. continued to have problems and her symptoms worsened. A.F. returned to her physician and, at that time, blood work and a muscle biopsy were conducted. A.F. was eventually diagnosed with LGMD.

On this day, A.F. presents to the MD clinic per recommendation of her primary care physician. The occupational therapist evaluates A.F. It was revealed that A.F. has had significant functional decline in the last year. She was previously walking with a walker for household distances. She is now using a borrowed wheelchair for all ambulation. A.F. can independently complete a stand-pivot transfer from her wheelchair to the examining table with increased time allotted. Manual muscle testing scores as follows: grossly 3/5 bilateral shoulder strength, 3+/5 strength at bilateral elbows, and 4/5 in the wrists and hands.

A.F. currently has a shower chair in the bathtub that she borrowed from her grandmother. However, A.F. further reports that she is no longer able to step over the side of the tub. She is now wearing a diaper due to her inability to get to the toilet quickly enough. She attempts to dress herself seated at the edge of the bed, but is unable to don her socks or shoes as a result of leg weakness and poor sitting balance. A.F. currently lives alone and does not have family close by to assist her. She has hired a maid to keep the house clean and assist with weekly laundry. She recently had to quit her job as a school teacher due to her physical decline. She is now significantly concerned about her finances.

She reports that she is feeling isolated at home. She does not identify any leisure interests other than watching television. She states that it is too much work to get out of the house, so she just stays home. A.F. is anxious about her recent decline, and is not knowledgeable about her condition or prognosis. She is not currently taking any medications except an over-the-counter analgesic, as needed.

Case 2

H.M. is a 12-year-old male diagnosed with DMD. He is currently an inpatient at a children's hospital. He presented to the ER with complaints of difficulty breathing. He subsequently required intubation and eventually a tracheostomy.

Occupational therapy was consulted to evaluate H.M. and to provide recommendations to his family. A review of the medical record reveals that H.M. was diagnosed with MD at the age of 3. He is currently on prednisone, digitalis, a multivitamin, a diuretic, and an analgesic as needed. He is the oldest of four children, with two other brothers also diagnosed with DMD. He had spinal stabilization surgery approximately 1 year ago and releases of bilateral knee contractures about 6 months ago.

Upon entering H.M.'s hospital room, the occupational therapist completes a parent interview and receives the following information: H.M. is currently in the 7th grade in a POHI classroom. He lives in a two-story home, with first-floor bedroom and bathroom. They have a ramp outside to enter the home. H.M. has not received therapy in almost a year. Parents are concerned that H.M. has outgrown his current wheelchair and is not properly supported by his seating system. Parents also report that H.M. has been gaining weight, making all wheelchair and surface transfers increasingly difficult. Prior to admission, H.M. required variable assistance for all ADL, IADL, and transfers. There is no current home exercise program in place.

Upon interviewing H.M., he appears to be delayed cognitively, requiring simple questions and multiple cues to follow one-step commands. He reports no pain throughout his day. He spends his time watching television, playing video games, and texting his friends on his cell phone. H.M. states that he would like to be more independent within his school and home environments.

Evaluation findings as follows: H.M. presents with decreased upper extremity active ROM and strength, as he is unable to raise his arms over his head or fully straighten his elbows. He also presents with contractures of bilateral shoulders, elbows, and wrists. H.M. demonstrates the ability to isolate all fingers and thumb movements. He presents with decreased grip strength bilaterally. He currently demonstrates the ability to feed himself with a spoon, but he is observed to lower his head to the plate. H.M. is coughing and choking during meals with minimal chewing observed. He currently requires maximal assistance for all bathing/dressing tasks which is being completed in bed at this time. Bed mobility is impaired. He requires maximum assistance to transfer from supine to edge of bed, and is unable to maintain sitting balance without support.

The inpatient occupational therapist made the following recommendations to H.M. and his family. Referrals were made to outpatient occupational and physical therapy following discharge. A thorough feeding evaluation is recommended with possible feeding tube placement, as he is showing signs/symptoms of aspiration. A new wheelchair and seating system evaluation is to be completed. H.M.'s parents were also provided an initial home exercise program for safe positioning, daily stretching, and mobilization. The social work department was contacted to address possible psychosocial and coping needs.

REFERENCES

Ashraf, E. A., & Wong, B. L. (2005). The diagnosis of muscular dystrophy. *The Pediatric Annals, 34,* 525–528.

Biggar, W. D. (2006). Duchenne muscular dystrophy. *Pediatrics in Review, 27,* 83–88.

Bonnemann, C. G. (2005). Limb girdle muscular dystrophy in childhood. *The Pediatric Annals, 34,* 569–577.

Bostrom, K., & Ahlstrom, G. (2005). Living with a hereditary disease: persons with muscular dystrophy and their next of kin. *American Journal of Medical Genetics, 136A,* 17–24.

Brown, S., Piercy, R., Muntoni, F., & Sewry, C. (2008). Investigating the pathology of Emery-Dreifuss muscular dystrophy. *Biochemical Society, 36,* 1335–1338.

Cardamone, M., Darras, B., & Ryan, M. (2008). Inherited myopathies and muscular dystrophies. *Seminars in Neurology, 28,* 250–259.

Chen, Jih-Yuan. (2008). Mediators affecting family function in families of children with Duchenne muscular dystrophy. *Kaohsiung Journal of Medical Science, 24,* 514–521.

Diseases. (2011). *Welcome to MDA, helping Jerry's kids.* Retrieved January 5, 2010, from http://www.mda.org

Donders, J., & Taneja, C. (2009). Neurobehavioral characteristics of children with Duchenne muscular dystrophy. *Child Neuropsychology, 15,* 295–304.

Emery, Alan E. H. (2001). *The muscular dystrophies.* New York, NY: Oxford University Press.

Emery, Alan E. H. (1994). *Muscular dystrophy: the facts.* New York, NY: Oxford University Press.

Gayathri, N., Taly, A. B., Sinha, S., Suresh, T. G., & Gorai, D. (2006). Emery Dreifuss muscular dystrophy: a clinico-pathological study. *Neurology India, 54,* 197–199.

Iosa, M., Mazza, C., Frusciante, R., Zok, M., Aprile, I., Ricci, E., et al. (2007). Mobility assessment of patients with fascioscapulohumeral dystrophy. *Journal of Clinical Biomechanics, 22,* 1074–1082.

Kohler, M., Clarenbach, C. F., Bahler, C., Brack, T., Russi, E. W., & Bloch, K. E. (2009). Disability and survival in Duchenne muscular dystrophy. *Journal of Neurology, Neurosurgery, and Psychology, 80,* 320–325.

McNally, E. M., & Pytel, P. (2007). Muscle diseases: the muscular dystrophies. *The Annual Review of Pathology: Mechanisms of Disease, 2,* 87–109.

Padberg, G.W., & van Engelen, B. G. M. (2009). Fascioscapulohumeral muscular dystrophy. *Current Opinion in Neurology, 22,* 539–542.

Poysky, J., & Kinnett, K. (2008). Facilitating family adjustment to a diagnosis of Duchenne muscular dystrophy. *Neuromuscular Disorders, 19,* 733–738.

Stockley, T., Akber, S., Bulgin, N., & Ray, P. (2006). Strategy for comprehensive molecular testing for Duchenne and Becker muscular dystrophies. *Genetic Testing, 10,* 229–243.

Thompson, C. E. (1999). *Raising a child with a neuromuscular disorder. A guide for parents, grandparents, friends, and professionals.* New York, NY: Oxford University Press.

Van der Maarel, S. M., Frants, R. R., & Padberg, G. (2007). Facioscapulohumeral muscular dystrophy. *Biochimica et Biophysica Acta, 1772,* 186–194.

Wohlgemuth, M., de Swart, B. J. M., Kalf, J. G., Joosten, F. B. M., Van der Vliet, A. M., & Padberg, G. W. (2006). Dysphagia in fascioscapulohumeral muscular dystrophy. *Neurology, 66,* 1926–1928.

Wren, T. A. L., Blumi, S., Tseng-Ong, L., & Gilsanz, V. (2007). Three-point technique of fat quantification of muscle tissue as a marker of disease progression in Duchenne muscular dystrophy: preliminary study. *American Journal of Radiology, 190,* W8–W12.

Yazdanpanah, P., Javan, A., Nadimi, B., & Ghaffarain Shirazi, H. R. (2007). Genetic pattern of 3 cases of Emery-Dreifuss muscular dystrophy in a family. *Eastern Mediterranean Health Journal, 13,* 201–205.

Glossary

Activity demands: The aspects of the task that influence the performance by the person. These demands include the objects used and their properties, space demands, social demands, sequencing and timing, required actions, required body functions, and required body structures.

Affect: Observable facial expressions of a feeling or emotion. Patients may be described as having a flat or blunt affect.

Affective and physiologic dysregulation: Behaviors include difficulty with arousal regulation and modulation and toleration and recovery from extreme affective states such as fear, anger, and shame that emerge from chronic trauma exposure, manifested by prolonged and extreme emotional tantrums on one side of the spectrum to catatonic-like immobilization.

Age-related macular degeneration (AMD): A low vision disorder that results from loss of function of the macula, which is the center of the retina. There are two types of AMD including dry AMD (atrophic) and wet AMD (neovascular/exudative). Dry AMD is atrophy of the macula and wet AMD is an ingrowth of new blood vessels that bleed into the subretinal space.

Agnosia: Inability to recognize the import of sensory impressions despite being able to recognize the elemental sensation of the stimulus. Language deficits must be absent for this diagnosis. Various agnosias correspond to several senses and may be distinguished as auditory, gustatory, olfactory, tactile, and visual. Specific sensory agnosias can occur when the connections are disrupted between the primary cortical receptor region for a stimulus and the memory of prior stimuli. For example, the inability to recognize familiar objects by sight or touch.

Agoraphobia: "A mental disorder characterized by an irrational fear of leaving the familiar setting of home, or venturing into the open; often associated with panic attacks." Commonly referred to as fear of the marketplace.

Alexithymia: The impaired capacity to describe emotions or bodily states; is a persistent sign of affective dysregulation.

Algorithms: A step-by-step approach to treatment based upon controlled clinical trials.

Allograft: An allograft (also referred to as a *homograft* or *cadaver skin*) is donor skin taken from another person.

Alogia: Absence of speech because of mental illness

Altruism: The unselfish concern for the welfare of others. This concept is reflected in actions and attitudes of commitment, caring, dedication, responsiveness, and understanding.

Alveoli: Small sacs in the lungs which perform the gas exchange. Oxygen is moved into the blood stream from the alveoli to be carried to cells throughout the body

Ambiguous hand preference: Absence of a dominant hand preference; the switching of hands within the same activity.

Aminobutyric acid (GABA): "A constituent of the central nervous system; quantitatively the principal inhibitory neurotransmitter."

Amotivation: Lacking in motivation.

Amygdala: A structure that is part of the limbic system and is involved in the emotions of aggression and fear.

Amyloid plaques: Insoluble shards of amyloid that stick to dead and dying neurons.

Amyloid precursor protein (APP): A benign substance that lives in various parts of the body, including the brain, and whose role in cellular function is unknown.

Amyotrophic lateral sclerosis (ALS): A progressive neurological disorder characterized by degeneration of motor neurons located in the ventral horn of the spinal cord.

Analgesic: A pain medication.

Anemia: Decrease in the number of red blood cells (RBC) or less than the normal quantity of hemoglobin in the blood

Aneurysm: Localized abnormal dilatation of the wall of a blood vessel, usually an artery, or in the heart, resulting in the formation of a sac. Usual causes are the weakness of the vessel wall, resulting from atherosclerosis, or a congenital defect. However, any injury to the middle or muscular layer of the arterial wall can predispose the stretching of the vessel wall.

Angioplasty: is a procedure where a small mesh tube is inserted into the coronary artery to widen the opening, thus increasing the blood flow.

Angle-closure glaucoma: The obstruction by the iris to the outflow pathway of aqueous humor at the angle between the peripheral cornea and the iris aqueous humor.

Anhedonia: A lack of interest in previously pleasurable activities.

Anhedonia: Reduced ability or inability to experience pleasure.

Ankylosis: the fusion of a joint, often in an abnormal position, usually resulting from destruction of articular cartilage and subchondral bone, as occurs in rheumatoid arthritis.

Anomia: Inability to name objects.

Anterograde amnesia: The inability to learn new long-term declarative information.

Antibodies: A specialized immune protein produced because of the introduction of an antigen into the body. The production of antibodies is a major function of the immune system.

Anticholinergic side effects: Most commonly dry mouth or constipation.

Antigen: A microorganism that is a uniquely configured protein that attaches to the pathogen and stimulates the body's production of antibodies.

Antipsychotic medications: Medications designed to reduce positive and negative symptoms.

Anxiety: "Apprehension of danger, and dread accompanied by restlessness, tension, tachycardia, and dyspnea unattached to a clearly identifiable stimulus."

Anxiolytic: A sedative or mild tranquilizer used to treat anxiety or alcohol withdrawal.

Apathy: An absence or suppression of emotion, feeling, or concern.

Aphasia: Difficulty with expressive and/or receptive language.

Apophyseal: Refers to the articulations between the articular facets of adjacent vertebrae, or facet joints. These joints are a frequent site of degenerative joint disease, or osteoarthritis, spondylitic and traumatic diseases.

Apraxia: Loss of skilled purposeful movement that cannot be attributed either to deficits in primary motor skills or problems in comprehension. It can affect ideation and concept formation as well as programming and planning of movement.

Arthroplasty: Joint replacement.

Arteriovenous: Referring both to an artery and a vein. An arteriovenous malformation, or AVM, is a congenital malformation characterized by an abnormal collection of blood vessels near the surface of the brain. AVM can lead to subarachnoid hemorrhage.

Asperger's disorder: A neurobiologic disorder of unknown etiology in which cognitive and communication skills develop normally or nearly normally during the first few years of life. However, social impairment is evident, repetitive and stereotypical behaviors are observed, and communication, though not delayed, is marked by unusual topics of interest and rigidity.

Aspiration: Pathological inhalation of food or mucus into the respiratory tract.

Associated reactions: Involuntary movements or reflexive increases in tone on the affected side of individuals with hemiplegia. These movements replicate synergy patterns and often appear when the individual is trying new or stressful activities, for example, a resisted grasp by the noninvolved hand causes a grasp reaction in the involved hand.

Associality: A negative symptom characterized by decreased interest in socialization and maintenance of relationships.

Astereognosis: Inability to recognize objects by touch (also called tactile agnosia; see Agnosia).

Asterixis: A hand-flapping tremor.

Ataxia: Inability to coordinate muscle activity during voluntary movement. In posterior column damage of the spinal cord, incoordination and a loss of proprioception is caused by misjudgment of limb position with balance problems. Cerebellar ataxia produces a reeling, wide-based gait.

Attentional and behavioral dysregulation: Signs and symptoms include impairment in those competencies related to sustained attention, learning, or coping with stress. An inability to sustain goal-directed behavior may include a lack of curiosity, difficulties with planning or completing tasks, or avolition.

Athetoid (dyskinetic): Resembling athetosis or repetitive involuntary, slow, sinuous, writhing movements. Classification of cerebral palsy in which involuntary purposeless movement occurs when an individual attempts purposeful motion. The abnormal movements may not only occur in the limb being moved but also involve an "overflow" of activity to all the other limbs with an exaggeration of reflexes.

Atherosclerosis: A widespread form of arteriosclerosis in which deposits of plaques (atheromas) containing cholesterol and other lipid material are formed within the inner layer (intima) of large- and medium-sized arteries.

Atheromas: An abnormal mass of fatty or lipid material with a fibrous covering, which forms a discrete raised plaque within the inner layer (intima) of an artery.

Arthritis: Inflammation or infection of a joint.

Atrophy: A wasting of tissue that results in decreased muscle mass.

Auditory processing: The process of the brain recognizing and interpreting sounds in the environment. This process is responsible for the comprehension of language.

Autistic disorder: A neurobiologic disorder with an unknown etiology, characterized by significant delay or deviation in social interaction, communication, and repetitive or stereotyped behaviors.

Autograft: The surgical transplantation of the patient's own skin from one area to another.

Autonomic dysreflexia (hyperreflexia): An uninhibited and exaggerated reflex of the autonomic nervous system to stimulation. The response occurs in about 85% of all patients who have spinal cord injury above the level of the 6th thoracic vertebra. It is potentially dangerous because of attendant vasoconstriction and immediate elevation of blood pressure, which in turn can bring about hemorrhagic retinal damage or cerebrovascular accident. Less serious effects include severe headache, changes in heart rate, sweating and flushing above the level of the spinal cord injury, and pallor and goose bumps below that level.

Autonomic neuropathy: A form of peripheral neuropathy. A group of symptoms that occur when there is damage to the nerves that manage every day body functions such as blood pressure, heart rate, bowel and bladder emptying, and digestion.

Autosomal dominant: A disease that occurs when a child inherits a normal gene from one parent and an affected gene from the other parent.

Autosomal recessive: A disease that occurs when both parents carry and pass on the affected gene.

Babinski's reflex: Dorsiflexion (extension) of the great toe and outspreading of the outer toes when the sole of the foot is stroked. Normally present in infants under the age of 6 months, in adults this reflex occurs in lesions of the pyramidal tract.

Benign tumor: Noncancerous, which do not invade other body tissues or spread to other body parts. However, may become life threatening as they cause increasing deficits with cell growth, because they press upon nearby structures and tissues.

Beta-amyloid plaques: An accumulation of amyloid precursor proteins that have not been correctly broken down in the body.

Boutonniere deformity: A common hand deformity secondary to the pathologic effects of rheumatoid arthritis resulting in a combination of PIP joint flexion and DIP joint hyperextension

Bradykinesia: Slowness of all voluntary movement and speech.

Brain attack: Synonym for stroke, or cerebrovascular accident.

Brainstem: connects the cerebrum with the spinal cord and includes the midbrain, medulla oblongata, and the pons. Motor and sensory neurons travel via the brainstem which allows for communication between brain and spinal cord. The brainstem also controls life-supporting autonomic functions of the peripheral nervous system.

Bronchopulmonary dysplasia: A chronic lung disease of babies, which most commonly develops in the first 4 weeks after birth and most often affects babies born at least 4 weeks before term.

Burden of disease: A situation in which a group experiences an illness to a greater degree than other subgroups.

Burn scar contracture: Forms due to the shortening and tightening of the burn scar. Burn scar contracture deformities are the most problematic over large joints.

Bursitis: Inflammation of the fluid-filled sac (bursa) that lies between a tendon and skin, or between a tendon and bone.

Carotid endarterectomy: Excision of thickened atheromatous areas of the innermost layer of an artery (intima) to improve circulation.

Carpal tunnel syndrome: Resulting from compression on the volar aspect of the wrist, which then impinge upon the median nerve. This causes paresthesia of the palmar aspect of the thumb, the second and third digits, and the radial aspect of the fourth digit.

Casein: A protein found in cow's milk. A theory in the field of autism suggests that children with autism do not digest this protein appropriately, leading to a buildup of morphine-like substances in the body and causing social withdrawal and abnormal behaviors.

Cataracts: Opacifications of the crystalline lens of the eye, which result in a decreased amount of light reaching the retina.

Catatonia: Extreme psychomotor agitation or retardation.

Catatonic behavior: Loss of responsiveness to environmental cues. A person with catatonic behavior may assume rigid or bizarre postures and resist attempts made to move or reposition him or her. Excessive, nonpurposeful motor activity may also be observed. In extreme cases, the individual appears to be completely unresponsive, as in a catatonic stupor.

Catheterization: Passage of a catheter into a body channel or cavity, especially introduction of a catheter via the urethra into the urinary bladder.

Cauda equina: The collection of dorsal and ventral nerve roots descending from the lower spinal cord and occupying the vertebral canal below the cord at the L1 region.

Central scotomas: Diminished vision or visual loss in the center of the visual field.

Central vision: Sharp, foveal vision used for reading, watching television, driving or any activity for which visual detail is of primary importance.

Cerebellum: A region of the brain that is found at the rear of the head and is above the brainstem. It has been traditionally known for its role in the coordination of movement, but recent research suggests the cerebellum may also have a role in cognitive, sensory, language, and abstract-thinking skills.

Cerebrovascular accident (CVA, stroke, brain attack): Disorder of the blood vessels serving the brain, resulting in disruption of blood flow to parts of the brain leading to neuronal death. Impact of CVA varies according to the cause of the disruption (blockages or hemorrhages) and location of the insult, as well as a variety of premorbid and psychosocial conditions.

Cerebrospinal fluid assays: A diagnostic tool that measures biomarkers in cerebrospinal fluid.

Charcot-Marie-Tooth (CMT): An inherited neurological disorder that results in motor and sensory peripheral neuropathy.

Childhood disintegrative disorder: A rare neurobiologic disorder that develops in children who had appeared completely normal during their first few years of life. Following its onset, language, social interaction, and self-care skills are lost and autistic-like symptoms appear.

Chronic bronchitis: Inflammation of the bronchial tubes resulting in a thickening of the walls, making it difficult to breathe.

Chronic obstructive pulmonary disease (COPD): A term that includes chronic bronchitis, asthma, emphysema, and bronchiectasis. The condition is irreversible and characterized by progressive limitation in the flow of air in and out of the lungs.

Cilia: Hair-like structures in the lungs airways that help to move the mucus out and clean the airways.

Circumlocution: The use of pantomime, nonverbal communication, or word substitution to avoid revealing an inability to say or remember a word.

Client factors: The body functions and the body structures that reside within the person.

Clonus: Alternate involuntary muscular contraction and relaxation in rapid succession.

Closed fracture: Refers to a fracture that has not broken through the skin.

Cogwheel rigidity: Stiff movement in one direction in small evenly spaced segments. The tension in muscle gives way in little jerks when the muscle is passively stretched.

Collagen: A basic structural fibrous protein found in all tissue. Excessive deposition of tissue collagen leads to a thickening of the burn scar.

Collateral circulation: Secondary circulation that continues to an area of the brain following obstruction of a primary blood vessel and may prevent major ischemia.

Colles' fracture: Fracture resulting in dorsal displacement, dorsal comminuting, and radius shortening; often referred to as a dinner fork deformity given its resemblance to an upside down fork.

Coma: A nonsleep loss of consciousness associated with unresponsiveness to touch, pain, sound, or movement that lasts for an extended period.

Complex regional pain syndrome (CRPD): Also referred to as reflex sympathetic dystrophy (RSD) is a chronic pain condition in which high levels of nerve impulses are sent to an affected site.

Comminuted fracture: A fracture in which a bone in broken, splintered, or crushed into a number of pieces.

Compensation: The use of one system or muscle group to complete the work not capable of being completed by the usual system.

Compound fracture: Also referred to as an open fracture as the fractured bone breaks through the skin surface and are more prone to infection.

Compression garment: Compression garments are the preferred conservative method to treat hypertrophic scars and have been in use since the early 1970s. Compression garments are thought to reduce oxygen flow to the scar thereby decreasing collagen production.

Compulsion: "Uncontrollable impulses to perform an act, often repetitively, as an unconscious mechanism to avoid unacceptable ideas and desires which, by themselves, arouse anxiety; the anxiety becomes fully manifest if performance of the compulsive act is prevented; may be associated with obsessive thoughts."

Concrete thinking: Literal interpretation of words without understanding abstract meanings.

Congenital: A condition existing before birth, at birth, or that develops during the first month of life.

Congestive heart failure: The inability of the heart to function as a pump, which results in a decreased blood flow to the tissues and congestion in the pulmonary and circulatory systems.

Constructional apraxia: Apraxia caused by loss of visuospatial skills; for example, difficulty drawing a clock face.

Contracture: Abnormal shortening of muscle tissue that renders the muscle highly resistant to stretching, which can lead to permanent disability. In many cases, contractures can be prevented by range of motion (ROM) exercises (active or passive) and by adequate support of the joints to eliminate constant shortening or stretching of the muscles and surrounding tissue.

Context: The conditions that surround the person. Those conditions include cultural, physical, social, personal, spiritual, temporal, and virtual contexts.

Contrast sensitivity: The ability to visually discern the edges or luminance of an object to strike the skull at an opposite location (contrecoup).

Coronary artery bypass grafting (CABG): A process in which arteries or vein from other parts of the body (often the legs) are "harvested" and then surgically attached to bypass the blocked arteries near the heart.

Coronary artery disease: Tied very closely to atherosclerosis where plaque, made of cholesterol, fat, calcium, and other substances, sticks to the inner lining of arteries that are taking oxygen-rich blood from the heart to the body.

Cortical atrophy: Birth defect with a nongenetic origin that can contribute to or cause ID due to shrinkage of the posterior part of the brain.

Corticobulbar: Refers to the pathway connecting the cerebral cortex to the brainstem. Bulbar refers to the nerves and tracts connected to the medulla; muscles innervated include those of the tongue, pharynx, and larynx.

Corticospinal: Also referred to as the pyramidal tracts; are descending tracts which conduct motor impulses from the brain to the spinal cord.

Corticosteroids: A class of steroids that are produced in the adrenal cortex. Synthetic versions are produced to closely resemble these steroids and are used for medicinal purposes.

Coup-contrecoup injury: Situation in which direct brain damage is incurred in traumatic event as the cerebrum rotates on the more stable brainstem while accelerating from the force of impact. The cerebrum strikes the skull (coup), and then accelerates in the opposite direction.

Craniostenosis: Birth defect with a nongenetic origin that can contribute to or cause ID due to premature fusion of the skull resulting in a reduction in space for the brain to grow and in increased intracranial pressure.

Creatine kinase: An enzyme expressed by various tissues and cells in the body.

Credé's method: Use of manual pressure on the bladder to express urine, particularly in bladder training for individuals with paralysis. The hands are held flat against the abdomen, just below the umbilicus. A firm downward stroke toward the bladder is repeated six or seven times, followed by pressure from both hands placed directly over the bladder to manually remove all urine.

Cyclothymia: Characterized by a chronic course of hypomania and mild depression, this disorder presents as a mild form of bipolar disorder (BPD).

Cytomegalovirus: A herpesvirus that can result in a congenital infection.

Debridement: The cleansing and removal of nonadherent and nonviable tissue.

Decerebrate rigidity: An extensor posture of all limbs and/or the trunk.

Decorticate rigidity: Flexion of the upper, but extension of the lower, limbs.

Decubitus ulcers: An ulcer caused by local interference with the circulation, usually occurring over a bony prominence at the sacrum, hip (trochanter), heel, shoulder, or elbow. It begins as a reddened area and can quickly involve deeper structures and become an ulcer, also called a bedsore or a pressure sore.

Decussation: An X-shaped crossing, especially of nerves or bands of nerve fibers, connecting parts on opposite sides of the brain or spinal cord.

Deep vein thrombosis (DVT): A thrombosis, commonly seen in the legs or pelvis, that results from phlebitis, vein injury, or prolonged bed rest.

Deformity: Distortion of any part or general disfigurement of the body.

Delayed union: A delayed union is when the bone takes more time to heal than is expected; it heals slowly. It may be suspected when pain and tenderness persist at the fracture site 3 months to 1 year after the injury.

Delusions: Atypical and well-organized beliefs not explained by evidence or culture.

Delusions of grandeur: Self-inflated views usually present in conversation.

Delusions of persecution: Individuals have consistent and organized beliefs about other people intending to harm them.

Demyelination: Destruction, removal, or loss of the myelin sheath of a nerve or nerves.

De Quervain's disease: Pathologic process that involves extensors at the thumb, causes severe pain and discomfort, resulting in a decrease in hand function and the ability to grip.

Developmental trauma disorder: Describes clinically significant patterns of behavior or syndromes that occur in an individual as a result of persistent and chronic exposure to violent episodes including physical, sexual, and emotional abuse resulting in functional impairment in one or more important areas.

Diabetic foot: A person who has diabetes is at increased risk for slow-healing injuries to distal extremities. It is caused by decreased vascularization; the risk of an infection that does not heal is higher. One possible intervention is limb amputation.

Diabetic ketoacidosis: State of medical emergency; life-threatening condition caused by a state of relative insulin deficiency, characterized by hyperglycemia, ketonemia, metabolic acidosis, and electrolyte depletion. Often the first presenting sign of type 1 diabetes.

Diarthroses: are the most mobile joints and are by far the most common articular pattern. Because these joints possess a synovial membrane and contain synovial fluid, these joints are more commonly referred to as synovial joints.

Diastolic blood pressure: The pressure in the arteries when the heart is at rest.

Dignity: The importance of valuing the inherent worth and uniqueness of each person. This value is demonstrated by an attitude of empathy and respect for self and others.

Diplegia: Paralysis of like parts on either side of the body. In cerebral palsy, diplegia describes involvement of the lower extremities predominantly, with only mildly affected upper extremities.

Diffusion-tensor imaging: A diagnostic tool that uses MRI methods to produce images of the structure and organization of the connections throughout the central nervous system.

Disease surveillance: An epidemiological practice by which the spread of disease is monitored in order to establish patterns of progression.

Disease trajectory: Patterns of progression and functional decline that result from a condition.

Disinhibition: Loss of inhibition, or the cultural and social sense of self restraint.

Disorganized behavior: Unpredictable, socially inappropriate behaviors that interfere with daily activities. Examples include agitated or angry outbursts with no known provocation; sexually acting out in public, that is, masturbation; and difficulties performing goal-directed tasks such as meal preparation or grooming.

Disorganized thinking: Thought processes that lack cohesive patterns. Speech, which can provide clues about disorganized thought processes, may include any of the following: loose associations (answers that begin to veer "off track" of the original questions), tangential (unrelated comments or answers) or incoherent (a mixture of words often referred to as a "word salad").

Dissociation: is essentially an "out-of-body experience" in which the person detaches from an event that is overwhelmingly stressful.

Distal radius fracture: Common fracture of the radius. Due to its proximity to the wrist joint, often referred to as a wrist fracture.

Dopamine: A neurotransmitter that helps regulate movement and emotional responses; a deficiency results in Parkinson's disease.

Down syndrome: A chromosomal condition caused by the presence or all or part of an extra 21st chromosome.

Dysarthria: Imperfect articulation of speech caused by disturbances of muscular control resulting from central or peripheral nervous system damage.

Dysesthesia: Impairment of any sense, especially of the sense of touch; a painful, persistent sensation induced by a gentle touch of the skin.

Dysgraphia: Inability to write a sentence.

Dysosmic aphasia: Difficulty naming objects.

Dysphagia: Difficulty in swallowing, which may range from mild discomfort to a seriously compromised ability to control the muscles needed for chewing and swallowing. Dysphagia may seriously interfere with a patient's nutritional status. Interventions, such as positioning the patient during feeding and use of foods of the proper consistency, are widely used.

Dysphoria: A mood disturbance resulting in a depressed mood.

Dyspnea: Difficult, labored, or painful breathing.

Dysthymia: Unlike individuals with depressive disorders, people with dysthymia report that they have always been depressed. Characterized by insidious onset frequently beginning in childhood, a persistent or intermittent course, and ongoing feelings of depression over a period of at least 2 years.

Dystophin: A protein that connects the cytoskeleton of a muscle fiber to the surrounding extracellular matrix through the cell membrane.

It is responsible for maintaining the shape and structure of the muscle fiber.

Ecchymosis: Skin discoloration caused by escape of blood into the tissues from ruptured blood vessels.

Echolalia: The automatic and meaningless repetition of another's words or phrases. In autism, this repetition may be either immediate or delayed, and often does not appear appropriate to the conversation or activity.

Electroconvulsive therapy: The induction of a brief seizure by passing electric current through the brain. This treatment is used mostly for depression.

Electroencephalogram: The record obtained during the amplification, recording, and subsequent analysis of the electrical activity of the brain using an instrument called an electroencephalograph.

Electromyography (EMG): A diagnostic tool used for testing the electrical activity of muscles.

Embolism: Sudden blockage of an artery by a moving clot of foreign material (embolus) lodged in place by the blood current. Emboli usually lodge at divisions of an artery, where the blood vessel narrows, and are typically blood clots. However, they may also be formed from globules of fat, air bubbles, pieces of tissue, or clumps of bacteria.

Emotional lability: Inability to regulate emotions appropriately, typically resulting in laughing or crying in unsuitable contexts.

Emphysema: The destruction of the walls of the bronchioles and alveoli, which results in abnormal and enlarged air spaces.

Epidemiology: A scientific discipline devoted to studying the patterns of communicable diseases.

Epiglottis: A thin flap of tissue in the esophagus that protects the lungs from foreign objects by covering the trachea during swallowing.

Epstein-Barr virus (EBV): A virus causing infection and is characterized by fatigue and general malaise. Infection with EBV is fairly common and is usually a transient and minor thing. However, in some individuals EBV can trigger chronic illness. It is a particular danger to people with compromised immune systems.

Equality: The value that all individuals are perceived as having the same fundamental human rights and opportunities. This value is demonstrated by an attitude of fairness and impartiality.

Equinovalgus: Deformity in which the foot is plantar flexed, everted, and abducted.

Equinovarus: Deformity in which the foot is planter flexed, inverted and adducted.

Eschar: The residual necrotic layers of skin destroyed by direct heat damage or the injury occurring secondary to heat damage.

Euphoria: A feeling or state of well-being or elation.

Euthymia: Normal range of mood.

Executive functioning: A broad band of skills that allow an individual to engage in independent, self-directed behavior. Includes volition, planning, purposeful action, and self-awareness. Executive functions involve the ability to formulate context-appropriate goals and to initiate, plan and organize, and sequence and adapt behavior based on anticipated or actual consequences of actions.

Extrapyramidal symptoms: Involuntary movement, changes in muscle tone, and abnormal posture.

Extrapyramidal syndrome: A side effect from medication that results in abnormal movements similar to Parkinson's disease.

Familial: A disease for which there is a family history.

Fixed ideas: An individual holds an unchangeable idea.

Flaccidity: Abnormally low muscle tone, which is felt as too little resistance to movement. Also known as hypotonus.

Flight of ideas: Accelerated speech with rapid changes in subject. Associations are understandable unlike the lack of connections that are associated with looseness of associations.

Fluid resuscitation: Medical practice of replenishing bodily fluid lost through sweating, bleeding, fluid shifts, or other pathologic processes.

Fragile X syndrome: is a genetic cause of ID that results from a mutation at what is known as the fragile site on the X chromosome.

Freedom: The value of allowing each individual the right to exercise choice and to demonstrate independence, initiative, and self-direction.

Frontal lobes: Region of the brain located at the front of the cerebrum. This region is responsible for social behavior, spontaneous production of language, initiation of motor activity, processing sensory stimuli and then planning reaction as a result of the input, abstract thinking, problem solving, and judgment.

Full thickness burn: Burn injury that destroys the entire epidermal and dermal layers of the skin and extends down into subcutaneous fat.

Gastrointestinal disorder: A disorder of the digestive system.

Gastroesophageal reflux: Caused by stomach acid coming up from the stomach into the esophagus. A typical symptom is heartburn.

Gaze shift: Sharing attention with another person by alternating gaze between an object and a person or following the gaze of.

Genes: A region of DNA that carries the genetic instructions for a cell.

Generalized anxiety disorder: Chronic, repeated episodes of anxiety or dread accompanied by autonomic changes.

Genotype: Genetic makeup of a living organism.

Glare sensitivity: Visual problem in which the person has difficulty discerning images in high light.

Gluten: A protein found in wheat products. A theory in the field of autism suggests that children with autism do not digest this protein appropriately, leading to a buildup of morphine-like substances in the body and causing social withdrawal and abnormal behaviors.

Gower's maneuver: The inability to rise off the floor without using the upper extremities to "walk up" the thighs to assist with hip extension.

Gower's sign: When a person is observed to use his or her upper extremities to "walk up" the thighs to assist with hip extension, it is a positive Gower's sign.

Grandiosity: An inflated sense of self-esteem or importance.

Graphesthesia: The ability by which outlines, numbers, words, or symbols traced or written on the skin are recognized.

Greenstick fracture: Often seen in children whose bones are still soft and growing. Rather than snapping into two, the bone breaks on one side and bends on the other. It is similar to how a young twig or tree limb breaks, thus the name greenstick fracture.

Hallucinations: Disorders of perception. Atypical auditory, visual, and/or olfactory sensory perceptions.

Health disparity: A situation in which a given population or group sharing a constellation of characteristics manifests lower health status and poorer health outcomes proportionate to the population as a whole.

Herd immunity: A phenomenon in which critical masses of people (or other animal species) are rendered immune to a communicable disease and the rampant spread of infection is curtailed.

Hematoma: A localized collection of extravasated blood, usually clotted, in an organ, space, or tissue. Familiar, typically benign forms of hematoma include contusions (bruises) and black eyes. Hematomas can occur almost anywhere in the body and are especially serious when they occur inside the skull, where they may produce pressure on the brain. The most common types affecting the brain are epidural (above the dura mater, between it and the skull) and subdural (beneath the dura mater, between the touch casing and the more delicate membranes covering the tissue of the brain, the pia-arachnoid).

Hemianopsia: Defective vision or blindness in one half of the visual field, usually referring to bilateral defects resulting from a single lesion, often as the result of a cerebrovascular accident (CVA). The individual is unable to perceive objects to the side of the visual midline. Visual loss is contralateral; that is, it is on the side opposite the brain lesion.

Hemiparesis: Paresis or weakness affecting one side of the body.

Hemiplegia: Paralysis of one side of the body, usually caused by a brain lesion, such as a tumor, or a cerebrovascular accident. Paralysis occurs on the side opposite the lesion, or infarct, because of decussation of most of the fibers in the motor tracts of the brain. For example, damage to the right hemisphere of the brain affects motor control of the left half of the body.

Hemoglobin A1c level: The average concentration of glucose in the blood over a 6-week to 3-month time period, with levels ≥6.5% diagnostic of diabetes.

Hemorrhagic stroke: A type of stroke resulting from blood that has escaped the normal vessels and entered brain tissue or the subarachnoid space. Intracerebral hemorrhage is a type of hemorrhagic stroke that occurs when blood leaking from a cerebral vessel directly enters the brain tissue.

Heterotopic ossification: The formation of bone in soft tissue and periarticular locations. Early clinical signs include warmth, swelling, pain, and decreased joint motion. Common joints for heterotopic ossification are the shoulder, elbow, hip, and knee.

Hippocampus: A structure that is part of the limbic system and is involved in long-term memory functions.

Homonymous hemianopsia: Loss of one half of the visual field, on the same side, in both eyes.

Human immunodeficiency virus (HIV): A retrovirus that causes acquired immunodeficiency syndrome (AIDS), a condition in humans in which progressive failure of the immune system allows life-threatening opportunistic infections and cancers to thrive.

Humeral fracture: A fracture that results in humeral displacement and malposition of the distal limb

Hydrocephalus: The abnormal accumulation of cerebrospinal fluid (CSF) in the brain.

Hydrocephaly: Birth defect with a nongenetic origin that can contribute to or cause ID due to an abnormal accumulation of cerebrospinal fluid in the ventricles of the brain causing increased intracranial pressure and progressive enlargement of the skull.

Hyperflexia: Overflexion of a limb.

Hyperglycemia: An abnormally high concentration of glucose (115 to 139 mg/dL) in the circulating blood, especially with reference to a fasting level.

Hyperlexia: The ability to read words above age-level expectation. Usually, children with this ability have difficulty understanding the meaning of the words they read.

Hyperphenylalaninemia: An environmental factor in the etiology of ID that is the result of the maternal condition in which the presence of blood phenylalanine levels exceed the limits of the upper reference range (2 mg/dL).

Hyperorality: Excessive overeating.

Hypersexuality: Disinhibition in regard to sexual impulses.

Hypertension: Persistent blood pressure measurements above the normal systolic (140 mm Hg) or diastolic (90 mm Hg) pressures.

Hypertonicity (spasticity): Abnormal muscle tone felt as too much resistance to movement as a result of hyperactive reflexes and loss of inhibiting influences from higher brain centers.

Hypertrophic scar: A cutaneous condition characterized by excess scar tissue, Hypertrophic scars occur when the body overproduces collagen, which causes the scar to be raised above the surrounding skin; these scars take the form of a red raised lump on the skin.

Hypervigilance: Autonomic and endocrine hyperarousal which are observed overreactions to stimuli. This may include being easily startled, craving high-risk, stimulating, or dangerous activity; all of which impair the balance of play, work, and rest.

Hypoglycemia: An abnormally small concentration of glucose in the circulating blood, that is, 50 mg/dL in men and <45 mg/dL in women.

Hypomania: An episode of manic symptoms that are not severe enough to meet the criteria for mania listed in *DSM IV-TR*.

Hypotonicity: Reduced tone; noted by minimal resistance to passive movement.

Hypoxemia: Insufficient oxygenation of the blood.

Hypoxia: A pathological condition that results in insufficient oxygenation of the blood.

Ideas of reference: Individuals believe that others are talking about or referring to them.

Immune response: A person's defense or resistance against infection.

Incentive spirometry: A machine that measures the amount (volume) of air inhaled. This machine is used to validate chronic obstructive pulmonary disease (COPD) as a diagnosis.

Incidence: A measure of the risk of developing a new condition within a specified period of time. It is usually expressed as a proportion or a rate.

Infectious diseases: A group of conditions that are characterized by a set of symptoms attributable to the introduction of a specific pathogen.

Inferior olive: Region of the brainstem that transmits error signals to the cerebellum.

Inflammation: The initial response of the body to harmful stimuli and is achieved by the increased movement of plasma and leukocytes from the blood into the injured tissues. A cascade of biochemical events propagates and matures the inflammatory response, involving the local vascular and immune system.

Inoculum dose: The amount of pathogen necessary to produce an infection.

Intraocular pressure (IOP): The fluid pressure of the aqueous humor inside the eye.

Ischemia: Deficiency of blood resulting from the functional constriction or actual obstruction of a blood vessel, often leading to the death (necrosis) of the surrounding tissue.

Joint attention: The ability to use eye contact and gestures in order to share experiences with others.

Justice: The value of upholding of such moral and legal principles as fairness, equity, truthfulness, and objectivity.

Juvenile rheumatoid arthritis: The most common rheumatic disease in childhood. The diagnostic criteria for JRA are onset at age younger than 16 years, persistent arthritis in one or more joints for at least 6 weeks, and exclusion of other types of childhood arthritis.

Kernicterus: A form of hemolytic jaundice of the newborn. The basal ganglia and other areas of the brain and spinal cord are infiltrated with bilirubin, a yellow-pigmented substance produced by the breakdown of hemoglobin. Develops during the 2nd to 8th day of life.

Ketonuria: Condition in which ketone bodies are present. Ketones are waste products from the body's breakdown of fat for energy.

Kinesthesia: The ability and sense by which position, weight, and movement are perceived.

Kyphosis: Abnormally increased convexity in the curvature of the thoracic spine viewed from the side, resulting from an acquired disease, an injury, or a congenital disorder or disease.

Lability: Rapidly shifting or changing emotions.

Latent tuberculosis: TB that exists in a dormant state.

Limbic system: This group of subcortical structures is involved in various emotions and memory functions.

Long-term memory: The ability to recall information for long periods of time without effort.

Lordosis: Forward curvature of the lumbar spine.

Lou Gehrig's disease: Common name for Amyotrophic Lateral Sclerosis (ALS) which is a fatal, progressive, degenerative motor neuron disease in which scars form on the neurons in the corticospinal pathways, the motor nuclei of the brainstem, and the anterior horn cells of the spinal cord.

Lower motor neuron: Injury to the ventral horn of the spinal cord results in lower motor neuron damage; sign include focal and multifocal weakness, atrophy, cramps, and muscle twitching as well as flaccid paralysis with loss of movement, tone, and reflex activity.

Macula: The visual structure at the center of the retina. It is responsible for the processing of the central vision.

Magnetic resonance imaging (MRI): A neuroimaging tool that uses radiology to visualize detailed internal structures.

Magnetic resonance spectroscopy: A diagnostic tool that measures the levels of different metabolites in body tissues.

Magnetic resonance volumetry: A diagnostic tool that measures the volume of the internal structures of the body.

Major depressive episode: A period of depressed or irritable mood lasting at least 2 weeks, resulting in severe impairments in functioning.

Malignant tumor: Composed of abnormal cells that multiply rapidly, with the ability to invade, or metastasize into other tissues.

Malunion: Refers to nonunion of a fractured bone.

Mania: An extremely elevated mood.

Manic episode: A highly elevated or irritable mood lasting at least 1 week, with or without psychotic symptoms such as delusions and hallucinations.

Melancholia: This term dates back to the 4th century and continues to be used in *DSM IV-TR*. Refers to the following signs: anhedonia, early morning awakening with depression worse in the morning, psychomotor agitation or retardation, weight loss, and feelings of guilt.

Mental disorders: *DSM IV-TR* characterizes a mental disorder as "a clinically significant behavioral or psychological syndrome or pattern that occurs in an individual and that is associated with present distress or disability or with significantly increased risk of suffering death, pain, disability, or an important loss of freedom."

Metabolic equivalent (MET): A MET is the amount of energy that an activity requires, with more sedentary tasks such as watching TV or doing computer work using 1.5 to 2 METS ranging up to some competitive sports requiring 11 or more METs.

Metamorphopsia: The visual distortion of objects.

Metastasis: is the spread of a disease from one organ or part to another nonadjacent organ or part.

Mild acquired TBI: Clinically identified as a loss of consciousness for <10 minutes or amnesia, a Glasgow Coma Scale (GCS) rating of 13 to 15, no skull fracture on physical examination, and a nonfocal neurological examination.

Mixed episode: The presence of both manic and major depressive symptoms almost daily for at least 1 week, resulting in rapid mood cycling with or without psychotic symptoms.

Moderate acquired TBI: Hospitalization of at least 48 hours, an initial GCS rating of 9 to 12 or higher.

Modified constraint-induced therapy: A treatment for hemiplegia characterized by restricted movement of the intact extremity to elicit movement of the involved extremity.

Morbidity: A diseased state, disability or poor health due to any cause.

Mortality: The condition of being susceptible to death. A mortality rate is a measure of the number of deaths in a given population.

MRSA: Methicillin-resistant Staphylococcus, a strain of staphylococcus that is resistant to customary antibiotics.

Muscle biopsy: A medical diagnostic tool used to examine the cellular makeup of the muscle tissue, and look at the differences in muscle fibers, fiber size, fiber splitting, and fiber necrosis.

Muscular dystrophy: A group of genetic conditions that results in progressive weakening of the muscles. Most types of MD are multisystem disorders that can affect the heart, gastrointestinal and nervous systems, endocrine glands, skin, eyes, and brain.

Mutism: Inability to speak.

Myelin: The lipid substance forming a sheath around the axons of certain nerve fibers, occurring predominantly in the cranial and spinal nerves that compose the white matter of the brain and spinal cord. The myelin sheath is formed by a glial cell, either an oligodendrocyte (in the central nervous system) or Schwann cell (in the peripheral nervous system).

Myelogram: A graphic representation of the differential count of cells found in a stained representation of bone marrow.

Myocardial infarction (MI): is caused by a lack of blood supply to the heart muscle and tissue death occurs.

Myoclonus: Spasm of a muscle or group of muscles.

Myopia: A condition of the eye where the light that comes in does not directly focus on the retina.

Negative symptoms: Decreases or deficits in typical behaviors, seen in mental illness.

Nonunion: A fracture in which the bone is not healing. A nonunion fracture may be caused by several factors such as vascular and tissue damage, poor alignment, stress to the fracture site, and infection.

Neovascular glaucoma: A secondary disorder that results from other diseases, such as diabetes mellitus or tumors, which cause new blood vessels to grow and obstruct the outflow of aqueous humor.

Nephropathy: Any disease of the kidney.

Neurobiologic: Of or relating to the biologic study of the nervous system. The cause of autism is considered to be an abnormality in the structure or function of the brain.

Neurodegenerative: Refers to degeneration of nervous tissue.

Neurofibrillary tangles: Contaminated tau protein that becomes twisted and causes eventual cell death.

Neurogenic bowel/bladder: Dysfunction resulting from congenital abnormality, injury, or disease process of the brain, spinal cord, or local nerve supply to the urinary bladder or rectum and their respective outlets. The dysfunction may manifest as partial or complete retention, incontinence, or frequency of elimination.

Neuroleptic: A medication having antipsychotic action, affecting sensorimotor, cognitive, and psychological functions.

Neuromuscular disorders: Diseases that affect the nerves that control voluntary muscles.

Neuron: A nerve cell that is specialized in transmitting and receiving electrical signals to communicate information between different regions of the body.

Neuropathy: Pathology of the nervous system.

Neurotransmitters: Chemical transmitters, such as dopamine and glutamate, secreted by neurons that bind receptors on nearby cells.

Nonreflex neurogenic bladder or bowel: Also called autonomic bladder/bowel. A neurogenic bladder/bowel resulting from a lesion or injury in the sacral portion of the spinal cord that interrupts the reflex arc that controls the bladder/bowel. The lesion may be in the cauda equina, conus medullaris, sacral roots, or pelvic nerve. It is marked by loss of normal bladder/bowel sensations and reflex activity, inability to initiate urination/elimination normally, and stress incontinence.

Nystagmus: Involuntary, rapid, rhythmic movement (horizontal, vertical, rotatory, or mixed, i.e., two types) of the eyeball.

Obsession: "A recurrent and persistent idea, thought, or impulse to carry out an act that is ego-dystonic, that is experienced as senseless or repugnant, and that the individual cannot voluntarily suppress."

Obsessive-compulsive disorder: "A type of anxiety disorder whose essential feature is recurrent thoughts, impulses or images or compulsions (repetitive, purposeful, and intentional behaviors performed in response to an obsession) sufficiently severe to cause marked distress, be time consuming or interfere significantly with the individual's normal routine, occupational functioning, or usual social activities or relationships with others."

Opacifications: Cloudy or opaque spots in the lens.

Open fracture: A fracture in which the bone breaks through the skin surface; also referred to as a compound fracture.

Open-angle glaucoma: A low vision disorder in which retinal damage occurs due to increased intraocular pressure.

Open reduction internal fixation (ORIF): A surgical procedure which involves the opening of and reducing the fracture site. Internal fixation is commonly done after an open reduction to secure the fracture. Internal fixation involves securing the fracture site with pins, rods, plates, and screws.

Optic neuritis: Inflammation of the optic nerve, affecting the part of the nerve within the eyeball (neuropapillitis) or the part behind the eyeball (retrobulbar neuritis), usually causing pain and partial blindness in one eye.

Orthostatic intolerance: An inability to tolerate sitting upright or standing, related to a fall in blood pressure that causes dizziness, syncope, and blurred vision.

Osteoarthritis: Also referred to as degenerative joint disease, is a noninflammatory joint disease that results in deterioration of articular cartilage and the formation of new bone or osteophytes on the joint surface.

Osteopenia: Low bone mass; reversible weakening of the bone that may be diagnosed through a bone density scan just as osteoporosis.

Osteoporosis: Disease characterized by low bone density and deterioration of bone. It is common in postmenopausal women due to the cessation of estrogen production.

Oxygen transport: The delivery of fully oxygenated blood to peripheral tissues, the cellular uptake of oxygen, the utilization of oxygen from the blood, and the return of partially desaturated blood to the lungs.

Panic: "Extreme and unreasoning anxiety and fear, often accompanied by disturbed breathing, increased heart activity, vasomotor changes, sweating and a feeling of dread."

Panic attack: "Sudden onset of intense apprehension, fear, terror or impending doom accompanied by increased autonomic nervous system activity and by various constitutional disturbances, depersonalization, and derealization."

Pannus: Activation of the synovial cells which accumulate and create pannus, a malignant mass over the cartilage, leading to cartilage breakdown. This granulation tissue continues to spread, the joint space is slowly effaced by fibrous adhesions, and eventually fibrous ankylosis appears.

Paranoia: Persecutory delusions.

Pathologic fracture: A weakening of bone that may result in it being unable to sustain normal forces experienced during daily activities. Thus, the bone may fracture while the person simply bends over or gets out of bed.

Paraphasia: A language disorder in which a person hears and comprehends words but is unable to speak correctly.

Paratonia: Involuntary resistance to passive movement of the extremities.

Parentification: A common occurrence among a group of siblings in an abusive and neglectful environment for one child, usually the oldest, to take on the role of a parent, as there is an absence of an adult care provider willing or able to provide care for others.

Parkinsonism: Characterized by tremor, muscle rigidity, slow shuffling gait, and other classic symptoms of Parkinson's disease.

Partial-thickness burn: Burn injury which involves part or all of the epidermis. Referred to as second-degree burns.

Pathogen: A microorganism that compromises the health of an individual. Most pathogens fall into three general categories: bacteria, viruses, and fungi.

Performance in areas of occupation: A broad category of human activity that are typically part of daily life. The areas include activities of daily living, instrumental activities of daily living, education, work, and play, leisure, and social participation.

Performance patterns: The habits, routines, and roles that a person adopts.

Performance skills: The features of what a person does during an activity. These skills are separated into the categories of motor skills, process skills, and communication/interaction skills.

Peripheral artery disease: Leads to impaired wound healing, tissue hypoxia, and decreased mobilization of white blood cells to infected tissues; occurs at an earlier age and at a rate of two to four times higher in people with diabetes.

Peripheral neuropathy: Most common symptoms include burning pain; stabbing, pricking, or tingling sensation; pathologic skin sensitivity; or deep aching pain; commonly diagnosed among people with diabetes.

Peripheral vision: Perception of images from the edges of the visual fields.

Peristalsis: The worm-like movement by which the alimentary canal or other tubular organs with both longitudinal and circular muscle fibers propel their contents, consisting of a wave of contraction passing along the tube.

Perseverative: Pertaining to the involuntary and pathologic repetition of verbal or motor response.

Personal episodic memory: Recall of time-related information about one's self, such as where and if one ate breakfast.

Person-first language: The identification of a person as the first descriptor and the disease as a secondary descriptor.

Phenotype: Genetic markers that show in observable characteristics in organisms.

Phobia: "Any objectively unfounded morbid dread or fear that arouses a state of panic."

Physiatrist: A physician specializing in rehabilitation medicine.

PICA: A medical disorder characterized by an appetite for nonfood substances.

Pneumonia: An inflammation of lung tissue, where the alveoli in the affected areas fill with fluid. The condition is caused by bacteria, viruses, aspiration, or immobility.

Polydipsia: Excessive thirst that occurs frequently.

Polyphagia: Excessive eating.

Polyuria: Excessive excretion of urine.

Positive symptoms: Observable behaviors of psychosis such as hallucinations and delusions.

Positron emission tomography: is a nuclear medicine imaging technique that produces a three-dimensional image of the functional processes of the body.

Posttraumatic stress disorder: Development of characteristic symptoms following a psychologically traumatic event that is generally outside the range of usual human experience; symptoms include numbed responsiveness to environmental stimuli, a variety of autonomic and cognitive dysfunctions, and dysphoria.

Premorbid functioning: The period of time before the onset of symptoms.

Prevalence: The total number of cases of the risk factor in the population divided by the number of individuals in the population. It is used to estimate how common a condition is within a population over a certain period of time.

Primitive reflexes: Innate primary reactions found in newborns and indicative of severe brain damage if present beyond their usual time of disappearance. Adult patients with closed head injury or stroke may manifest these signs; absence on reevaluation is a sign of progress in recovery. Examples include placing reactions, Moro reflex, grasp reflex, rooting reflex, and sucking reflex.

Procedural memory: Recall of information on how to perform a task such as knowing how to write or ride a bike.

Prodromal phase: The period of time when symptoms begin to emerge, which can range from weeks or months to years before the full onset of symptoms.

Prudence: The ability to govern and discipline oneself through the use of reason. To be prudent is to value judiciousness, discretion, vigilance, moderation, care, and circumspection in the management of one's affairs, to temper extremes, make judgments, and respond on the basis of intelligent reflection and rational thought.

Procedural learning: The ability to learn new motor, perceptual, or basic cognitive behaviors.

Progressive: Representing change. In the medical fields, it usually means a continual decline in function.

Psychomotor agitation: Repetitive and nonproductive motor activity. May present as pacing or fidgeting.

Psychomotor retardation: Movements, reactions, and speech that are slowed.

Psychosis: The inability to distinguish fantasy from reality; delusion or hallucinations that may be mood-congruent or mood-incongruent. Presence of psychotic features in major depressive disorders (MDDs) indicates a poor prognosis.

Pulse oximetry: Measures the oxygen concentration in arterial blood. The normal range is 95% to 100%. Measurements are taken to prevent hypoxia and to evaluate treatment.

Purkinje cells: Cells that form a layer near the surface of the cerebellum and convey signals away from the cerebellum.

Quadriplegia: Paralysis of all four limbs (also referred to as tetraplegia).

Rales: Crackling sounds or rumbling sound caused by increased mucus which the physician diagnoses by way of listening to the chest during breathing is.

Rapid-cycling: Four or more episodes of some type of mood disturbance within the past year episodes meet criteria for mania, hypomania, mixed, or depressed episodes as identified in *DSM IV-TR*.

Recent memory: The cognitive ability to temporarily store and manage information that is required to carry out cognitive tasks such as learning and reasoning. It is also referred to as short-term or working memory.

Reflex arc: A reflex, which is built in and does not need conscious thought to take effect, is the total of any particular automatic response mediated by the nervous system. A reflex arc is usually a simple reflex such as a knee jerk, which involves only two nerves and one synapse. Other arcs may involve an interneuron. When the sensory nerve ending is stimulated, a nerve impulse travels along a sensory (afferent) neuron to the spinal cord. An association neuron or interneuron then transfers the impulse to a motor (efferent) neuron, which carries the impulse to a muscle, which then contracts and moves a body part.

Relapse: Return of symptoms, resulting in rehospitalization for mental illness.

Remodeling: The final stage of bone healing in which the bone is ideally reshaped to its original form to enable it to resume its intended function as best as possible.

Remote memory: The cognitive ability to recall information from the past. It is also referred to as long-term memory.

Resiliency: The ability of an individual to recover from adverse or traumatic events in a manner that is adaptive and nonpathologic.

Retina: A structure of the central nervous system that consists of a multilayered, light-sensitive tissue that lines the rear inner surface of the eye.

Retinopathy: Noninflammatory degenerative disease of the retina.

Retrograde amnesia: Loss of memory of events that occurred prior to the injury.

Rett's disorder: A rare neurobiologic disorder that primarily affects females and is caused by a deviation on the methyl-CpG-binding protein 2 (MECP2) gene. This disorder has a distinctive course since early development in children is typical, followed by the deceleration of head growth, loss of purposeful hand movements, and appearance of autistic-like symptoms.

Rheumatoid arthritis: Arthritis refers to joint inflammation; "rheum" in rheumatoid refers to the stiffness, general aching, weakness, and fatigue that is experienced throughout the body.

Rheumatoid factor (RF): An antibody that is measurable in the blood. Antibodies are normal proteins in our blood that are important parts of our immune system; however, rheumatoid factor is an antibody that is not usually present in the normal individual. The prognosis for those with an RF positive factor is that they are at higher risk for erosions, nodules, growth retardation, lack of adequate bone mineralization, anemia, and poor functional status.

Rheumatologist: A physician who specializes in treatment of rheumatic diseases.

Risk factors: A variable associated with an increased risk of disease or infection.

Rote memory: The process of memorizing and using language overheard from others rather than producing spontaneously generated language.

Self and relational dysfunction: One of the most significant signs of the developmental impact of trauma; is a disruption of attachment. The type of relationship between a child and a caregiver influences how a child responds to present and future emotional and physical experiences.

Spina bifida: Birth defect with a nongenetic origin that can contribute to or cause ID due to an incomplete closing of the embryonic neural tube.

Scoliosis: Lateral curvature of the vertebral column. This deviation of the normally straight vertical line of the spine may or may not include rotation or deformity of the vertebrae.

Semantic memory: Ability to remember the name of an object.

Severe acquired brain injury: Loss of consciousness and/or posttraumatic amnesia for more than 24 hours, a GCS rating of 1 to 8.

Short-term memory: The ability to recall information after a short period of time.

Sjogren's syndrome: is a chronic disease of unknown etiology causing corneal and conjunctival lesions and is characterized by dry eyes and mouth.

Smith's fracture: Opposite of Colles' fracture in that the displacement from the break is positioned toward the volar or palmar aspect of the wrist rather than the dorsal aspect.

Social phobia: "A persistent pattern of significant fear of a social or performance situation, manifested by anxiety or panic on exposure to the situation or in anticipation of it, which the person realizes is unreasonable or excessive and interferes significantly with the person's functioning."

Somatization: occurs when mental and emotional stresses become physical complaints in the absence of an explained diagnosis.

Spasticity (hypertonicity): Abnormally high muscle tone, i.e., tone which is felt as too much resistance to movement, resulting from hyperactive reflexes or the loss of inhibiting influences from higher brain centers.

Sphygmomanometer: The instrument used to measure blood pressure.

Spinal muscular atrophy (SMA): A neuromuscular disease characterized by degeneration of motor neurons resulting in progressive muscular atrophy and weakness.

Spinal shock: Result of an acute transverse lesion of the spinal cord that causes immediate flaccid paralysis and loss of all sensation and reflex activity (including autonomic functions) below the level of injury. On return of reflex activity, there is increased spasticity of muscles and exaggerated tendon reflexes.

Stereotyped behavior: A pattern of behavior, such as hand flapping or nonproductive exploration of objects, that is often seen in autism.

Strabismus: Deviation of the eye in which the visual axes assume a position relative to each other different from that required by the physiological conditions; also called squint.

Stretch reflex: Reflex contraction of a muscle in response to passive longitudinal stretching.

Subdural hematoma: An accumulation of blood in the subdural space of the brain, usually caused by an injury.

Substantia nigra: Located in the basil ganglia, this structure produces dopamine, a neurotransmitter, and transports it to the striatum.

Sundowning: A condition in which a person with cognitive impairment becomes confused or disoriented at the end of the day.

Superficial burn: refers to the depth of the burn; also referred to as a first-degree burn, occurs when the top layer of skin, called the epidermis, is burned.

Swan-neck deformity: A deformity which results from contractures of the interosseus and flexor muscles and tendons, which in turn produce a flexor contracture of the MCP joint, compensatory hyperextension of the PIP joint, and flexion of the DIP joint.

Synovial: Pertaining to, consisting of, or secreting synovia, the lubricating fluid of the joints, bursae, and tendon sheaths.

Systolic blood pressure: The amount of force used to pump blood out of the heart into the arterial circulation.

Tachycardia: Abnormal rapid heart rate which may indicate inefficient heart function, reducing circulation integrity and diminishing oxygenation of other body structures.

Tactile defensiveness: A type of sensory defensiveness in which a person overreacts or avoids touching certain textures.

Tangential thinking: Rapid shifting from one thought to a closely related thought.

Tangentiality: Pattern of communicating in which the person moves off the central point and, unlike circumstantiality, is unable to return to the point.

Tardive dyskinesia: A side effect from medication that results in motor abnormalities such as writhing movements.

Tau: A type of protein.

Tay-Sachs disease: An autosomal, recessive, single gene disorder that can cause ID.

Temporal lobes: This region of the brain is located at the side of the cerebrum, below the frontal lobe. Its functions include auditory processing, comprehension, naming, verbal memory, and high-level visual processing including object and facial recognition.

Tenosynovitis: Inflammation of the synovial lining of the tendon sheath.

Teratogenic: Environmental factors that cause malformations of an embryo or fetus.

Theory of mind: The ability to understand another person's thoughts, feelings, or intentions.

Thrombus: A blood clot comprising such blood factors as platelets and fibrin; frequently the cause of obstructions in the vascular system resulting in medical problems such as stroke.

Tissue plasminogen activator (tPA): Medications used for dissolution of an occluding thrombus.

Topagnosia: Loss of ability to localize site of tactile sensations.

Topographic orientation: Orientation of the self within the environment.

Toxemia: An environmental factor in the etiology of ID that is the result of the maternal condition in which high blood pressure and protein in the urine develop after the 20th week of pregnancy (also known as preeclampsia).

Trabecular meshwork: An area of tissue in the eye at the base of the cornea that is responsible for draining the aqueous humor from the eye via the anterior chamber.

Transgenerational: Caregiver's actions are based on his or her own previous parenting experiences.

Transient ischemic attacks (TIA): A sudden episode of temporary symptoms, typically due to diminished blood flow through the carotid arteries or sometimes related to impaired circulation through the vertebrobasilar vessels. TIA is a powerful warning sign of stroke, and symptoms can range from obvious loss of sensation or motor function to more subtle signs. See Cerebrovascular accident.

Trauma: From the Greek word meaning *wound*, has been traditionally used in medicine to indicate a serious physical injury but it is more widely used to refer to emotional shock following a stressful event or to chronic experience that is deeply distressing.

Truth: Faithful to facts and reality. Truthfulness or veracity is demonstrated by being accountable, honest, forthright, accurate, and authentic in our attitudes and actions.

Tuberculosis (TB): A serious and highly contagious, airborne infection usually affecting the lungs. It is caused by mycobacterium tuberculosis.

Type 1 diabetes: A disease in which the pancreas stops producing insulin as a result of autoimmune destruction of cells.

Type 2 diabetes: A disease where the body cells are insulin resistant.

Unipolar: Refers to the syndrome that consists only of major depressive episodes without manic episodes.

Unilateral spatial neglect: Inattention to visual stimuli presented on the individual's side contralateral to a cerebral lesion. It may occur independently of visual deficits or with hemianopsia.

Utilization behavior: Touching, grasping, or manipulating anything that is within sight.

Valley Sign: A diagnostic observation in which two bulges are visible on either side of a depression on the back of the shoulder when a person is asked to abduct the shoulders to 90 degrees with 90-degree flexion of the elbows so that hands are pointing upward.

Vegetative signs: Physiologic signs that develop in the areas of sexual activity, sleep, appetite, and other biologic rhythms.

Visuospatial: Pertaining to the ability to comprehend visual representations and their spatial relationships.

Volkmann's deformity: An orthopedic deformity that results from severe damage to tissues and muscles caused by increased pressure in the forearm compartments.

Winged scapulae: A condition in which the shoulder blade protrudes from a person's back in an abnormal position.

X-linked: A disease that occurs when a mother who carries the affected gene passes it onto her son. Although the mother carries the affected gene on one of her X chromosomes, she may never show symptoms since it is a recessive trait.

Zoonotic infection: A condition that can cross species.

Index

Page numbers followed by *f* or *t* refer to illustrations or tables, respectively.